A Clinical Guide to Pulmonary Hypertension

A Clinical Guide to Pulmonary Hypertension

Editor: Jim Foster

AMERICAN
MEDICAL PUBLISHERS
www.americanmedicalpublishers.com

AMERICAN
MEDICAL PUBLISHERS
www.americanmedicalpublishers.com

Cataloging-in-Publication Data

A clinical guide to pulmonary hypertension / edited by Jim Foster.
p. cm.
Includes bibliographical references and index.
ISBN 978-1-63927-840-4
1. Pulmonary hypertension. 2. Hypertension. 3. Pulmonary circulation.
4. Pulmonary hypertension--Diagnosis. 5. Pulmonary hypertension--Treatment.
I. Foster, Jim.
RC776.P87 C55 2023
616.24--dc23

American Medical Publishers,
41 Flatbush Avenue,
1st Floor, New York,
NY 11217, USA

ISBN 978-1-63927-840-4 (Hardback)

Contents

Preface

Pulmonary hypertension (PH) is a condition in which the blood pressure in the pulmonary arteries becomes too high. Pulmonary arteries are responsible for carrying oxygen-poor blood from the heart to the lungs. Some common symptoms of pulmonary hypertension are shortness of breath, chest pain, fatigue, swelling in ankles, racing heartbeat and decreased hunger. Various risk factors associated with it are heart disease, lung disease, hypoxia, Down syndrome, and presence of blood clots in pulmonary arteries. There are many different kinds of tests for the diagnosis of pulmonary hypertension, such as right heart catheterization and Doppler echocardiogram tests. The common tests to examine the underlying cause of pulmonary hypertension include blood tests, chest CT scan, chest X-ray, and pulmonary ventilation/perfusion scan. The treatment methods for pulmonary arterial hypertension are diuretics, oxygen therapy, and pulmonary vasodilators. This book explores the clinical aspects of pulmonary hypertension in detail. It consists of contributions made by international experts. This book will prove immensely beneficial to professionals and students involved in the study and management of this medical condition at various levels.

Various studies have approached the subject by analyzing it with a single perspective, but the present book provides diverse methodologies and techniques to address this field. This book contains theories and applications needed for understanding the subject from different perspectives. The aim is to keep the readers informed about the progresses in the field; therefore, the contributions were carefully examined to compile novel researches by specialists from across the globe.

Indeed, the job of the editor is the most crucial and challenging in compiling all chapters into a single book. In the end, I would extend my sincere thanks to the chapter authors for their profound work. I am also thankful for the support provided by my family and colleagues during the compilation of this book.

Editor

1

The Selective Angiotensin II Type 2 Receptor Agonist, Compound 21, Attenuates the Progression of Lung Fibrosis and Pulmonary Hypertension in an Experimental Model of Bleomycin-Induced Lung Injury

Anandharajan Rathinasabapathy[1,2], Alana Horowitz[1,3], Kelsey Horton[1], Ashok Kumar[4,5], Santhi Gladson[2], Thomas Unger[6], Diana Martinez[1], Gaurav Bedse[7], James West[2], Mohan K. Raizada[4], Ulrike M. Steckelings[8], Colin Sumners[4], Michael J. Katovich[1*] and Vinayak Shenoy[1,9*]*

[1] Department of Pharmacodynamics, University of Florida, Gainesville, FL, United States, [2] Allergy, Pulmonary and Critical Care Medicine, Vanderbilt University Medical Center, Nashville, TN, United States, [3] Anatomy, University of California at San Francisco, San Francisco, CA, United States, [4] Department of Physiology and Functional Genomics, University of Florida, Gainesville, FL, United States, [5] Cardiopulmonary Vascular Biology Lab, Providence VA Medical Center, Brown University, Providence, RI, United States, [6] Cardiovascular Research Institute Maastricht School for Cardiovascular Diseases, Maastricht University, Maastricht, Netherlands, [7] Psychiatry and Behavioral Sciences, Vanderbilt University Medical Center, Nashville, TN, United States, [8] Department of Cardiovascular and Renal Research, Institute for Molecular Medicine, University of Southern Denmark, Odense, Denmark, [9] Department of Pharmaceutical and Biomedical Sciences, California Health Sciences University, Clovis, CA, United States

***Correspondence:**
Anandharajan Rathinasabapathy
anandharajan.rathinasabapathy@vanderbilt.edu
Michael J. Katovich
katovich@cop.ufl.edu
Vinayak Shenoy
vshenoy@chsu.org

Idiopathic Pulmonary Fibrosis (IPF) is a chronic lung disease characterized by scar formation and respiratory insufficiency, which progressively leads to death. Pulmonary hypertension (PH) is a common complication of IPF that negatively impacts clinical outcomes, and has been classified as Group III PH. Despite scientific advances, the dismal prognosis of IPF and associated PH remains unchanged, necessitating the search for novel therapeutic strategies. Accumulating evidence suggests that stimulation of the angiotensin II type 2 (AT_2) receptor confers protection against a host of diseases. In this study, we investigated the therapeutic potential of Compound 21 (C21), a selective AT_2 receptor agonist in the bleomycin model of lung injury. A single intra-tracheal administration of bleomycin (2.5 mg/kg) to 8-week old male Sprague Dawley rats resulted in lung fibrosis and PH. Two experimental protocols were followed: C21 was administered (0.03 mg/kg/day, ip) either immediately (prevention protocol, BCP) or after 3 days (treatment protocol, BCT) of bleomycin-instillation. Echocardiography, hemodynamic, and Fulton's index assessments were performed after 2 weeks of bleomycin-instillation. Lung tissue was processed for gene expression, hydroxyproline content (a marker of collagen deposition), and histological analysis. C21 treatment prevented as well as attenuated the progression of lung fibrosis, and accompanying PH. The beneficial effects of C21 were associated with decreased infiltration of macrophages in the lungs, reduced lung inflammation and diminished pulmonary collagen accumulation. Further, C21 treatment also improved pulmonary pressure, reduced muscularization of the pulmonary vessels and normalized cardiac function in both the experimental protocols. However, there were no major differences in any of the outcomes measured from the two experimental protocols. Collectively, our findings indicate that stimulation of the AT_2 receptor by C21 attenuates bleomycin-induced lung injury and associated cardiopulmonary pathology, which needs to be further explored as a promising approach for the clinical treatment of IPF and Group III PH.

Keywords: pulmonary fibrosis, pulmonary hypertension, C21, AT_2 receptor, bleomycin, rats

INTRODUCTION

Idiopathic Pulmonary Fibrosis (IPF) is a chronic, progressive interstitial lung disease with a median survival of 3 years after diagnosis (Raghu et al., 2011). The origin of IPF remains unknown; however, smoking, viral infections, pollutants, and aging have been identified as potential risk factors (Wolters et al., 2014). Pulmonary hypertension (PH) is a common comorbidity in patients with IPF where it is classified as Group III PH by the World Health Organization (WHO). In fact, PH associated with IPF is considered as one of the principal predictors of mortality (Collum et al., 2017). The prevalence of IPF is growing at an alarming rate worldwide (Ley and Collard, 2013) and the available medical options are very limited. Currently, nintedanib (inhibits multiple tyrosine kinase) and pirfenidone (downregulates transforming growth factor β) are the only drugs approved for IPF treatment (Raghu and Selman, 2015). However, they provide little therapeutic efficacy, fail to prolong survival, and are associated with increased incidence of side effects (Canestaro et al., 2016). All these factors necessitate the search for novel strategies to effectively combat IPF and associated cardiopulmonary symptoms.

The renin angiotensin system (RAS) is a major driving force in maintaining renal, metabolic, and cardiovascular homeostasis. The members of the RAS family have been recently characterized into two major arms that exert opposing actions to one another (Iwai and Horiuchi, 2009)—(a) the deleterious ACE/Ang II/AT_1 receptor axis, which comprises of Angiotensin converting enzyme (ACE), Angiotensin II (Ang II), and the Angiotensin type 1 (AT_1) receptor; and, (b) the protective ACE2/Ang-(1-7)/Mas axis, consisting of Angiotensin converting enzyme 2 (ACE2), Angiotensin-(1-7) [Ang-(1-7)], and the Mas receptor. Interestingly, the beneficial effects of activating the ACE2/Ang-(1-7)/Mas axis have been associated with a concomitant increase in the expression of Angiotensin type 2 (AT_2) receptor (Shenoy et al., 2014), suggesting an active role for this receptor against tissue/organ damage.

Consistent with the aforementioned observations, stimulation of the AT_2 receptor by a selective ligand, Compound 21 (C21) was shown to confer protection against experimental models of kidney damage (Patel et al., 2016), myocardial infarction (Kaschina et al., 2008), ischemic stroke (Joseph et al., 2014), and islet cell injury (Wang L. et al., 2017). C21 is a highly selective angiotensin II AT_2 receptor agonist with a K_i value of 0.4 nM for the AT_2 receptor and a $K_i >$ 10 mM for the AT_1 receptor (Wan et al., 2004). We have recently reported that treatment with C21 (0.03 mg/kg/day, ip) after the establishment of disease pathogenesis effectively arrests the progression of monocrotaline-induced PH, and these beneficial effects are abolished by co-administration of the AT_2 receptor antagonist, PD123319 (Bruce et al., 2015). Though the effects of C21 have been evaluated against a wide variety of disease conditions and organ fibrosis (Wang Y. et al., 2017), its actions against PF and Group III PH are yet to be investigated. Hence, in this study, we investigated the therapeutic potential of C21 against lung fibrosis and associated cardiopulmonary complications in the bleomycin-model of lung injury. The bleomycin animal model mimics key pathophysiological features of human IPF and associated PH following intra-tracheal challenge (Nogueira-Ferreira et al., 2016).

MATERIALS AND METHODS

Reagents and Chemicals

Bleomycin sulfate (BLEO) was purchased from EMD Millipore (Billerica, MA). C21 was a kind gift from Vicore Pharma (Gothenburg, Sweden). α-smooth muscle actin (α-SMA) and CD68 antibodies were purchased from Abcam (Cambridge, MA, USA) and Dako (Santa Clara, CA, USA), respectively.

Animals

All animal procedures were approved by the Institutional Animal Care and Use Committee at the University of Florida, complied with National Institutes of Health guidelines and were performed in accordance with the Guide for the Care and Use of Laboratory Animals (Eight Edition, 2011, published by National Academics Press, 500 Fifth Street NW, Washington, DC 20001, USA).

Abbreviations: Agtr2, angiotensin type 2 receptor; Ang-(1-7), Angiotensin-(1-7); AT_1, angiotensin type 1; AT_2, angiotensin type 2; BLEO, bleomycin; BCP, bleomycin + compound 21 (prevention); BCT, bleomycin + compound 21 (treatment); Col1a1, Collagen, type 1, a1; Col3a1, Collagen, type3, a1; Ctgf, Connective Tissue Growth Factor; C21, compound 21; ECHO, echocardiography; ECM, extracellular matrix; EDA, end diastolic area; EF, ejection fraction; Il-6, Interleukin 6; Il-13, Interleukin 13; IPF, Idiopathic Pulmonary Fibrosis; LV, left ventricle; MMP, matrix metalloproteinases; MCP-1, monocyte chemoattractant protein 1; PF, pulmonary fibrosis; PH, Pulmonary Hypertension; RAS, renin angiotensin system; RVH, right ventricular hypertrophy; RVSP, right ventricular systolic pressure; TIMP, tissue inhibitor of metalloproteinase; TLR4, Toll Like Receptor 4.

Study Design

Two different protocols were followed in this study—Prevention and Treatment. For both the protocols, 8-week old male Sprague Dawley rats were used (Charles River Laboratories, Wilmington, MA). A pilot experiment was initially performed to determine the best time to initiate C21 injection for the treatment protocol. In this pilot study, PF and accompanying PH (Group III) was induced by a single intra-tracheal injection of BLEO (2.5 mg/kg ≡ 4U/kg, $n = 4$), while control animals received saline ($n = 4$). Three days after BLEO instillation, right ventricular (RV) hemodynamics was measured, and lung tissues were processed for histological examination. Based on this pilot study, it was decided to initiate C21 treatment (0.03 mg/kg/day, ip) after 3 days of bleomycin-instillation (treatment protocol, BCT). However, for the prevention protocol C21 was administered immediately after bleomycin injection (prevention protocol, BCP). For both the protocols, ECHO assessment of RV function and hemodynamics were performed after 2 weeks of BLEO instillation. Lung and heart tissues were harvested for RNA and histological analysis. A subsequent experiment (both prevention and treatment) was performed to obtain all the five lung lobes for estimation of total lung collagen deposition. We have previously demonstrated that C21 was therapeutically active in the monocrotaline model of PH at a dose, 0.03 mg/kg/day (Bruce et al., 2015). At this dose, C21 did not alter any of the following parameters - basal systemic blood pressure, basal right ventricular systolic pressure, cardiac function, and gene expression in normal animals. Both C21 and BLEO were dissolved in sterile deionized water. The terminology AT_2 (human) has been used throughout the article to denote angiotensin type 2 receptor, except for gene expression studies, wherein, Agtr2 (rat) has been used.

TABLE 1 | Rat primers used for RT-PCR experiment.

No	Gene	Sequence
1.	Col1a1	Rn01463848_m1
2.	Col3a1	Rn01437681_m1
3.	Ctgf	Rn01537279_g1
4.	Mmp12	Rn00588640_m1
5.	Timp1	Rn01430873_g1
6.	IL-13	Rn00587615_m1
7.	Ccl2	Rn00580555_m1
8.	IL-6	Rn01410330_m1
9.	Tlr4	Rn00569848_m1
10.	Agtr2	Rn00560677_s1
11.	18S	Hs99999901_s1

Echocardiography and Hemodynamic Assessments

Transthoracic echocardiography was performed after 2 weeks of BLEO instillation to assess ventricular dimensions and cardiac function using a GE Vivid7 ultrasound machine with a 12-MHz transducer (GE Healthcare, NJ, USA). Following echocardiography, the right ventricular systolic

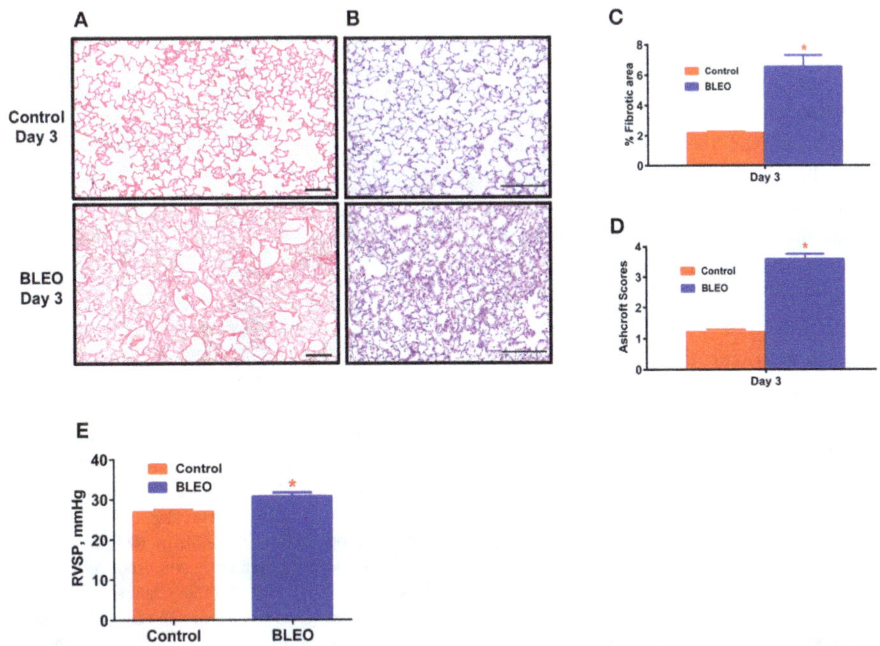

FIGURE 1 | Early onset of lung tissue remodeling and pulmonary hypertension in BLEO animals. **(A,B)** Representative images demonstrating picro-sirius and hematoxylin-eosin staining. **(C,D)** Summary data showing the lung tissue remodeling and fibrosis. **(E)** Summary data showing RVSP after 3 days of BLEO instillation. The data presented in **(C–E)** are mean ± SEM ($n = 4$). *Represents a p-value of ≤ 0.05 when comparing BLEO animals against the controls. **(A)** Scale bar = 100 μm and **(B)** Scale bar = 200 μm.

pressure (RVSP) was measured as described previously (Rathinasabapathy et al., 2016). Subsequently, animals were sacrificed and organs were harvested for RNA, histology and hypertrophy assessments. Right ventricular hypertrophy [RVH = RV/(LV+S)] was calculated as the ratio of wet weight of right ventricle (RV) and left ventricle + intra-ventricular septum (LV+S).

Real-Time Quantitative RT-PCR Analysis

Real time qRT-PCR was performed using Taqman Gene Expression System (Life Technologies, USA) to evaluate gene expression of cytokines, fibrotic and extracellular matrix (ECM) markers *viz.* collagen type 1 (Col1a1), collagen type 3 (Col3a1), connective tissue growth factor (Ctgf), interleukin 13 (Il-13), matrix metalloproteinases 12 (Mmp12), tissue inhibitor of metalloproteinases 1 (Timp1), monocyte chemotactic protein 1 (Ccl2), interleukin 6 (Il-6), toll like receptor 4 (Tlr4), and angiotensin receptor type 2 (Agtr2). Total RNA and cDNA preparation was performed as described previously (Anandharajan et al., 2009). Gene expression was calculated by the ΔΔCT method and data was presented as relative fold change from that of control animals. The rat primers have been listed in **Table 1**.

Histochemical Analysis

Following hemodynamic measurements, the left lobe of the lung was inflated with phosphate-buffered saline (PBS), followed by 10% neutral buffered formalin and stored in formalin overnight. Subsequently, the fixed lung tissue was processed (4 μm section) and stained with picro-sirius red. Images were photographed at 10X magnification using an Aperio Imagescope (Leica Biosystems, US). Using Image-J software, the percent of fibrotic area was assessed. To determine remodeling of the lung tissue, sectioned lung specimens (4 μm) were stained with hematoxylin-eosin (H&E) and imaged. Blinded Ashcroft scoring system was performed to grade the tissue remodeling across all experimental groups (Ashcroft et al., 1988). A minimum of 10 non-overlapping images was randomly chosen from each lung section for picro-sirius and H&E staining. For macrophage and muscularization analysis, lung sections (5 μm) were stained with CD68 (1:100) and α-smooth muscle actin (1:200) antibody, respectively, and imaged at 10X (15 random fields/lung section). The degree of muscularization was determined by quantifying the amount of α-smooth muscle actin in different sized vessels (vessel inner diameter—0–25, 25–50, and 50–100 μm). Briefly, when more than 70% of the pulmonary vessel wall is stained by smooth muscle actin, it is classified as completely muscularized, while if it is <70%, it is classified as partially muscularized. Results from each animal was averaged for the subsequent statistical analysis.

Collagen Estimation—Hydroxyproline Assay

Hydroxyproline assay was performed to estimate lung collagen deposition, as an index of fibrosis. In a separate set of experiments, all the five lung lobes were harvested from each animal, and dried at 65°C for 3 h. Subsequently, the dried lungs were weighed and subjected to collagen estimation according to the protocol provided in the assay kit (Biovisions, CA).

Statistics

Graph Pad Prism, version 5.0 (La Jolla, CA) was used for statistical analysis. A simple student *t*-test was performed to analyze the data presented in **Figure 1**. One-way ANOVA followed by Newman-Keuls *post-hoc* analysis test was carried out for all the other end point experimental parameters. Values are represented as means ± SEM, *p*-values ≤ 0.05 were considered statistically significant.

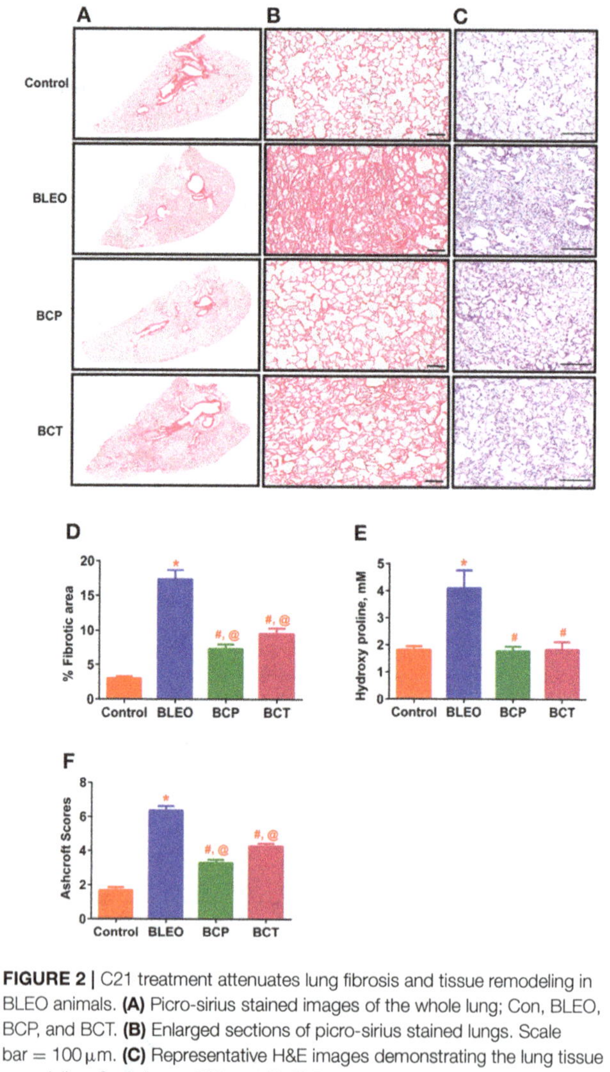

FIGURE 2 | C21 treatment attenuates lung fibrosis and tissue remodeling in BLEO animals. **(A)** Picro-sirius stained images of the whole lung; Con, BLEO, BCP, and BCT. **(B)** Enlarged sections of picro-sirius stained lungs. Scale bar = 100 μm. **(C)** Representative H&E images demonstrating the lung tissue remodeling. Scale bar = 200 μm. **(D,F)** Summary data showing the improvement in lung fibrosis and tissue remodeling in BLEO animals in presence of C21. **(E)** Summary data showing the collagen synthesis estimated by measuring hydroxyproline. The data presented in **(D–F)** are mean ± SEM, from 5, 4–6, and 7–8 animals, respectively. *Indicates a *p*-value of ≤ 0.05, comparing BLEO animals against the controls. #Indicates a *p*-value of ≤ 0.05, comparing BCP and BCT vs. BLEO. @ Indicates a *p*-value of ≤ 0.05, comparing BCP and BCT vs. control.

RESULTS

C21 Treatment Attenuates Lung Fibrosis and Tissue Remodeling

A pilot 3-day study revealed considerable lung damage in BLEO animals compared to controls, as evidenced by picro-sirius red and H&E staining (p $\leq$ 0.05, **Figures 1A–D**). In addition, BLEO instilled animals showed significant increase in RVSP (**Figure 1E**). Based on these histological and hemodynamic assessments, we decided to initiate C21 treatment after 3 days of BLEO insult in the treatment protocol (BCT group, $n = 8$). On the other hand, C21 was injected immediately after BLEO instillation in the prevention (BCP) protocol. It is evident from **Figures 2A,B** that BLEO lungs are stained intense red (represents lung collagen accumulation) as compared to controls, and that this pattern is significantly attenuated by C21 in both BCP and BCT groups. Quantification of the red color collagen staining is provided in **Figure 2D**. Likewise, hydroxyproline analysis revealed that C21 treatment normalized BLEO-induced increase in hydroxyproline levels in both BCP and BCT groups ($p \leq 0.05$, **Figure 2E**). Further, Ashcroft scoring of the H&E stained lung sections showed considerable disruption of the lung architecture (especially collapsed alveoli) upon bleomycin instillation, which was attenuated by C21 administration ($p \leq 0.05$, **Figures 2C,F**).

C21 Treatment Improves Ventricular Remodeling and Hemodynamics in Bleomycin Animals

Following 2 weeks of BLEO instillation, RVSP was significantly increased in the BLEO group as compared to controls ($p \leq 0.05$, **Figure 3A**). This increase in pressure was associated with development of RVH ($p \leq 0.05$, **Figure 3B**). However, administration of C21 substantially attenuated the altered hemodynamics and RVH in both the experimental protocols ($p \leq 0.05$, **Figures 3A,B**). Further, analysis of the ECHO images revealed a shift in the intra-ventricular septum toward the left ventricle in BLEO-instilled animals, which could be due to elevated RVSP. An increase in RV/LV end diastolic area (EDA) was also observed in BLEO animals that was accompanied with decreased ejection fraction (EF) ($p \leq 0.05$, **Figures 3C,E**). In line with the hemodynamics and RVH data, C21 treatment significantly improved the cardiac function in both the experimental protocols ($p \leq 0.05$, **Figures 3D,E**). Although C21

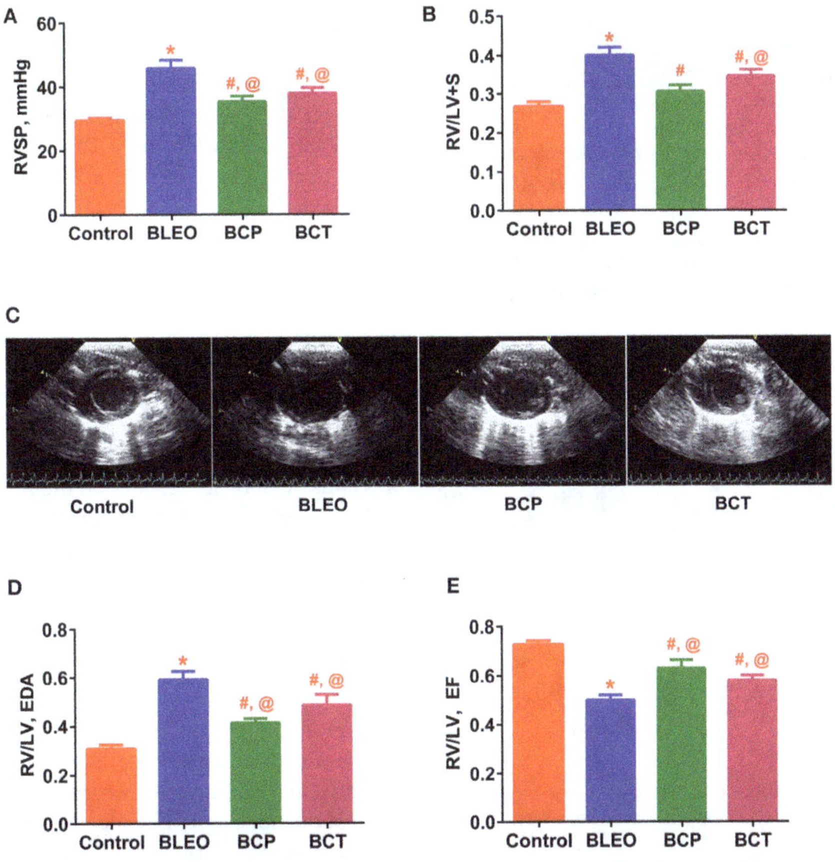

FIGURE 3 | C21 treatment attenuates the right ventricular remodeling in BLEO animals. **(A,B,D,E)** Summary data showing the improvement of RVSP, RVH, RV/LV EDA, and RV/LV EF in BLEO animals in presence of C21. **(C)** Representative images of parasternal short axis view of the ventricles on Day-14. Data represented in **(A,B,D,E)** are mean ± SEM (n = 6–8). *Indicates a p-value of $\leq$ 0.05, comparing BLEO animals against the controls. # Indicates a p-value of $\leq$ 0.05, comparing BCP and BCT vs. BLEO. @ Indicates a p-value of $\leq$ 0.05, comparing BCP and BCT vs. control.

treatment was beneficial in improving hemodynamic and all cardiac parameters in the prevention protocol, statistical analysis revealed that only RVH was completely prevented (BCP group), while all other parameters showed partial attenuation in both the experimental groups.

C21 Treatment Improves Pulmonary Vascular Remodeling in Bleomycin Animals

In order to investigate remodeling of the pulmonary vasculature, we performed α-smooth muscle actin staining and quantified the degree of muscularization. We observed extensive remodeling of the BLEO lungs as evidenced by an increase in the number of completely muscularized pulmonary vessels (0–100 μm, $p \leq 0.05$, **Figures 4A–E**), as well as muscularization of the smaller vessels ($p \leq 0.05$, **Figures 4F–H**). In agreement with the hemodynamics and cardiac function data, C21 treatment significantly reduced muscularization of the pulmonary vessels in both the experimental groups, when compared against the BLEO group ($p \leq 0.05$, **Figures 4E–G**). However, a detailed statistical analysis revealed that there was total prevention of the completely muscularized vessels, while other muscularization outcomes were partially prevented in the prevention protocol. Likewise, though statistically significant only partial attenuation of muscularization was observed in the BCT group.

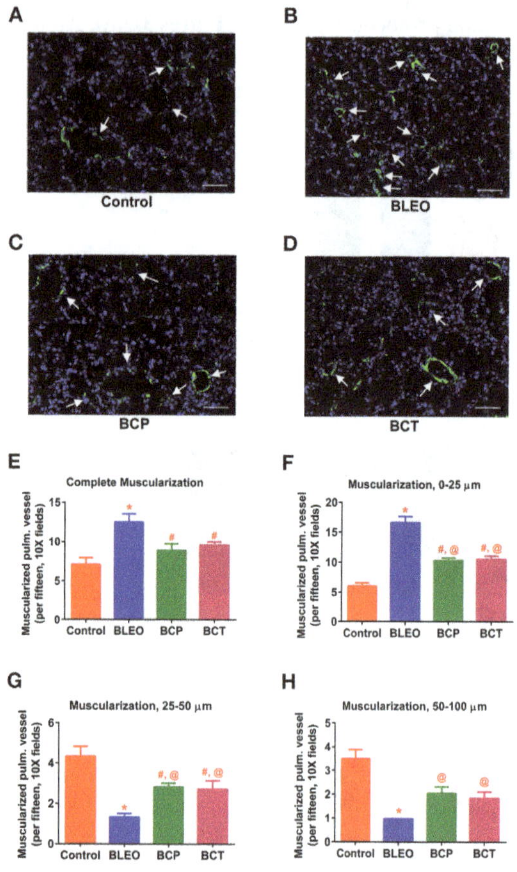

FIGURE 4 | C21 treatment attenuates pulmonary vascular remodeling in BLEO animals. **(A–D)** Representative images of α-smooth muscle actin stained pulmonary vessel wall (white arrows). **(E–H)** Summary data showing the improvement of muscularization by C21 in BLEO animals for the complete, 0–25, 25–50, and 50–100 μm category, respectively. Data represented in **(E–H)** are mean ± SEM ($n = 3$). *Indicates a p-value of ≤ 0.05, comparing BLEO animals against the controls. # Indicates a p-value of ≤ 0.05, comparing BCP and BCT vs. BLEO. @ indicates a p-value of ≤ 0.05, comparing BCP and BCT vs. control. Scale = 50 μm.

C21 Treatment Attenuates the Expression of ECM and Inflammatory Markers, Along With Decreasing Macrophage Infiltration in Bleomycin Animals

To investigate the possible mechanism (or pathways) by which C21 attenuates lung fibrosis, real time qRT-PCR determinations and immunohistochemical staining of the lung macrophages were performed. Gene expression of Col1a1 and Col3a1 was found to be significantly upregulated in BLEO animals, but was attenuated by C21 treatment ($p \leq 0.05$, **Figures 5A,B**). Similarly, C21 treatment significantly attenuated the gene expression of Ctgf, Mmp12, Timp1 and Il-13) in both the experimental protocols ($p \leq 0.05$, **Figures 5C–F**). Further, the key markers of inflammation, (Ccl2 and Il-6) and innate immune system (Tlr4) were also significantly upregulated in the BLEO animals, but significantly attenuated by C21 ($p \leq 0.05$, **Figures 6A–C**). As a next step, we performed immunohistochemical staining to estimate the infiltration of macrophages in the lungs. In line with our gene expression results, BLEO lungs exhibited significant infiltration of $CD68^{+}$ macrophages, which was attenuated by C21 treatment in both the experimental groups ($p \leq 0.05$, **Figures 7A–E**). However, statistical analysis revealed that macrophage infiltration was normalized only in the BCP group, while it was partially attenuated in the BCT group.

C21 Treatment Alters the Expression of Angiotensin Type 2 Receptor in Bleomycin Animals

qRT-PCR determinations revealed that the expression of Agtr2 was considerably upregulated in the BLEO animals as compared with controls ($p \leq 0.05$, **Figure 8**). However, C21 treatment significantly reduced the expression of Agtr2 in both the experimental groups ($p \leq 0.05$, **Figure 8**).

DISCUSSION

The most significant finding of the present work is that pharmacological activation of the AT_2 receptor by C21 effectively mitigates PF, and improves cardiopulmonary complications in an experimental model of bleomycin-induced lung injury. We observed that C21 treatment of BLEO animals significantly: (1) reduces PH and decreases muscularization of the pulmonary vessels, along with restoring cardiac function; (2) prevents as well as attenuates the progression of PF by reducing ECM remodeling and lung collagen accumulation, and; (3) alleviates inflammatory stress by reducing the infiltration of lung macrophages. Collectively, these data suggest a potential role

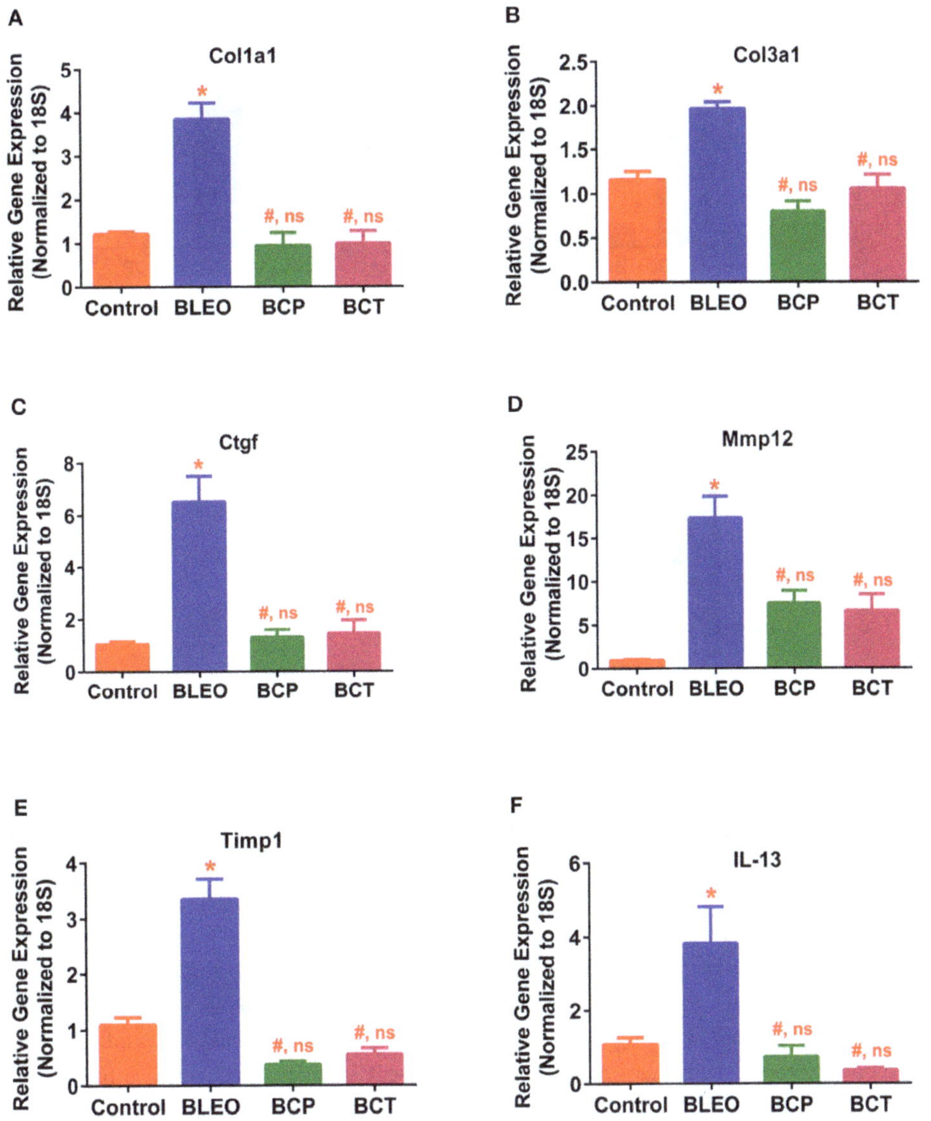

FIGURE 5 | C21 treatment attenuates the expression of markers of fibrosis and ECM in BLEO animals. **(A)** Col1a1, **(B)** Col3a1, **(C)** Ctgf, **(D)** Mmp12, **(E)** Timp1, and **(F)** IL-13. Data represented in **(A–F)** are mean ± SEM, $n = 5$ animals/group. *Indicates a p-value of ≤ 0.05, comparing BLEO animals against the controls. # Indicates a p-value of ≤ 0.05, comparing BCP and BCT vs. BLEO. ns indicates a p-value of non-significant, comparing BCP and BCT vs. control.

of the AT_2 receptor and its synthetic activator (C21) in the treatment of patients with PF and associated Group III PH.

PH due to interstitial lung disease (IPF and chronic obstructive pulmonary disease) has been classified as Group III PH by the WHO. There is an increased incidence of PH and right heart failure in patients with IPF, which adversely affects disease outcomes and survival. To our knowledge, this is the first report to show that stimulation of the AT_2 receptor using a synthetic activator (C21) renders protection against bleomycin-induced cardiopulmonary injury, which could open up novel therapeutic avenues to tackle lung fibrosis and Group III PH. We chose to evaluate the effects of C21 in the BLEO-model since it mimics key pathological features of human IPF and associated PH. We have previously demonstrated that a single intra-tracheal injection of BLEO induces fibrosis and alters pulmonary hemodynamics within 14 days of insult (Shenoy et al., 2013; Rathinasabapathy et al., 2016). In our experience, remodeling of the lung tissue and changes in pulmonary hemodynamics commence as early as 3 days, which worsens over time, causing considerable mortality after 15 days of intra-tracheal BLEO injection. For this reason, we terminate our experiments after 2-weeks of BLEO instillation. It was interesting to observe that markers of fibrosis and pulmonary pressure were elevated just after 3 days of bleomycin instillation. Thus, it appears that the pathology of PF and PH occur simultaneously in the bleomycin model. Though it is logical to believe that PH follows fibrotic lung injury, it is possible that both the pathological conditions might occur concurrently. From our study, it is difficult to figure out which pathology comes first—PF or PH. Additional studies in the bleomycin model are warranted to evaluate and clarify these points.

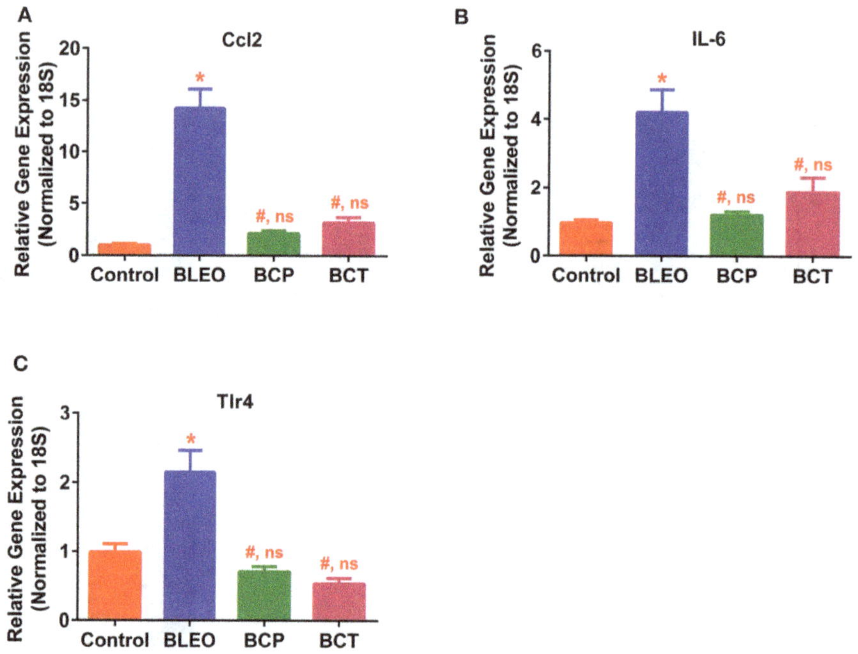

FIGURE 6 | C21 treatment attenuates the expression of inflammatory markers in BLEO animals **(A)** Ccl2, **(B)** IL-6, and **(C)** Tlr4. Data represented in **(A–C)** are mean $\pm$ SEM, $n = 5$ animals/group. *Indicates a p-value of ≤ 0.05, comparing BLEO animals against the controls. # Indicates a p-value of ≤ 0.05, comparing BCP and BCT vs. BLEO. ns indicates a p-value of non-significant, comparing BCP and BCT vs. control.

Right ventricular structure and function is often altered in patients with IPF because of increased pulmonary vascular resistance and cardiac overload (Han et al., 2013; Rivera-Lebron et al., 2013). In our animal study, bleomycin-instillation was associated with ventricular hypertrophy and right heart dysfunction. Interestingly, treatment with C21 not only attenuated bleomycin-induced cardiac hypertrophy but also improved right heart function in both the experimental protocols. It is conceivable that the protective effects of C21 on the heart may be secondary to a reduction in fibrotic lung injury. However, it is also possible that C21 may exhibit direct actions on the heart. In fact, C21 has been shown to exert protective actions against experimental models of cardiovascular injury (Kaschina et al., 2008; Rehman et al., 2012). With regards to pirfenidone and nintedanib (the approved anti-fibrotic drugs), there exists limited data in the literature on the cardioprotective effects of these agents in the bleomycin model. However, pirfenidone, has been shown to produce beneficial actions on the heart (Avila et al., 2014). It would be interesting to evaluate the cardiopulmonary effects of a combination therapy with C21 and pirfenidone/nintedanib. In conjunction to improving the heart function, C21 treatment also improved pulmonary vascular remodeling by reducing the muscularization of smaller vessels, as evidenced by histology. A potential limitation of our study is that the lungs of BLEO-injected animals at the onset of C21 administration in the treatment protocol (Day 4) resembles early stage of IPF, and not an advanced disease stage. Further studies are warranted to evaluate the effects of C21 on the advanced stage of lung fibrosis by commencing C21 treatment after 7 or 10 days of BLEO instillation. One another limitation is that we have not conducted antagonist experiments with an AT_2 receptor blocker (PD123319) to convincingly show that C21 mediates its anti-fibrotic effects via stimulation of the AT_2 receptor. Additional studies need to be performed with an AT_2 receptor blocker to address this deficiency. However, at this point we contend that the significant findings observed in the present investigation overrules the above mentioned potential limitations and ascertains that C21 could indeed be an effective strategy for the treatment of IPF and Group III PH.

Accumulating evidence indicate that the RAS has important functions within the cardiopulmonary system. While the role of the AT_1 receptor has been well-recognized, little is known about the functional significance of the AT_2 receptor. The reason being, there is a relatively lower expression of AT_2 receptor in the adult tissue. However, during injury, the receptor expression levels increase significantly (Matavelli and Siragy, 2015). There have been conflicting reports on whether the observed increase in AT_2 receptor during injury contributes to tissue damage, or that it plays a compensatory protective role. With regards to fibrotic lung injury, Konigshoff et al., reported an upregulation of the AT_2 receptor in the lungs of IPF patients (Königshoff et al., 2007). Similarly, animal models of lung fibrosis were associated with increased pulmonary AT_2 receptor levels (Königshoff et al., 2007; Rey-Parra et al., 2012). Consistent with these reports, we also observed an elevation in the expression of lung AT_2 receptor in BLEO animals.

AT_2 receptor is primarily expressed by lung epithelial cells (Bullock et al., 2001), fibroblasts, and activated myofibroblasts

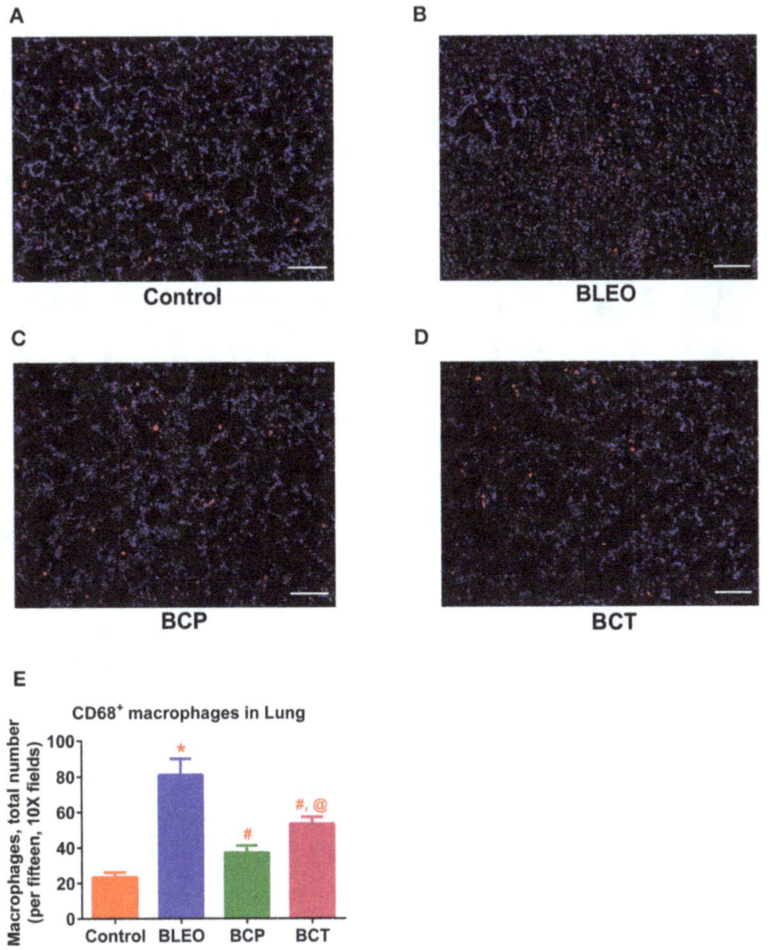

FIGURE 7 | C21 treatment reduces the infiltration of pulmonary macrophages in BLEO animals **(A–D)** Representative images of $CD68^+$ macrophages. **(E)** Summary data showing the reduction of $CD68^+$ pulmonary macrophages (red) in BLEO animals in presence of C21. Data represented in **(E)** is mean ± SEM ($n = 3$). *Indicates a p-value of ≤ 0.05, comparing BLEO animals against the controls. # Indicates a p-value of ≤ 0.05, comparing BCP and BCT vs. BLEO. @ indicates a p-value of ≤ 0.05, comparing BCP and BCT vs. control. Scale = 100 μm.

(Königshoff et al., 2007). We propose that the observed upregulation of AT_2 receptor in BLEO animals could arise from increased numbers of lung fibroblast/myofibroblast, a common feature of fibrotic lung injury (Pardo and Selman, 2016). However, the AT_2 receptor levels were significantly lower in C21 treated animals, which correlated with reduced pathology. Further support that the AT_2 receptors are found on the myofibroblasts comes from a recent report by Kumar et al. (2016) who demonstrated that in cultured human lung fibroblasts (MRC5 cells), BLEO (5 μg/ml) triggered the differentiation of fibroblasts into myofibroblasts with a marked elevation of expression level of fibrotic markers, fibronectin, alpha smooth muscle actin, collagen type1, and collagen type 3. Co-treatment of these cells with C21 (10 μg/ml) blocked the expression of these markers (Kumar et al., 2016). Thus, a plausible explanation for our *in vivo* findings is that C21 may inhibit fibroblast proliferation or differentiation, and/or reduce the influx of circulating fibrocytes. Since there is less fibroblast/myofibroblast with C21 treatment, there is less AT_2 receptor in the treated group. On the contrary, in the monocrotaline-induced PH model, we have reported that the AT_2 levels increase with C21 treatment. These contrasting findings could be attributed to differences in disease models (monocrotaline vs. bleomycin), the time of C21 treatment initiation, and/or the different lung cell-types involved in the disease pathology. We believe that identification of cell-types that express the AT_2 receptor in these two varied models of lung injury (Bleomycin and Monocrotaline) would be beneficial and help to resolve some of the observed discrepancy.

Lung fibroblasts are actively involved in the secretion of collagen type I, type III, and fibronectin, thus contributing to the accumulation of ECM proteins and fibrogenesis (Shimbori et al., 2013). The synthesis rates of types I and III collagen are regulated by the mRNA expression levels of Col1a1 and Col3a1, respectively. We observed that the gene expression of Col1a1 and Col3a1 are significantly upregulated in BLEO lungs, but normalized with C21 treatment in both the experimental protocols. Our results are in agreement with the recent findings,

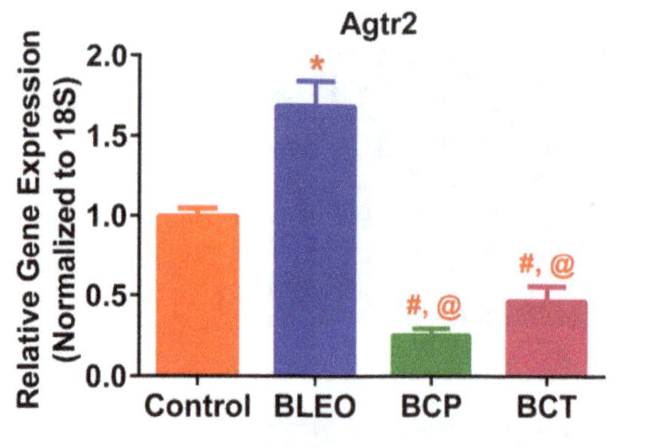

FIGURE 8 | C21 treatment attenuates the expression of Angiotensin type 2 receptor in BLEO animals. Treatment of BLEO animals with C21 attenuated the expression of Agtr2 in the lungs. Data represented is mean ± SEM, $n = 5$ animals/group. *Indicates a p-value of ≤ 0.05, comparing BLEO animals against the controls. #Indicates a p-value of ≤ 0.05, comparing BCP and BCT vs. BLEO. @ indicates a p-value of ≤ 0.05, comparing BCP and BCT vs. control.

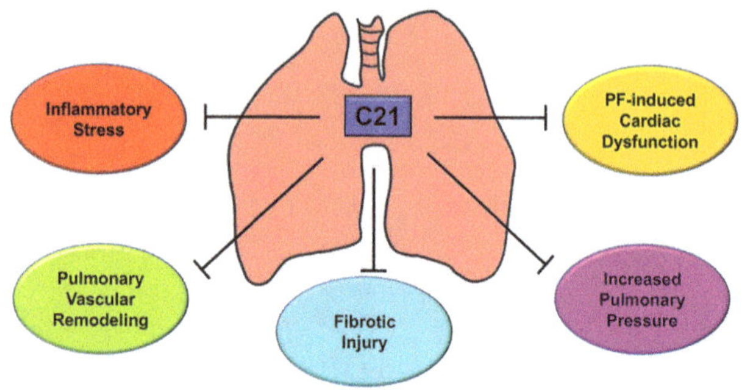

FIGURE 9 | Putative mechanism of action - AT_2R stimulation by C21. C21 exerts a host of actions on the cardiopulmonary system that include decrease in lung inflammatory stress, reduction of pulmonary vascular remodeling, attenuation of fibrotic lung injury, lowering of pulmonary pressure, and improvement of cardiac function. All these properties are responsible for the protective actions of C21 against pulmonary fibrosis and associated cardiac damage.

which demonstrated that stimulation of the AT_2 receptor with C21 suppresses collagen synthesis to exhibit anti-fibrotic actions in diverse models of organ fibrosis (Castoldi et al., 2016; Chow et al., 2016). Apart from collagen, a wide variety of matrix metalloproteinases (MMPs) and endogenous inhibitors of metalloproteinases (TIMPs, tissue inhibitor of MMPs) are involved in lung fibrogenesis (Giannandrea and Parks, 2014). In addition, upregulation of Il-13 and Ctgf (Guo et al., 2015; Yang et al., 2015) expression levels contribute to fibrotic lung diseases. Hence, we wanted to investigate the effects of C21 on the gene expression of Mmp 12, Timp1, Il-13, and Ctgf. Interestingly, stimulation of the AT_2 receptor by C21 decreased levels of Mmp12, Timp1, Il-13, and Ctgf in both the experimental protocols. Our results are in line with the published literature (Koulis et al., 2015). Thus, the anti-fibrotic effects of C21 may be partly mediated by modulation of MMP's, TIMP's, Il-13, and CTGF.

Increasing evidence suggests that pharmacological activation of the AT_2 receptor attenuates inflammation and oxidative stress to exert anti-fibrotic actions (Koulis et al., 2015). In the present study, treatment of BLEO animals with C21 resulted in significant downregulation of Ccl2, Il-6, and Tlr4 in combination with reduced recruitment or infiltration of macrophages to the injured lung, could contribute to the observed protective effects. A recent review on AT_2 receptor agonists summarizes that the receptor activation by C21 mechanistically arrests and attenuates the multiple process of fibrosis by: (i) the direct inhibition of pro-inflammatory and fibrotic factors; (ii) inhibition of remodeling of macrophages and fibroblasts to myofibroblasts; and (iii) inhibition of secretion or synthesis of ECM or collagen by myofibroblasts (Wang Y. et al., 2017). Overall, these findings strongly support our contention that the activation of the AT_2 receptor by C21 has a direct role in providing anti-inflammatory and anti-fibrotic actions.

To improve life expectancy in patients with Group III PH due to fibrotic lung injury, it is preemptive to treat cardiovascular complications since fibrosis is an irreversible process. In this investigation, we have demonstrated that activation of the AT_2 receptor by C21 significantly decreased inflammatory stress, reduced pulmonary vascular remodeling, mitigated fibrotic lung injury, restored pulmonary hemodynamics, and attenuated cardiac dysfunction as represented in **Figure 9**. Collectively, our study provides the necessary experimental evidence to attempt the strategy of utilizing AT_2 receptor agonist for the treatment of IPF and Group III PH.

AUTHOR CONTRIBUTIONS

AR, MK, MR, and VS: Conceived and designed the experiment; AR, AH, KH, AK, DM, SG, GB, and VS: Performed the experiment; AR, TU, MR, JW, US, CS, MK, and VS: Analyzed the data; AR, US, CS, MK, and VS: Wrote the paper.

REFERENCES

Anandharajan, R., Sayyed, S. G., Doshi, L. S., Dixit, P., Chandak, P. G., Dixit, A. V., et al. (2009). 18F9 (4-(3,6-bis (ethoxycarbonyl)-4,5,6,7-tetrahydrothieno (2,3-c) pyridin-2-ylamino)-4-oxobutanoic acid) enhances insulin-mediated glucose uptake *in vitro* and exhibits antidiabetic activity *in vivo* in db/db mice. *Metab. Clin. Exp.* 58, 1503–1516. doi: 10.1016/j.metabol.2009.04.036

Ashcroft, T., Simpson, J. M., and Timbrell, V. (1988). Simple method of estimating severity of pulmonary fibrosis on a numerical scale. *J. Clin. Pathol.* 41, 467–470. doi: 10.1136/jcp.41.4.467

Avila, G., Osornio-Garduño, D. S., Ríos-Pérez, E. B., and Ramos-Mondragón, R. (2014). Functional and structural impact of pirfenidone on the alterations of cardiac disease and diabetes mellitus. *Cell Calcium* 56, 428–435. doi: 10.1016/j.ceca.2014.07.008

Bruce, E., Shenoy, V., Rathinasabapathy, A., Espejo, A., Horowitz, A., Oswalt, A., et al. (2015). Selective activation of angiotensin AT2 receptors attenuates progression of pulmonary hypertension and inhibits cardiopulmonary fibrosis. *Br. J. Pharmacol.* 172, 2219–2231. doi: 10.1111/bph.13044

Bullock, G. R., Steyaert, I., Bilbe, G., Carey, R. M., Kips, J., De Paepe, B., et al. (2001). Distribution of type-1 and type-2 angiotensin receptors in the normal human lung and in lungs from patients with chronic obstructive pulmonary disease. *Histochem. Cell Biol.* 115, 117–124. doi: 10.1007/s004180000235

Canestaro, W. J., Forrester, S. H., Raghu, G., Ho, L., and Devine, B. E. (2016). Drug

Treatment of Idiopathic Pulmonary Fibrosis: Systematic Review and Network Meta-Analysis. *Chest* 149, 756–766. doi: 10.1016/j.chest.2015.11.013

Castoldi, G., di Gioia, C. R., Carletti, R., Roma, F., Zerbini, G., and Stella, A. (2016). Angiotensin Type-2 (AT-2)-Receptor activation reduces renal fibrosis in cyclosporine nephropathy: evidence for blood-pressure independent effect. *Biosci. Rep.* 36, e00403. doi: 10.1042/BSR20160278

Chow, B. S., Koulis, C., Krishnaswamy, P., Steckelings, U. M., Unger, T., Cooper, M. E., et al. (2016). The angiotensin II type 2 receptor agonist compound 21 is protective in experimental diabetes-associated atherosclerosis. *Diabetologia* 59, 1778–1790. doi: 10.1007/s00125-016-3977-5

Collum, S. D., Amione-Guerra, J., Cruz-Solbes, A. S., DiFrancesco, A., Hernandez, A. M., Hanmandlu, A., et al. (2017). Pulmonary Hypertension Associated with Idiopathic Pulmonary Fibrosis: Current and Future Perspectives. *Can. Respir. J.* 2017:1430350. doi: 10.1155/2017/1430350

Giannandrea, M., and Parks, W. C. (2014). Diverse functions of matrix metalloproteinases during fibrosis. *Dis. Model. Mech.* 7, 193–203. doi: 10.1242/dmm.012062

Guo, J., Yao, H., Lin, X., Xu, H., Dean, D., Zhu, Z., et al. (2015). IL-13 induces YY1 through the AKT pathway in lung fibroblasts. *PLoS ONE* 10:e0119039. doi: 10.1371/journal.pone.0119039

Han, M. K., Bach, D. S., Hagan, P. G., Yow, E., Flaherty, K. R., Toews, G. B., et al. (2013). Sildenafil preserves exercise capacity in patients with idiopathic pulmonary fibrosis and right-sided ventricular dysfunction. *Chest* 143, 1699–1708. doi: 10.1378/chest.12-1594

Iwai, M., and Horiuchi, M. (2009). Devil and angel in the renin-angiotensin system: ACE-angiotensin II-AT1 receptor axis vs. ACE2-angiotensin-(1-7)-Mas receptor axis. *Hypertens Res.* 32, 533–536. doi: 10.1038/hr.2009.74

Joseph, J. P., Mecca, A. P., Regenhardt, R. W., Bennion, D. M., Rodríguez, V., Desland, F., et al. (2014). The angiotensin type 2 receptor agonist Compound 21 elicits cerebroprotection in endothelin-1 induced ischemic stroke. *Neuropharmacology* 81, 134–141. doi: 10.1016/j.neuropharm.2014.01.044

Kaschina, E., Grzesiak, A., Li, J., Foryst-Ludwig, A., Timm, M., Rompe, F., et al. (2008). Angiotensin II type 2 receptor stimulation: a novel option of therapeutic interference with the renin-angiotensin system in myocardial infarction? *Circulation* 118, 2523–2532. doi: 10.1161/CIRCULATIONAHA.108.784868

Königshoff, M., Wilhelm, A., Jahn, A., Sedding, D., Amarie, O. V., Eul, B., et al. (2007). The angiotensin II receptor 2 is expressed and mediates angiotensin II signaling in lung fibrosis. *Am. J. Respir. Cell Mol. Biol.* 37, 640–650. doi: 10.1165/rcmb.2006-0379TR

Koulis, C., Chow, B. S., McKelvey, M., Steckelings, U. M., Unger, T., Thallas-Bonke, V., et al. (2015). AT2R agonist, compound 21, is reno-protective against type 1 diabetic nephropathy. *Hypertension* 65, 1073–1081. doi: 10.1161/HYPERTENSIONAHA.115.05204

Kumar, A., Rathinasabapathy, A., Horowitz, A., Horton, K., Martinez, D., Raizada, M., et al. (2016). Stimulation of AT2 receptor decreases collagen expression and inhibits myofibroblast differentiation to protect against bleomycin-induced pulmonary fibrosis. *FASEB J.* 30(1 Suppl), lb586. doi: 10.1096/fasebj.30.1_supplement.lb586

Ley, B., and Collard, H. R. (2013). Epidemiology of idiopathic pulmonary fibrosis. *Clin. Epidemiol.* 5, 483–492. doi: 10.2147/CLEP.S54815

Matavelli, L. C., and Siragy, H. M. (2015). AT2 receptor activities and pathophysiological implications. *J. Cardiovasc. Pharmacol.* 65, 226–232. doi: 10.1097/FJC.0000000000000208

Nogueira-Ferreira, R., Faria-Costasup, G., Ferreira, R., and Henriques-Coelho, T. (2016). Animal models for the study of pulmonary hypertension: potential and limitations. *Cardiol. Cardiovasc. Med.* 1, 1–22. doi: 10.26502/fccm.9292001

Pardo, A., and Selman, M. (2016). Lung fibroblasts, aging, and idiopathic pulmonary fibrosis. *Ann. Am. Thorac Soc.* 13(Suppl. 5), S417–S421. doi: 10.1513/AnnalsATS.201605-341AW

Patel, S. N., Ali, Q., and Hussain, T. (2016). Angiotensin II type 2-receptor agonist C21 reduces proteinuria and oxidative stress in kidney of high-salt-fed obese zucker rats. *Hypertension* 67, 906–915. doi: 10.1161/HYPERTENSIONAHA.115.06881

Raghu, G., Collard, H. R., Egan, J. J., Martinez, F. J., Behr, J., Brown, K. K., et al. (2011). An official ATS/ERS/JRS/ALAT statement: idiopathic pulmonary fibrosis: evidence-based guidelines for diagnosis and management. *Am. J. Respir. Crit. Care Med.* 183, 788–824. doi: 10.1164/rccm.2009-040GL

Raghu, G., and Selman, M. (2015). Nintedanib and pirfenidone. New antifibrotic treatments indicated for idiopathic pulmonary fibrosis offer hopes and raises questions. *Am. J. Respir. Crit. Care Med.* 191, 252–254. doi: 10.1164/rccm.201411-2044ED

Rathinasabapathy, A., Bruce, E., Espejo, A., Horowitz, A., Sudhan, D. R., Nair, A., et al. (2016). Therapeutic potential of adipose stem cell-derived conditioned medium against pulmonary hypertension and lung fibrosis. *Br. J. Pharmacol.* 173, 2859–2879. doi: 10.1111/bph.13562

Rehman, A., Leibowitz, A., Yamamoto, N., Rautureau, Y., Paradis, P., and Schiffrin, E. L. (2012). Angiotensin type 2 receptor agonist compound 21 reduces vascular injury and myocardial fibrosis in stroke-prone spontaneously hypertensive rats. *Hypertension* 59, 291–299. doi: 10.1161/HYPERTENSIONAHA.111.180158

Rey-Parra, G. J., Vadivel, A., Coltan, L., Hall, A., Eaton, F., Schuster, M., et al. (2012). Angiotensin converting enzyme 2 abrogates bleomycin-induced lung injury. *J. Mol. Med.* 90, 637–647. doi: 10.1007/s00109-012-0859-2

Rivera-Lebron, B. N., Forfia, P. R., Kreider, M., Lee, J. C., Holmes, J. H., and Kawut, S. M. (2013). Echocardiographic and hemodynamic predictors of mortality in idiopathic pulmonary fibrosis. *Chest* 144, 564–570. doi: 10.1378/chest.12-2298

Shenoy, V., Gjymishka, A., Jarajapu, Y. P., Qi, Y., Afzal, A., Rigatto, K., et al. (2013). Diminazene attenuates pulmonary hypertension and improves angiogenic progenitor cell functions in experimental models. *Am. J. Respir. Crit. Care Med.* 187, 648–657. doi: 10.1164/rccm.201205-0880OC

Shenoy, V., Kwon, K. C., Rathinasabapathy, A., Lin, S., Jin, G., Song, C., et al. (2014). Oral delivery of Angiotensin-converting enzyme 2 and Angiotensin-(1-7) bioencapsulated in plant cells attenuates pulmonary hypertension. *Hypertension* 64, 1248–1259. doi: 10.1161/HYPERTENSIONAHA.114.03871

Shimbori, C., Gauldie, J., and Kolb, M. (2013). Extracellular matrix microenvironment contributes actively to pulmonary fibrosis. *Curr. Opin. Pulm. Med.* 19, 446–452. doi: 10.1097/MCP.0b013e328363f4de

Wan, Y., Wallinder, C., Plouffe, B., Beaudry, H., Mahalingam, A. K., Wu, X., et al. (2004). Design, synthesis, and biological evaluation of the first selective nonpeptide AT2 receptor agonist. *J. Med. Chem.* 47, 5995–6008. doi: 10.1021/jm049715t

Wang, L., Wang, Y., Li, X. Y., and Leung, P. S. (2017). Angiotensin II type 2 receptor activation with compound 21 augments islet function and regeneration in streptozotocin-induced neonatal rats and human pancreatic progenitor cells. *Pancreas* 46, 395–404. doi: 10.1097/MPA.0000000000000754

Wang, Y., Del Borgo, M., Lee, H. W., Baraldi, D., Hirmiz, B., Gaspari, T. A., et al. (2017). Anti-fibrotic potential of AT2 receptor agonists. *Front. Pharmacol.* 8:564. doi: 10.3389/fphar.2017.00564

Wolters, P. J., Collard, H. R., and Jones, K. D. (2014). Pathogenesis of idiopathic pulmonary fibrosis. *Annu. Rev. Pathol.* 9, 157–179. doi: 10.1146/annurev-pathol-012513-104706

Yang, Z., Sun, Z., Liu, H., Ren, Y., Shao, D., Zhang, W., et al. (2015). Connective tissue growth factor stimulates the proliferation, migration and differentiation of lung fibroblasts during paraquat-induced pulmonary fibrosis. *Mol. Med. Rep.* 12, 1091–1097. doi: 10.3892/mmr.2015.3537

2

Incremental Shuttle Walking Test Distance is Reduced in Patients with Pulmonary Hypertension in World Health Organisation Functional Class I

*Catherine G. Billings[1], Robert Lewis[1], Iain J. Armstrong[1], Judith A. Hurdman[1], Ian A. Smith[1], Matthew Austin[1], Charlie A. Elliot[1], Athanasios Charalampopoulos[1], Ian Sabroe[2], Allan Lawrie[2], A. A. Roger Thompson[2], Robin Condliffe[1] and David G. Kiely[1,2,3]**

[1] Sheffield Pulmonary Vascular Disease Unit, Sheffield Teaching Hospitals NHS Foundation Trust, Royal Hallamshire Hospital, Sheffield, United Kingdom, [2] Department of Infection, Immunity and Cardiovascular Disease, University of Sheffield, Medical School, Sheffield, United Kingdom, [3] Insigneo Institute for in Silico Medicine, University of Sheffield, Sheffield, United Kingdom

***Correspondence:**
David G. Kiely
david.kiely@sth.nhs.uk

Background: There is increasing interest in screening for and diagnosing pulmonary hypertension earlier in the course of disease. However, there is limited data on cardiopulmonary abnormalities in patients with pulmonary hypertension newly diagnosed in World Health Organization Function Class (WHO FC) I.

Methods: Data were retrieved from the ASPIRE registry (Assessing the Spectrum of Pulmonary hypertension Identified at a REferral center) for consecutive treatment naïve patients diagnosed with pulmonary hypertension by cardiac catheterization between 2001 and 2010 who underwent incremental shuttle walk exercise testing.

Results: Eight hundred and ninety-five patients were diagnosed with Group 1-5 pulmonary hypertension. Despite the absence of symptoms, patients in WHO FC I ($n = 9$) had a significant reduction in exercise capacity (Incremental shuttle walk distance percent predicted (ISWD%pred) $65 \pm 13\%$, Z score -1.77 ± 1.05), and modest pulmonary hypertension with a median (interquartile range) pulmonary artery pressure 31(20) mmHg and pulmonary vascular resistance 2.1(8.2) Wood Units, despite a normal diffusion of carbon monoxide adjusted for age and sex (DLco)%pred $99 \pm 40\%$. Compared to patients in WHO FC I, patients in WHO FC II ($n = 162$) had a lower ISWD%pred 43 $\pm$ 22 and lower DLco%pred $65 \pm 21\%$.

Conclusion: Our results demonstrate that patients with newly diagnosed pulmonary hypertension with no or minimal symptomatic limitation have a significant reduction of exercise capacity.

Keywords: incremental shuttle walk test, pulmonary hypertension, WHO functional class, screening, early diagnosis, hemodynamics, exercise testing

INTRODUCTION

Despite advances in treatment, pulmonary hypertension (PH) remains a progressive life-limiting disease (1). Studies have suggested that earlier intervention results in better outcomes (2, 3). However, patients are usually diagnosed when the disease is advanced (4, 5) and consequently there is interest in developing strategies to enable earlier diagnosis (6). To diagnose pulmonary hypertension prior to the development of significant disease, it is recommended that people at increased risk of developing pulmonary hypertension such as patients with systemic sclerosis should be screened (7). These international guidelines emphasize the importance of echocardiography in the screening process. In systemic sclerosis where the prevalence of pulmonary arterial hypertension is particularly high, investigators have also recommended the use of diffusion capacity of the lung for carbon monoxide percent predicted (DLco%pred) which is frequently reduced in patients with systemic sclerosis and pulmonary arterial hypertension (8–10). More recently a cross-sectional, international study looked at a large number of candidate biomarkers in systemic sclerosis to construct a model to aid decisions to proceed to cardiac catheterisation (the DETECT study) (11).

At rest the pulmonary circulation has large microcirculatory reserves. These are recruited during exercise, increasing the capillary surface area available for gas exchange and maintaining a low pulmonary artery pressure despite increased flow (12). Any reduction in pulmonary vasculature reserves may therefore be first detected during exercise. Although exercise testing using the 6-min walk test was included as a candidate marker in the DETECT study, and may have been expected to contribute to an early diagnostic model, it had no utility in the model constructed to diagnose pulmonary arterial hypertension. This may reflect the inability of the 6-min walk test to identify the presence of early pulmonary vascular disease given its ceiling effect where in mild disease 6 min walking test distance no longer reflects maximal oxygen aerobic capacity (13–15) or disease severity (16) or be due to an inability of patients with systemic sclerosis to exercise as a consequence of musculoskeletal disease. In addition, a systematic review of studies looking at the correlation of the New York Heart Association (NYHA) Classification and the 6-min walk distance (6MWD) in patients with heart failure without musculoskeletal disease (17) also found no significant difference between asymptomatic/mildly symptomatic patients (NYHA I and II).

The incremental shuttle walking test (ISWT) has no ceiling effect (18) and correlates better with peak exercise capacity than the 6-min walking test (19). We have hypothesized that the incremental shuttle walking test will be reduced in patients with pulmonary hypertension in World Health Organization functional class I (WHO FC I) when the patients have either no or minor symptoms of breathlessness.

METHODS

Data were retrieved from the ASPIRE registry (Assessing the Spectrum of Pulmonary hypertension Identified at a REferral center) for consecutive, treatment naïve patients diagnosed with pulmonary hypertension between 2001 and 2010 (4). The systematic assessment of the patients has previously described in detail (4). Patients included in this retrospective study were diagnosed as Group 1–5 PH and were required to have mean pulmonary artery pressure at right heart catheterisation of at least 25 mmHg and had a baseline ISWT within 3 months of cardiac catheterization.

Incremental Shuttle Walk Test

The ISWT was performed according to the method of Singh et al. (20). Patients were asked to walk as far as possible around the 10 m course keeping in time to an audio signal until they were too breathless or could no longer keep up with the speed. The initial walking speed was 0.50 m/s and this increased incrementally every minute to a maximum of 2.37 m/s. Breathlessness was measured at rest and at the end of the test using the modified Borg scale. Heart rate was measured throughout the test. ISWT distance (ISWD) percent predicted (ISWD%pred) and z score were calculated for each patient based on sex, age and BMI using the equation derived by Probst et al. (21). No supplemental oxygen was used during testing. If patients could not walk or could not walk without oxygen the distance was recorded as 0 m.

Lung Function Tests

Lung function tests were performed in accordance to the European Respiratory Society guidelines (22–25). Predicted DLco (DLco%pred) and z score were calculated for each patient

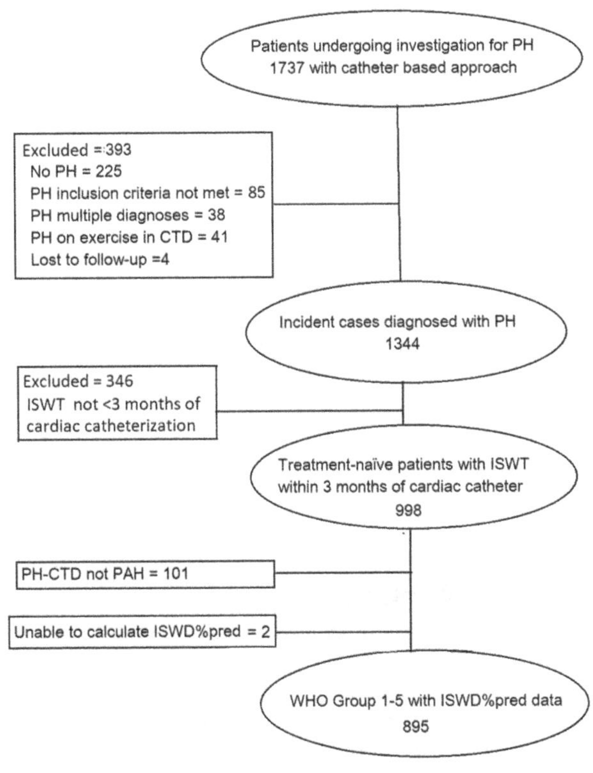

FIGURE 1 | Patient flow diagram.

TABLE 1 | Patient characteristics and hemodynamic parameters.

	WHO functional class			
	I	II	III	IV
n	9	162	592	132
Sex male/female %	44/56	46/54	38/62	37/63
Age years	51 ± 13	56 ± 16	61 ± 16*	64 ± 16
BMI kg/m2	28.2 ± 4.7	28.0 ± 6.1	27.7 ± 6.2	27.1 ± 6.6
Smoking % Never/Ex/Current	43/57/0	48/44/8	38/51/12	36/57/7
Pack years	10 ± 16	12 ± 19	17 ± 20	25 ± 30†
Oxygen therapy % None/LTOT/Other	100/0/0	89/6/5	62/32/7	26/68/6
HEMODYNAMICS				
mRAP mmHg	8(8)	8(7)	9(8)	12(8)†
mPAP mmHg	31(20)	37(16)	45(17)	47(12)
sPAP mmHg	51(38)	58(25)	74(29)	75(24)
Wedge mmHg	16 ± 9	13 ± 6	12 ± 6	11 ± 5
CI L/min/m^2	3.4 ± 1.8	3.1 ± 0.8	2.7 ± 0.8*	2.1 ± 0.6†
PVR Wood Unit	2.1(8.2)	3.6(3.8)	7.0(6.9)*	11.5(6.8)†
SmvO2 %	67 ± 6	67 ± 7	63 ± 9*	58 ± 9†
ISWT				
ISWD m	450(150)	280(258)▲	120(140)*	10(58)†
ISWD%pred	65(20)	42(28)▲	20(21)*	3(9) †
ISWD Z score	−1.77 ± 1.05	−2.36 ± 1.36▲	−3.11 ± 1.14*	−3.48 ± 1.10†
Starting SaO2 %	96.7 ± 2.1	93.8 ± 4.2▲	91.0 ± 6.3*	85.0†
Lowest SaO2 %	84.2 ± 10.5	83.4 ± 11.0	82.6 ± 11.2	79.1 ± 11.6†
Starting HR bpm	85. ± 14	82 ± 17	83 ± 17	85 ± 18
Highest HR bpm	144 ± 37	125 ± 30	114 ± 23*	110 ± 23
Resting SBP mmHg	125 ± 25	131 ± 22	127 ± 20*	117 ± 19†
Highest SBP mmHg	159 ± 11	158 ± 25	145 ± 27*	128 ± 24†
Borg dyspnea score				
Pre-test	0.6 ± 0.7	0.7 ± 1.0	1.1 ± 1.3*	1.8 ± 1.4†
Post-test	3.8 ± 1.6	4.2 ± 1.9	4.3 ± 1.9	4.7 ± 2.0†
LUNG FUNCTION				
FEV1%pred	97 ± 14	75 ± 23▲	74 ± 21	67 ± 23†
FVC%pred	103 ± 17	87 ± 23	87 ± 23	81 ± 27
DLco mmol/min/kPa	7.6 ± 3.2	5.6 ± 2.2▲	4.3 ± 2.0*	2.9 ± 1.7†
DLco%pred	99 ± 40	72 ± 24▲	59 ± 22*	41 ± 21†
DLco Z score	−0.57 ± 3.43	−2.22 ± 1.96▲	−3.45 ± 2.37*	−5.69 ± 3.10†

*Presented as mean ± SD for parametric data and median(interquartile range) for nonparametric data. Categorical variables were presented as %. ISWT, incremental shuttle walk test; WHO FC, World Health Organisation functional class; BMI, body mass index; mRAP, mean right atrial pressure; mPAP, mean pulmonary arterial pressure; sPAP, systolic pulmonary arterial pressure; CI, cardiac index; PVR, pulmonary vascular resistance; SmvO2, mixed venous oxygen saturation; ISWD, incremental shuttle walk test distance; %pred: percent predicted; SaO2, oxygen saturation; HR, heart rate; SBP, systolic blood pressure; FEV1, forced expiratory volume in 1 second; FVC, forced vital capacity; DLco, diffusion factor across the lung for carbon monoxide; z score, standardized score; ▲$p < 0.05$ WHO FC I vs. WHO FC II; *$p < 0.05$ WHO FC II vs. WHO FC III; †$p < 0.05$ WHO FC III vs. WHO FC IV.*

using the Global Lung Function Initiative (GLI) reference equations (26).

Statistical Analysis

Statistical analysis was performed using IBM SPSS Statistics v19 (SPSS, Chicago, IL, USA). Data is presented as mean ± SD for parametric data and median (interquartile range) for nonparametric data. Categorical variables were presented as %. To evaluate our hypothesis that the incremental shuttle walking test will be reduced in WHO FC I, the main outcome variable was ISWD%pred. DLco%pred was a secondary outcome to be used in comparison to the ISWD. Pearson's correlation test was used to assess correlations between these parameters and WHO FC and hemodynamic parameters. The student *t*-test and Mann Whitney U-test and Kruskal-Wallis test were used to compare groups. Event (death or transplantation) free survival from date of diagnosis was estimated using the Kaplan–Meier method with comparison between groups performed by the log-rank test. Cox proportional hazards regression analysis was used to assess the effect of ISWD%pred, age, sex, BMI, mPAP and DLco on survival time. As left to right shunt is known to result in high DLco%pred (27),

TABLE 2 | Correlation of ISWD%pred with WHO FC, hemodynamics, dyspnea score and DLco%pred.

	N	r	95% CI		p
WHO FC	895	−0.576	−0.598	−0.553	< 0.001
mRAP	778	−0.238	−0.301	−0.175	< 0.001
sPAP	762	−0.145	−0.214	−0.075	< 0.001
mPAP	777	−0.171	−0.239	−0.103	< 0.001
PVR	755	−0.263	−0.327	−0.195	< 0.001
CI	754	0.271	0.139	0.336	< 0.001
Smv02	762	0.284	0.217	0.348	< 0.001
Wedge	724	0.014	−0.059	0.087	0.697
Borg Pre	631	−0.366	−0.432	−0.297	< 0.001
Borg Post	617	0.032	0.111	−0.047	0.433
DLco%pred	815	0.371	0.311	0.413	< 0.001

ISWD%pred, Incremental Shuttle Walk Test distance percent predicted; WHO FC, World Health Organization functional class; mRAP, mean right atrial pressure; sPAP, systolic pulmonary arterial pressure; mPAP, mean pulmonary arterial pressure; PVR, pulmonary vascular resistance; CI, cardiac index; SmvO2, mixed venous oxygen saturation; ISWD, Incremental Shuttle Walk Test distance; %pred, percent predicted; DLco%pred, diffusion factor across the lung for carbon monoxide percent predicted.

separate analyses were also performed omitting patients with congenital heart disease. Post-hoc analyses were also performed on the group of patients in WHO FC I and II with pulmonary hypertension related to systemic sclerosis who had undergone screening for PH. A p-value of <0.05 was deemed statistically significant. Ethical approval was granted by the North Sheffield Research Ethics Committee (Reference No. 06/Q2308/8).

RESULTS

During the duration of the study 895 patients were diagnosed with pulmonary hypertension and met the entry criteria (**Figure 1**). At diagnosis 9 patients (1%) were in WHO functional class 1, and 162 (18%), 592 (66%), and 132 (15%) in WHO Functional Class II, III, and IV, respectively. Of those in WHO FC I, 3 had systemic sclerosis (one of whom had a PAWP > 15 mmHg), 3 had congenital heart disease with left to right shunts, 1 left heart disease, 1 chronic thromboembolic pulmonary hypertension and 1 hereditary pulmonary arterial hypertension.

Demographics and Pulmonary Hemodynamics

Patients' characteristics are shown in **Table 1**. Patients in WHO FC I were not significantly different to patients in the other WHO FC's with respect to age, sex distribution or smoking history. No patients in WHO FC I were on oxygen therapy compared with 6% in WHO FC II. Patients in WHO FC I had modest pulmonary hypertension: mPAP median(Interquartile range) 31(20) mmHg, preserved cardiac index (CI): mean ± standard deviation 3.4 ± 1.8 l/min/m^2 with no significant difference compared to WHO FC II.

Incremental Shuttle Walking Test and Lung Function Testing

Incremental shuttle walking distances (absolute, %pred and standardized (z) score) were all significantly higher in WHO FC I compared to WHO FC II. In addition, resting oxygen saturation pre-test was significantly higher in WHO FC I compared to WHO FC II. There was no significant difference in Borg dyspnea score between these 2 groups either pre- or post-ISWT and no significant difference in highest heart rate or highest systolic blood pressure measured. ISWD%pred correlated significantly (p all <0.05) with WHO FC, mRAP, mPAP, sPAP, CI, PVR, and SmVO_2 (**Table 2**).

There were also significant differences in lung function between WHO FC I and II. DLco, DLco%pred, DLco z score and FVC were all significantly higher in WHO FC I. DLco%pred correlated with WHO FC, CI, PVR, and SmVO_2 but not mRAP, mPAP, or sPAP. There was a stronger correlation of WHO FC with ISWD%pred compared with correlation to DLco%pred, −0.576 and −0.382, respectively.

Although there were significant correlations between WHO FC and ISWD%pred and DLco%pred, there was heterogeneity in ISWD%pred and particularly DLco%pred within each WHO FC (**Figure 2**). **Figures 3A,B** show the median and interquartile range of results for ISWD%pred and DLco%pred, respectively, for all patients by WHO FC. A large interquartile range was noted for DLco%pred in WHO FC I. When patients with congenital heart disease were omitted from analysis (**Figures 3C,D**) the interquartile range of DLco%pred in WHO FC I was reduced. However, although ISWD%pred still discriminated between patients in WHO FC I and II (63 ± 15 vs. 45 ± 23 $p = 0.02$), DLco%pred (74 ± 14 vs. 69 ± 17) and FVC%pred (96 ± 12 vs. 89 ± 23) were no longer significantly different ($p > 0.05$). Similar patterns of heterogeneity was seen in the frequency of standardized scores.

To assess the suitability of the ISWT as a screening tool, cut-off points using %pred and z-score were investigated. **Figure 4** shows the percentage of patients with an ISWD%pred of <80%. A greater percentage of patients were identified using a cut-off of <80 ISWD%pred than by using the DLco%pred <80 cut-off. **Figure 2** shows that for any given %pred cut-off point, ISWD%pred will positively identify more of the PH patients than DLco%pred. Using z scores, ISWD is again a better discriminator than DLco (**Figure 5**). In WHO FC 1 44% of patients had an ISWD below the 5th percentile and 78% were below the 10th percentile. Overall 73% of patients in WHO FC I and II are below the 5th percentile for ISWD compared to only 58% below the 5th percentile for DLco. Eighty four percent vs. 66% respectively were below the 10th percentile.

Survival Analysis

Kaplan-Meier survival analysis demonstrated that WHO FC was a significant predictor of outcome with decreasing survival with increasing WHO FC ($p < 0.0001$) (**Figure 6**). Multivariate Cox survival analysis including the parameters ISWD%pred, age, sex, BMI, mPAP and DLco showed that ISWD%pred remained a significant predictor ($p < 0.001$) (**Table 3**).

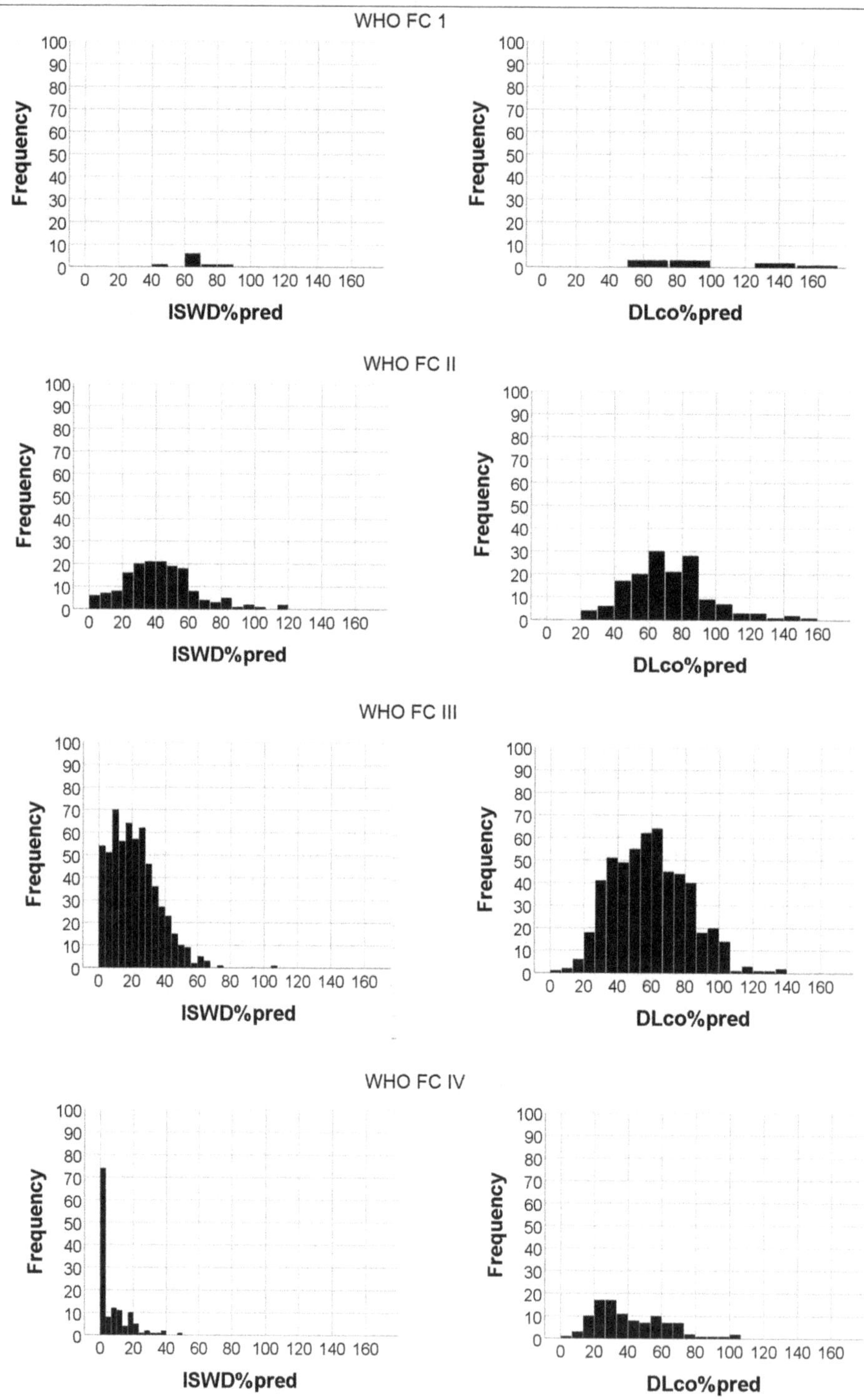

FIGURE 2 | Histogram of Incremental shuttle walk distance percent predicted (ISWD%pred) and Diffusing capacity across the lung for carbon monoxide percent predicted (DLco%pred) frequencies by World Health Organization functional class.

DISCUSSION

To our knowledge we have shown for the first time that patients with pulmonary hypertension in WHO FC I have a significant reduction in exercise capacity compared to predicted values. We have also demonstrated that exercise capacity is more sensitive than measurements of gas transfer made at rest in identifying patients with pulmonary hypertension in WHO FC I and WHO FC II. A single cut-off point is often suggested for screening as it is easy to remember and apply. We evaluated the use of a cut-off

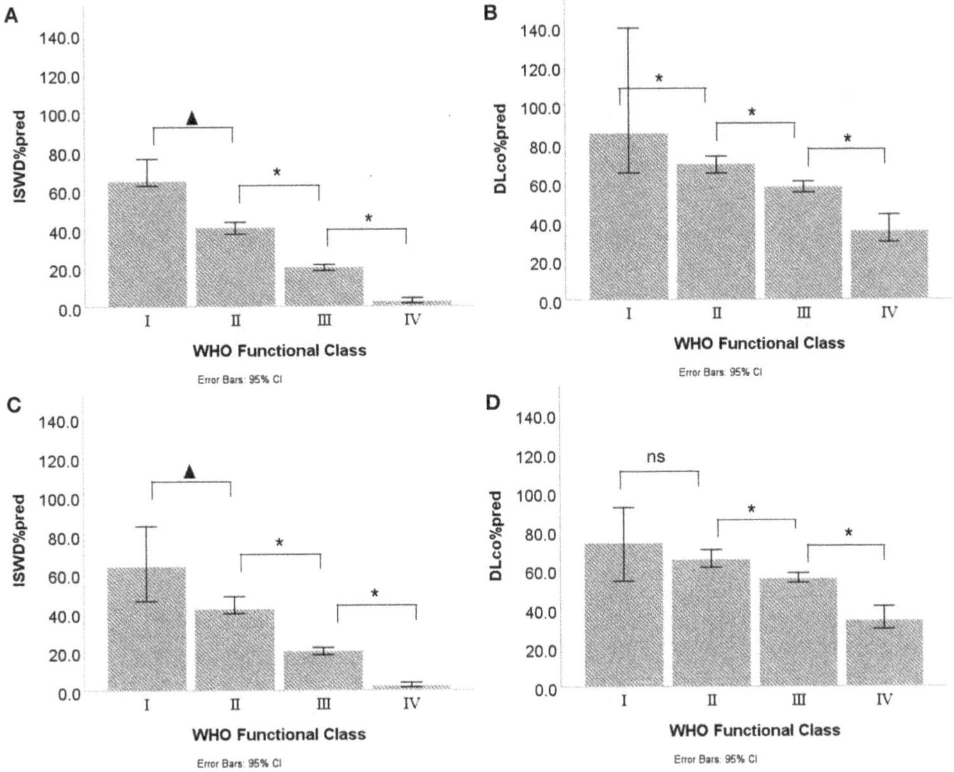

FIGURE 3 | Median and interquartile ranges for Incremental shuttle walk distance percent predicted (ISWD%pred) and Diffusing capacity across the lung for carbon monoxide percent predicted (DLco%pred) by World Health Organization Functional Class (WHO FC) in **(A,B)** all patients and **(C,D)** with congenital heart disease patients excluded. $p < 0.05$; $^*p < 0.005$; ns, not significant.

point of 80%pred looking for early changes and found that 89% of patients in WHO FCI were below this cut-off point. Whilst traditionally the normal range for a lung function parameters was considered as being between 80 and 120%pred it is known now that this could lead to misdiagnosis (28). We therefore also examined percentile scores as cut-off points and again found that the ISWT was a sensitive test with 73% of patients in WHO FC I and II below the 5th percentile for ISWD.

In addition to confirming the findings of previous studies (4, 29, 30) that WHO FC has a significant impact on survival, we have also demonstrated that in the absence of symptoms of breathlessness or in the presence of mild symptoms (i.e. patients in WHO FC 1/II) patients have a modest elevation of pulmonary artery pressure at initial diagnosis. In contrast patients with more severe symptoms of breathlessness (WHO FC III and IV) had significantly higher mean pulmonary artery pressure elevation. Therefore strategies to diagnose patients earlier when they have less symptomatic limitation is likely to identify patient with less severe pulmonary haemodynamic disease. Patients in WHO FC I included 3 patients with systemic sclerosis who had been identified from screening regimens and these patients had only mild elevation of mean pulmonary artery pressure, median 27 mmHg. Patients not undergoing regular screening, may also have been referred on the basis of echocardiograms performed for the assessment of incidental murmurs or on the basis of morphological changes consistent with pulmonary hypertension seen on cross sectional imaging.

It could be possible that there is some misclassification of the patients as classification into WHO FC is limited by patient and physician subjectivity and agreement between observers is often poor (31). There are however significant differences in ISWD%pred and DLco%predicted between FC I and II and there is a trend for increased survival. Breathlessness post ISWT is no greater in WHO FC I suggesting that the increased distance walked is not due to increased effort. This study, therefore, does emphasize that if we are to rely on self-reported symptoms of breathlessness to diagnose pulmonary hypertension then patients will have established hemodynamic changes of pulmonary hypertension at the time of diagnosis.

Current ESC/ERS guidelines recommend the use of Doppler echocardiography for screening for pulmonary hypertension in at risk patients. Like all screening tools echocardiography has limitations. In 10–20% of patients it is not possible to obtain interpretable results and the precision of echocardiography estimation of systolic pulmonary artery pressure can be poor (32). To overcome these difficulties other data, using lung function tests and utilizing gas transfer (which is reduced as a consequence of vascular involvement), have been used inscreening algorithms.

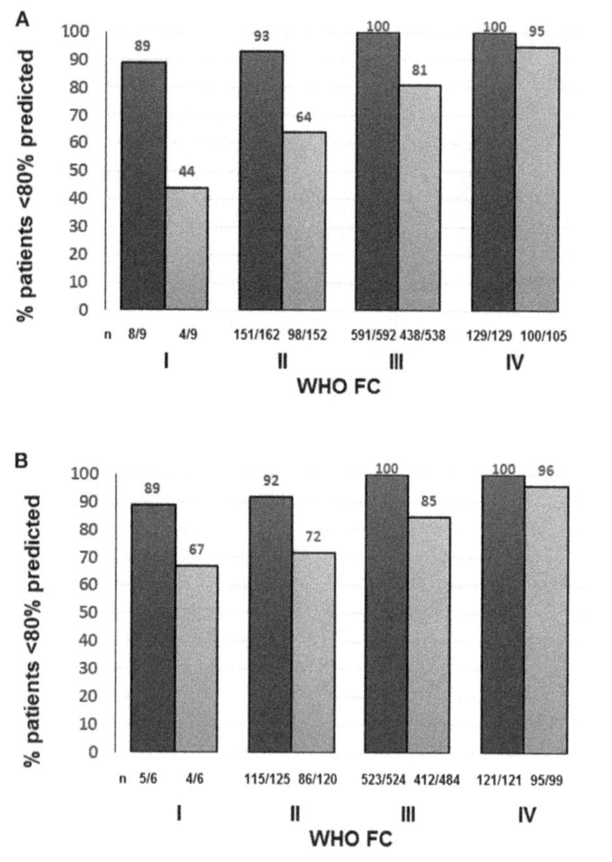

FIGURE 4 | Percentage of patients with Incremental shuttle walk distance percent predicted (ISWD%pred) ■ and Diffusing capacity across the lung for carbon monoxide percent predicted (DLco%pred) ■ less than 80% predicted in **(A)** All patients **(B)** Patients with congenital heart disease excluded by World Health Organization Functional Class (WHO FC).

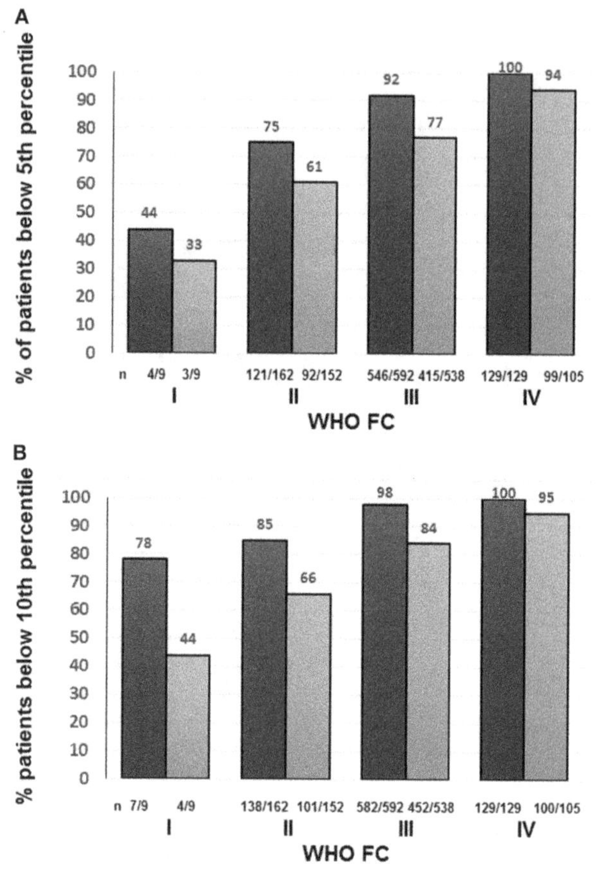

FIGURE 5 | Percentage of all patients with Incremental shuttle walk distance percent predicted (ISWD%pred) ■ and Diffusing capacity across the lung for carbon monoxide percent predicted (DLco%pred) ■ less than **(A)** the 5th percentile and **(B)** the 10th percentile World Health Organization Functional Class (WHO FC).

Most work has been done in systemic sclerosis using DLco%pred. Hanchulla et al. (9) in a French multi-center trial found that a low DLco of <60% predicted was associated with a higher probability of PAH with only 30% of the newly diagnosed patients having a DLco > 60%pred. A UK study among 243 systemic sclerosis-associated PH patients found that <10% had a DLco >60%pred (10). Guidelines now suggest using a cut-off of DLco%pred <60% as part of the screening algorithm indicative of possible pulmonary hypertension in systemic sclerosis (33). This strategy has been shown to successfully enrich this population of patients undergoing right heart catheter to investigate possible pulmonary hypertension (11). However, whilst this algorithm has been used with some success in systemic sclerosis it is not applicable in patients with pulmonary hypertension associated with other aetiologies (34). Our study highlights the large range of DLco%pred found in WHO FC I, even when omitting patients with congenital heart disease. In contrast ISWD%pred correlated well with WHO FC with <10% of patients in WHO FC I and II having an ISWD >80%pred.

A number of studies have looked at the use of exercise testing including cardiopulmonary exercise testing, exercise Doppler echocardiography or diffusion capacity during exercise (35–39) to try to detect loss of compliance in the cardiopulmonary circulation earlier than parameters measured at rest but the tests used are complex. The advantage of the ISWT for screening is that it is a very simple test to perform and has been shown to reflect disease severity without a ceiling effect (8). Data from this study suggest it might be suited to detecting early disease. Pulmonary arterial hypertension and chronic thromboembolic pulmonary hypertension, for which specific therapies exist, are rare and therefore early identification relies on having a high degree of awareness in patients at risk and deploying appropriate disease specific strategies. Reducing the time to diagnosis and institution of treatment for patients with pulmonary hypertension requires a number of complimentary approaches and screening for pulmonary hypertension in at risk groups is only one approach. In addition to considering pulmonary hypertension in high risk groups (e.g., systemic sclerosis, portal hypertension, HIV, family history of PAH), there needs to be an increased awareness amongst patients to seek advice when they have exercise limitation and for physicians

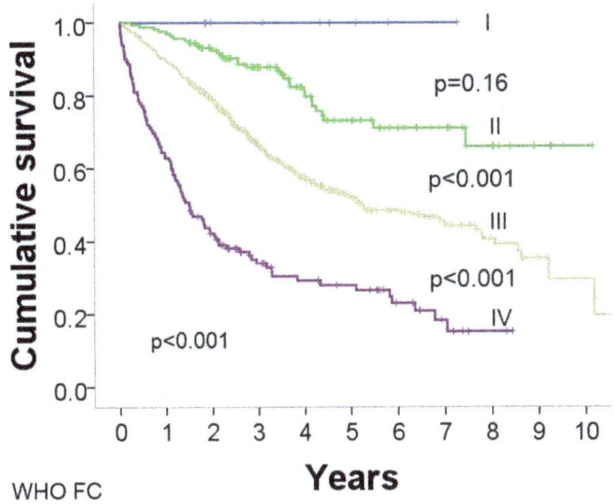

WHO FC											
I	9	9	6	6	5	3	1				
II	162	158	130	98	64	44	28	20	12	4	1
III	592	530	423	287	204	133	88	54	28	10	3
IV	132	83	63	32	24	21	12	6	2		
All	895	780	622	423	297	201	129	80	42	14	4

FIGURE 6 | Kaplan Meier survival analysis by World Health Organisation functional class.

TABLE 3 | Multivariate Cox survival analysis.

	HR	95% CI	*p*
ISWD%pred	0.983	0.975 – 0.990	<0.0001
Age	1.017	1.007 – 1.026	<0.0001
BMI	0.980	0.961 – 0.999	0.044
mPAP	1.022	1.011 – 1.032	<0.0001
DLco%pred	0.974	0.967 – 0.980	<0.0001

ISWD%pred, Incremental shuttle walk test percent predicted; BMI, body mass index; mPAP, mean pulmonary arterial pressure; DLco%pred, diffusion factor across the lung for carbon monoxide percent predicted; HR, hazard ratio; CI, confidence interval.

to more systematically assess the breathless patient. Our results suggest that exercise limitation (identified using a maximal exercise test) is an almost universal finding in patients with pulmonary hypertension even in patients who are asymptomatic. Further study is required to assess whether the incremental shuttle walking test could be used as a first line investigation or as part of a battery of tests to screen at risk patients, proceeding to more complex testing if abnormal.

LIMITATIONS

This was a retrospective, single center study. Within the studied population only 1% of patients were diagnosed in WHO FC I and 18% in WHO FC II. These percentages are small (but are very similar to those found in the Geissen Pulmonary Hypertension Registry, which has 1.0% patients in WHO FC I, and confirm the findings in other registries (4, 26) that the majority of patients are diagnosed with PH in WHO FC III when symptomatic and haemodynamic severity are advanced. Given the small number of patients in WHO FC I, interpretation of negative results must be viewed with caution Classification of WHO FC may be limited by patient and physician subjectivity and agreement between observers is often poor (31). However in this study there appears to be a trend to increased survival in WHO FC 1 patients and ISWD is significantly higher in patients in WHO FC I. Although patient motivation could affect distance walked, the ISWT is externally paced which limits the effect of motivation and patients in WHO FC I did not report a higher dyspnoea score post-test suggesting that the difference in distance walked was not due to greater patient effort.

CONCLUSION

Our results demonstrate that patients with newly diagnosed pulmonary hypertension with no or minimal symptomatic limitation have a significant reduction of exercise capacity.

AUTHOR CONTRIBUTIONS

CB, IA, RC, and DK: study design; JH, RL, CB, IAS, MA, AC, CE, RC, and DK: performance of the research; CB, AT, CE, IS, AC, AL, and DK: data analysis; CB and DK: writing of the paper; All authors: revision of manuscript.

FUNDING

None of the authors has a financial relationship with a commercial entity that has an interest in the subject of the presented manuscript. JH 's research fellowship during the period of the study was part-funded by an unrestricted educational grant from Actelion Pharmaceuticals Ltd. The funding bodies had no involvement in the development of this research or manuscript.

Financial Relationships to commercial entities not related to submitted manuscript. In the past 3 years AC, CE, DK, and RC have received have received honoraria for participation in advisory boards and for giving lectures and have received funding to attend educational meetings from personal fees and non-financial support to attend educational meetings from Actelion Pharmaceuticals Ltd and GSK. CE, DK, and RC also received honoraria for participation in advisory boards and for giving lectures and non-financial support from Bayer. In addition, RC received fees and support from United Therapeutics. IAS has received an unrestricted educational grant from GSK to support a clinical teaching meeting, an unrestricted educational grant from Triniti Chiesi Ltd. to support medical humanities research and projects, and funding to attend educational meetings from Boehringer Ingelheim and Actelion Pharmaceuticals Ltd. JH received funding from GSK and Pfizer to attend educational meetings. AT received funding from Actelion Pharmaceuticals Ltd. to attend educational meetings. IAS and CB received support from the Pulmonary Hypertension Association UK to attend educational meetings.

REFERENCES

1. Kiely DG, Elliot CA, Sabroe I, Condliffe R. Pulmonary hypertension: diagnosis and management. *BMJ* (2013) 346:f2028. doi: 10.1136/bmj.f2028
2. Humbert M, Yaici A, de Groote P, Montani D, Sitbon O, Launay D, et al. Screening for pulmonary arterial hypertension in patients with systemic sclerosis: clinical characteristics at diagnosis and long-term survival. *Arthr Rheumatism* (2011) 63:3522–30. doi: 10.1002/art.30541
3. Vizza CD, Badagliacca R, Messick CR, Rao Y, Nelsen AC, Benza RL. The impact of delayed treatment on 6-minute walk distance test in patients with pulmonary arterial hypertension: a meta-analysis. *Int J Cardiol.* (2018) 254:299–301. doi: 10.1016/j.ijcard.2017.12.016
4. Hurdman J, Condliffe R, Elliot CA, Davies C, Hill C, Wild JM, et al. ASPIRE registry: assessing the Spectrum of Pulmonary hypertension Identified at a REferral centre. *Eur Respir J.* (2012) 39:945–55. doi: 10.1183/09031936.00078411
5. Gall H, Felix JF, Schneck FK, Milger K, Sommer N, Voswinckel R, et al. The Giessen Pulmonary Hypertension Registry: Survival in pulmonary hypertension subgroups. *J Heart Lung Transp.* (2017) 36:957–67. doi: 10.1016/j.healun.2017.02.016
6. Lau EM, Manes A, Celermajer DS, Galiè N. Early detection of pulmonary vascular disease in pulmonary arterial hypertension: time to move forward. *Eur Heart J.* (2011) 32:2489–98. doi: 10.1093/eurheartj/ehr160
7. Galiè N, Humbert M, Vachiery JL, Gibbs S, Lang I, Torbicki A, et al. 2015 ESC/ERS Guidelines for the diagnosis and treatment of pulmonary hypertension: The Joint Task Force for the Diagnosis and Treatment of Pulmonary Hypertension of the European Society of Cardiology (ESC) and the European Respiratory Society (ERS): Endorsed by: Association for European Paediatric and Congenital Cardiology (AEPC), International Society for Heart and Lung Transplantation (ISHLT). *Eur Heart J.* (2016) 37:67–119. doi: 10.1093/eurheartj/ehv317
8. Elliot CA, KielyDG. Pulmonary hypertension: diagnosis and treatment. *Clin Med.* (2004) 4:211–5. doi: 10.7861/clinmedicine.4-3-211
9. Hachulla E, Gressin V, Guillevin L, Carpentier P, Diot E, Sibilia J, et al. Early detection of pulmonary arterial hypertension in systemic sclerosis: a French nationwide prospective multicenter study. *Arthr Rheum* (2005) 52:3792–3800. doi: 10.1002/art.21433
10. Schwaiger JP, Khanna D, Gerry Coghlan J. Screening patients with scleroderma for pulmonary arterial hypertension and implications for other at-risk populations. *Eur Respir Rev.* (2013) 22:515–25. doi: 10.1183/09059180.00006013
11. Coghlan JG, Denton CP, Grünig E, Bonderman D, Distler O, Khanna D, et al. DETECT study group. Evidence-based detection of pulmonary arterial hypertension in systemic sclerosis: the DETECT study. *Ann Rheum Dis* (2014) 73:1340–9. doi: 10.1136/annrheumdis-2013-203301
12. Lee G, DuBois AB. Pulmonary capillary blood flow in man. *J Clin Invest* (1955) 34:1380–90. doi: 10.1172/JCI103187
13. Lipkin DP, Scriven AJ, Crake T, Poole-Wilson PA. Six minute walking test for assessing exercise capacity in chronic heart failure. *Br Med J.* (1986) 292:653–5.
14. Deboeck G, Taboada D, Hagan G, Treacy C, Page K, Sheares K, et al. Maximal cardiac output determines 6 minutes walking distance in pulmonary hypertension. *PLoS ONE* (2014) 9:e92324. doi: 10.1371/journal.pone.0092324
15. van der Plas MN, Duffels MGJ, Ponse D, Mulder BJM, Bresser P. Bosentan in mild pulmonary hypertension. *Lancet* (2008) 372:1730. doi: 10.1016/S0140-6736(08)61725-0
16. Degano B, Sithon O, Savale L, Garcia G, O'Callaghan DS, Jaïs X, et al. Characterization of pulmonary arterial hypertension patients walking more than 450 m in 6 min at diagnosis. *Chest* (2010) 137:1297–303. doi: 10.1378/chest.09-2060
17. Yap J1, Lim FY, Gao F, Teo LL, Lam CS, Yeo KK. Correlation of the New York Heart association classification and the 6-minute walk distance: a systematic review. *Clin Cardiol.* (2015) 38:621–8. doi: 10.1002/clc.22468
18. Billings CG, Hurdman JA, Condliffe R, Elliot CA, Smith IA, Austin M, et al. Incremental shuttle walk test distance and autonomic dysfunction predict survival in pulmonary arterial hypertension. *J Heart Lung Trans.* (2017) 36:871–9. doi: 10.1016/j.healun.2017.04.008
19. Irisawa H, Takeuchi K, Inui N, Miyakawa S, Morishima Y, Mizushima T, et al. Incremental shuttle walk test as a valuable assessment of exercise performance in patients with pulmonary hypertension. *Circ J.* (2014) 78:215–21. doi: 10.1253/circj.CJ-13-0238
20. Singh SJ, Morgan MDL, Scott S, Walters D, Hardman AE. Development of a shuttle walking test of disability in patients with chronic airways obstruction. *Thorax* (1992) 47:1019–24.
21. Probst VS, Hernandes NA, Teixeira DC, Felcar JM, Mesquita RB, Gonçalves CG, et al. Reference values for the incremental shuttle walking test. *Respir Med.* (2012) 106:243–8. doi: 10.1016/j.rmed.2011.07.023
22. Quanjer PH, Tammeling GJ, Cotes JE, Pedersen OF, Peslin R, Yernault JC. Lung volumes and forced ventilatory flows. Report Working Party Standardization of Lung Function Tests, European Community for Steel and Coal. Official Statement of the European Respiratory Society. *Eur Respir J.* (1993) 6(Suppl. 16):S5–S40.
23. Cotes JE, Chinn DJ, Quanjer PH, Roca J, Yernault JC. Standardization of the measurement of transfer factor (diffusing capacity). Report Working Party Standardization of Lung Function Tests, European Community for Steel and Coal. Official Statem ent of the European Respiratory Society. *Eur Respir J.* (1993) 6(Suppl. 16), S41–S52.
24. Miller MR, Hankinson J, Brusasco V, Burgos F, Casaburi R, Coates A, et al. ATS/ERS Task Force. Standardisation of spirometry. *Eur Respir J.* (2005) 26:319–38. doi: 10.1183/09031936.05.00034805
25. Macintyre N, Crapo RO, Viegi G, Johnson DC, van der Grinten CP, Brusasco V, et al. Standardisation of the single-breath determination of carbon monoxide uptake in the lung. *Eur Respir J.* (2005) 26:720–35. doi: 10.1183/09031936.05.00034905
26. Stanojevic S, Graham BL, Cooper BG, Thompson BR, Carter KW, Francis RW, et al. On behalf of the Global Lung Function Initiative TLCO working group. Official ERS technical standards: Global Lung Function Initiative reference values for the carbon monoxide transfer factor for Caucasians. *Eur Respir J.* (2017) 50:170001. doi: 10.1183/13993003.00010-2017
27. Burgess JH. Pulmonary diffusing capacity in disorders of the pulmonary circulation. *Circulation* (1974) 49:541–50.
28. Miller MR, Quanjer PH, Swanney MP, Ruppel G, Enright PL. Interpreting lung function data using 80% predicted and fixed thresholds misclassifies more than 20% of patients. *Chest* (2011) 139:52–9. doi: 10.1378/chest.10-0189
29. Farber HW, Miller DP, Poms AD, Badesch DB, Frost AE, Muros-Le Rouzic E, et al. Five-Year outcomes of patients enrolled in the REVEAL Registry. *Chest* (2015) 148:1043–54. doi: 10.1378/chest.15-030
30. Humbert M, Sitbon O, Chaouat A, Bertocchi M, Habib G, Gressin V, et al. Survival in patients with idiopathic, familial, and anorexigen-associated pulmonary arterial hypertension in the modern management era. *Circulation* (2010) 122:156–63. doi: 10.1161/CIRCULATIONAHA.109.911818
31. Taichman DB, McGoon MD, Harhay MO, Archer-Chicko C, Sager JS, Murugappan M, et al. Wide variation in clinicians' assessment of New York Heart Association/World Health Organization functional class in patients with pulmonary arterial hypertension. *Mayo Clin Proc.* (2009) 84:586–92. doi: 10.1016/S0025-6196(11)60747-7
32. Fisher MR, Forfia PR, Chamera E, Housten-Harris T, Champion HC, Girgis RE, et al. Accuracy of Doppler echocardiography in the hemodynamic assessment of pulmonary hypertension. *Am J Respir Crit Care Med.* (2009) 179:615–21. doi: 10.1164/rccm.200811-1691OC
33. Khanna D, Gladue H, Channick R, Chung L, Distler O, Furst DE, et al. Scleroderma Foundation and Pulmonary Hypertension Association. Recommendations for screening and detection of connective-tissue disease associated pulmonary arterial hypertension. *Arthritis Rheum.* (2013) 65:3194–201. doi: 10.1002/art.38172
34. Lau EMT, Humbert M, Celermajer DS. Early detection of pulmonary arterial hypertension. *Nat Rev. Cardiol.* (2015) 12:143–155. doi: 10.1038/nrcardio.2014.191
35. Dumitrescu D, Nagel C, Kovacs G, Bollmann T, Halank M, Winkler J, et al. Cardiopulmonary exercise testing for detecting pulmonary arterial hypertension in systemic sclerosis. *Heart* (2017) 103:774–82. doi: 10.1136/heartjnl-2016-309981
36. Mueller J, Heck PB, Ewert P, HagerA. Noninvasive screening for pulmonary hypertension by exercise testing in congenital heart disease. *Ann Thorac Surg.* (2017) 103:1544–49. doi: 10.1016/j.athoracsur.2016.09.038
37. Trip P, Vonk-Noordegraaf A, Bogaard HJ. Cardiopulmonary exercise testing reveals onset of disease and response to treatment in a case of heritable pulmonary arterial hypertension. *Pulm Circ.* (2012) 2:387–9. doi: 10.4103/2045-8932.101658

38. Baptista R, Serra S, Martins R, Teixeira R, Castro G, Salvador MJ, et al. Exercise echocardiography for the assessment of pulmonary hypertension in systemic sclerosis: a systematic review. *Arthr Res Ther.* (2016) 18:153. doi: 10.1186/s13075-016-1051-9
39. Legnani D, Rizzi M, Sarzi-Puttini P, Cristiano A, La Spina T, Frassanito F, et al. Diffusing pulmonary capacity measured during effort: a possible early marker of pulmonary involvement in Systemic Sclerosis. *Isr Med Assoc J.* (2015) 17:739–43.

3

Circulating MicroRNA Markers for Pulmonary Hypertension in Supervised Exercise Intervention and Nightly Oxygen Intervention

Gabriele Grunig[1,2], Christina A. Eichstaedt[3], Jeremias Verweyen[3], Nedim Durmus[1], Stephanie Saxer[4], Greta Krafsur[5], Kurt Stenmark[5], Silvia Ulrich[4], Ekkehard Grünig[3] and Serhiy Pylawka[2]*

[1] Department of Environmental Medicine and Division of Pulmonary Medicine, Department of Medicine, New York University School of Medicine, New York, NY, United States, [2] Mirna Analytics LLC, New York, NY, United States, [3] Thoraxklinik, Heidelberg University Hospital, Heidelberg, Germany, [4] Clinic for Pulmonology, University Hospital Zürich, Zurich, Switzerland, [5] Department of Medicine, University of Colorado, Aurora, CO, United States

***Correspondence:**
Gabriele Grunig
ggrunig1@earthlink.net;
grunig01@nyu.edu

Rationale: Therapeutic exercise training has been shown to significantly improve pulmonary hypertension (PH), including 6-min walking distance and right heart function. Supplemental nightly oxygen also has therapeutic effects. A biomarker tool that could query critical gene networks would aid in understanding the molecular effects of the interventions.

Methods: Paired bio-banked serum (n = 31) or plasma (n = 21) samples from the exercise or oxygen intervention studies, respectively, and bio-banked plasma samples (n = 20) from high altitude induced PH in cattle were tested. MicroRNAs (miRNAs) markers were chosen for study because they regulate gene expression, control the function of specific gene networks, and are conserved across species.

Results: miRNAs that control muscle (miR-22-3p, miR-21-5p) or erythrocyte function (miR-451a) were chosen based on pilot experiments. Plasma samples from cattle that developed PH in high altitude had significantly higher miR-22-3p/(relative to) miR-451a values when compared to control cattle tolerant to high altitude. Measurements of miR-22-3p/miR-451a values in serum from patients receiving exercise training showed that the values were significantly decreased in 74.2% of the samples following intervention and significantly increased in the remainder (25.8%). In samples obtained after exercise intervention, a higher composite miRNA value, made of miR-22-3p and miR-21-5p/miR-451a and spike RNA, was significantly decreased in 65% of the samples and significantly increased in 35% of the samples. In the study of nightly oxygen intervention, when comparing placebo and oxygen, half of the samples showed a significant down-ward change and the other half a significant up-ward change measuring either of the miRNA markers. Samples that had a downward change in the miRNA marker following either intervention originated from patients who had a significantly higher 6-min-walking-distance at baseline (mean difference of 90 m or 80 m following exercise or oxygen intervention, respectively) when compared to samples that had an upward change in the miRNA marker.

Conclusion: These natural animal model and human sample studies further highlight the utility of miRNAs as future biomarkers. The different directional changes of the miRNA markers following supervised exercise training or nightly oxygen intervention could indicate different PAH molecular pathomechanisms (endotypes). Further studies are needed to test this idea.

Keywords: pulmonary hypertension, MicroRNA, circulating biomarker, high altitude pulmonary hypertension, supervised exercise training, nightly oxygen intervention

INTRODUCTION

Pulmonary hypertension (PH) is a progressive disease for which there is no cure. PH is characterized by increased blood pressure in the pulmonary vasculature and the right heart, and can occur as a primarily vascular disease, or associated with conditions that cause pulmonary vascular remodeling and constriction. In all instances, PH leads to adverse clinical outcomes relative to the respective disease or healthy control groups that have no PH, and can be the cause of early mortality with 2–5 years life expectancy. The current World Symposium on Pulmonary Hypertension (WSPH) classification of PH is based on a combination of patient characteristics, clinical features and cardiopulmonary hemodynamics and these WHO groups are used to inform drug treatment options (Simonneau et al., 2013). Recently, PH interventions based on supervised exercise training and nightly oxygen have been developed that have significant therapeutic effect to a degree that is expected from adding another drug for multi-drug treatment of PH (Mereles et al., 2006; Grunig et al., 2011, 2012a,b; Nagel et al., 2012; Becker-Grunig et al., 2013; Schumacher et al., 2014; Pandey et al., 2015; Ulrich et al., 2015; Ehlken et al., 2016; Gonzalez-Saiz et al., 2017; Keusch et al., 2017; Moreira-Goncalves et al., 2017; Richter et al., 2017; Leggio et al., 2018). Already after a 3-week period, supervised exercise training improved, for example, the 6MWD and hemodynamics, which are important signs for PH prognosis (Grunig et al., 2012a,b). Nightly oxygen, even after 1 week, likewise, significantly improved the 6MWD (Schumacher et al., 2014; Ulrich et al., 2015).

Aside from genetic testing and the measurement of the right-heart stress markers B-type natriuretic peptide biomarkers that would identify the molecular or cellular pathobiologic mechanism that identify the cause of PH are not established (Hoffmann et al., 2016). Further, biomarkers that could explain the effects of therapeutic interventions like supervised exercise training or nightly oxygen, would aid in the understanding of the causes of PH, and represent optimal monitoring tools for the disease. Additionally, biomarkers that could identify underlying molecular mechanisms would be important to understand the diversity of PH by characterizing subtypes of PH that are distinguished by molecular pathomechanisms [endotypes (Lotvall et al., 2011)] (Hemnes et al., 2017). This is important for personalized medicine for PH patients. The diverse molecular nature of PH is underscored by our recent understanding of mutations that can cause heritable PH. For example, recent work has identified multiple genes in multiple different molecular pathways that have gene-function altering mutations and confer greatly increased risk for developing PH. Examples include BMPR2 gene and other genes in the BMPR – transforming growth factor signaling networks, potassium channel dysfunction (KCNK3 gene), transcription factors, water channel (aquaporin gene) (Eichstaedt et al., 2017; Kimura et al., 2017; Ma and Chung, 2017; Olschewski et al., 2017; Gräf et al., 2018). Further evidence for the complex molecular cause of PH is that several risk factors have to come together to trigger disease (Viales et al., 2015; Evans et al., 2016).

MicroRNAs (miRNAs) function as epigenetic regulators of gene expression. miRNAs are small non-coding RNAs that negatively regulate gene expression by binding to the 3′UTR (untranslated region) of target messenger RNAs (mRNAs), thereby promoting mRNA degradation or suppressing the translation of the mRNA, in both cases, limiting or suppressing protein production from that specific gene. Currently, several thousands of miRNAs have been identified, each miRNA binding to several mRNAs, to control the function of several genes. In contrast to mRNA, miRNAs are actively excreted by cells and occur in the circulation (blood), miRNAs are very stable in bodily fluids, and are conserved among species. The importance of miRNA for PH has been established in recent studies (Bockmeyer et al., 2012; Brock et al., 2012; White et al., 2012). miRNAs are known for their critical function in gene-reprogramming that occurs in response to hypoxia (Hale et al., 2012), and hypoxia is an important cause for PH. Additionally, miR-204 has been identified as a critical pathogenic mediator in experimental PH, and it is down-regulated in human PH (Courboulin et al., 2011). Several miRNAs, among them miR-21 or miR-20, have been shown to target BMPR2 (Qin et al., 2009; Brock et al., 2012) and to also have critical function for the hypoxia mediated reprogramming of the pulmonary vasculature (Sarkar et al., 2010; Brock et al., 2012; Yang et al., 2012).

The current studies were designed to test the idea that circulating miRNA marker levels measured in the serum or plasma would be associated with PH in an animal model (Newman et al., 2015), and demonstrate significant change following PH-alleviating supervised exercise training (Grunig et al., 2012; Ehlken et al., 2016) or nightly oxygen

Abbreviations: 6MWD, 6-min walking distance; BMI, body mass index; BMPR2, bone morphogenetic protein receptor 2; miRNA, MicroRNA; PAP, pulmonary artery pressure; PH, pulmonary hypertension.

(Schumacher et al., 2014; Ulrich et al., 2015) interventions in human patients.

MATERIALS AND METHODS

Ethics Statement

All samples were from bio-repositories at the collaborating institutions. Serum and plasma samples were obtained for studies unrelated to the current experiments and then stored in respective bio-repositories at the University of Colorado (cattle plasma samples), or Universities of Zürich or Heidelberg (human samples). The previous studies (Grunig et al., 2012a; Schumacher et al., 2014; Newman et al., 2015; Ulrich et al., 2015; Ehlken et al., 2016) were performed under the supervision of the respective ethics committees at the collaborating institutions with the consent that bio-repositories can be instituted. The human participants gave written informed consent for blood sample studies for the supervised exercise intervention (Ehlken et al., 2016) and the nocturnal oxygen intervention (Ulrich et al., 2015) studies, respectively. The blood samples were obtained for other outcomes, unrelated to our study. For the current studies, the samples were sent to us from our collaborators in a de-identified manner, by persons not directly involved in the current study, such that we would never be able to access the link to the identifying data. For this reason, our research falls under the category 'no human or animal subjects involvement' and therefore ethics approval was not required for this research as per our Institution's guidelines and national regulations.

Cattle Plasma Samples

Plasma samples were analyzed from groups of cattle that were kept at high altitude (2300 m and higher) and that had received approval by the Institutional Animal Use and Care Committee at the University of Colorado (Newman et al., 2015). One group of cattle remained healthy and tolerant of the altitude with mean pulmonary artery pressures (mean PAP) of 50 mmHg and less (Newman et al., 2015). The other group had exhibited signs of intolerance to high altitude with mean PAP of 79 mmHg and more. A few cattle had an intermediate response with mean PAP of 50–79 mmHg.

Human Plasma and Serum Samples

De-identified, plasma and serum samples from bio-repositories were received from two different centers at the Universities of Heidelberg (Grunig et al., 2012a; Ehlken et al., 2016) and Zürich (Schumacher et al., 2014; Ulrich et al., 2015), respectively. The baseline characteristics of the sample donors are listed in **Table 1**, and the diagnoses are summarized in **Table 2**. The study from the Thoraxclinic, University of Heidelberg, had the goal to test the treatment effects of a supervised exercise program that was administered for the duration of 3 weeks in PH patients (Grunig et al., 2012a; Ehlken et al., 2016). Paired serum samples had been obtained before and after the supervised exercise program for outcomes unrelated to our study. The samples were sent to us from a repository. The study from the University of Zürich had been designed to test the effects of nightly oxygen that was administered in a randomized, double blinded manner to PH patients (Schumacher et al., 2014; Ulrich et al., 2015). Each patient was randomly assigned to placebo (air) or oxygen first, and then was crossed-over to receive the other intervention. Paired plasma samples were obtained from the placebo and the oxygen parts of the study, respectively, for outcomes unrelated to our study, each taken after 1-week duration of the placebo or oxygen periods, respectively. Samples were sent to us from a repository.

RNA Isolation

The same volume (200 μl) plasma or serum was used for total RNA purification for all samples. Total RNA was purified using miRNAeasy Mini Kit according to the protocol of the manufacturer (Qiagen, Valencia, CA, United States) and eluted into 35 μl of water. During RNA isolation process, after the lysis and homogenization step of the manufacturer's protocol, 1 μl of UniSp6 RNA Spike-in template (representing 10^8 copies) was added. The Spike RNA was used as an exogenous reference for the miRNA measurements. The UniSp6 RNA Spike-in template was provided with the miRCURY LNA^{TM} Universal cDNA synthesis kit II (Exiqon, Woburn, MA, United States).

For all human plasma samples, we performed a heparinase step following RNA purification. Thirty nanograms of RNA was treated with the following mix: 0.3U of heparinase (H2519-50UN, Sigma-Aldridge, St. Louis, MO, United States) and 22U RNAse inhibitor (Invitrogen) re-suspended in 1xRT buffer from miRCURY LNA^{TM} Universal cDNA synthesis kit II, for 1 h at 25°C to remove heparin.

The cattle RNA was isolated in the same manner with addition of dialysis step prior RNA isolation, because the cattle samples were thought to contain citrate and heparin. Briefly,

TABLE 1 | Characteristics of sample populations.

		U. Heidelberg (Grunig et al., 2012a; Ehlken et al., 2016) exercise intervention	**U. Zürich (Schumacher et al., 2014; Ulrich et al., 2015) oxygen intervention**
Number of pairs		31	21
Age		50.68 ± 2.935[1]	65.14 ± 2.205
Gender	Female	21	13
	Male	10	8
NYHA class[2]	II	16	5
	III	9	16
BMI (kg/m^2)		28.28 ± 1.239	27.33 ± 0.892
6MWD (m)		459.5 ± 23.03	438.30 ± 19.79
PH with additional diagnosis[3]		87%	100%
Mean PA pressure (mmHg)		50.54 ± 3.383	40.50 ± 3.801

*[1]Means ± SEM are indicated. [2]Information was not available for each of the variables [e.g., NYHA (New York Heart Association) class of heart failure and mean pulmonary artery (PA) pressure]. Of the patients with missing NYHA classification (n = 6) the mean pulmonary artery pressures at rest were between 50 and 80 mmHg in three patients, and 40 mmHg in one patient. [3]PH classifications and Additional Diagnoses are listed in **Table 2**.*

TABLE 2 | Diagnoses for PH Patients.

	U. Heidelberg (exercise intervention)	U. Zürich (oxygen intervention)
Total number of PH patients	31 (100%)	21 (100%)
	Primary diagnosis[1]	
Idiopathic PAH	19 (61%)	12 (57%)
Heritable PAH	7 (22.6%)	
Associated PAH		
connective tissue disease	2 (6.5%)	1 (4.8%)
portal hypertension	2 (6.5%)	1 (4.8%)
congenital heart disease	1 (3.2%)	
Chronic thromboembolic PH		7 (33%)
	Additional diagnosis[2]	
Number of patients who had additional diagnoses	27 (87%)	21 (100%)
Transient embolic episodes of the pulmonary artery	6 (19%)	
Peripheral vascular disease (hypertension, subdural hematoma, arterial blockage, chronic venous disease)	9 (29%)	8 (38%)
Chronic lung disease (COPD, airway hyperreactivity, airway obstruction, asthma)	8 (26%)	6 (28%)
Left heart disease and/or heart rhythm abnormalities	7 (23%)	6 (28%)
Anemia, or iron therapy	8 (26%)	2 (9.5%)
Auto-immune disease (e.g., insulin dependent diabetes, or autoimmune thyroiditis)	3 (9.7%)	2 (9.5%)
Kidney disease	5 (16%)	5 (24%)
Tumor	2 (6.5%)	1 (4.8%)

[1] *One primary diagnosis per patient. All patients received PH specific medication.*
[2] *One or more additional diagnoses per patient. The patients received diagnosis specific medication as needed.*

200 μl of sample in dialysis tube [Slide-A-Lyser Mini Dialysis Unit, 2000 MWCO] (Thermo Fisher Scientific, Waltham, MA, United States) was dialyzed against 200 ml of 1xTE (10 mM Tris-HCl pH 8.0, 1 mM EDTA) at room temperature for 1 h. This was followed by miRNAeasy Mini Kit extraction with addition of 10^8 copies UniSp6-Spike RNA and heparinase treatment.

Reverse transcriptase reaction was performed with miRCURY LNA™ Universal cDNA synthesis kit II accordingly to manufacturer's instructions. RNA concentrations were measured with DS-11 spectrophotometer (DeNovix, Wilmington, DE, United States).

miRNA Expression

Real time PCR was performed in triplicate with 0.1 ng of cDNA per reaction using a 7900HT Fast Real-Time PCR instrument (Applied Biosystems/Life Technologies, Grand Island, NY, United States) in a 10 μl volume. The PCR reactions were run with LNA-modified primers and SYBR Green master mix (Exiqon, Denmark/now Qiagen) in 384-well plate under the following conditions: 95°C for 10 min, followed by 45 cycles of 95°C for 10 s and 60°C for 1 min, followed by a hold at 4°C. The following LNA-modified primers were used: hsa-miR-451a (target 5′AAACCGUUACCAUUACUGAGUU); hsa-miR-22-3p (target 5′AAGCUGCCAGUUGAAGAACUGU); hsa-miR-21-5p (target 5′UAGCUUAUCAGACUGAUGUUGA); Spike6 (target the synthetic spike RNA, UniSP6, supplied in the cDNA kit).

For the pilot study, we purchased LNA-modified primers specific for 16 additional miRNAs (hsa-let-7g-5p, hsa-miR-17-5p, hsa-miR-20a-5p, hsa-miR-20b-5p, hsa-miR-26a-5p, hsa-miR-27a-3p, hsa-miR-27b-5p, hsa-miR-30e-3p, hsa-miR-30e-5p, hsa-miR-93-5p, hsa-miR-103a-3p, hsa-miR-135a-5p, hsa-miR-142-5p, hsa-miR-150-5p, hsa-miR-204-5p, Exiqon) and performed real time PCR exactly as described above.

Raw data were then analyzed with SDS Relative Quantification Software version 2.4.1 (Applied Biosystems) to determine cycle threshold (Ct). The miRNA values that were calculated relative to synthetic spike RNA used the following equation: 1.98 to the power of [Ct of spike6 RNA − Ct of miRNA determinant], and then multiplied by 10,000 (human data) or multiplied by 10 (cattle data). The composite miRNA values were calculated as follows: 1.98 to the power of [Ct of miRNA reference(s) − Ct of miRNA determinant(s)], and then multiplied by 10,000. The miRNA values were calculated without knowledge of the characteristics of the sample donors. The full data sets that were calculated relative to synthetic spike RNA are shown in Excel data files (Supplementary Files: cattle_data.xlsx; human_large_sample_set.xlsx; human_large_mir_set.xlsx).

Statistical Analysis

Group comparisons were performed with the two-tailed, independent Mann–Whitney *U* test, or the Wilcoxon matched pairs signed rank test as indicated. Correlations were calculated with the Spearman's Rank Correlation test. Statistics were calculated and graphs were generated using Prism 6 (GraphPad, La Jolla, CA, United States). A p-value < 0.05 was considered to be statistically significant.

Hierarchical clustering was performed to calculate principal component analysis and to generate heatmaps with the freely available online R-based tool ClustVis[1] (Metsalu and Vilo, 2015). Unsupervised hierarchical clustering was performed using Euclidean distance and complete linkage for columns (miRNA value relative to spike RNA) and rows (sample ID). The heat map graphs were re-oriented (columns and rows transposed) for best display of the data.

RESULTS

Choice of miRNAs

Pilot studies were performed with RNA from whole blood and serum (n = 12 and n = 6, respectively) from paired samples from patients who had received exercise training intervention. We utilized RNA sequencing of whole blood RNA (data not shown) and literature mining to choose 18 miRNAs for a pilot study in serum samples

[1] https://biit.cs.ut.ee/clustvis/

(**Supplementary Figure S1**). Specific LNA-modified primers to hsa-let-7g-5p, hsa-miR-17-5p, hsa-miR-20a-5p, hsa-miR-20b-5p, hsa-miR-21-5p, hsa-miR-22-3p, hsa-miR-26a-5p, hsa-miR-27a-3p, hsa-miR-27b-5p, hsa-miR-30e-3p, hsa-miR-30e-5p, hsa-miR-93-5p, hsa-miR-103a-3p, hsa-miR-135a-5p, hsa-miR-142-5p, hsa-miR-150-5p, hsa-miR-204-5p, and hsa-miR-451a were detected by quantitative PCR and were calculated relative to synthetic spike RNA (**Supplementary Figure S1a**). We performed hierarchical cluster analysis to identify miRNAs that would show changed levels when comparing samples taken after and before training. We focused on the magnitude of the change, irrespectively, of the direction of the change (increased or decreased). Three miRNAs were most interesting: miR-22-3p, miR-451a, and miR-21-5p (**Supplementary Figure S1b**). We also searched for endogenous reference miRNAs that would show little, if any variations among the samples, and did not find clear candidates. However, a literature review indicated that miR-451a had been considered as a reference miRNA (Song et al., 2012), although in our samples this was not the case when miR-451a was measured against the extrinsically added spike RNA (**Supplementary Figure S1**).

Cattle Model of High Altitude Induced PH

Because the human PH condition is heterogeneous, we wanted to test the miRNAs that we had identified in the pilot studies with human samples (with focus on miR-22-3p and miR-451a) in an animal model. High altitude induced PH was chosen because this is a natural disease in cattle that has clearly identified etiology (high altitude, with the decreased oxygen tension and hypoxia challenge) with genetic predisposition in the EPAS-1 (Endothelial PAS Domain-Containing Protein 1) gene, also known as hypoxia inducible factor 2-alpha. Additional reasons to choose the cattle model included the possibility to measure pulmonary arterial pressures (PAP) by catheterization, even in the clinical setting, and the cross-species conservation of the miRNAs between cattle and human. Plasma samples from cattle that were tolerant to high altitude (mean PAP less than 50 mmHg), cattle that had developed PH (mean PAP more than 79 mmHg) and cattle with intermediate mean PAP values were analyzed. The data showed significantly decreased miR-22-3p determined relative to miR-451a values in the plasma samples from the tolerant (control) cattle, as compared to the intolerant and intermediate groups (**Figure 1**). miR-22-3p and miR-451a are of molecular interest in PH, particularly in PH associated with oxygen consumption, because miR-22-3p has been shown to regulate muscle function, including skeletal (Eisenberg et al., 2007; Schweisgut et al., 2017), heart and smooth muscle (Huang et al., 2013; Huang and Wang, 2014; Zhao et al., 2015), control estrogen signaling by targeting the estrogen receptor (Pandey and Picard, 2009), while miR-451a controls erythrocyte function (Dore et al., 2008; Yu et al., 2010) and skeletal muscle function (Davidsen et al., 2011).

Choice of Reference miRNAs for the Human Test

Having confirmed the utility of miR-22-3p and miR-451a as potential biomarkers for PH in the cattle model, we wanted to further understand the relationships between the miRNA measurements, including also miR-21-5p. Hierarchical cluster analysis was performed on all data from both intervention studies (exercise or oxygen, respectively, with 52 donors and 104 samples in total). The results are presented in a heatmap display (**Supplementary Figure S2**). The cluster analysis showed that miR-21-5p and miR-22-3p clustered together, separately from miR-451a, Additionally, the clustered miRNA's separated the before and after intervention measurements in 46 donors, and only 6 donor data clustered together (**Supplementary Figure S2**).

For miR-22-3p relative to miR-451a and additionally for each of the studied miRNA's we calculated the miRNA level values relative to spike RNA and determined the fold change after training or oxygen, respectively. We then determined correlations of the fold-change values (**Table 3**). The calculations showed that the fold change determined in miR-22-3p (relative to spike) was significantly correlated with the fold change in miR-21-5p (relative to spike) in both the training and the oxygen intervention studies, respectively (**Table 3**). This prompted us to also compare the fold-change in composite miRNA values, combining miR-22-3p and miR-21-5p, as a way to diminish the significance of technical variations (minute pipetting errors for example) as causes for variations in the qPCR quantification

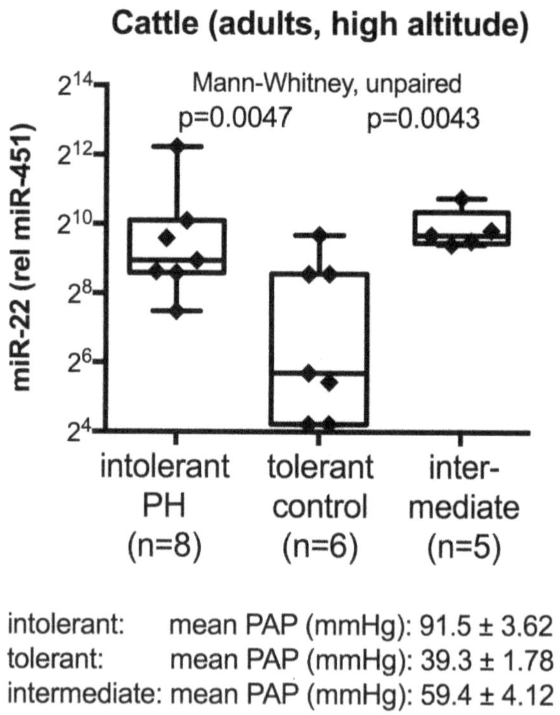

FIGURE 1 | Circulating plasma miRNA values in cattle at high altitude. Box-plots with whiskers and individual points show miR-22-3p relative to miR-451a (10,000×) values in plasma samples from control cattle that were tolerant to high altitude [mean pulmonary artery pressure, mean PAP, <50 mm Hg (Newman et al., 2015)], or that developed PH (mean PAP ≥79 mmHg), or that had intermediate mean PAP. Groups were compared with the unpaired, 2-tailed Mann–Whitney test; $p < 0.05$ was considered significant.

values. As for the reference miRNA composite choice, we used miR-451a plus spike RNA, because spike RNA is the invariant component of our test, as the same number of copies (10^8) of spike RNA were added to each 200 μl of sample used for the RNA isolation. The composite miRNA marker was then calculated as miR-22-3p + miR-21-5p relative to miR-451a + spike RNA. The composite marker (miR-22-3p + miR-21-5p relative to miR-451a + spike RNA) was significantly correlated with the values for miR-22-3p relative to miR-451a in both the exercise training and oxygen intervention studies, respectively (**Table 3**).

TABLE 3 | Correlations between different types of miRNA measurement readouts.

(A) miRNA marker change following exercise training intervention (*n* = 31 pairs).						
X – Variable	miR-22/miR451	miR-22/miR451	miR-22/miR451	miR-22/spike	miR-451/spike	miR-22/miR451
Y – Variable	miR-22/spike	miR-451/spike	miR-21/spike	miR-21/spike	miR-21/spike	miR-22 + miR-21/miR-451 + spike
Spearman's *R*	0.3156	−0.348	0.09699	0.704	0.629	0.5986
P-Value	0.0838	0.055	0.6037	**<0.0001**	**0.0002**	**0.0004**
(B) miRNA marker change following nightly oxygen intervention (*n* = 21 pairs).						
X – Variable	miR-22/miR451	miR-22/miR451	miR-22/miR451	miR-22/spike	miR-451/spike	miR-22/miR451
Y – Variable	miR-22/spike	miR-451/spike	miR-21/spike	miR-21/spike	miR-21/spike	miR-22 + miR-21/miR-451 + spike
Spearman's *R*	0.7636	−0.2558	0.3143	0.5221	0.2494	0.8688
P-Value	**<0.0001**	0.2630	0.1653	**0.0152**	0.2757	**<0.0001**

Correlations and significance were calculated with Spearman's rank correlation test on the fold-change after training relative to baseline, or oxygen relative to placebo, respectively. A p < 0.05 was considered significant (bold).

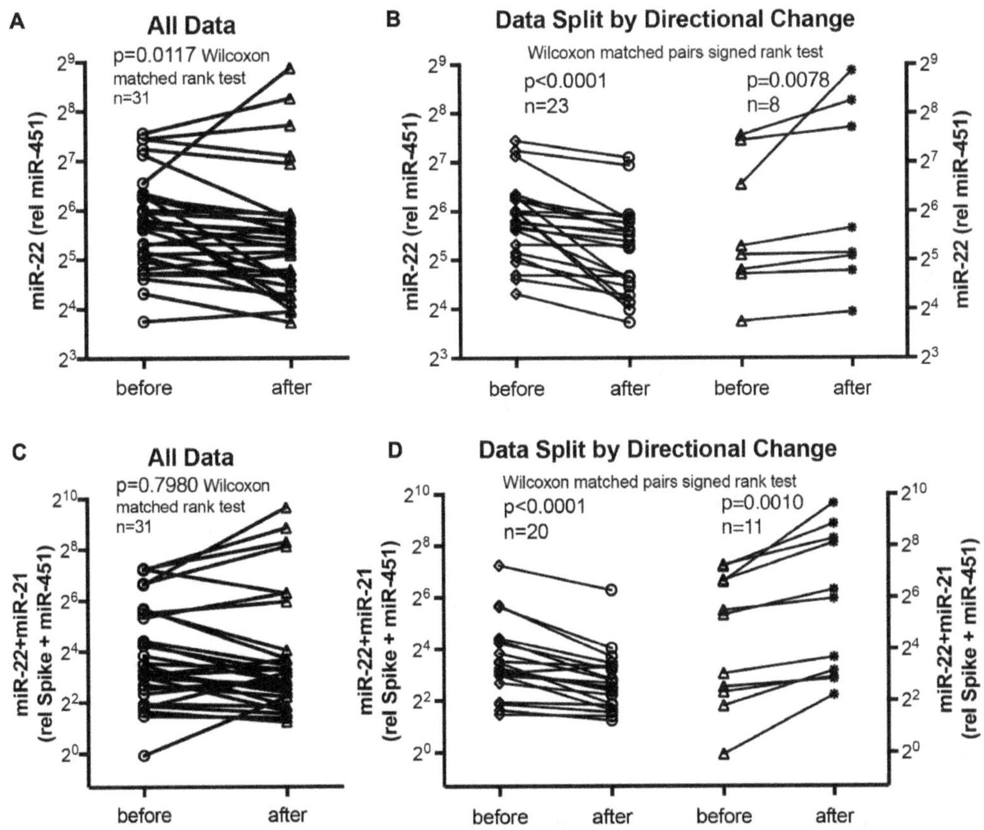

FIGURE 2 | Circulating serum miRNA values in the supervised exercise training intervention study. Symbols and lines graphs show miR-22-3p relative to miR-451a (10,000×) values **(A,B)**, or miR-22-3p + miR-21-5p relative to spike-RNA + miR-451a (10,000×) values **(C,D)** in serum samples obtained from patients (Ehlken et al., 2016; Grunig et al., 2012a) before and after exercise training intervention. All of the data are plotted in **(A,C)**; in **(B,D)** the data are separated by the directional change in the samples after exercise training intervention. Groups before and after intervention were compared with the Wilcoxon matched pairs signed rank test; $p < 0.05$ was considered significant.

miRNA Value Changes After Supervised Exercise Training or Oxygen Interventions

We used miR-22-3p relative to miR-451a and miR-22-3p + miR-21-5p relative to miR-451a + spike RNA values to compare changes following supervised exercise training (**Figures 2, 3**) or nightly oxygen (**Figures 4, 5**), respectively. In the exercise intervention, the serum levels of miR-22-3p relative to miR-451a were significantly decreased ($p = 0.012$) following training, however, the direction of change was clearly increased in some of the samples (**Figure 2A**). The divergence of the direction of the change in miRNA values could be clearly shown by dividing the samples based on the direction of the fold change (**Figure 2B**). The divergence of the direction of change in miRNA values was even more pronounced when miR-22-3p + miR-21-5p relative to miR-451a + spike RNA was calculated (**Figures 2C,D**). Comparing miRNA directional changes to baseline disease characteristics we found a significant difference in the 6-min-walking distance (**Figure 3**). Samples that showed a decreased directional change in the miRNA marker [miR-22-3p + miR-21-5p relative to miR-451a + spike RNA] (**Figure 2D**) were obtained from patients who had a significantly longer 6-min-walking distance at baseline (**Figure 3**). For this analysis, we omitted samples from 3 patients who had a BMI greater that 40 kg/m^2 and who achieved 6-min-walking-distances between 150 and 190 m.

The data from the nightly oxygen intervention study showed that we measured higher miRNA marker values as compared to the values measured in the exercise intervention study (**Figure 4** compared to **Figure 2**). This is likely due to the different materials being studied: serum in the exercise intervention study (**Figure 2**), plasma in the oxygen intervention study (**Figure 4**).

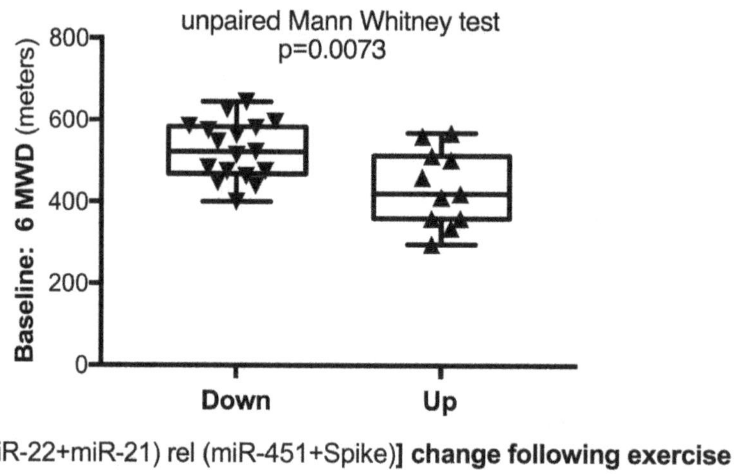

MiRNA biomarker change following exercise

	Down	Up	
N	17	11	
Gender (female / male)	13 / 4	6 / 5	
Age (Y)	47.6 ± 4.10	52.4 ± 5.09	ns
BMI (kg/m^2)	27.1 ± 1.22	26.20 ± 1.67	ns
6MWD (m)	525.4 ± 17.2	435.5 ± 27.9	p=0.0073
NYHA class (II / III)	11 / 3	5 / 4	
Mean PA pressure (mmHg)	50.2 ± 4.35 (n=15)	53.7 ± 6.44 (n=10)	ns

FIGURE 3 | Baseline 6-min walking distance in the exercise training intervention study - comparison with directional change of the miRNA marker. Box-plots with whiskers and individual points show 6-min-walking-distance (6MWD, m) measured at baseline examination from patients in the exercise training intervention study. The data were grouped by the directional change of the miR-22-3p + miR-21-5p relative to spike-RNA + miR-451a (10,000×) values after versus before exercise training intervention: down or up, as shown in **Figure 2D**. Groups were compared with the unpaired, 2-tailed Mann–Whitney test; $p < 0.05$ was considered significant, ns is not significant. The table graph lists the characteristics of the sample donors for each group. For this analysis, samples from three patients who had a body mass index (BMI) greater that 40 kg/m^2 and who achieved 6-min-walking-distances between 150 and 190 m were omitted; two of these three patients were NYHA class III, one was NYHA class not determined.

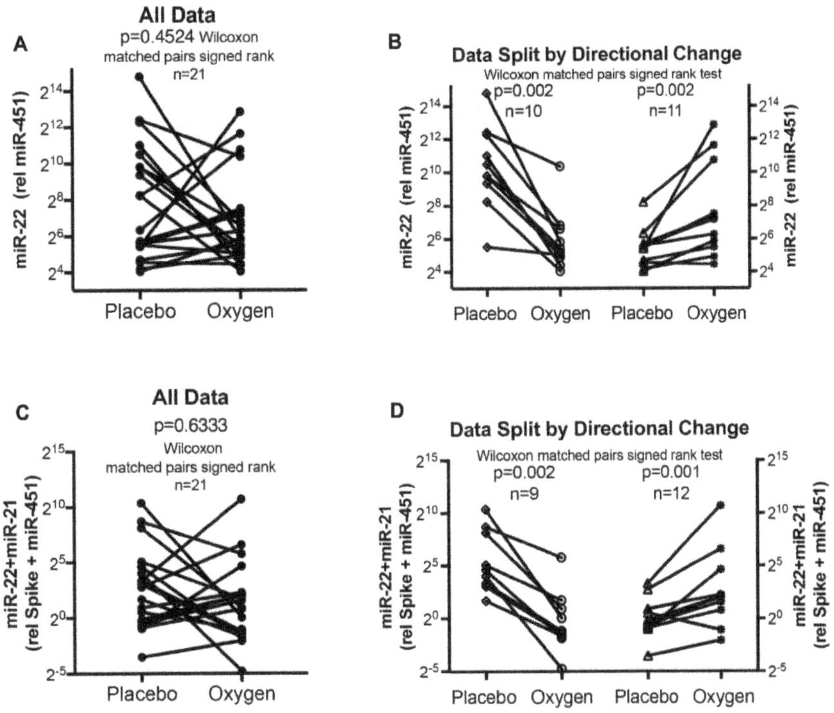

FIGURE 4 | Circulating serum miRNA values in the oxygen intervention study. Symbols and lines graphs show miR-22-3p relative to miR-451a (10,000×) values **(A,B)**, or miR-22-3p + miR-21-5p relative to spike-RNA + miR-451a (10,000×) values **(C,D)** in plasma samples obtained from patients (Schumacher et al., 2014; Ulrich et al., 2015) given placebo (air) or oxygen in a cross-over design. All of the data are plotted in **(A,C)**; in **(B,D)** the data are separated by the directional change in the samples after oxygen intervention. Groups before and after intervention were compared with the Wilcoxon matched pairs signed rank test; $p < 0.05$ was considered significant.

This idea is supported by the data from cattle plasma samples that show miRNA marker values in a similar range as the human plasma samples (**Figure 1** compared to **Figure 4**). As observed in the exercise intervention study (**Figure 2**), the oxygen intervention study showed that significant changes in the direction of the miRNA values followed individual variation, with approximately half demonstrating decreased, and the other half increased miRNA marker values (**Figure 4**). This was found both with miRNA marker values being calculate by miR-22-3p relative to miR-451a, or miR-22-3p + miR-21-5p relative to miR-451a + spike RNA (**Figures 4B,D**). To understand if the fold change difference could represent different PH endotypes, we compared the groups of patients whose miRNA value was either significantly decreased or increased following oxygen intervention. We found a significant difference between these groups in the 6MWD recorded at baseline (**Figure 5**). As we had already seen in the data from the exercise intervention study (**Figure 3**), the group that had an upward change in the miRNA marker following oxygen intervention had a significantly lower 6-min-walking-distance at baseline (**Figure 5**). Further, in both intervention studies, there was a higher percentage of males in the group with an upward direction of the miRNA marker change, but the difference to the group that had a down-ward change was not significant (**Figures 3, 5**). To further confirm the possibility that the 6-min-walking-distance at baseline could predict, or be correlated, with the directional, fold-change of the miRNA marker following intervention, we plotted fold-change of serum or plasma miR-22-3p + miR-21-5p relative to miR-451a + spike RNA (**Figure 6**). The data from the exercise training and the nightly oxygen intervention studies were combined to increase the number of observations for analysis and to query for generalizable impact (**Figure 6**). For this analysis, we omitted samples from three patients who had a BMI greater that 40 kg/m^2 and who achieved 6-min-walking-distances between 150 and 190 m. The analysis showed a significant correlation calculated with Spearman's rank correlation test between 6MWD at baseline and the fold change of the miRNA marker (miR-22-3p + miR-21-5p relative to miR-451a + spike RNA, **Figure 6**).

DISCUSSION

Our studies identified circulating miRNA markers composed of miR-21, miR-22, and miR-451 that showed significant change in a natural animal model (Newman et al., 2015), and in two intervention studies [supervised exercise training (Grunig et al., 2012a; Ehlken et al., 2016) and nightly oxygen (Schumacher et al., 2014; Ulrich et al., 2015)] in human PH patients. In the human studies, the change in miRNA value following intervention was significantly correlated with the 6MWD at baseline. While the present study did not evaluate the genes (mRNA) controlled by the miRNAs, a literature search shows that, for example,

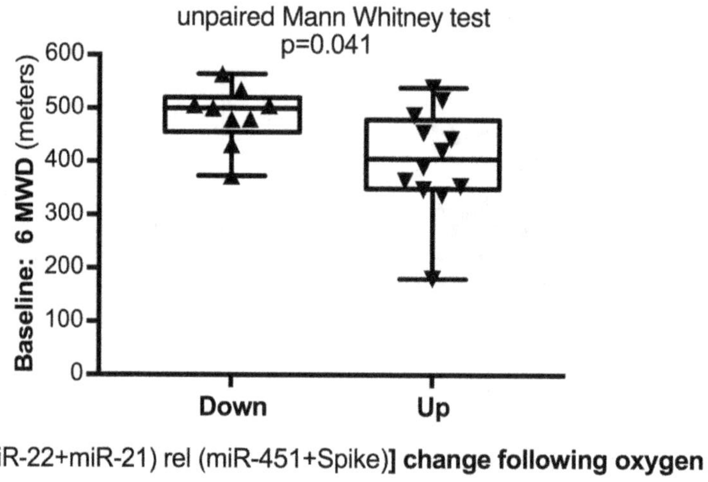

MiRNA biomarker change following Oxygen

	Down	Up	
N	9	12	
Gender (female / male)	6 / 3	7 / 5	
Age (Y)	66.44 ± 2.76	64.17 ± 3.33	ns
BMI (kg/m ^{2})	27.47 ± 1.49	27.24 ± 1.15	ns
6MWD (m)	485.8 ± 18.72	402.7 ± 28.04	p=0.041
NYHA class (II / III)	2 / 7	3 / 9	
Mean PA pressure (mmHg)	39.56 ± 4.82 (n=8)	44.86 ± 4.61 (n=11)	ns

FIGURE 5 | Baseline 6-min walking distance in the oxygen intervention study – comparison with directional change of the miRNA marker. Box-plots with whiskers and individual points show 6-min-walking-distance (6MWD, m) measured at baseline examination from patients in the oxygen intervention study. The data were grouped by the directional change of the miR-22-3p + miR-21-5p relative to spike-RNA + miR-451a (10,000×) values after oxygen versus placebo: down or up, as shown in **Figure 4D**. Groups were compared with the unpaired, 2-tailed Mann–Whitney test; $p < 0.05$ was considered significant, ns is not significant. The table graph lists the characteristics of the sample donors for each group.

miR-21 directly targets BMPR2 (Qin et al., 2009). Both miR-21 and miR-22 control fibrosis in the lungs (Liu et al., 2010), or kidney, respectively (Long et al., 2013). Further, miR-21 and miR-22 are dysregulated in some primary muscle diseases (Eisenberg et al., 2007) and miR-451 is differentially regulated in low and high responders of a specific muscle training program of healthy volunteers (Davidsen et al., 2011). miR-22 is also a critical regulator of cardiac muscle health, and smooth muscle differentiation (Huang et al., 2013; Huang and Wang, 2014; Zhao et al., 2015). miR-451a is a critical regulator of erythropoiesis and erythrocyte function (Dore et al., 2008; Yu et al., 2010).

Our data add to the knowledge of miRNA function in PH (Bockmeyer et al., 2012; White et al., 2012; Deng et al., 2015; Caruso et al., 2017) that has thus far mainly focused on miRNA control of endothelial cells (Huertas et al., 2018), vascular smooth muscle cells, the right heart, the important PH risk factor gene, BMPR2, and the PH inducing hypoxia miRNAs (hypoxamirs), with particular significance of miR-204 (Courboulin et al., 2011), miR-20 (Brock et al., 2012), and miR-21 (Qin et al., 2009; Sarkar et al., 2010; Yang et al., 2012). miRNAs have been further shown to have critical significance for the dysfunction of endothelial cell metabolism and function (miR-124) in PH and mitochondrial dysfunction of fission and calcium transport causing hyper-proliferation of smooth muscle cells (miR-34a-3p, miR-138, miR-25) in PH (Caruso et al., 2017; Hong et al., 2017; Chen et al., 2018).

Our studies highlight the significance of skeletal muscle function in PH as miR-21, miR-22, and miR-451a share skeletal muscle as one of their cellular targets (Eisenberg et al., 2007; Davidsen et al., 2011; Schweisgut et al., 2017). Furthermore, miR-451 is known for its control of erythrocyte function (Dore et al., 2008; Yu et al., 2010). This may be the reason why the composite miRNA marker value that contained miR-22, miR-21, miR-451a, and spike-RNA was correlated with the 6-min-walking distance

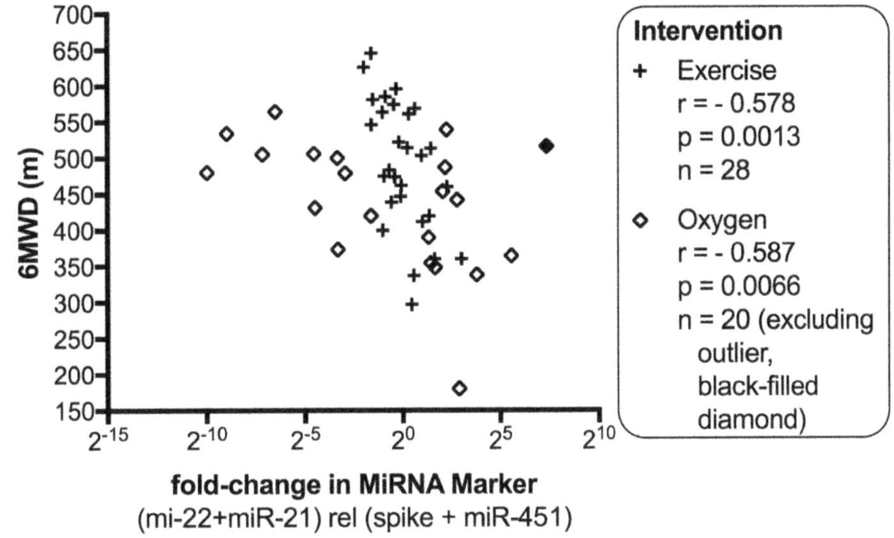

FIGURE 6 | Correlation between change in miRNA marker and 6-min-walking-distance, supervised exercise training and nightly oxygen intervention data combined. The fold-change in miR-22-3p + miR-21-5p relative to spike-RNA + miR-451a (10,000×) values (after/before exercise, or oxygen/placebo, respectively) were plotted against 6-min walking distance (m) measured at baseline examination from the patients. The data from the exercise training intervention study were plotted with × symbols, and the data from the nightly oxygen intervention study were plotted as clear/black-filled diamond symbols. The black-filled diamond represents one outlier data point, and correlations were calculated with and without the outlier point as indicated. The correlation was calculated with Spearman's rank correlation test; $p < 0.05$ was considered significant. For this analysis, samples from three patients who had a body mass index (BMI) greater that 40 kg/m^2 and who achieved 6-min-walking-distances between 150 and 190 m were omitted.

measured at baseline by the patients who participated in the exercise training intervention or oxygen intervention studies, respectively. Skeletal muscle function and optimal erythrocyte transport of oxygen are critical for achieving optimal walking distances, and muscle wasting has been described in PH patients (Marra et al., 2015). Optimized erythrocyte function is an important adaptation to high altitude hypoxia (Song et al., 2017). It is intriguing that miR-451a has been described as one of the miRNAs that demonstrate differential response directions in healthy young men who underwent resistance exercise training and had varying degrees of muscle mass gain (Davidsen et al., 2011). Therefore, future studies have to be designed to distinguish between the possibilities that the divergent directional changes in miRNA marker values that we observed, are already an intrinsic personal trait due to skeletal muscle responsiveness prior to the development of PH, or are developed as consequence of the PH disease.

Our studies provide an example for the importance of using animal models for biomarker discovery in PH because of the variations intrinsic to human disease. In our case, there was no optimal experimental mouse or rat model of exercise or oxygen intervention in PH available. The cattle model has the advantages of being a natural disease, and, importantly, control as well as PH cattle are perfectly matched (Newman et al., 2015). Control animals share the same environment as the animals that develop to PH including high altitude, food, pasture, animal housing (Newman et al., 2015). In contrast, in experimental models of hypoxia induced PH, the experimental group is exposed to hypoxia, the control group is not. In our case where the goal was to identify miRNA markers that track PH, it was essential that the control animal group was also exposed to hypoxia, as hypoxia itself induces changes in the expression of a large set of miRNA markers, called hypoxamirs (Hale et al., 2012). Furthermore, our data in cattle may be hypothesis generating to further develop the understanding of the regulation of PAP at high altitude in humans by miRNAs (Blissenbach et al., 2018).

Our study in samples from human patients was designed with the heterogeneity of PH in focus, although all patients responded favorably to the supervised exercise training intervention (Grunig et al., 2012a; Ehlken et al., 2016), or nightly oxygen (Schumacher et al., 2014; Ulrich et al., 2015) intervention, respectively. The heterogeneity of PH is highlighted by the heterogeneity of gene mutations in heritable PH (Eichstaedt et al., 2017; Ma and Chung, 2017; Gräf et al., 2018). The heterogeneity of the underlying molecular mechanisms that cause disease has prompted the development of tools for personalized medicine (Hemnes et al., 2017). Big data, OMICS studies are currently conducted to fine-map clinical, physiological, imaging and molecular parameters that are then used to better define clinical subtypes and to identify disease endotypes (Hemnes et al., 2017). One example in PH is the pulmonary vascular disease OMICS (PVDOMICS) study (Hemnes et al., 2017). Our study, in contrast, did not have the power based on thousands of individual data points to draw this fine-map of PH. Instead we used three different sample cohorts to identify miRNA markers that would demonstrate significant changes in the biomarker: a high altitude animal model of PH (Newman et al., 2015), and PH interventions in humans consisting either of supervised exercise training (Grunig et al., 2012a; Ehlken et al., 2016) or nightly oxygen (Schumacher et al., 2014; Ulrich et al., 2015). The significant difference in the homogenous animal model, in contrast to the individual differences in the direction of the change of the miRNA marker together with differences among groups with respect to baseline 6-min-walking-distance in human PH, implies that the biomarker may have distinguished PH endotypes. However, further studies using large patient cohorts are needed to confirm this idea.

CONCLUSION

Our analysis identified circulating miRNAs that control muscle and erythrocyte function (miR-22-3p, miR-21-5p, miR-451a) that may have utility as biomarkers of PH progression and responses to intervention. The strength of our data is in the consistency across different patient groups given supervised exercise training or oxygen intervention, respectively, consistency across sample processes (serum versus plasma), and confirmation in a natural animal model. Further research in larger patient groups and in additional data sets is needed to validate our data and to test the idea that different PH endotypes are, in part, the cause for the individual variation in the direction of the miRNA marker changes in response to the training or oxygen interventions. Future studies will also need to address the relationship between the miRNA markers and commonly used markers in PH (e.g.,) B-type natriuretic peptide). Furthermore, future studies will need to be designed to identify the molecular mechanisms by which exercise training or oxygen interventions provide feedback signals via the changed levels of circulating miRNAs to the pulmonary vasculature, and the clinical PH phenotype, because miR-21 and miR-22 also have functions in the pulmonary vasculature (Sarkar et al., 2010; Yang et al., 2012; Zhao et al., 2015 and in the heart (Huang et al., 2013; Huang and Wang, 2014).

AUTHOR CONTRIBUTIONS

GG and SP conceived the study, performed the experiments, and wrote and edited the manuscript. CE, JV, SS, GK, KS, SU, and EG established and maintained the sample bio-repositories. JV and SS sent samples to GG and SP for study. CE, ND, SU, and EG edited the figures and manuscript.

SUPPLEMENTARY MATERIAL

FIGURE S1 | Hierarchical clustering of serum miRNA levels determined relative to synthetic spike RNA from samples obtained before (B) or after (A) exercise intervention. **(a)** Full pilot study miRNA panel. Note that miR-22-3p and miR-21-5p are in clusters distinct from miR-451a. Also note that samples from a single donor are listed together (box) but not clustered together. **(b)** Selected miRNAs. Note that miR-22-3p and miR-21-5p are clustered together apart from miR-451a. Note that none of the paired samples are listed together.

FIGURE S2 | Hierarchical clustering of serum or plasma miRNA levels determined relative to synthetic spike RNA from $n = 52$ paired samples, total $n = 104$. The samples were obtained before (B) or after (A) exercise intervention at the University of Heidelberg (HD), or following placebo (P) or oxygen (O) intervention at the University of Zurich (ZH), respectively. Samples from 46 donors clustered apart; the samples from 6 donors were either listed or clustered together and are indicated (boxes).

REFERENCES

Becker-Grunig, T., Klose, H., Ehlken, N., Lichtblau, M., Nagel, C., Fischer, C., et al. (2013). Efficacy of exercise training in pulmonary arterial hypertension associated with congenital heart disease. *Int. J. Cardiol.* 168, 375–381. doi: 10.1016/j.ijcard.2012.09.036

Blissenbach, B., Nakas, C. T., Kronke, M., Geiser, T., Merz, T. M., and Pichler Hefti, J. (2018). Hypoxia-induced changes in plasma micro-RNAs correlate with pulmonary artery pressure at high altitude. *Am. J. Physiol. Lung Cell. Mol. Physiol.* 314, L157–L164. doi: 10.1152/ajplung.00146.2017

Bockmeyer, C. L., Maegel, L., Janciauskiene, S., Rische, J., Lehmann, U., Maus, U. A., et al. (2012). Plexiform vasculopathy of severe pulmonary arterial hypertension and microRNA expression. *J. Heart Lung Transplant.* 31, 764–772. doi: 10.1016/j.healun.2012.03.010

Brock, M., Samillan, V. J., Trenkmann, M., Schwarzwald, C., Ulrich, S., Gay, R. E., et al. (2012). AntagomiR directed against miR-20a restores functional BMPR2 signalling and prevents vascular remodelling in hypoxia-induced pulmonary hypertension. *Eur. Heart J.* 35, 3203–3211. doi: 10.1093/eurheartj/ehs060

Caruso, P., Dunmore, B. J., Schlosser, K., Schoors, S., Dos Santos, C., Perez-Iratxeta, C., et al. (2017). Identification of MicroRNA-124 as a major regulator of enhanced endothelial cell glycolysis in pulmonary arterial hypertension via PTBP1 (polypyrimidine tract binding protein) and pyruvate kinase m2. *Circulation* 136, 2451–2467. doi: 10.1161/CIRCULATIONAHA.117.028034

Chen, K. H., Dasgupta, A., Lin, J., Potus, F., Bonnet, S., Iremonger, J., et al. (2018). Epigenetic dysregulation of the Drp1 binding partners MiD49 and MiD51 increases mitotic mitochondrial fission and promotes pulmonary arterial hypertension: mechanistic and therapeutic implications. *Circulation* doi: 10.1161/CIRCULATIONAHA.117.031258 [Epub ahead of print].

Courboulin, A., Paulin, R., Giguere, N. J., Saksouk, N., Perreault, T., Meloche, J., et al. (2011). Role for miR-204 in human pulmonary arterial hypertension. *J. Exp. Med.* 208, 535–548. doi: 10.1084/jem.20101812

Davidsen, P. K., Gallagher, I. J., Hartman, J. W., Tarnopolsky, M. A., Dela, F., Helge, J. W., et al. (2011). High responders to resistance exercise training demonstrate differential regulation of skeletal muscle microRNA expression. *J. Appl. Physiol.* 110, 309–317. doi: 10.1152/japplphysiol.00901.2010

Deng, L., Blanco, F. J., Stevens, H., Lu, R., Caudrillier, A., McBride, M., et al. (2015). MicroRNA-143 activation regulates smooth muscle and endothelial cell crosstalk in pulmonary arterial hypertension. *Circ. Res.* 117, 870–883. doi: 10.1161/CIRCRESAHA.115.306806

Dore, L. C., Amigo, J. D., Dos Santos, C. O., Zhang, Z., Gai, X., Tobias, J. W., et al. (2008). A GATA-1-regulated microRNA locus essential for erythropoiesis. *Proc. Natl. Acad. Sci. U.S.A.* 105, 3333–3338. doi: 10.1073/pnas.071231 2105

Ehlken, N., Lichtblau, M., Klose, H., Weidenhammer, J., Fischer, C., Nechwatal, R., et al. (2016). Exercise training improves peak oxygen consumption and haemodynamics in patients with severe pulmonary arterial hypertension and inoperable chronic thrombo-embolic pulmonary hypertension: a prospective, randomized, controlled trial. *Eur. Heart J.* 37, 35–44. doi: 10.1093/eurheartj/ehv337

Eichstaedt, C. A., Song, J., Viales, R. R., Pan, Z., Benjamin, N., Fischer, C., et al. (2017). First identification of Kruppel-like factor 2 mutation in heritable pulmonary arterial hypertension. *Clin. Sci.* 131, 689–698. doi: 10.1042/CS20160930

Eisenberg, I., Eran, A., Nishino, I., Moggio, M., Lamperti, C., Amato, A. A., et al. (2007). Distinctive patterns of microRNA expression in primary muscular disorders. *Proc. Natl. Acad. Sci. U.S.A.* 104, 17016–17021. doi: 10.1073/pnas.0708115104

Evans, J. D., Girerd, B., Montani, D., Wang, X. J., Galie, N., Austin, E. D., et al. (2016). BMPR2 mutations and survival in pulmonary arterial hypertension:

an individual participant data meta-analysis. *Lancet Respir. Med.* 4, 129–137. doi: 10.1016/S2213-2600(15)00544-5

Gonzalez-Saiz, L., Fiuza-Luces, C., Sanchis-Gomar, F., Santos-Lozano, A., Quezada-Loaiza, C. A., Flox-Camacho, A., et al. (2017). Benefits of skeletal-muscle exercise training in pulmonary arterial hypertension: the WHOLEi+12 trial. *Int. J. Cardiol.* 231, 277–283. doi: 10.1016/j.ijcard.2016.12.026

Gräf, S., Haimel, M., Bleda, M., Hadinnapola, C., Southgate, L., Li, W., et al. (2018). Identification of rare sequence variation underlying heritable pulmonary arterial hypertension. *Nat. Commun.* 9:1416. doi: 10.1038/s41467-018-03672-4

Grunig, E., Ehlken, N., Ghofrani, A., Staehler, G., Meyer, F. J., Juenger, J., et al. (2011). Effect of exercise and respiratory training on clinical progression and survival in patients with severe chronic pulmonary hypertension. *Respiration* 81, 394–401. doi: 10.1159/000322475

Grunig, E., Lichtblau, M., Ehlken, N., Ghofrani, H. A., Reichenberger, F., Staehler, G., et al. (2012a). Safety and efficacy of exercise training in various forms of pulmonary hypertension. *Eur. Respir J.* 40, 84–92. doi: 10.1183/09031936.00123711

Grunig, E., Maier, F., Ehlken, N., Fischer, C., Lichtblau, M., Blank, N., et al. (2012b). Exercise training in pulmonary arterial hypertension associated with connective tissue diseases. *Arthritis Res. Ther.* 14:R148. doi: 10.1186/ar3883

Hale, A. E., White, K., and Chan, S. Y. (2012). Hypoxamirs in pulmonary hypertension: breathing new life into pulmonary vascular research. *Cardiovasc. Diagnosis Ther.* 2, 200–212.

Hemnes, A. R., Beck, G. J., Newman, J. H., Abidov, A., Aldred, M. A., Barnard, J., et al. (2017). PVDOMICS: a multi-center study to improve understanding of pulmonary vascular disease through phenomics. *Circ. Res.* 121, 1136–1139. doi: 10.1161/CIRCRESAHA.117.311737

Hoffmann, J., Wilhelm, J., Olschewski, A., and Kwapiszewska, G. (2016). Microarray analysis in pulmonary hypertension. *Eur. Respir. J.* 48, 229–241. doi: 10.1183/13993003.02030-2015

Hong, Z., Chen, K. H., DasGupta, A., Potus, F., Dunham-Snary, K., Bonnet, S., et al. (2017). MicroRNA-138 and MicroRNA-25 down-regulate mitochondrial calcium uniporter, causing the pulmonary arterial hypertension cancer phenotype. *Am. J. Respir. Crit. Care Med.* 195, 515–529. doi: 10.1164/rccm.201604-0814OC

Huang, Z. P., Chen, J., Seok, H. Y., Zhang, Z., Kataoka, M., Hu, X., et al. (2013). MicroRNA-22 regulates cardiac hypertrophy and remodeling in response to stress. *Circ. Res.* 112, 1234–1243. doi: 10.1161/CIRCRESAHA.112.300682

Huang, Z. P., and Wang, D. Z. (2014). miR-22 in cardiac remodeling and disease. *Trends Cardiovasc. Med.* 24, 267–272. doi: 10.1016/j.tcm.2014.07.005

Huertas, A., Guignabert, C., Barberà, J. A., Bärtsch, P., Bhattacharya, J., and Bhattacharya, S. (2018). Pulmonary vascular endothelium: orchestra conductor in respiratory diseases highlights from basic research to therapy. *Eur. Respir. J.* 51, 1700745. doi: 10.1183/13993003.00745-2017

Keusch, S., Turk, A., Saxer, S., Ehlken, N., Grunig, E., Ulrich, S., et al. (2017). Rehabilitation in patients with pulmonary arterial hypertension. *Swiss. Med. Wkly.* 147:w14462. doi: 10.4414/smw.2017.14462

Kimura, M., Tamura, Y., Guignabert, C., Takei, M., Kosaki, K., Tanabe, N., et al. (2017). A genome-wide association analysis identifies PDE1A| DNAJC10 locus on chromosome 2 associated with idiopathic pulmonary arterial hypertension in a Japanese population. *Oncotarget* 8, 74917–74926. doi: 10.18632/oncotarget.20459

Leggio, M., Fusco, A., Armeni, M., D'Emidio, S., Severi, P., Calvaruso, S., et al. (2018). Pulmonary hypertension and exercise training: a synopsis on the more recent evidences. *Ann. Med.* 50, 226–233. doi: 10.1080/07853890.2018.1432887

Liu, G., Friggeri, A., Yang, Y., Milosevic, J., Ding, Q., Thannickal, V. J., et al. (2010). miR-21 mediates fibrogenic activation of pulmonary fibroblasts and lung fibrosis. *J. Exp. Med.* 207, 1589–1597. doi: 10.1084/jem.2010 0035

Long, J., Badal, S. S., Wang, Y., Chang, B. H., Rodriguez, A., and Danesh, F. R. (2013). MicroRNA-22 is a master regulator of bone morphogenetic protein-7/6 homeostasis in the kidney. *J. Biol. Chem.* 288, 36202–36214. doi: 10.1074/jbc.M113.498634

Lotvall, J., Akdis, C. A., Bacharier, L. B., Bjermer, L., Casale, T. B., Custovic, A., et al. (2011). Asthma endotypes: a new approach to classification of disease entities within the asthma syndrome. *J. Allergy Clin. Immunol.* 127, 355–360. doi: 10.1016/j.jaci.2010.11.037

Ma, L., and Chung, W. K. (2017). The role of genetics in pulmonary arterial hypertension. *J. Pathol.* 241, 273–280. doi: 10.1002/path.4833

Marra, A. M., Arcopinto, M., Bossone, E., Ehlken, N., Cittadini, A., and Grunig, E. (2015). Pulmonary arterial hypertension-related myopathy: an overview of current data and future perspectives. *Nutr. Metab. Cardiovasc. Dis.* 25, 131–139. doi: 10.1016/j.numecd.2014.10.005

Mereles, D., Ehlken, N., Kreuscher, S., Ghofrani, S., Hoeper, M. M., Halank, M., et al. (2006). Exercise and respiratory training improve exercise capacity and quality of life in patients with severe chronic pulmonary hypertension. *Circulation* 114, 1482–1489. doi: 10.1161/CIRCULATIONAHA.106.618397

Metsalu, T., and Vilo, J. (2015). ClustVis: a web tool for visualizing clustering of multivariate data using principal component analysis and heatmap. *Nucleic Acids Res.* 43, W566–W570. doi: 10.1093/nar/gkv468

Moreira-Goncalves, D., Ferreira-Nogueira, R., Santos, M., Silva, A. F., Ferreira, R., Leite-Moreira, A., et al. (2017). Exercise training in pulmonary hypertension and right heart failure: insights from pre-clinical studies. *Adv. Exp. Med. Biol.* 999, 307–324. doi: 10.1007/978-981-10-4307-9_17

Nagel, C., Prange, F., Guth, S., Herb, J., Ehlken, N., Fischer, C., et al. (2012). Exercise training improves exercise capacity and quality of life in patients with inoperable or residual chronic thromboembolic pulmonary hypertension. *PLoS One* 7:e41603. doi: 10.1371/journal.pone.0041603

Newman, J. H., Holt, T. N., Cogan, J. D., Womack, B., Phillips, J. A. III, Li, C., et al. (2015). Increased prevalence of EPAS1 variant in cattle with high-altitude pulmonary hypertension. *Nat. Commun.* 6:6863. doi: 10.1038/ncomms7863

Olschewski, A., Veale, E. L., Nagy, B. M., Nagaraj, C., Kwapiszewska, G., Antigny, F., et al. (2017). TASK-1 (KCNK3) channels in the lung: from cell biology to clinical implications. *Eur. Respir. J.* 50, 1700754. doi: 10.1183/13993003.00754-2017

Pandey, A., Garg, S., Khunger, M., Garg, S., Kumbhani, D. J., Chin, K. M., et al. (2015). Efficacy and Safety of Exercise Training in Chronic Pulmonary Hypertension: Systematic Review and Meta-Analysis. *Circ Heart Fail* 8, 1032–1043. doi: 10.1161/CIRCHEARTFAILURE.115.002130

Pandey, D. P., and Picard, D. (2009). miR-22 inhibits estrogen signaling by directly targeting the estrogen receptor alpha mRNA. *Mol. Cell. Biol.* 29, 3783–3790. doi: 10.1128/MCB.01875-08

Qin, W., Zhao, B., Shi, Y., Yao, C., Jin, L., and Jin, Y. (2009). BMPRII is a direct target of miR-21. *Acta Biochim. Biophys. Sin.* 41, 618–623. doi: 10.1093/abbs/gmp049

Richter, M. J., Grimminger, J., Kruger, B., Ghofrani, H. A., Mooren, F. C., Gall, H., et al. (2017). Effects of exercise training on pulmonary hemodynamics, functional capacity and inflammation in pulmonary hypertension. *Pulm. Circ.* 7, 20–37. doi: 10.1086/690553

Sarkar, J., Gou, D., Turaka, P., Viktorova, E., Ramchandran, R., and Raj, J. U. (2010). MicroRNA-21 plays a role in hypoxia-mediated pulmonary artery smooth muscle cell proliferation and migration. *Am. J. Physiol. Lung Cell. Mol. Physiol.* 299, L861–L871. doi: 10.1152/ajplung.00201.2010

Schumacher, D. S., Muller-Mottet, S., Hasler, E. D., Hildenbrand, F. F., Keusch, S., Speich, R., et al. (2014). Effect of oxygen and acetazolamide on nocturnal cardiac conduction, repolarization, and arrhythmias in precapillary pulmonary hypertension and sleep-disturbed breathing. *Chest* 146, 1226–1236. doi: 10.1378/chest.14-0495

Schweisgut, J., Schutt, C., Wust, S., Wietelmann, A., Ghesquiere, B., Carmeliet, P., et al. (2017). Sex-specific, reciprocal regulation of ERalpha and miR-22 controls muscle lipid metabolism in male mice. *EMBO J.* 36, 1199–1214. doi: 10.15252/embj.201695988

Simonneau, G., Gatzoulis, M. A., Adatia, I., Celermajer, D., Denton, C., Ghofrani, A., et al. (2013). Updated clinical classification of pulmonary hypertension. *J. Am. Coll. Cardiol.* 62, D34–D41. doi: 10.1016/j.jacc.2013.10.029

Song, A., Zhang, Y., Han, L., Yegutkin, G. G., Liu, H., Sun, K., et al. (2017). Erythrocytes retain hypoxic adenosine response for faster acclimatization upon re-ascent. *Nat. Commun.* 8:14108. doi: 10.1038/ncomms14108

Song, J., Bai, Z., Han, W., Zhang, J., Meng, H., Bi, J., et al. (2012). Identification of suitable reference genes for qPCR analysis of serum microRNA in gastric cancer patients. *Dig. Dis. Sci.* 57, 897–904. doi: 10.1007/s10620-011-1981-7

Ulrich, S., Keusch, S., Hildenbrand, F. F., Lo Cascio, C., Huber, L. C., Tanner, F. C., et al. (2015). Effect of nocturnal oxygen and acetazolamide on exercise performance in patients with pre-capillary pulmonary hypertension and sleep-disturbed breathing: randomized, double-blind, cross-over trial. *Eur. Heart J.* 36, 615–623. doi: 10.1093/eurheartj/eht540

Viales, R. R., Eichstaedt, C. A., Ehlken, N., Fischer, C., Lichtblau, M., Grunig, E., et al. (2015). Mutation in BMPR2 promoter: a 'second hit' for manifestation of pulmonary arterial hypertension? *PLoS One* 10:e0133042. doi: 10.1371/journal.pone.0133042

White, K., Loscalzo, J., and Chan, S. Y. (2012). Holding our breath: The emerging and anticipated roles of microRNA in pulmonary hypertension. *Pulm. Circ.* 2, 278–290. doi: 10.4103/2045-8932.101395

Yang, S., Banerjee, S., Freitas, A., Cui, H., Xie, N., Abraham, E., et al. (2012). miR-21 regulates chronic hypoxia-induced pulmonary vascular remodeling. *Am. J. Physiol. Lung Cell. Mol. Physiol.* 302, L521–L529. doi: 10.1152/ajplung.00316.2011

Yu, D., dos Santos, C. O., Zhao, G., Jiang, J., Amigo, J. D., Khandros, E., et al. (2010). miR-451 protects against erythroid oxidant stress by repressing 14-3-3zeta. *Genes Dev.* 24, 1620–1633. doi: 10.1101/gad.1942110

Zhao, H., Wen, G., Huang, Y., Yu, X., Chen, Q., Afzal, T. A., et al. (2015). MicroRNA-22 regulates smooth muscle cell differentiation from stem cells by targeting methyl CpG-binding protein 2. *Arterioscler. Thromb. Vasc. Biol.* 35, 918–929. doi: 10.1161/ATVBAHA.114.305212

4

Divergent Roles for TRAIL in Lung Diseases

Adam T. Braithwaite, Helen M. Marriott and Allan Lawrie*

Department of Infection, Immunity and Cardiovascular Disease, University of Sheffield, Medical School, Sheffield, United Kingdom

***Correspondence:**
Adam T. Braithwaite
a.braithwaite@sheffield.ac.uk

The tumour necrosis factor-related apoptosis-inducing ligand (TRAIL) is a widely expressed cytokine that can bind five different receptors. TRAIL has been of particular interest for its proposed ability to selectively induce apoptosis in tumour cells. However, it has also been found to regulate a wide variety of non-canonical cellular effects including survival, migration and proliferation via kinase signalling pathways. Lung diseases represent a wide range of conditions affecting multiple tissues. TRAIL has been implicated in several biological processes underlying lung diseases, including angiogenesis, inflammation, and immune regulation. For example, TRAIL is detrimental in pulmonary arterial hypertension—it is upregulated in patient serum and lungs, and drives the underlying proliferative pulmonary vascular remodelling in rodent models. However, TRAIL protects against pulmonary fibrosis in mice models—by inducing apoptosis of neutrophils—and reduced serum TRAIL is found in patients. Conversely, in the airways TRAIL positively regulates inflammation and immune response. In COPD patients and asthmatic patients challenged with antigen, TRAIL and its death receptors are upregulated in serum and airways. Furthermore, TRAIL-deleted mouse models have reduced airway inflammation and remodelling. In the context of respiratory infections, TRAIL assists in immune response, e.g., via T-cell toxicity in influenza infection, and neutrophil killing in S. pneumoniae infection. In this mini-review, we examine the functions of TRAIL and highlight the diverse roles TRAIL has in diseases affecting the lung. Disentangling the facets of TRAIL signalling in lung diseases could help in understanding their pathogenic processes and targeting novel treatments.

Keywords: TRAIL, TNF-related apoptosis-inducing ligand, pulmonary arterial hypertension, immune regulation, pulmonary vascular disease, pulmonary fibrosis, respiratory tract infections, chronic obstructive pulmonary diseases

INTRODUCTION

The tumour necrosis factor-related apoptosis-inducing ligand (TRAIL), also known as Apo2 ligand is an apoptosis-inducing cytokine that is expressed in most cell types. As its name suggests, TRAIL was primarily of particular interest for its ability to selectively induce apoptosis in tumour cells *in vitro* and *in vivo*, while apparently exhibiting minimal off-target effects (1–3). TRAIL-deficient mice are also more susceptible to tumour formation and metastasis (4), suggesting TRAIL has a protective role in cancer suppression. Consequently TRAIL signalling has been targeted for use in several anticancer therapies (5), however several types of cancer cells are resistant to TRAIL-induced apoptosis. In these cells, TRAIL can activate pro-inflammatory signalling pathways (6, 7), proliferation (8–10) and metastasis (11). The purpose of this mini-review is to discuss how the known function of TRAIL has evolved beyond apoptosis to these alternative effects and highlight the different roles TRAIL has in diseases affecting the lung (**Figure 1**), where TRAIL is widely expressed (12, 13). The better understanding of the diverse roles for TRAIL in lung disease could lead to the development of more effective, and novel treatments.

TRAIL MOLECULAR SIGNALLING

TRAIL, a type II transmembrane protein, is a member of the death receptor ligand family; a subclass of the tumour necrosis factor family (14) and is widely expressed in a variety of human tissues, most predominantly in lung, spleen and prostate (14). TRAIL is proteolytically-cleaved and its extracellular domain can bind five TRAIL receptors: membrane-bound death receptors DR4 (TRAIL-R1) and DR5 (TRAIL-R2), membrane-bound decoy receptors DcR1 (TRAIL-R3), and DcR2 (TRAIL-R4) and the soluble decoy osteoprotegerin (OPG) (15–21) [TRAIL is conserved in mice—they have two decoy receptors and a single TRAIL death receptor, mDR5, which is more similar to DR5 than DR4 (22)].

TRAIL is composed of 281 amino acids and forms a homotrimeric structure upon binding three receptor molecules (23). The death receptors DR4 and DR5 are type I transmembrane proteins containing a cytoplasmic death domain. In the canonical TRAIL apoptosis signalling pathway (**Figure 2A**), binding of death receptors by TRAIL leads to recruitment of Fas-associated protein with death domain (FADD), formation of a complex known as death-inducing signalling complex (DISC), activation of caspase-8 and subsequently downstream caspase-3 dependent apoptosis of the cell [**Figure 1**; (24–26)]. Unlike the TRAIL death receptors, the decoy receptor DcR1 has no death domain (15, 18) and DcR2 has a truncated, non-functional death domain (15, 17, 27). These decoy receptors, and additionally binding with lower affinity, the soluble OPG, are suggested to suppress apoptotic signalling by competitively binding TRAIL (28, 29).

Conversely, TRAIL can also stimulate pathways promoting cell survival, proliferation and migration via activation of kinase signalling pathways (**Figure 2B**) (30). This non-canonical signalling may depend on the formation of a secondary signalling complex after initial DISC assembly (31), recruiting other factors including FADD, Caspase 8, RIPK1, TNF receptor-associated factor 2 (TRAF2) and inhibitor of NF-κB kinase subunit gamma (IKK-γ). Activation of non-canonical TRAIL signalling pathways may also be regulated by expression of DcR1, as antibody neutralisation of this decoy receptor can inhibit TRAIL-induced cell proliferation (30). Downstream non-canonical signalling by TRAIL has been shown to be effected by activation of kinase signalling e.g., NF-κB, p38, c-Jun N-terminal kinase (JNK), phosphatidylinositide 3-kinases (PI3K), Akt, and extracellular signal-regulated kinases (ERK); leading to activation of gene transcription (32). By activating NF-κB, TRAIL can also modulate levels of FADD-like interleukin-1β-converting enzyme)-inhibitory protein [c-FLIP; (33)], a negative regulator of caspase-mediated apoptosis—a further mechanism by which a cell may deviate from pro-apoptotic to pro-survival signalling in response to TRAIL.

PULMONARY ARTERIAL HYPERTENSION

TRAIL has been implicated in the pathobiology of pulmonary arterial hypertension (30, 34). This is indicated by elevated levels of soluble TRAIL found in the serum of PAH patients, and increased abundance of serum TRAIL, which is associated with worsened clinical severity (35). The pulmonary vasculature is complex, and many aberrant processes can lead to disease. PAH is a multifactorial disorder characterised by remodelling of the pulmonary arteries and a progressive increase in pulmonary vascular resistance, leading to raised afterload on the right ventricle and ultimately right heart failure (36). The most frequent alterations are sustained pulmonary vasoconstriction and remodelling of the pulmonary arteries and arterioles. The arterial remodelling is characterised by medial hypertrophy, intimal fibrosis and often the development of thrombotic or plexiform lesions (37). Together, these processes cause the occlusion of small pulmonary arteries. Combined with the muscularisation and progressive obliteration of distal vessels, the subsequent loss of cross-sectional area generates increased right ventricular afterload. At the cellular level, the neoplastic pathologies of PAH are thought to be driven by excessive proliferation of apoptosis-resistant endothelial cells (ECs), together with proliferation and migration of medial smooth muscle cells (SMCs) and fibroblasts.

TRAIL immunoreactivity has been shown in pulmonary vascular lesions from idiopathic PAH patients (13) and increased TRAIL mRNA expression is detected in the lungs of rodent models of PAH (35, 38). Furthermore, TRAIL has been demonstrated—by knockout and by inactivation—as necessary for the development of PAH in multiple pre-clinical models of PAH (30). Reversal of established PAH in rodent models was also demonstrated by administration of an anti-TRAIL antibody (30). TRAIL knockout also had a similar protective effect in a Sugen5416 and hypoxia mouse model of PAH (34). Increased TRAIL, DR4 and DcR1 mRNA levels have been detected in explanted pulmonary artery SMCs from idiopathic PAH patients, compared to healthy control cells (30). Additionally, TRAIL depletion or blockade in rodent models of PAH is associated with reduced pulmonary arterial remodelling with fewer proliferating pulmonary artery SMCs (30, 34). This evidence indicates that TRAIL is a key promoter of the pulmonary arterial SMC proliferation associated with the pathogenic vascular remodelling in PAH. Recombinant TRAIL was also shown to induce proliferation and migration of idiopathic PAH patient pulmonary artery SMCs *in vitro*, via phosphorylation of ERK1/2 (30). The

---

Abbreviations: COPD, Chronic obstructive pulmonary disease; DcR1/2, Decoy receptor 1/2; DISC, Death-inducing signalling complex; DR4/5, Death receptor 4/5; EC, Endothelial cell; PAH, Pulmonary arterial hypertension; PF, Pulmonary fibrosis; SMC, Smooth muscle cell; SSc, Systemic sclerosis.

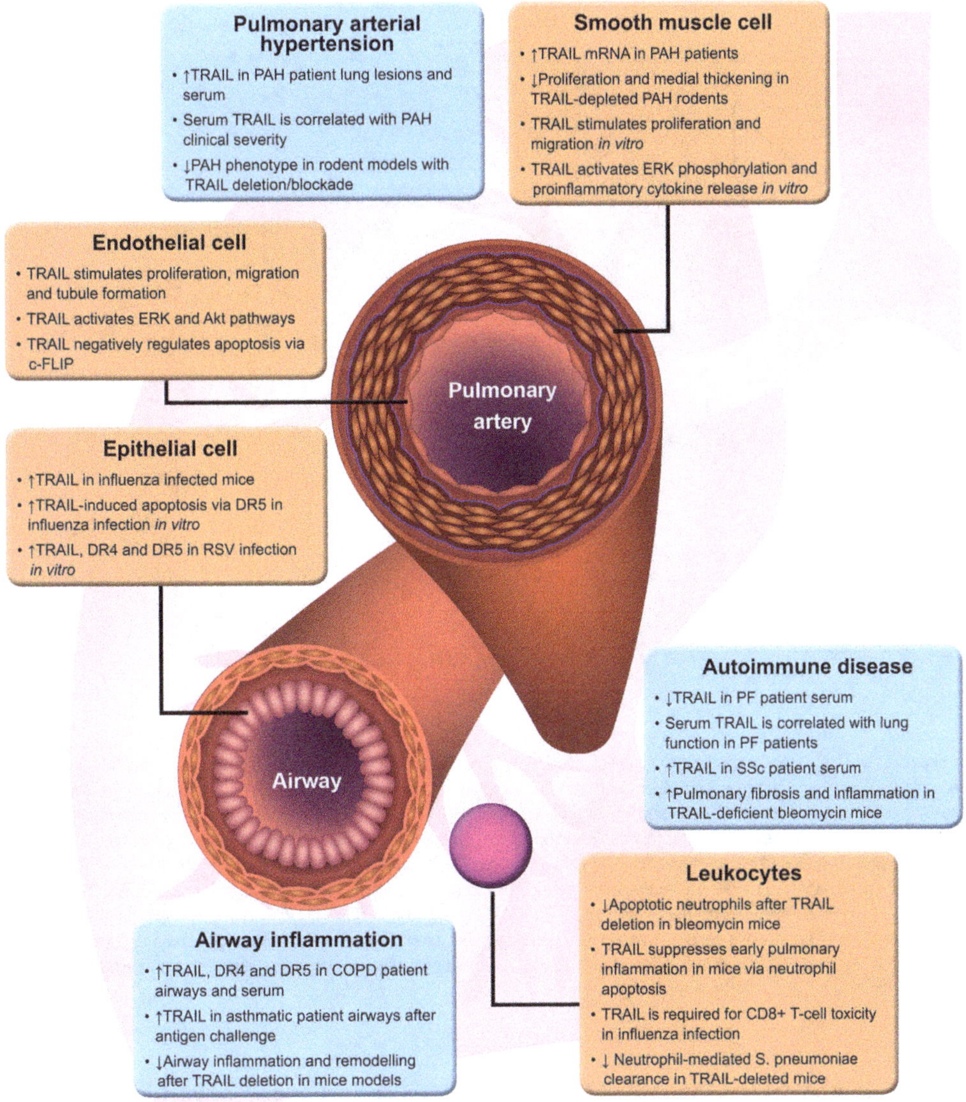

FIGURE 1 | TRAIL functions in lung disease. A brief summary of evidence for the varied roles of TRAIL in different lung diseases. ↑ and ↓ represent up- and down-regulation, respectively. Akt, protein kinase B; COPD, chronic obstructive pulmonary disease; DR4/5, TRAIL death receptor 4/5; ERK, extracellular signal-regulated kinase; PAH, pulmonary arterial hypertension; PF, pulmonary fibrosis; RSV, respiratory syncytial virus; SSc, systemic sclerosis; TRAIL, tumour necrosis factor-related apoptosis-inducing ligand.

pro-proliferative effect of TRAIL was reversed by the addition of DcR1 neutralising antibody, suggesting this decoy receptor is essential to non-canonical TRAIL signalling in pulmonary artery SMCs. Other studies have similarly demonstrated that TRAIL can stimulate proliferation and migration of vascular SMCs via non-canonical kinase signalling cascades (39, 40). Additionally, following activation of NF-κB, TRAIL has been shown to stimulate production and release of pro-inflammatory cytokines in vascular SMCs (41).

EC dysfunction is another key aspect of the angioproliferative state of pulmonary arteries in PAH. Several studies have demonstrated that TRAIL can stimulate angiogenic processes in vascular ECs *in vitro*, including proliferation (33, 42, 43), migration (33, 43, 44) and tubule formation (43). Similarly to non-canonical TRAIL signalling in SMCs, its angioproliferative effect in ECs has been linked to activation of Akt and ERK pathways (42), as well as upregulation of DcR2 (45). Conversely, TRAIL has also been demonstrated to have apoptotic (12, 46) and anti-angiogenic (47) effects on vascular ECs. The reason for this disparity is unclear, although each of these studies used a relatively high concentration of recombinant TRAIL (100 ng/ml), suggesting the pro-angiogenic signalling in endothelium may preferentially occur at lower TRAIL concentrations. In Cantarella et al. (33), high levels of TRAIL were shown to induce caspase

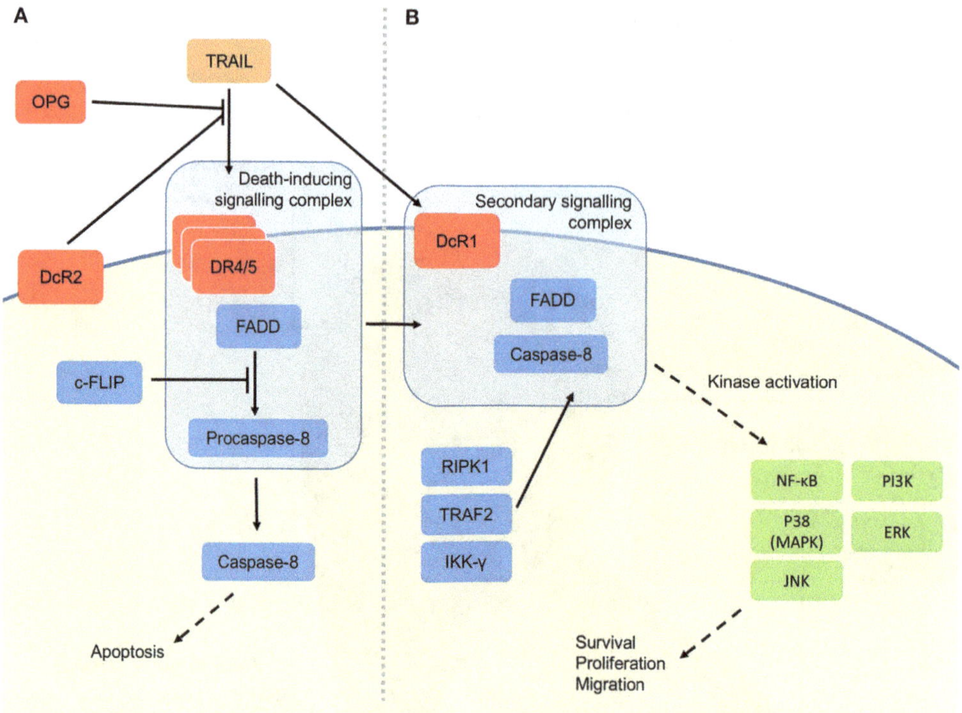

FIGURE 2 | Molecular signalling of TRAIL. **(A)** Three proteolytically-cleaved tumour necrosis factor-related apoptosis-inducing ligand (TRAIL) proteins form a homotrimeric structure when binding death receptor 4 (DR4) or death receptor 5 (DR5) at the cell membrane. These are joined by Fas-associated death domain (FADD) and procaspase-8 to form the so-called death-inducing signalling complex (DISC). The DISC causes activation of the caspase cascade, leading to apoptosis of the cell. TRAIL may also bind the membrane decoy receptors (DcR1/2) or soluble osteoprotegerin (OPG), which do not contain a death domain, thus preventing TRAIL-induced apoptosis. Apoptosis can also be suppressed by (FADD-like interleukin-1β-converting enzyme)-inhibitory protein (c-FLIP), which inhibits the function of the DISC. **(B)** In the non-canonical signalling pathway, the receptor and ligand are thought to be lost, leaving FADD and caspase-8 to be joined by receptor-interacting serine/threonine-protein kinase 1 (RIPK1), TNF receptor-associated factor 2 (TRAF2) and inhibitor of NF-κB kinase subunit gamma (IKK-γ). This secondary signalling complex initiates protein kinase signalling pathways, leading to activation of kinases including nuclear factor kappa-light-chain-enhancer of activated B cells (NF-κB), p38 (mitogen-activated protein kinase; MAPK), c-Jun N-terminal kinase (JNK), phosphatidylinositide 3-kinases (PI3K) and extracellular signal-regulated kinase (ERK). The effects of these kinases include survival, proliferation and migration.

8-mediated apoptosis of ECs, whereas low levels of TRAIL were pro-angiogenic. Interestingly, these dose-dependent opposing effects of TRAIL in ECs were linked to modulation of levels of c-FLIP, a procaspase-8 homolog and negative regulator of apoptosis (33).

AUTOIMMUNE DISEASE

TRAIL is now known to have crucial functions in regulation of inflammation and immune response. These systems are significant in the pathogenesis of many forms of lung disease, including autoimmune disorders and respiratory infection in addition to pulmonary vascular disease (**Figure 2**). A role for TRAIL in regulating inflammation via apoptosis was highlighted in a knockout of the mouse TRAIL death receptor, as in addition to tumour formation, the mice were prone to chronic inflammation (48). Additionally, TRAIL has been demonstrated to suppress the early inflammatory response via apoptosis of neutrophils (49).

PAH is an associated complication in autoimmune disease, e.g., 7–12% of patients with systemic sclerosis (SSc) develop PAH (50, 51). SSc is a heterogeneous autoimmune disorder, characterised by tissue fibrosis and vascular injury. Pulmonary fibrosis (PF) is a condition often found in interstitial lung disease and autoimmune disorders of the connective tissue, including SSc and rheumatoid arthritis. Elevated serum TRAIL levels have been found in SSc patients compared to healthy controls, in addition to being elevated in SSc patients with either PAH or PF compared to those without pulmonary involvement (52), suggesting that TRAIL may also may play a key role. In contrast, soluble TRAIL has been found at lower levels in the serum of patients with the idiopathic form of PF than health controls (53). Within the idiopathic PF patient group, lung function—shown by transfer factor of the lung for carbon monoxide—was correlated with serum levels of TRAIL, suggesting it may have a protective role in idiopathic PF (53). Furthermore, a direct link to PF pathobiology is illustrated in TRAIL-deficient mice, where fibrosis in the bleomycin model of PF was enhanced in comparison to wild-type mice (53). In this model, TRAIL deletion also increased pulmonary inflammation (neutrophil counts in bronchoalveolar lavage fluid). The inflammatory phenotype in TRAIL knockout mice was accompanied by a reduced number of apoptotic cells in lung tissue, with a corresponding reduction of apoptotic neutrophils in bronchoalveolar lavage fluid. This suggests that TRAIL-mediated apoptosis of neutrophils is a protective process in this form of PF.

AIRWAY INFLAMMATION

Contrary to its protective effect in idiopathic PF, TRAIL appears to have a detrimental role in the context of both acute and chronic airway inflammation, by upregulating inflammation and autoimmune responses (**Figure 2**). TRAIL is elevated in bronchoalveolar lavage fluid from asthmatic patients following antigen challenge, and isolated eosinophils express more TRAIL and DcR2, but less DR4 and DR5 (54). Deletion of the TRAIL gene in mice diminishes airway hyper-reactivity, inflammation and remodelling in an ovalbumin-induced model of allergic asthma (55, 56) and a rhinovirus-induced asthma model (57). Additionally, chronic asthmatic inflammation, remodelling and lung function are worsened by TRAIL deletion in mice infected as neonates with chlamydia (58).

Prolonged exposure to irritants and inflammation can lead to chronic obstructive pulmonary disease (COPD). A role for TRAIL in COPD has been highlighted by its elevated levels in the lungs of COPD patients. One study found increased TRAIL, DR4, DR5, and DcR1 protein in lung parenchyma from COPD patients (59). Higher levels of TRAIL, DR4, and DR5 mRNA were also found in airway epithelial brushing of COPD patients compared to healthy controls (60). Another study found increased levels of serum TRAIL and DR5 in COPD patients compared to healthy controls (61). Additionally, with the COPD patient group serum levels of TRAIL and DR5 were found to be inversely correlated with forced expiratory volume (61). Inflammation and alveolar cell apoptosis are key processes in many forms of COPD. A pro-apoptotic function of TRAIL in COPD was originally suggested, as emphysematous lung tissue is more sensitive to TRAIL-induced apoptosis than health lung (62). However, a pro-inflammatory element may also be important. In a chronic cigarette smoke-exposure mouse model of COPD, TRAIL mRNA, and protein expression was increased in the airway epithelium and parenchyma, and in mice with TRAIL deletion, airway inflammation—as well as remodelling—was reduced (60). The activation by TRAIL of both apoptotic and inflammatory pathways within COPD highlights its varied roles and how specific cell types are targeted—whether or not this is this mediated by differential receptor expression or some other mechanism remains unclear.

RESPIRATORY INFECTION

In lower respiratory tract infections, TRAIL has differing roles in immune response and damage to host tissues (**Figure 2**). Apoptosis of virus-infected cells is a key mechanism for clearance of viral infection and *in vitro*. In the context of influenza infection, TRAIL-induced apoptosis of human lung alveolar epithelial cells is enhanced; an effect which is inhibited by blocking DR5 (63). Similarly, TRAIL, DR4, and DR5 are strongly upregulated in response to respiratory syncytial virus infection in pulmonary epithelial cells, leading to increased sensitivity to apoptosis (64). In animal models, TRAIL expressed by CD8+ T-cells has been demonstrated as essential for viral immunity, with TRAIL knockout mice exhibiting increased influenza-associated morbidity and reduced CD8+ T-cell cytotoxicity (65–67). DR5 expression was also shown to be upregulated in influenza-infected pulmonary epithelial cells *in vivo* (63 65).

In opposition to its protective role in viral clearance, other studies have shown that TRAIL expressed by macrophages is instrumental in damage to airways caused by apoptosis of alveolar epithelial cells in influenza infection (68, 69). Deletion of TRAIL in mice led to a reduction in mortality and the alveolar epithelial apoptosis and alveolar leakage associated with influenza virus pneumonia (68). This highlights an interesting situation whereby TRAIL death signalling may be used for host for viral clearance, while also assisting in viral infection via tissue damage. TRAIL has also been demonstrated as important in immune response to bacterial respiratory infection. In the context of Streptococcus pneumoniae infection, deletion of TRAIL in mice reduces bacterial clearance in the lungs and worsens survival—an effect that is reversed by treatment with TRAIL or DR5 agonist antibody (70). In the same study, neutrophils were found to be the key source of TRAIL (70).

CONCLUSIONS

As highlighted in this mini-review, TRAIL is multifaceted in a variety of lung diseases. TRAIL also has the ability to function as either pro-apoptotic or pro-survival depending on the cells type, and receptor expression on local tissue to mediate either protective or pathogenic mechanisms. The exact mechanism by which TRAIL modulates these functions is not fully understood, although regulation of TRAIL, and its cleavage, as well as the expression of receptors by specific cell types is clearly important in determining its effects. Further work is required to fully elucidate the divergent roles of TRAIL to gain a better understanding of the role it plays in underlying processes of lung disease, and its potential as a therapeutic agent—or target—depending on disease context.

AUTHOR CONTRIBUTIONS

AB was involved in conception and design of the work, drafting the article and final approval of the version to be published. HM and AL were involved in critical revision of the article and final approval of the version to be published.

REFERENCES

1. Ashkenazi A, Pai RC, Fong S, Leung S, Lawrence DA, Marsters SA, et al. Safety and antitumor activity of recombinant soluble Apo2 ligand. *J Clin Invest.* (1999) 2:155–62. doi: 10.1172/JCI6926
2. Walczak H, Miller RE, Ariail K, Gliniak B, Griffith TS, Kubin M, et al. Tumoricidal activity of tumor necrosis factor-related apoptosis-inducing ligand *in vivo* *Nat Med.* (1999) 2:157–63. doi: 10.1038/5517

3. Chinnaiyan AM, Prasad U, Shankar S, Hamstra DA, Shanaiah M, Chenevert TL, et al. Combined effect of tumor necrosis factor-related apoptosis-inducing ligand and ionizing radiation in breast cancer therapy. *Proc Natl Acad Sci USA.* (2000) 4:1754–9. doi: 10.1073/pnas.030545097
4. Cretney E, Takeda K, Yagita H, Glaccum M, Peschon JJ, Smyth MJ. Increased susceptibility to tumor initiation and metastasis in TNF-related apoptosis-inducing ligand-deficient mice. *J Immunol.* (2002) 3:1356–61. doi: 10.4049/jimmunol.168.3.1356
5. Johnstone RW, Frew AJ, Smyth MJ. The TRAIL apoptotic pathway in cancer onset, progression and therapy. *Nat Rev Cancer* (2008) 10:782–98. doi: 10.1038/nrc2465
6. Berg D, Stuhmer T, Siegmund D, Muller N, Giner T, Dittrich-Breiholz O, et al. Oligomerized tumor necrosis factor-related apoptosis inducing ligand strongly induces cell death in myeloma cells, but also activates proinflammatory signaling pathways. *FEBS J.* (2009) 23:6912–27. doi: 10.1111/j.1742-4658.2009.07388.x
7. Nguyen V, Cudrici C, Zernetkina V, Niculescu F, Rus H, Drachenberg C, et al. TRAIL, DR4 and DR5 are upregulated in kidneys from patients with lupus nephritis and exert proliferative and proinflammatory effects. *Clin Immunol.* (2009) 1:32–42. doi: 10.1016/j.clim.2009.02.011
8. Ehrhardt H, Fulda S, Schmid I, Hiscott J, Debatin KM, Jeremias I. TRAIL induced survival and proliferation in cancer cells resistant towards TRAIL-induced apoptosis mediated by NF-kappa B. *Oncogene* (2003) 25:3842–52. doi: 10.1038/sj.onc.1206520
9. Baader E, Toloczko A, Fuchs U, Schmid I, Beltinger C, Ehrhardt H, et al. Tumor necrosis factor-related apoptosis-inducing ligand-mediated proliferation of tumor cells with receptor-proximal apoptosis defects. *Cancer Res.* (2005) 17:7888–95. doi: 10.1158/0008-5472.CAN-04-4278
10. Azijli K, Yuvaraj S, Peppelenbosch MP, Wurdinger T, Dekker H, Joore J, et al. Kinome profiling of non-canonical TRAIL signaling reveals RIP1-Src-STAT3-dependent invasion in resistant non-small cell lung cancer cells. *J Cell Sci.* (2012) (Pt 19):4651–61. doi: 10.1242/jcs.109587
11. Trauzold A, Siegmund D, Schniewind B, Sipos B, Egberts J, Zorenkov D, et al. TRAIL promotes metastasis of human pancreatic ductal adenocarcinoma. *Oncogene* (2006) 56:7434–39. doi: 10.1038/sj.onc.1209719
12. Gochuico BR, Zhang J, Ma BY, Marshak-Rothstein A, Fine A. TRAIL expression in vascular smooth muscle. *Am J Physiol Lung Cell Mol Physiol.* (2000) 5:L1045–50. doi: 10.1152/ajplung.2000.278.5.L1045
13. Lawrie A, Waterman E, Southwood M, Evans D, Suntharalingam J, Francis S, et al. Evidence of a role for osteoprotegerin in the pathogenesis of pulmonary arterial hypertension. *Am J Pathol.* (2008) 1:256–64. doi: 10.2353/ajpath.2008.070395
14. Wiley SR, Schooley K, Smolak PJ, Din WS, Huang CP, Nicholl JK, et al. Identification and characterization of a new member of the TNF family that induces apoptosis. *Immunity* (1995) 6:673–82. doi: 10.1016/1074-7613(95)90057-8
15. Degli-Esposti MA, Smolak PJ, Walczak H, Waugh J, Huang CP, DuBose RF, et al. Cloning and characterization of TRAIL-R3, a novel member of the emerging TRAIL receptor family. *J Exp Med.* (1997) 7:1165–70. doi: 10.1084/jem.186.7.1165
16. MacFarlane M, Ahmad M, Srinivasula SM, Fernandes-Alnemri T, Cohen GM, Alnemri ES. Identification and molecular cloning of two novel receptors for the cytotoxic ligand TRAIL. *J Biol Chem.* (1997) 41:25417–20. doi: 10.1074/jbc.272.41.25417
17. Marsters SA, Sheridan JP, Pitti RM, Huang A, Skubatch M, Baldwin D, et al. A novel receptor for Apo2L/TRAIL contains a truncated death domain. *Curr Biol.* (1997) 12:1003–6. doi: 10.1016/S0960-9822(06)00422-2
18. Pan G, Ni J, Wei YF, Yu G, Gentz R, Dixit VM. An antagonist decoy receptor and a death domain-containing receptor for TRAIL. *Science* (1997) 5327:815–8.
19. Pan G, O'Rourke K, Chinnaiyan AM, Gentz R, Ebner R, Ni J, et al. The receptor for the cytotoxic ligand TRAIL. *Science* (1997) 5309:111–3.
20. Screaton GR, Mongkolsapaya J, Xu XN, Cowper AE, McMichael AJ, Bell JI. TRICK2, a new alternatively spliced receptor that transduces the cytotoxic signal from TRAIL. *Curr Biol.* (1997) 9:693–6.
21. Emery JG, McDonnell P, Burke MB, Deen KC, Lyn S, Silverman C, et al. Osteoprotegerin is a receptor for the cytotoxic ligand TRAIL. *J Biol Chem.* (1998) 23:14363–7. doi: 10.1074/jbc.273.23.14363
22. Schneider P, Olson D, Tardivel A, Browning B, Lugovskoy A, Gong D, et al. Identification of a new murine tumor necrosis factor receptor locus that contains two novel murine receptors for tumor necrosis factor-related apoptosis-inducing ligand (TRAIL). *J Biol Chem.* (2003) 7:5444–54. doi: 10.1074/jbc.M210783200
23. Hymowitz SG, Christinger HW, Fuh G, Ultsch M, O'Connell M, Kelley RF, et al. Triggering cell death: the crystal structure of Apo2L/TRAIL in a complex with death receptor 5. *Mol Cell.* (1999) 4:563–71. doi: 10.1016/S1097-2765(00)80207-5
24. Pitti RM, Marsters SA, Ruppert S, Donahue CJ, Moore A, Ashkenazi A. Induction of apoptosis by Apo-2 ligand, a new member of the tumor necrosis factor cytokine family. *J Biol Chem.* (1996) 22:12687–90. doi: 10.1074/jbc.271.22.12687
25. Suliman A, Lam A, Datta R, Srivastava RK. Intracellular mechanisms of TRAIL: apoptosis through mitochondrial-dependent and -independent pathways. *Oncogene* (2001) 17:2122–33. doi: 10.1038/sj.onc.1204282
26. Dickens LS, Boyd RS, Jukes-Jones R, Hughes MA, Robinson GL, Fairall L, et al. A death effector domain chain DISC model reveals a crucial role for caspase-8 chain assembly in mediating apoptotic cell death. *Mol Cell.* (2012) 2:291–305. doi: 10.1016/j.molcel.2012.05.004
27. Pan G, Ni J, Yu G, Wei YF, Dixit VM. TRUNDD, a new member of the TRAIL receptor family that antagonizes TRAIL signalling. *FEBS Lett.* (1998) 1–2:41–45. doi: 10.1016/S0014-5793(98)00135-5
28. Miyashita T, Kawakami A, Nakashima T, Yamasaki S, Tamai M, Tanaka F, et al. Osteoprotegerin (OPG) acts as an endogenous decoy receptor in tumour necrosis factor-related apoptosis-inducing ligand (TRAIL)-mediated apoptosis of fibroblast-like synovial cells. *Clin Exp Immunol.* (2004) 2:430–6. doi: 10.1111/j.1365-2249.2004.02534.x
29. Daniels RA, Turley H, Kimberley FC, Liu XS, Mongkolsapaya JP, Ch'En, et al. Expression of TRAIL and TRAIL receptors in normal and malignant tissues. *Cell Res.* (2005) 6:430–8. doi: 10.1038/sj.cr.7290311
30. Hameed AG, Arnold ND, Chamberlain J, Pickworth JA, Paiva C, Dawson S, et al. Inhibition of tumor necrosis factor-related apoptosis-inducing ligand (TRAIL) reverses experimental pulmonary hypertension. *J Exp Med.* (2012) 11:1919–35. doi: 10.1084/jem.20112716
31. Varfolomeev E, Maecker H, Sharp D, Lawrence D, Renz M, Vucic D, et al. Molecular determinants of kinase pathway activation by Apo2 ligand/tumor necrosis factor-related apoptosis-inducing ligand. *J Biol Chem.* (2005) 49:40599–608. doi: 10.1074/jbc.M509560200
32. Russo M, Mupo A, Spagnuolo C, Russo GL. Exploring death receptor pathways as selective targets in cancer therapy. *Biochem Pharmacol.* (2010) 5:674–82. doi: 10.1016/j.bcp.2010.03.011
33. Cantarella G, Di Benedetto G, Ribatti D, Saccani-Jotti G, Bernardini R. Involvement of caspase 8 and c-FLIPL in the proangiogenic effects of the tumour necrosis factor-related apoptosis-inducing ligand (TRAIL). *FEBS J.* (2014) 5:1505–13. doi: 10.1111/febs.12720
34. Dawson S, Arnold N, Pickworth J, Francis S, and Lawrie A. TRAIL deficient mice are protected from sugen/hypoxia induced pulmonary arterial hypertension. *Diseases* (2014) 3:260. doi: 10.3390/diseases2030260
35. Liu H, Yang E, Lu X, Zuo C, He Y, Jia D, et al. Serum levels of tumor necrosis factor-related apoptosis-inducing ligand correlate with the severity of pulmonary hypertension. *Pulm Pharmacol Ther.* (2015) 33:39–46. doi: 10.1016/j.pupt.2015.06.002
36. Hoeper MM, Bogaard HJ, Condliffe R, Frantz R, Khanna D, Kurzyna M, et al. Definitions and diagnosis of pulmonary hypertension. *J Am Coll Cardiol.* (2013) 25 (Suppl.):D42–50. doi: 10.1016/j.jacc.2013.10.032
37. Pietra GG, Edwards WD, Kay JM, Rich S, Kernis J, Schloo B, et al. Histopathology of primary pulmonary hypertension. A qualitative and quantitative study of pulmonary blood vessels from 58 patients in the National Heart, Lung, and Blood Institute, Primary Pulmonary Hypertension Registry. *Circulation* (1989) 5:1198–206. doi: 10.1161/01.CIR.80.5.1198
38. Lawrie A, Hameed AG, Chamberlain J, Arnold N, Kennerley A, Hopkinson K, et al. Paigen diet-fed apolipoprotein E knockout mice develop severe pulmonary hypertension in an interleukin-1-dependent manner. *Am J Pathol* (2011) 4:1693–705. doi: 10.1016/j.ajpath.2011.06.037

39. Secchiero P, Zerbinati C, Rimondi E, Corallini F, Milani D, Grill V, et al. TRAIL promotes the survival, migration and proliferation of vascular smooth muscle cells. *Cell Mol Life Sci.* (2004) 15:1965–74. doi: 10.1007/s00018-004-4197-6
40. Kavurma MM, Schoppet M, Bobryshev YV, Khachigian LM, Bennett MR. TRAIL stimulates proliferation of vascular smooth muscle cells via activation of NF-kappaB and induction of insulin-like growth factor-1 receptor. *J Biol Chem.* (2008) 12:7754–62. doi: 10.1074/jbc.M706927200
41. Song S, Choi K, Ryu SW, Kang SW, Choi C. TRAIL promotes caspase-dependent pro-inflammatory responses via PKCdelta activation by vascular smooth muscle cells. *Cell Death Dis.* (2011) 2:e223. doi: 10.1038/cddis.2011.103
42. Secchiero P, Gonelli A, Carnevale E, Milani D, Pandolfi A, Zella D, et al. TRAIL promotes the survival and proliferation of primary human vascular endothelial cells by activating the Akt and ERK pathways. *Circulation* (2003) 17:2250–56. doi: 10.1161/01.CIR.0000062702.60708.C4
43. Cartland SP, Genner SW, Zahoor A, Kavurma MM. Comparative evaluation of TRAIL, FGF-2 and VEGF-a-induced angiogenesis *in vitro* and *in vivo*. *Int J Mol Sci.* (2016) 12:E2025. doi: 10.3390/ijms17122025
44. Zauli G, Pandolfi A, Gonelli A, Di Pietro R, Guarnieri S, Ciabattoni G, et al. Tumor necrosis factor-related apoptosis-inducing ligand (TRAIL) sequentially upregulates nitric oxide and prostanoid production in primary human endothelial cells. *Circ Res.* (2003) 7:732–40. doi: 10.1161/01.RES.0000067928.83455.9C
45. Harith HH, Di Bartolo BA, Cartland SP, Genner S, Kavurma MM. Insulin promotes vascular smooth muscle cell proliferation and apoptosis via differential regulation of tumor necrosis factor-related apoptosis-inducing ligand. *J Diabetes.* (2016) 4:568–78. doi: 10.1111/1753-0407.12339
46. Alladina SJ, Song JH, Davidge ST, Hao C, Easton AS. TRAIL-induced apoptosis in human vascular endothelium is regulated by phosphatidylinositol 3-kinase/Akt through the short form of cellular FLIP and Bcl-2. *J Vasc Res* (2005) 4:337–47. doi: 10.1159/000086599
47. Cantarella G, Risuglia NR, Dell'eva, Lempereur L, Albini A, Pennisi G, et al. TRAIL inhibits angiogenesis stimulated by VEGF expression in human glioblastoma cells. *Br J Cancer* (2006) 10:1428–35. doi: 10.1038/sj.bjc.6603092
48. Finnberg N, Klein-Szanto AJ, El-Deiry W S. TRAIL-R deficiency in mice promotes susceptibility to chronic inflammation and tumorigenesis. *J Clin Invest.* (2008) 1:111–23. doi: 10.1172/JCI29900
49. McGrath EE, Marriott HM, Lawrie A, Francis SE, Sabroe I, Renshaw SA, et al. TNF-related apoptosis-inducing ligand (TRAIL) regulates inflammatory neutrophil apoptosis and enhances resolution of inflammation. *J Leukoc Biol* (2011) 5:855–65. doi: 10.1189/jlb.0211062
50. Mukerjee D, St George D, Coleiro B, Knight C, Denton CP, Davar J, et al. Prevalence and outcome in systemic sclerosis associated pulmonary arterial hypertension: application of a registry approach. *Ann Rheum Dis.* (2003) 11:1088–93. doi: 10.1136/ard.62.11.1088
51. Hachulla E, Gressin V, Guillevin L, Carpentier P, Diot E, Sibilia J, et al. Early detection of pulmonary arterial hypertension in systemic sclerosis: a French nationwide prospective multicenter study. *Arthritis Rheum.* (2005) 12:3792–800. doi: 10.1002/art.21433
52. Azab NA, Rady HM, Marzouk S A. Elevated serum TRAIL levels in scleroderma patients and its possible association with pulmonary involvement. *Clin Rheumatol.* (2012) 9:1359–64. doi: 10.1007/s10067-012-2023-3
53. McGrath EE, Lawrie A, Marriott HM, Mercer P, Cross SS, Arnold N, et al. Deficiency of tumour necrosis factor-related apoptosis-inducing ligand exacerbates lung injury and fibrosis. *Thorax.* (2012) 9:796–803. doi: 10.1136/thoraxjnl-2011-200863
54. Robertson NM, Zangrilli JG, Steplewski A, Hastie A, Lindemeyer RG, Planeta MA, et al. Differential expression of TRAIL and TRAIL receptors in allergic asthmatics following segmental antigen challenge: evidence for a role of TRAIL in eosinophil survival. *J Immunol.* (2002) 10:5986–96. doi: 10.4049/jimmunol.169.10.5986
55. Weckmann M, Collison A, Simpson JL, Kopp MV, Wark PA, Smyth MJ, et al. Critical link between TRAIL and CCL20 for the activation of TH2 cells and the expression of allergic airway disease. *Nat Med.* (2007) 11:1308–15. doi: 10.1038/nm1660
56. Collison A, Li JA, Pereira de Siqueira, Zhang J, Toop HD, Morris JC, et al. Tumor necrosis factor-related apoptosis-inducing ligand regulates hallmark features of airways remodeling in allergic airways disease. *Am J Respir Cell Mol Biol.* (2014) 1:86–93. doi: 10.1165/rcmb.2013-0490OC
57. Girkin JL, Hatchwell LM, Collison AM, Starkey MR, Hansbro PM, Yagita H, et al. TRAIL signaling is proinflammatory and proviral in a murine model of rhinovirus 1B infection. *Am J Physiol Lung Cell Mol Physiol.* (2017) 1:L89–99. doi: 10.1152/ajplung.00200.2016
58. Starkey MR, Nguyen DH, Essilfie AT, Kim RY, Hatchwell LM, Collison AM, et al. Tumor necrosis factor-related apoptosis-inducing ligand translates neonatal respiratory infection into chronic lung disease. *Mucosal Immunol.* (2014) 3:478–88. doi: 10.1038/mi.2013.65
59. Morissette MC, Vachon-Beaudoin G, Parent J, Chakir J, Milot J. Increased p53 level, Bax/Bcl-x(L) ratio, and TRAIL receptor expression in human emphysema. *Am J Respir Crit Care Med.* (2008) 3:240–7. doi: 10.1164/rccm.200710-1486OC
60. Haw TJ, Starkey MR, Nair PM, Pavlidis S, Liu G, Nguyen DH, et al. A pathogenic role for tumor necrosis factor-related apoptosis-inducing ligand in chronic obstructive pulmonary disease. *Mucosal Immunol.* (2016) 4:859–72. doi: 10.1038/mi.2015.111
61. Wu Y, Shen Y, Zhang J, Wan C, Wang T, Xu D, et al. Increased serum TRAIL and DR5 levels correlated with lung function and inflammation in stable COPD patients. *Int J Chron Obstruct Pulmon Dis.* (2015) 2015:2405–2412. doi: 10.2147/COPD.S92260
62. Morissette MC, Parent J, Milot J. The emphysematous lung is abnormally sensitive to TRAIL-mediated apoptosis. *Respir Res.* (2011) 12:105. doi: 10.1186/1465-9921-12-105
63. Brincks EL, Kucaba TA, Legge KL, Griffith TS. Influenza-induced expression of functional tumor necrosis factor-related apoptosis-inducing ligand on human peripheral blood mononuclear cells. *Hum Immunol.* (2008b) 10:634–46. doi: 10.1016/j.humimm.2008.07.012
64. Kotelkin A, Prikhod'ko EA, Cohen JI, Collins PL, Bukreyev A. Respiratory syncytial virus infection sensitizes cells to apoptosis mediated by tumor necrosis factor-related apoptosis-inducing ligand. *J Virol.* (2003) 17:9156–72. doi: 10.1128/JVI.77.17.9156-9172.2003
65. Ishikawa E, Nakazawa M, Yoshinari M, Minami M. Role of tumor necrosis factor-related apoptosis-inducing ligand in immune response to influenza virus infection in mice. *J Virol.* (2005) 12:7658–63. doi: 10.1128/JVI.79.12.7658-7663.2005
66. Brincks EL, Katewa A, Kucaba TA, Griffith TS, Legge KL. CD8 T cells utilize TRAIL to control influenza virus infection. *J Immunol.* (2008) 7:4918–25. doi: 10.4049/jimmunol.181.7.4918
67. Brincks EL, Gurung P, Langlois RA, Hemann EA, Legge KL, Griffith TS. The magnitude of the T cell response to a clinically significant dose of influenza virus is regulated by TRAIJL. *J Immunol.* (2011) 9:4581–8. doi: 10.4049/jimmunol.1002241
68. Herold S, Steinmueller M, von Wulffen W, Cakarova L, Pinto R, Pleschka S, et al. Lung epithelial apoptosis in influenza virus pneumonia: the role of macrophage-expressed TNF-related apoptosis-inducing ligand. *J Exp Med.* (2008) 13:3065–77. doi: 10.1084/jem.20080201
69. Peteranderl C, Morales-Nebreda L, Selvakumar B, Lecuona E, Vadasz I, Morty RE, et al. Macrophage-epithelial paracrine crosstalk inhibits lung edema clearance during influenza infection. *J Clin Invest.* (2016) 4:1566–80. doi: 10.1172/JCI83931
70. Steinwede K, Henken S, Bohling J, Maus R, Ueberberg B, Brumshagen C, et al. TNF-related apoptosis-inducing ligand (TRAIL) exerts therapeutic efficacy for the treatment of pneumococcal pneumonia in mice. *J Exp Med.* (2012) 11:1937–52. doi: 10.1084/jem.20120983

5

Pulmonary Arterial Hypertension: Iron Matters

Latha Ramakrishnan, Sofia L. Pedersen, Quezia K. Toe, Gregory J. Quinlan†* and Stephen J. Wort*†*

Cardiorespiratory Interface – Vascular Biology, The National Heart and Lung Institute, Faculty of Medicine, Imperial College London, London, United Kingdom

***Correspondence:**
Gregory J. Quinlan
g.quinlan@imperial.ac.uk
Stephen J. Wort
s.wort@imperial.ac.uk

†These authors have contributed equally to this work.

The interplay between iron and oxygen is longstanding and central to all aerobic life. Tight regulation of these interactions including homeostatic regulation of iron utilization ensures safe usage of this limited resource. However, when control is lost adverse events can ensue, which are known to contribute to an array of disease processes. Recently, associations between disrupted iron homeostasis and pulmonary artery hypertension (PAH) have been described with the suggestion that there is a contributory link with disease. This review provides a background for iron regulation in humans, describes PAH classifications, and discusses emerging literature, which suggests a role for disrupted iron homeostatic control in various sub-types of PAH, including a role for decompartmentalization of hemoglobin. Finally, the potential for therapeutic options to restore iron homeostatic balance in PAH are discussed.

Keywords: iron, hepcidin and ferroportin 1 (Fpn1), pulmonary arterial hypertension, pulmonary arterial remodeling, pulmonary hypertension

BACKGROUND OF IRON HANDLING IN HEALTH

Iron and Oxygen

Iron is the principal catalyst that allows for oxygen utilization. The electronic structure of ground state molecular oxygen provides inherent stability (two unpaired electrons with parallel spin); so called spin restriction. Ground state molecular oxygen is, therefore, a relatively unreactive molecule. In order to facilitate oxygen utilization for metabolism, conversion to a reactive state (activation) is achieved via single electron transfer reactions. Iron, as a classical transition metal, has the ability to exist in different states of valence and, therefore, the ability to donate or accept electrons singly, enabling it to convert oxygen to a reactive and therefore metabolically active state. Consequently, body iron requirements are almost exclusively involved with some aspect of oxygen utilization. Notable examples include: respiration, molecular transport, molecular storage, antioxidant protection and biosynthesis.

Mammalian Iron Requirements

Healthy human adults contain between 2 and 4 g of iron; daily iron requirements for metabolism and biosynthesis are 20 mg, largely for heme biosynthesis, to satisfy the daily requirement for the production of 200 billion red blood cells. However, iron utilization is not limited to these processes; for instance, all cells require iron to proliferate, iron being essential for DNA biosynthesis as well as for cell cycle progression (Yu et al., 2007). In addition, many proteins and particularly those involved in oxygen metabolism have an essential requirement for iron, which is usually localized to heme and non- heme containing active centers. Mitochondria are principal cellular sites for heme and iron–sulfur cluster biosynthesis and therefore require an adequate supply of iron to maintain these activities.

Iron uptake from the diet is largely facilitated by enterocytes localized to the duodenum but these can provide only 1–2 mg of iron on a daily basis. Moreover, daily iron losses are similar; although no specific iron excretory mechanisms exist in mammals, losses do occur through shedding of intestinal epithelial cells and skin cells, blood loss and, in addition, via bile and urine excretion. Iron uptake from the gut therefore balances these losses but cannot accommodate the daily requirement of 20 mg. The majority of this essential iron requirement is therefore supplied by recycling endogenous iron resources and stores rather than by intestinal uptake, and is under strict regulatory control, not least because iron is a limited and precious resource.

Iron Homeostatic Control

Cellular Regulation

Regulation of cellular iron requirements are chiefly facilitated by post-transcriptional feedback mechanisms directed by the activity of two cytosolic iron regulatory proteins, IRP-1 and IRP-2, which, when active, bind to key regulatory motifs termed iron responsive elements (IREs) either located at the 5′ or 3′ ends in target mRNAs. IRP binding to 5′ IREs prevents ribosomal translation and hence biosynthesis, whereas 3′ binding stabilizes mRNA and supports translation. IRPs are activated by low cytosolic cellular iron levels. Under these circumstances synthesis of both light (L) and heavy (H) chains of the intracellular iron storage protein complex, ferritin, is down regulated (as is the synthesis of the transmembrane protein and iron exporter, ferroportin). Importantly, the translation of hypoxia inducible factor (Hif)-2α which is one component of the Hif complex, is also inhibited demonstrating the interplay between iron and oxygen homeostasis (see also section "Oxygen Sensing and Iron Regulation"). Conversely, IRP 3' IRE mRNA binding promotes the synthesis of transferrin receptor 1 (TFR-1), a transmembrane glycoprotein that facilitates the uptake of iron-loaded transferrin from the circulation via receptor mediated endocytosis. Additionally, divalent metal transporter 1 (DMT-1) a protein that binds to a variety of metals including cadmium, copper, zinc, and iron, provides an additional route for (direct) iron uptake by cells. Thus, in situations when cellular iron levels are low, active IRPs down-regulate iron storage and cellular export whilst facilitating cellular iron uptake. The opposite occurs when cellular iron levels are replete or overloaded- IRPs are inactivated. Operational within cells such as enterocytes, macrophages, and hepatocytes, and important for iron turnover and control, it is also apparent that such regulation is common to other cell types. In addition, IREs have been identified in mRNAs for numerous proteins beyond those described above indicating a more complex role for the IRPs in cellular regulation of iron and oxygen homeostasis; for reviews, see Kuhn (2015) and Simpson and McKie (2015).

Global Regulation: The Importance of the Hepcidin-Ferroportin Axis

Often described as the master regulator of iron homeostasis, hepcidin is a small peptide hormone (25 amino acids) synthesized in the main by liver hepatocytes; a process that is regulated by plasma and liver iron levels and which involves signaling via bone morphogenetic protein (BMP) and SMAD pathways, inflammation and, in particular, IL-6 levels via the JAK/stat pathway. In the circulation hepcidin targets and binds to cellular ferroportin causing it to be endocytosed and degraded hence halting cellular iron export (**Figure 1**).

Hypoxia and erythropoiesis are also important regulatory signals for hepcidin production (**Figure 2**). Consequences of such inhibition include prevention of intestinal iron absorption, limitation of release of liver iron stores and hindrance of recycling processes linked to macrophages. If hepcidin release is sustained, the accumulation of iron in tissues (hepatocytes, macrophages,

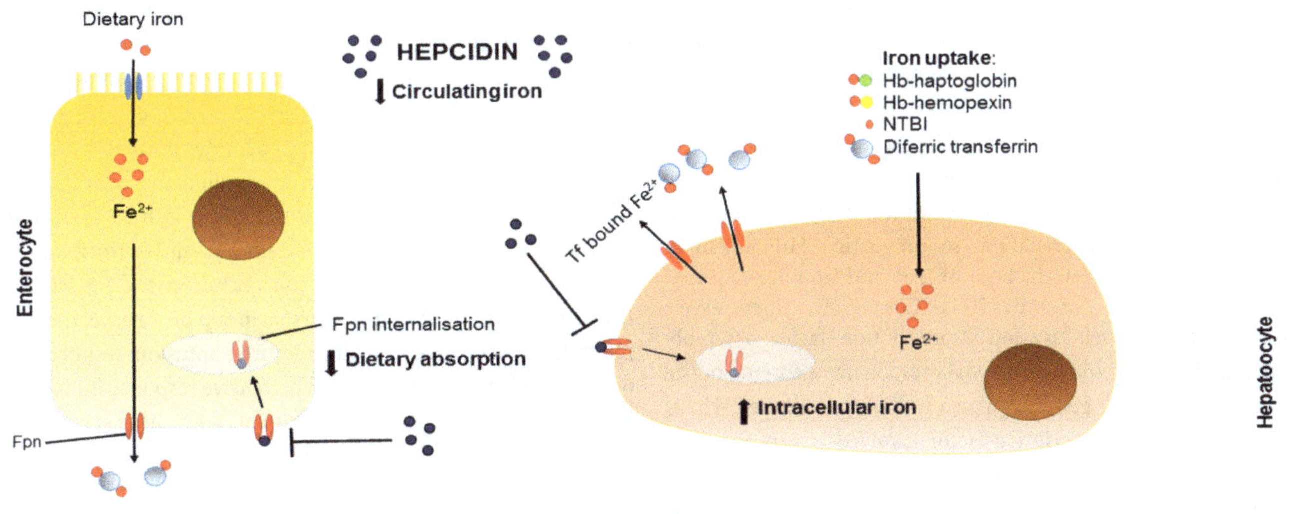

FIGURE 1 | Effects of hepcidin on iron homeostasis. Schematic representation of the effects of hepcidin on dietary absorption of iron (left) and intracellular iron stores (right). Fpn, ferroportin; Tf, transferrin; Fe, iron; Hb, hemoglobin; NTBI, non-transferrin-bound iron.

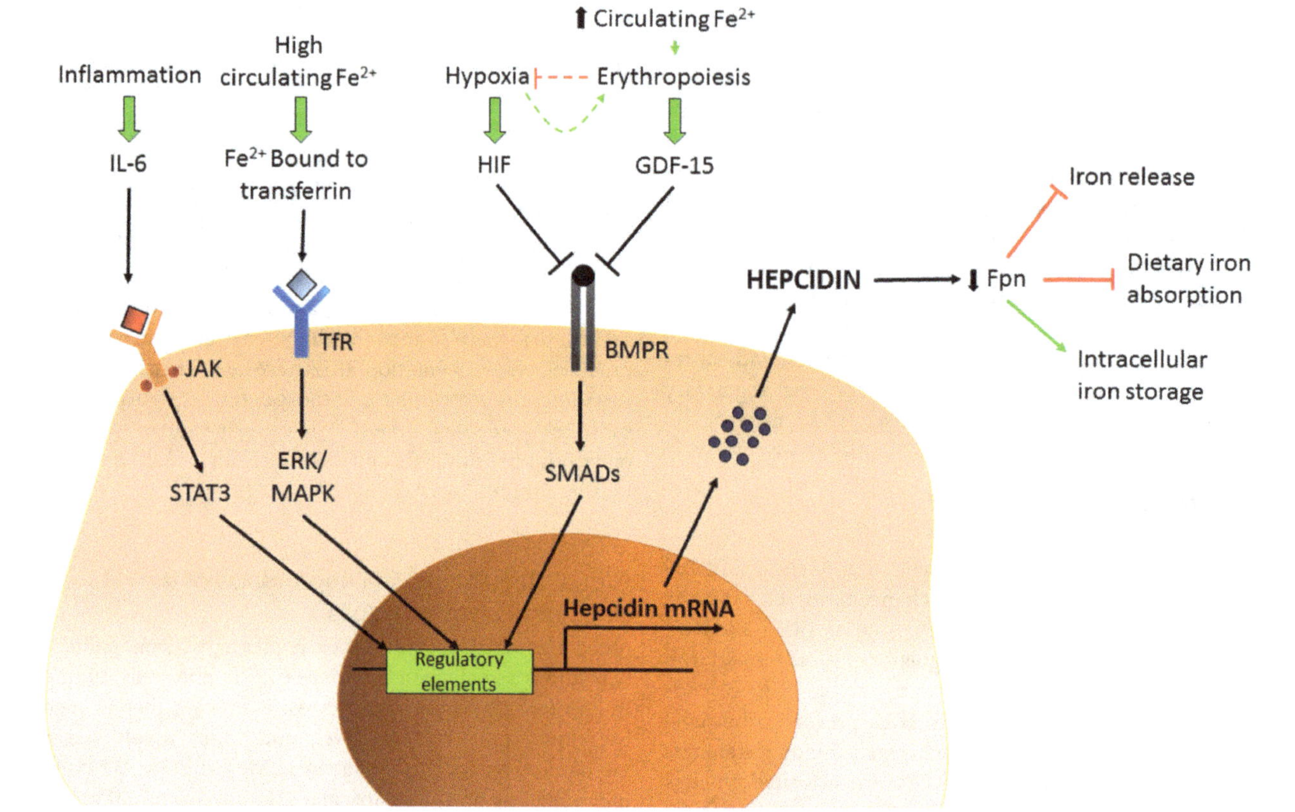

FIGURE 2 | Control of hepcidin expression. Schematic representation of the factors controlling hepcidin transcription. IL-6, interleukin 6; JAK/STAT3, Janus kinase/signal transducers and activator of transcription 3; Fe, iron; TfR, transferrin receptor; HIF, hypoxia-inducible factor; GDF-15, growth/differentiation factor 15; BMPR, bone morphogenetic protein receptor; Fpn, ferroportin.

and other cell types) coupled with limited iron uptake from the diet result in a negative iron balance and tissue iron loading. For a comprehensive review, see Drakesmith et al. (2015).

Oxygen Sensing and Iron Regulation

Iron and oxygen utilization are closely linked and longstanding in nature, being essential for all aerobic life. This relationship is aptly illustrated by the joint regulatory roles for both oxygen and iron in the control of the activity of Hif. Hif is composed of an oxygen-dependent subunit, Hif 2α, and a constitutively expressed β subunit. The prolyl hydroylases (PHDs) hydroxylate two key prolyl residues on Hif 2α which ultimately leads to ubiquitination and degradation, so preventing HiF assembly and activation. Importantly, both oxygen and iron are required for enzyme activity of the PHDs. Conversely, when either iron or oxygen levels are low, transcription factor assembly occurs and binding to target hypoxia responsive elements in the promoter regions of genes regulated by Hif is facilitated. Hif is a multifunctional transcription factor involved in expression of genes linked to cytoskeleton formation, energy metabolism, and erythropoiesis and importantly, in the context of this review: vasomotor function, migration, proliferation, angiogenesis, and the regulation of iron transport. For a general review of Hif, see Simpson and McKie (2015).

EVIDENCE FOR IMPORTANCE OF IRON AND RELATED MOLECULES IN THE NORMAL HUMAN VASCULATURE

Literature describing the role of iron in the maintenance of balanced vascular function is somewhat limited with most studies on iron homeostasis focusing on global aspects involved in control of erythropoiesis. However, some studies undertaken with healthy human volunteers have demonstrated that iron chelation with desferrioxamine promotes hypoxic vasoconstriction (HPV) and increases pulmonary artery systolic pressure (PASP) compared to iron replete individuals (Smith et al., 2008). Furthermore, the same group performed two randomized placebo controlled trials investigating the effect of iron on HPV and PASP. In the first, a group of sea-level dwelling individuals were taken to altitude; iron infusion resulted in a 6 mmHg fall in the pulmonary hypertensive response initiated by hypoxia. In the second protocol, patients with chronic mountain sickness received isovolaemic 2 l venesections followed 2 weeks later by an infusion of iron or placebo. Venesection resulted in a 25% increase in PASP. However, subsequent iron infusion did not ameliorate the increase in PASP (Smith et al., 2009). Additional support for the role of iron in HPV is provided by Frise et al. (2016). In 13 iron deficient individuals, 6 h of hypoxia led to an increase in PASP compared to iron replete controls. Intravenous iron (given before the hypoxic challenge) attenuated the rise in PASP in both groups but to a greater extent in the iron deficient group (Frise et al., 2016). The above findings indicate a key role for iron in the sensing and signaling response to hypoxia in normal pulmonary vascular function.

As for evidence of any role for iron regulation at the level of the pulmonary vascular cell, these studies are somewhat lacking but new findings from our own laboratory have recently demonstrated the presence of the iron exporter ferroportin in pulmonary artery smooth muscle cells (PASMCs) and pulmonary artery endothelial cells (PAECs) (Ramakrishnan et al., 2014) suggesting a potential dynamic role for the hepcidin-ferroportin axis and the regulation of cellular iron stores at the level of the pulmonary vasculature. Please see Section "Group 3: PH Related to Chronic Lung Disease and/or Hypoxia (Including High Altitude)" for further discussion of response of the pulmonary vasculature to hypoxia and relevance to the development of pulmonary hypertension (PH).

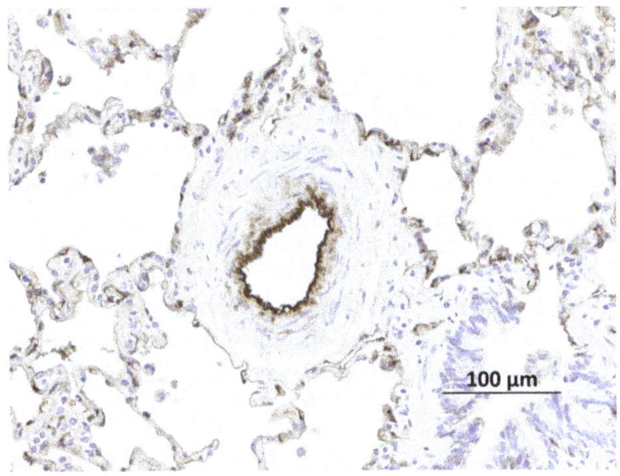

FIGURE 3 | Remodeled pulmonary arteriole from a patient with idiopathic pulmonary arterial hypertension taken after transplant. Remodeling in this case is characterized by an increase in the number of smooth muscle cells in the media. The endothelium is stained with an anti-vWF antibody (brown stain). vWF, von Willibrand Factor. Figure courtesy of Dr. Allan Lawrie and Dr. Roger Thompson, University of Sheffield, United Kingdom.

PULMONARY HYPERTENSION: DEFINITION AND CLASSIFICATION

Pulmonary hypertension encompasses a group of conditions characterized by raised blood pressure in the pulmonary arteries. The formal diagnosis requires right heart catheterization: PH is defined as a mean pulmonary arterial pressure $\geq$25 mmHg at rest. There is a further hemodynamic division into pre- and post- capillary PH depending on whether the pulmonary artery wedge pressure (a measure of left atrial pressure) is $\leq$15 mmHg (pre-capillary PH) or >15 mmHg (post-capillary PH). PH is divided into five clinical groups, each group of which shares similar pathophysiology and anticipated response to treatment (Galie et al., 2016). Group 1 PH is known as pulmonary arterial hypertension (PAH). All the conditions within this group have pre-capillary hemodynamics, a raised pulmonary vascular resistance (PVR) and no evidence of significant lung disease (Group 3 PH) or thromboembolic disease (Group 4). The main disorders presenting with PAH are congenital heart disease (predominantly Eisenmenger Syndrome), scleroderma associated PAH and idiopathic (i)PAH (a diagnosis of exclusion) (Humbert et al., 2006; Peacock et al., 2007). Within the clinical phenotype of Group 1 PAH, a small proportion will have a family history and most will carry a genetic abnormality in one of the genes associated with the condition, predominantly, bone morphogenetic protein receptor (BMPR) 2 (Rudarakanchana et al., 2002; Soubrier et al., 2013). All members of Group 1 have similar histology with remodeling of pulmonary arterioles (diameter < 500 μM). This involves hyperplasia of cells encompassing all three layers of the vessel wall, although predominantly smooth muscle (**Figure 3**). The resulting increase in PVR increases the afterload on the right ventricle (RV) provoking RV hypertrophy, enlargement and eventually failure (Tuder et al., 2013). PAH is always associated with increased morbidity and mortality, but with some heterogeneity depending on sub-type. Patients with iPAH have one of the worse prognoses with a pre-treatment era median survival of only 2.8 years, comparable to many advanced cancers (Barst et al., 1996). In addition, it has a female predominance and tends to affect younger adults (Peacock et al., 2007).

Pathophysiology of PAH

This review is predominantly involved with the pre-capillary remodeling observed in PAH, although pure vasoconstriction is likely to be involved in acute responses to hypoxia, described in other sections.

The exact sequence of events leading to pulmonary vascular remodeling remains unknown; however, the lung pulmonary vasculature does show a stereotypical response to insult(s) as histopathology of lesions remains very similar across sub-types of PAH, see **Figure 3** for a representative remodeled human pulmonary arteriole On the one hand, it is very likely that increased endothelial shear stress from left to right blood flow across an intra- or extra-cardiac defect is the initiating insult in Eisenmenger syndrome (D'Alto and Mahadevan, 2012). On the other, in heritable PAH, defects predominantly in the BMPR2 gene increase susceptibility to developing PAH. However, the penetrance of the genetic defect remains low, suggesting other "hits" are necessary. Additional insults are likely to include: infection, exposure to hypoxia, exposure to serotoninergic drugs and pregnancy related changes in female hormone levels (Tuder et al., 2013). Although not proven, one of the earliest abnormalities is probably endothelial cell dysfunction leading to an imbalance of vasoactive molecules: increased production of the vasoconstrictor and mitogen, endothelin (ET)-1 and reduced production of nitric oxide (NO) and prostacyclin (PGI_2), both vasodilators and anti-proliferative agents (Humbert et al., 2004). Damage to the endothelium may expose the underlying smooth muscle (SM) to cytokines and serum factors that promote proliferation.

The presence of BMPR2 mutations pre-dispose SM cells to increased proliferative rates and reduced apoptosis (Yang et al., 2011). Medial (SM) hypertrophy in resistance arterioles is one of the cardinal histological features of PAH (**Figure 3**). As the disease progresses, it is likely that apoptotic resistant endothelial cells lead to neointimal formation and fibrosis and the formation of plexiform lesions. The adventitia is also involved with increased numbers of fibroblasts and extra-cellular matrix protein deposition. Inflammatory changes are often observed surrounding remodeled vessels, although the exact contribution of inflammation (marker or mediator) remains unclear. However, circulating cytokines, such as IL-6, IL-8, and IL-10 are increased in patients with PAH and correlate with outcome (Soon et al., 2010). Other important mediators are growth factors such as platelet derived growth factor (PDGF) and transforming growth factor (TGF)- β. Most recently, it is clear that there are also epigenetic mechanisms involved (Pullamsetti et al., 2016). A more complete discussion, apart from reviewing the role of iron and iron-related molecules below is beyond the scope of the present review.

EVIDENCE FOR ABNORMAL IRON HANDLING IN PULMONARY HYPERTENSION

Most of the literature relating abnormal iron handling to the development of PH concentrates on iPAH and Eisenmenger syndrome, which will be the main focus of this section. However, there is good evidence to relate iron deficiency to an exaggerated response to hypoxia, which may of course relate to respiratory conditions associated with PH in Group 3 of the international classification as well as exposure to high altitude. Chronic exposure to hypoxia, and the development of high altitude PH has been the topic of several recent reviews (Wilkins et al., 2015). See also Section "Group 3: PH Related to Chronic Lung Disease and/or Hypoxia (Including High Altitude)" of this review.

Evidence for Abnormal Iron Handling in iPAH

Ruiter et al. (2011) reported the first data to support iron deficiency in patients with iPAH. In 70 patients, 30 (43%) had iron deficiency as determined by a serum iron $< 10\mu mol^{-1}$ and transferrin saturation < 15% in females and <20% in males; in normal individuals levels of iron saturation of transferrin are 25% and above; 50% saturation indicates iron overload. Six-minute walk test (6MWT) was reduced in iron-deficient patients compared with iron replete patients, irrespective as to whether they had anemia or not. In a sub-set of patients who received oral iron therapy, only eight out of 18 had ferritin levels restored to normal levels, suggesting impaired oral uptake in these patients (which has subsequently been proposed to be secondary to increased hepcidin levels). These findings were confirmed in a slightly later study where it was also demonstrated that iron deficiency was more prevalent in patients with iPAH compared to patients with chronic thromboembolic PH (CTEPH) (Soon et al., 2011). Interestingly, IL-6 levels were correlated with iron levels in iPAH patients but not in CTEPH patients. As described earlier, IL-6 is known to promote hepcidin production, but in this study there was no correlation of IL-6 with hepcidin in iPAH patients. Data from another United Kingdom group suggested that hepcidin levels may be inappropriately high in a subset of iPAH patients (Rhodes et al., 2011a). Furthermore, iron deficiency, this time defined by increased circulating soluble transferrin receptor levels, was associated with disease severity and poor clinical outcome.

There are also potential implications related to BMPR2 gene mutation or subsequent downstream pathway dysfunction and altered iron handling in PAH, as BMPR2/SMAD pathways, amongst other functions, are also involved in regulation of iron homeostasis, facilitated through the control of hepcidin production (**Figure 2**) (Finberg, 2013). As mentioned earlier, under normal circumstances iron availability directs such homeostatic control. In patients with iPAH this homeostasis is presumably lost, leading to iron deficiency and hepcidin excess (Rhodes et al., 2011b). Inflammation may impact further on dysfunctional BMPR2 signaling and loss of iron homeostasis, as plasma IL-6 levels are raised in patients with PAH (Selimovic et al., 2009); IL-6 is also known to up-regulate hepcidin expression via the JAK-STAT pathway (Soon et al., 2010) (**Figure 2**). Intriguingly, increased autophagy mediated by lysosomal action (where BMPR2 and ferroportin are both degraded) has been implicated in PAH (Long et al., 2013) suggesting a potential link with altered iron handling.

Further evidence for abnormal iron handling was demonstrated by Decker et al. (2011) who showed that zinc protoporphyrin (Zn-pp) levels are high in patients with PAH (mainly iPAH) indicating deficient iron incorporation to form heme suggestive of iron deficiency; levels were closely related to clinical severity (Decker et al., 2011). Zinc competes with iron for binding sites, therefore when iron levels are diminished zinc replaces iron at these sites. PAH patients also had a high red cell distribution width (RDW), again corresponding to markers of clinical severity, such as higher pulmonary arterial pressures and lower 6MWT. Most recently, using proteome analysis in the plasma of patients with PAH, Rhodes et al. (2017) were able to identify a combination of nine circulating proteins associated with a high risk of mortality, two of which, plasminogen and erythropoietin, are associated with abnormal iron metabolism (Rhodes et al., 2017).

Evidence for Abnormal Iron Handling in Eisenmenger Syndrome

Iron deficiency has been recognized in patients with cyanotic congenital heart disease for much longer than other forms of PAH. This is considered to be a direct response of increased secondary erythrocytosis (due to chronic cyanosis). However, the exact underlying mechanisms remain unclear. An additional factor, historically, was the routine use of venesection, which was associated with increased risk of hemoptysis, anemia and iron deficiency (Daliento et al., 1998). Iron deficiency is associated with adverse outcomes in Eisenmenger patients (Van De Bruaene et al., 2011). Venesection is now not recommended and iron deficiency actively corrected in this population (Dimopoulos et al., 2008).

Although very different diseases, pulmonary vascular remodeling in ES and iPAH is similar; however, dysfunctional BMP signaling linked to the gene defects in BMPR II has not been found in ES (Therrien et al., 2006) (although BMPRII protein levels have been reported to be reduced in this population). As for determinants of disrupted iron homoeostasis in these patients, data are limited but, in a small comparative observational study undertaken by ourselves (published in abstract form), there were significant increases in an array of plasma markers including: soluble transferrin receptor, free heme, iron saturation of transferrin, IL-6 and hepcidin; clearly demonstrating elevated levels of these iron indices in ES cohorts as compared to iPAH patients and healthy controls (Mumby et al., 2016).

Evidence for Abnormal Iron Handling in Other Forms of PH

Group 1: Associated Forms of PAH

With regards to associated forms of PAH in Group 1, only when in association with scleroderma has there been a link with iron deficiency described in the literature. Iron deficiency (as determined by soluble transferrin receptor) was present in 46% of patients with scleroderma-PH compared to 16% of patients with scleroderma but no PH (note that not all of these had PAH). Iron deficiency was associated with lower exercise capacity and worse survival. Hepcidin levels were overall high and related to transferrin receptor status but not to IL-6 levels (Ruiter et al., 2011).

Group 3: PH Related to Chronic Lung Disease and/or Hypoxia (Including High Altitude)

As described earlier, iron deficiency causes an exaggerated response, in terms of PASP, to acute hypoxia, compared to iron replete controls. Iron replacement reverses this response (Frise et al., 2016). Apart from periods when humans are exposed to hypoxia, these findings may be relevant to PH that develops in conjunction with respiratory conditions, which are characterized by alveolar hypoxia (Group 3). Indeed, iron deficiency has been shown to associate with echo derived PASP in non-anemic patients with COPD (Plesner et al., 2017). Potential relevant mechanisms are described next.

A role for Hif in hypoxia and normoxia

The molecular mechanisms underpinning the response to hypoxia are incompletely understood, although Hif is likely to be key. Mutations which lead to over activation of Hif in normoxia, a condition called Chuvash polycythemia, result in an exaggerated vasoconstrictor response under hypoxic conditions (Smith et al., 2006). Mouse models of the von Hippel-Lindau mutation, that characterizes Chuvash polycythemia, result in PH and fibrosis (Imtiyaz et al., 2010). Moreover, mouse models with heterozygous mutations in Hif components result in some protection from PH under conditions of hypoxia (Yu et al., 1999; Brusselmans et al., 2003). Furthermore, as Hif activity is both regulated by iron and itself regulates aspects of iron homeostatic control, an interactive role for iron and Hif in PH seems plausible. Indeed, for an increasing number of genes involved in iron homeostasis, the presence of IREs and hypoxic responsive elements (HREs) within the promoter region have been described. Expression at the level of mRNA is therefore regulated not just by the IRPs but also by the hypoxia inducible transcription factor component, Hif-2α. Moreover, as mentioned above, Hif-2α activity is controlled via the enzymatic activity of the iron and oxygen sensing prolyl hydroxylases, and depletion of either substrate leads to Hif activation and an array of transcriptional responses. Therefore, iron deficiency, in a similar fashion to hypoxia, can lead to Hif activity; but potentially under normoxic conditions.

Hif and regulation of cellular iron content

Importantly, the ferroportin gene contains both IREs and HREs; thus, hypoxia represents a further signal for ferroportin expression via Hif-2α (Simpson and McKie, 2015). As for any role for hypoxia in hepcidin expression/activity there are controversies in the literature with some studies suggesting an involvement for Hif-2α in hepcidin suppression, (Peyssonnaux et al., 2007) whereas more recent literature refutes this suggestion (Volke et al., 2009); however, other soluble factors may be involved (Ravasi et al., 2014). Reactive oxygen species (ROS) may also have a role as the redox sensitive transcription factor, NF-κB, has been shown to regulate hepcidin expression in part in macrophages (Sow et al., 2009). Given the role of hypoxia and ROS production in PAH it is likely that such perturbations will be influential in aspects of disrupted iron homeostasis of relevance to the pulmonary vasculature and will further modulate the hepcidin/ferroportin axis. Another iron homeostatic perturbation that may be of relevance to Hif activity is iron regulatory protein-1 (IRP-1) dysfunction; targeted deletion of IRP-1 in mice resulted in PH and polycythemia, responses, which were more apparent in animals, fed an iron-restricted diet. Hif-2α expression in pulmonary endothelial cells cultured from these animals was elevated in comparison to those from wild type controls (Ghosh et al., 2013); effects on the hepcidin/ferroportin axis were not described in this study. Additionally, iron–sulfur cluster deficiency linked to either hypoxic or genetic alterations in the microRNA-210-ISCU1/2 axis also contribute to PH in murine models, (White et al., 2015) all of which suggests a link to mitochondrial dysfunction, given that iron–sulfur synthesis occurs in this organelle and its function is dramatically affected by ischemia or hypoxia. Finally, there may also be implications in relation to IRP-1 activity which is regulated by iron–sulfur cluster assembly (Kuhn, 2015). The role of Hif, hypoxia and iron as potential drivers of PAH are therefore complex and still emerging.

Group 5: Miscellaneous Causes of PH: The Hemolytic Anemias

The last group to mention is the chronic hemolytic anemias, which sit in Group 5 of PH classification. Abnormal iron handling may clearly be a factor in conditions such as Sickle

Cell Disease (SCD) and the Thalassemias. Potential factors that may contribute to disease presentation in these circumstances are numerous and include consequences related to the release of free hemoglobin. The potential for a direct proliferative role linked to decompartmentalization of free iron/heme/hemoglobin is also of potential importance and is given consideration below. However, as for mechanisms of disease onset and progression, in addition to the more detailed descriptions presented below, consideration should also be given to high cardiac output-PH in very anemic patients, as well as direct myocardial involvement producing a post-capillary PH picture (Group 2 PH).

Hemoglobin and oxidative stress

Hemoglobin, once decompartmentalized, disassociates to the dimeric form, is subject to the release of free heme and is also likely to shed iron, which, in an extracellular setting of complete transferrin iron saturation, will remain free or loosely bound. This, in turn, will be available to catalyze damaging hydroxyl radical formation from hydrogen peroxide and initiate or propagate peroxidation of membrane polyunsaturated fatty acids causing damage that is not necessarily limited to endothelial targets. In addition, both hemoglobin and heme are redox catalysts and so can also contribute to damaging oxidant production and an overall altered redox balance. Thus, there are numerous iron breakdown products released or formed consequent to hemolysis, which may have implications for disease onset and progression.

Endogenous protection of a limited resource

Targeted binding by haptoglobin for hemoglobin, hemopexin and or albumin for heme and transferrin or lactoferrin for iron, followed by receptor mediated cellular uptake limits adverse aspects related to the release of these species in the extracellular setting. However, during prolonged or pronounced hemolytic episodes, such binding processes are saturated leading to extracellular accumulation of these products of hemolysis and also increased iron storage within cells and tissues. In this regard, it is now widely recognized that PH is a common co-morbidity for patients suffering from hemoglobinopathies resultant from hemolytic anemias (Souza et al., 2009) and consequently that endogenous protection is compromised in these patient groups.

A role for decompartmentalized hemoglobin in PAH

Decompartmentalization of hemoglobin and subsequent binding of NO that affects vascular reactivity and remodeling has been hypothesized as a functional component in PAH associated with hemoglobinopathies such as the Thalassemias and SCD (Mathew et al., 2016). In addition, hemoglobin/heme containing red cell microparticle formation also accompanies hemolysis with known effects on the endothelium and resultant vascular occlusion in SCD (Camus et al., 2015). In epidemiological terms for SCD populations, PAH is many orders of magnitude more common than in the normal population (Buehler et al., 2012) and additionally for SCD patients with PAH, hemolytic anemia is much more severe (Potoka and Gladwin, 2014); all of which strongly suggests active involvement of hemolysis in the development of PAH in SCD. A link which is also apparent for β-thalassemia major where PAH development is thought to be related to both the severity of hemolysis and also the need for repeated transfusions (leading to tissue iron overload); whereas for β-thalassemia intermedia, ongoing hemolysis without transfusion also causes iron loading and is associated with PAH (Fraidenburg and Machado, 2016). In a small study of non-transfusion dependent thalassemia patients, PAH was relatively common (10%) and was associated with previous multiple transfusions, splenectomy and non-transferrin bound iron (a marker of iron overload) (Inthawong et al., 2015). A role in PAH is also apparent for other hemolytic disorders such as hereditary spherocytosis, microangiopathic anemias, and paroxysmal nocturnal hemoglobinuria to name but a few (Machado and Farber, 2013). Importantly, recent studies in patients with iPAH and heritable PAH have demonstrated red cell abnormalities: specifically enhanced levels of zinc-protoporphyrin (Decker et al., 2011); elevated creatine (Fox et al., 2012) and plasma free hemoglobin, which was independently associated with increased risk for admission to hospital (Brittain et al., 2014) all of which are suggestive of iron deficiency and sub-clinical hemolysis. Moreover, decreased levels of haptoglobin are apparent across PAH phenotypes and demonstrates a negative correlation with mean pulmonary artery pressure for patients with connective tissue disease associated PAH (Nakamura et al., 2017). Given the role of haptoglobin as an extracellular hemoglobin binding protein these studies further support a role for hemolysis and decompartmentalized hemoglobin in PAH progression.

IN VITRO AND *IN VIVO* MODELS OF DISRUPTED IRON HOMEOSTASIS

There are a number of recently published studies, which have investigated the relationship between iron availability, or deficiency, and proliferative responses in settings of relevance to PAH. In one study the use of iron chelation via the administration of desferrioxamine to rats was found to inhibit chronic hypoxia induced PH and remodeling suggesting that iron is requisite for vascular proliferation in these circumstances; an assertion further supported by *in vitro* studies by the same authors which showed that an iron chelation strategy also inhibited proliferation of cultured PASMCs (Wong et al., 2012). In another study, use of plumbagin, an iron chelator, (Padhye et al., 2012) was found to limit proliferation in human PASMCs and decrease distal pulmonary artery remodeling in a rat model of PAH (Courboulin et al., 2012). Additionally, iron was found to induce remodeling in cultured rat PAECs (Gorbunov et al., 2012). Together, these studies indicate a role for iron availability in proliferation and remodeling. However, in other recent studies, opposing responses have been reported; for instance, iron deficient (iron restricted diet) monocrotaline treated rats were somewhat protected from pulmonary vascular remodeling and right ventricular failure; however, the low levels of hepcidin shown in these animals compared to controls (iron replete) is at variance with elevated hepcidin as observed in clinical PAH and also suggests that cellular iron retention is less likely in these circumstances (Naito et al., 2013). In a related rat model, iron deficiency alone of 4 weeks duration was shown to contribute to in pulmonary vascular remodeling, raised pulmonary artery pressure and right ventricular hypertrophy. All these changes were reversed on restoration of a dietary iron (Cotroneo et al., 2015) suggesting that iron deficiency contributes to vascular remodeling. Whilst not in absolute agreement, collectively, these studies do indicate that iron availability or otherwise is a key component of vascular remodeling in experimental PAH.

As for any role for iron retention or release at the level of the cell, these studies are fledgling in nature and largely limited to published abstracts. Our own studies in this regard have established that ferroportin is present on both human PAMSCs (Ramakrishnan et al., 2014) and human PAECs (Ramakrishnan et al., 2013) and that hepcidin treatment of human PASMCs causes a proliferative response most likely linked to cellular iron retention. Moreover, treatment with IL-6 also promotes human PASMC proliferation (Ramakrishnan et al., 2015). Interestingly, the hemoglobin-haptoglobin receptor/scavenger molecule, CD163, has been shown to be expressed and regulated in both human PAECs as well as PASMCs (Ramakrishnan et al., 2015, 2016) suggesting a means for cellular uptake of iron by these cells. In related studies, an *in vivo* model of vascular remodeling linked to cellular iron accumulation was reversed with haptoglobin therapy (Irwin et al., 2015) indicating a potential role for free hemoglobin in these processes. Thus there may be a generalized functional impact related to decompartmentalization of hemoglobin of relevance to PAH which given our observational data (Mumby et al., 2016) may be of greater relevance in condition such as Eisenmenger syndrome.

TREATMENTS: SUMMARY OF CLINICAL EVIDENCE WITH IRON REPLACEMENT IN PAH

There are very few clinical trials investigating the effect of iron replacement in patients with PAH. Viethen et al. (2014) presented the results of 20 iron deficient patients with mixed PAH etiology, given IV ferric carboxymaltose (1,000 mg) in an open label fashion. Compared to a non-treated group, there was an improvement in iron status, significant increase in 6-min walk test and quality of life score (Viethen et al., 2014). There have been two trials in specific PAH sub-types, described below.

Iron Therapy in Cyanotic Congenital Heart Disease

There are no randomized, placebo controlled studies investigating the effect of iron replacement in the cyanotic congenital heart disease population. However, Tay et al. (2011) studied 25 iron-deficient cyanotic CHD patients, 14 of which had Eisenmenger Syndrome, who received oral iron replacement in a prospective open label manner (Tay et al., 2011). Oral ferrous fumarate was titrated to a maximum of 200 mg tds. After 3 months of treatment, hemoglobin, ferritin and transferrin saturation had all significantly increased. Significant improvements were also seen in quality of life and 6MWT, although peak VO_2 was unchanged. Oral treatment was well tolerated with no complications. In clinical practice in the cyanotic CHD population treatment of iron deficiency (as a complication of secondary erythrocytosis) is managed quite aggressively, usually with intravenous iron replacement. In 142 consecutive cyanotic CHD patients of which 49% were ES, treatment with IV ferrous carboxymaltose (500 mg; Ferrinject^{TM}) resulted in improvement in hemoglobin, hematocrit, ferritin, and transferrin saturation. There were no cases of excessive erythrocytosis with very few complications (personal communication).

Iron Therapy and Idiopathic Pulmonary Arterial Hypertension

There is only one published study on the use of iron replacement in patients with iPAH (Gerrina et al., 2015). Fifteen patients with iPAH and iron deficiency received a single, high dose of IV iron in an open label fashion. After 12 weeks, the primary endpoint, 6MWT, was not changed. However, exercise endurance time and aerobic capacity increased significantly without change in cardiac function. There was improved quadriceps muscle oxygen handling. IV iron was well tolerated and there was an improvement in quality of life. A randomized, placebo controlled trial is currently active and the results are eagerly awaited (Howard et al., 2013).

Iron Therapy in Other Forms of PH

There are no other studies investigating the use of iron replacement in other forms of PH apart from experimental studies in acute hypoxia driven PH. Bart et al. (2016) investigated the effect of 1 g IV iron (or saline) on increases in PASP associated with 6 h of hypoxia in 22 subjects. Patients receiving iron before hypoxia had a 50% reduction in PASP rise which was sustained up to 43 days after iron therapy (Bart et al., 2016).

Future Treatments

Clearly from the literature presented above, it is apparent that protocols are under development and in use involving iron supplementation therapies in order to correct perceived iron patient deficits. Whilst this ultimately may help restore iron homeostasis there is nevertheless the potential to for cellular iron-loading to occur particularly in a setting of hepcidin excess as is seen in PAH; in which case shorter term benefits may be outweighed by longer term effects on pulmonary vascular remodeling. Other potential solutions that would aim to restore iron homeostatic control could involve targeted inhibition (modulation) of the hepcidin/ferroportin axis. In fact, there are several treatment options under development/developed which either seek to stabilize ferroportin expression and activity in spite of hepcidin excess or that target hepcidin directly (Sebastiani et al., 2016). Such approaches will thereby allow for iron uptake from the gut and also cellular iron excretion, which may be of relevance for the pulmonary vasculature and any links with iron retention and remodeling in PAH. Finally, given the relationship between IL-6 and hepcidin expression and release, therapies that selectively target this cytokine would also be expected to influence iron homeostatic control. Indeed such approaches are already underway in PAH groups (TRANSFORM UK study) albeit not specifically to correct iron imbalance.

SUMMARY

Presently the field of disrupted iron homeostasis in PAH is poorly understood, not least because most studies of iron regulatory control have centered on global mechanisms and cells principally involved in recycling body iron resources.

However, emerging literature does suggest similar regulatory controls are also operational across other cell types including, potentially, in the vasculature. Links between disrupted iron homeostatic control and sub-types of PH, especially PAH, PH associated to hemolytic anemias and hypoxia may therefore well have implications for iron turnover and control in pulmonary artery vascular cells. Debate centered on the role of iron deficits or overload in PAH and models thereof may merely serve to strengthen the supposition that loss of iron homeostatic control is an important contributory factor to disease onset and progression. Additional studies may well confirm these suggestions and ultimately offer much needed alternative therapeutic options.

AUTHOR CONTRIBUTIONS

SW and GQ were responsible for the conception of idea and design and wrote most of the manuscript. LR was responsible for the contribution of ideas, design, figures, and copy-editing. SP was responsible for the contribution of ideas, figures, and contents research. QT contributed ideas, copy-editing, and contents research. All authors contributed to the manuscript revision, read and approved the final version.

REFERENCES

Barst, R. J., Rubin, L. J., Long, W. A., Mcgoon, M. D., Rich, S., Badesch, D. B., et al. (1996). A comparison of continuous intravenous Epoprostenol (Prostacyclin) with conventional therapy for primary pulmonary hypertension. *N. Engl. J. Med.* 334, 296–301. doi: 10.1056/NEJM199602013340504

Bart, N. K., Curtis, M. K., Cheng, H.-Y., Hungerford, S. L., Mclaren, R., Petousi, N., et al. (2016). Elevation of iron storage in humans attenuates the pulmonary vascular response to hypoxia. *J. Appl. Physiol.* 121, 537–544. doi: 10.1152/japplphysiol.00032.2016

Brittain, E. L., Janz, D. R., Austin, E. D., Bastarache, J. A., Wheeler, L. A., Ware, L. B., et al. (2014). Elevation of plasma cell-free hemoglobin in pulmonary arterial hypertension. *Chest* 146, 1478–1485. doi: 10.1378/chest.14-0809

Brusselmans, K., Compernolle, V., Tjwa, M., Wiesener, M. S., Maxwell, P. H., Collen, D., et al. (2003). Heterozygous deficiency of hypoxia-inducible factor-2α protects mice against pulmonary hypertension and right ventricular dysfunction during prolonged hypoxia. *J. Clin. Invest.* 111, 1519–1527. doi: 10.1172/JCI15496

Buehler, P. W., Baek, J. H., Lisk, C., Connor, I., Sullivan, T., Kominsky, D., et al. (2012). Free hemoglobin induction of pulmonary vascular disease: evidence for an inflammatory mechanism. *Am. J. Physiol. Lung Cell. Mol. Physiol.* 303, L312–L326. doi: 10.1152/ajplung.00074.2012

Camus, S. M., De Moraes, J. A., Bonnin, P., Abbyad, P., Le Jeune, S., Lionnet, F., et al. (2015). Circulating cell membrane microparticles transfer heme to endothelial cells and trigger vasoocclusions in sickle cell disease. *Blood* 125, 3805–3814. doi: 10.1182/blood-2014-07-589283

Cotroneo, E., Ashek, A., Wang, L., Wharton, J., Dubois, O., Bozorgi, S., et al. (2015). Iron homeostasis and pulmonary hypertension: iron deficiency leads to pulmonary vascular remodeling in the rat. *Circ. Res.* 116, 1680–1690. doi: 10.1161/CIRCRESAHA.116.305265

Courboulin, A., Barrier, M., Perreault, T., Bonnet, P., Tremblay, V. L., Paulin, R., et al. (2012). Plumbagin reverses proliferation and resistance to apoptosis in experimental Pah. *Eur. Respir. J.* 40, 618–629. doi: 10.1183/09031936.00084211

Daliento, L., Somerville, J., Presbitero, P., Menti, L., Brach-Prever, S., Rizzoli, G., et al. (1998). Eisenmenger syndrome. Factors relating to deterioration and death. *Eur. Heart J.* 19, 1845–1855. doi: 10.1053/euhj.1998.1046

D'Alto, M., and Mahadevan, V. S. (2012). Pulmonary arterial hypertension associated with congenital heart disease. *Eur. Respir. Rev.* 21, 328–337. doi: 10.1183/09059180.00004712

Decker, I., Ghosh, S., Comhair, S. A., Farha, S., Tang, W. H., Park, M., et al. (2011). High levels of zinc-protoporphyrin identify iron metabolic abnormalities in pulmonary arterial hypertension. *Clin. Transl. Sci.* 4, 253–258. doi: 10.1111/j.1752-8062.2011.00301.x

Dimopoulos, K., Giannakoulas, G., Wort, S. J., and Gatzoulis, M. A. (2008). Pulmonary arterial hypertension in adults with congenital heart disease: distinct differences from other causes of pulmonary arterial hypertension and management implications. *Curr. Opin. Cardiol.* 23, 545–554. doi: 10.1097/HCO.0b013e3283126954

Drakesmith, H., Nemeth, E., and Ganz, T. (2015). Ironing out Ferroportin. *Cell Metab.* 22, 777–787. doi: 10.1016/j.cmet.2015.09.006

Finberg, K. E. (2013). Regulation of systemic iron homeostasis. *Curr. Opin. Hematol.* 20, 208–214. doi: 10.1097/MOH.0b013e32835f5a47

Fox, B. D., Okumiya, T., Attas-Fox, L., Kassirer, M., Raviv, Y., and Kramer, M. R. (2012). Raised erythrocyte creatine in patients with pulmonary arterial hypertension–evidence for subclinical hemolysis. *Respir. Med.* 106, 594–598. doi: 10.1016/j.rmed.2011.12.005

Fraidenburg, D. R., and Machado, R. F. (2016). Pulmonary hypertension associated with thalassemia syndromes. *Ann. N. Y. Acad. Sci.* 1368, 127–139. doi: 10.1111/nyas.13037

Frise, M. C., Cheng, H.-Y., Nickol, A. H., Curtis, M. K., Pollard, K. A., Roberts, D. J., et al. (2016). Clinical iron deficiency disturbs normal human responses to hypoxia. *J. Clin. Invest.* 126, 2139–2150. doi: 10.1172/JCI85715

Galie, N., Humbert, M., Vachiery, J. L., Gibbs, S., Lang, I., Torbicki, A., et al. (2016). 2015 ESC/ERS guidelines for the diagnosis and treatment of pulmonary hypertension: the joint task force for the diagnosis and treatment of pulmonary hypertension of the European society of cardiology (ESC) and the European respiratory society (ERS): endorsed by: association for European paediatric and congenital cardiology (AEPC), international society for heart and lung transplantation (ISHLT). *Eur. Heart J.* 37, 67–119. doi: 10.1093/eurheartj/ehv317

Gerrina, R., Emmy, M., Chris, M. H., Ingrid, S., Herman, G., Luke, S. H., et al. (2015). Intravenous iron therapy in patients with idiopathic pulmonary arterial hypertension and iron deficiency. *Pulm. Circ.* 5, 466–472. doi: 10.1086/682217

Ghosh, M. C., Zhang, D. L., Jeong, S. Y., Kovtunovych, G., Ollivierre-Wilson, H., Noguchi, A., et al. (2013). Deletion of iron regulatory protein 1 causes polycythemia and pulmonary hypertension in mice through translational derepression of HIF2ALPHA. *Cell Metab.* 17, 271–281. doi: 10.1016/j.cmet.2012.12.016

Gorbunov, N. V., Atkins, J. L., Gurusamy, N., and Pitt, B. R. (2012). Iron-induced remodeling in cultured rat pulmonary artery endothelial cells. *Biometals* 25, 203–217. doi: 10.1007/s10534-011-9498-2

Howard, L. S., Watson, G. M., Wharton, J., Rhodes, C. J., Chan, K., Khengar, R., et al. (2013). Supplementation of iron in pulmonary hypertension: Rationale and design of a phase II clinical trial in idiopathic pulmonary arterial hypertension. *Pulm. Circ.* 3, 100–107. doi: 10.4103/2045-8932.109923

Humbert, M., Sitbon, O., Chaouat, A., Bertocchi, M., Habib, G., Gressin, V., et al. (2006). Pulmonary arterial hypertension in France. *Am. J. Respir. Crit. Care Med.* 173, 1023–1030. doi: 10.1164/rccm.200510-1668OC

Humbert, M., Sitbon, O., and Simonneau, G. (2004). Treatment of pulmonary arterial hypertension. *N. Engl. J. Med.* 351, 1425–1436. doi: 10.1056/NEJMra040291

Imtiyaz, H. Z., Williams, E. P., Hickey, M. M., Patel, S. A., Durham, A. C., Yuan, L.-J., et al. (2010). Hypoxia-inducible factor 2α regulates macrophage function in mouse models of acute and tumor inflammation. *J. Clin. Invest.* 120, 2699–2714. doi: 10.1172/JCI39506

Inthawong, K., Charoenkwan, P., Silvilairat, S., Tantiworawit, A., Phrommintikul, A., Choeyprasert, W., et al. (2015). Pulmonary hypertension in non-transfusion-dependent thalassemia: correlation with clinical parameters, liver iron concentration, and non-transferrin-bound iron. *Hematology* 20, 610–617. doi: 10.1179/1607845415Y.0000000014

Irwin, D. C., Baek, J. H., Hassell, K., Nuss, R., Eigenberger, P., Lisk, C., et al. (2015). Hemoglobin induced lung vascular oxidation, inflammation, and remodeling contributes to the progression of hypoxic pulmonary hypertension and is attenuated in rats with repeat dose haptoglobin administration. *Free Radic. Biol. Med.* 82, 50–62. doi: 10.1016/j.freeradbiomed.2015.01.012

Kuhn, L. C. (2015). Iron regulatory proteins and their role in controlling iron metabolism. *Metallomics* 7, 232–243. doi: 10.1039/C4MT00164H

Long, L., Yang, X., Southwood, M., Lu, J., Marciniak, S. J., Dunmore, B. J., et al. (2013). Chloroquine prevents progression of experimental pulmonary hypertension via inhibition of autophagy and lysosomal bone morphogenetic protein type II receptor degradation. *Circ. Res.* 112, 1159–1170. doi: 10.1161/CIRCRESAHA.111.300483

Machado, R. F., and Farber, H. W. (2013). Pulmonary hypertension associated with chronic hemolytic anemia and other blood disorders. *Clin. Chest Med.* 34, 739–752. doi: 10.1016/j.ccm.2013.08.006

Mathew, R., Huang, J., Wu, J. M., Fallon, J. T., and Gewitz, M. H. (2016). Hematological disorders and pulmonary hypertension. *World J. Cardiol.* 703–718. doi: 10.4330/wjc.v8.i12.703

Mumby, S., Aleksander Kempny, L. R., Quinlan, G., and Wort, J. (2016). Omalizumab, airway obstruction and remodeling. *Eur. Respir. J.* 48:PA4901. doi: 10.1183/13993003.congress-2015.PA4901

Naito, Y., Hosokawa, M., Hao, H., Sawada, H., Hirotani, S., Iwasaku, T., et al. (2013). Impact of dietary iron restriction on the development of monocrotaline-induced pulmonary vascular remodeling and right ventricular failure in rats. *Biochem. Biophys. Res. Commun.* 436, 145–151. doi: 10.1016/j.bbrc.2013.05.059

Nakamura, H., Kato, M., Nakaya, T., Kono, M., Tanimura, S., Sato, T., et al. (2017). Decreased haptoglobin levels inversely correlated with pulmonary artery pressure in patients with pulmonary arterial hypertension: a cross-sectional study. *Medicine* 96:e8349. doi: 10.1097/MD.0000000000008349

Padhye, S., Dandawate, P., Yusufi, M., Ahmad, A., and Sarkar, F. H. (2012). Perspectives on medicinal properties of plumbagin and its analogs. *Med. Res. Rev.* 32, 1131–1158. doi: 10.1002/med.20235

Peacock, A. J., Murphy, N. F., Mcmurray, J. J. V., Caballero, L., and Stewart, S. (2007). An epidemiological study of pulmonary arterial hypertension. *Eur. Respir. J.* 30, 104–109. doi: 10.1183/09031936.00092306

Peyssonnaux, C., Zinkernagel, A. S., Schuepbach, R. A., Rankin, E., Vaulont, S., Haase, V. H., et al. (2007). Regulation of iron homeostasis by the hypoxia-inducible transcription factors (HIFS). *J. Clin. Invest.* 117, 1926–1932. doi: 10.1172/JCI31370

Plesner, L. L., Schoos, M. M., Dalsgaard, M., Goetze, J. P., Kjøller, E., Vestbo, J., et al. (2017). Iron deficiency in Copd associates with increased pulmonary artery pressure estimated by echocardiography. *Heart Lung Circ.* 26, 101–104. doi: 10.1016/j.hlc.2016.04.020

Potoka, K. P., and Gladwin, M. T. (2014). Vasculopathy and pulmonary hypertension in sickle cell disease. *Am. J. Physiol. Lung Cell. Mol. Physiol.* 308, L314–L324. doi: 10.1152/ajplung.00252.2014

Pullamsetti, S. S., Perros, F., Chelladurai, P., Yuan, J., and Stenmark, K. (2016). Transcription factors, transcriptional coregulators, and epigenetic modulation in the control of pulmonary vascular cell phenotype: therapeutic implications for pulmonary hypertension (2015 Grover Conference series). *Pulm. Circ.* 6, 448–464. doi: 10.1086/688908

Ramakrishnan, L., Anwar, A., Wort, J. S., and Quinlan, G. J. (2016). Haemoglobin mediated proliferation and Il-6 release in human pulmonary artery endothelial cells: a role for Cd163 and implications for pulmonary vascular remodelling. *Thorax* 71, A220–A220. doi: 10.1136/thoraxjnl-2016-209333.387

Ramakrishnan, L., Mumby, S., Meng, C., Wort, S. J., and Quinlan, G. (2013). IL6 mediated proliferative responses in human pulmonary vascular cells (PVCs) are differentially modulated by iron/heme/hemoglobin. *Eur. Respir. J.* 42:P5152.

Ramakrishnan, L., Mumby, S., Wort, J. S., and Quinlan, G. (2014). Ferroportin is expressed in human pulmonary artery smooth muscle cells: implications for pulmonary arterial hypertension. *Thorax* 69, A21–A21. doi: 10.1136/thoraxjnl-2014-206260.42

Ramakrishnan, L., Mumby, S., Wort, J. S., and Quinlan, G. J. (2015). Cd163 is expressed and modulated in human pulmonary artery smooth muscle cells: Implications for pulmonary artery hypertension. *Eur. Respir. J.* 46:PA4901. doi: 10.1183/13993003.congress-2015.PA4901

Ravasi, G., Pelucchi, S., Greni, F., Mariani, R., Giuliano, A., Parati, G., et al. (2014). Circulating factors are involved in hypoxia-induced hepcidin suppression. *Blood Cells Mol. Dis.* 53, 204–210. doi: 10.1016/j.bcmd.2014.06.006

Rhodes, C. J., Howard, L. S., Busbridge, M., Ashby, D., Kondili, E., Gibbs, J. S. R., et al. (2011a). Iron deficiency and raised hepcidin in idiopathic pulmonary arterial hypertension: clinical prevalence, outcomes, and mechanistic insights. *J. Am. Coll. Cardiol.* 58, 300–309. doi: 10.1016/j.jacc.2011.02.057

Rhodes, C. J., Wharton, J., Howard, L., Gibbs, J. S., Vonk-Noordegraaf, A., and Wilkins, M. R. (2011b). Iron deficiency in pulmonary arterial hypertension: a potential therapeutic target. *Eur. Respir. J.* 38, 1453–1460. doi: 10.1183/09031936.00037711

Rhodes, C. J., Wharton, J., Ghataorhe, P., Watson, G., Girerd, B., Howard, L. S., et al. (2017). Plasma proteome analysis in patients with pulmonary arterial hypertension: an observational cohort study. *Lancet Respir. Med.* 5, 717–726. doi: 10.1016/S2213-2600(17)30161-3

Rudarakanchana, N., Flanagan, J. A., Chen, H., Upton, P. D., Machado, R., Patel, D., et al. (2002). Functional analysis of bone morphogenetic protein type II receptor mutations underlying primary pulmonary hypertension. *Hum. Mol. Genet.* 11, 1517–1525. doi: 10.1093/hmg/11.13.1517

Ruiter, G., Lankhorst, S., Boonstra, A., Postmus, P. E., Zweegman, S., Westerhof, N., et al. (2011). Iron deficiency is common in idiopathic pulmonary arterial hypertension. *Eur. Respir. J.* 37, 1386–1391. doi: 10.1183/09031936.00100510

Sebastiani, G., Wilkinson, N., and Pantopoulos, K. (2016). Pharmacological Targeting of the Hepcidin/Ferroportin Axis. *Front. Pharmacol.* 7:160. doi: 10.3389/fphar.2016.00160

Selimovic, N., Bergh, C. H., Andersson, B., Sakiniene, E., Carlsten, H., and Rundqvist, B. (2009). Growth factors and interleukin-6 across the lung circulation in pulmonary hypertension. *Eur. Respir. J.* 34, 662–668. doi: 10.1183/09031936.001

Simpson, R. J., and McKie, A. T. (2015). Iron and oxygen sensing: a tale of 2 interacting elements? *Metallomics* 7, 223–231. doi: 10.1039/C4MT00225C

Smith, T. G., Balanos, G. M., Croft, Q. P. P., Talbot, N. P., Dorrington, K. L., Ratcliffe, P. J., et al. (2008). The increase in pulmonary arterial pressure caused by hypoxia depends on iron status. *J. Physiol.* 586, 5999–6005. doi: 10.1113/jphysiol.2008.160960

Smith, T. G., Brooks, J. T., Balanos, G. M., Lappin, T. R., Layton, D. M., Leedham, D. L., et al. (2006). Mutation of von Hippel–Lindau tumour suppressor and human cardiopulmonary physiology. *PLoS Med.* 3:e290. doi: 10.1371/journal.pmed.0030290

Smith, T. G., Talbot, N. P., Privat, C., et al. (2009). Effects of iron supplementation and depletion on hypoxic pulmonary hypertension: Two randomized controlled trials. *JAMA* 302, 1444–1450. doi: 10.1001/jama.2009.1404

Soon, E., Holmes, A. M., Treacy, C. M., Doughty, N. J., Southgate, L., Machado, R. D., et al. (2010). Elevated levels of inflammatory cytokines predict survival in idiopathic and familial pulmonary arterial hypertension. *Circulation* 122, 920–927. doi: 10.1161/CIRCULATIONAHA.109.933762

Soon, E., Treacy, C. M., Toshner, M. R., Mackenzie-Ross, R., Manglam, V., Busbridge, M., et al. (2011). Unexplained iron deficiency in idiopathic and heritable pulmonary arterial hypertension. *Thorax* 66, 326–332. doi: 10.1136/thx.2010.147272

Soubrier, F., Chung, W. K., Machado, R., Grünig, E., Aldred, M., Geraci, M., et al. (2013). Genetics and Genomics of Pulmonary Arterial Hypertension. *J. Am. Coll. Cardiol.* 62, D13–D21. doi: 10.1016/j.jacc.2013.10.035

Souza, R., Fernandes, C. J., and Jardim, C. V. (2009). Other causes of PAH (schistosomiasis, porto-pulmonary hypertension and hemolysis-associated pulmonary hypertension). *Semin. Respir. Crit. Care Med.* 30, 448–457. doi: 10.1055/s-0029-1233314

Sow, F. B., Alvarez, G. R., Gross, R. P., Satoskar, A. R., Schlesinger, L. S., Zwilling, B. S., et al. (2009). Role of STAT1, NF-kappaB, and C/EBPbeta in the macrophage transcriptional regulation of hepcidin by mycobacterial infection and Ifn-gamma. *J. Leukoc. Biol.* 86, 1247–1258. doi: 10.1189/jlb.1208719

Tay, E. L., Peset, A., Papaphylactou, M., Inuzuka, R., Alonso-Gonzalez, R., Giannakoulas, G., et al. (2011). Replacement therapy for iron deficiency improves exercise capacity and quality of life in patients with cyanotic congenital heart disease and/or the Eisenmenger syndrome. *Int. J. Cardiol.* 151, 307–312. doi: 10.1016/j.ijcard.2010.05.066

Therrien, J., Rambihar, S., Newman, B., Siminovitch, K., Langleben, D., Webb, G., et al. (2006). Eisenmenger syndrome and atrial septal defect: nature or nurture? *Can. J. Cardiol.* 22, 1133–1136. doi: 10.1016/S0828-282X(06)70950-3

Tuder, R. M., Archer, S. L., Dorfmüller, P., Erzurum, S. C., Guignabert, C., Michelakis, E., et al. (2013). Relevant issues in the pathology and pathobiology of pulmonary hypertension. *J. Am. Coll. Cardiol.* 62, D4–D12. doi: 10.1016/j.jacc.2013.10.025

Van De Bruaene, A., Delcroix, M., Pasquet, A., De Backer, J., De Pauw, M., Naeije, R., et al. (2011). Iron deficiency is associated with adverse outcome in Eisenmenger patients. *Eur. Heart J.* 32, 2790–2799. doi: 10.1093/eurheartj/ehr130

Viethen, T., Gerhardt, F., Dumitrescu, D., Knoop-Busch, S., Ten Freyhaus, H., Rudolph, T. K., et al. (2014). Ferric carboxymaltose improves exercise capacity and quality of life in patients with pulmonary arterial hypertension and iron deficiency: a pilot study. *Int. J. Cardiol.* 175, 233–239. doi: 10.1016/j.ijcard.2014.04.233

Volke, M., Gale, D. P., Maegdefrau, U., Schley, G., Klanke, B., Bosserhoff, A. K., et al. (2009). Evidence for a lack of a direct transcriptional suppression of the iron regulatory peptide hepcidin by hypoxia-inducible factors. *PLoS One* 4:e7875. doi: 10.1371/journal.pone.0007875

White, K., Lu, Y., Annis, S., Hale, A. E., Chau, B. N., Dahlman, J. E., et al. (2015). Genetic and hypoxic alterations of the microrna-210-Iscu1/2 axis promote iron–sulfur deficiency and pulmonary hypertension. *EMBO Mol. Med.* 7, 695–713. doi: 10.15252/emmm.201404511

Wilkins, M. R., Ghofrani, H. A., Weissmann, N., Aldashev, A., and Zhao, L. (2015). Pathophysiology and treatment of high-altitude pulmonary vascular disease. *Circulation* 131, 582–590. doi: 10.1161/CIRCULATIONAHA.114.006977

Wong, C. M., Preston, I. R., Hill, N. S., and Suzuki, Y. J. (2012). Iron chelation inhibits the development of pulmonary vascular remodeling. *Free Radic. Biol. Med.* 53, 1738–1747. doi: 10.1016/j.freeradbiomed.2012.08.576

Yang, X., Long, L., Reynolds, P. N., and Morrell, N. W. (2011). Expression of mutant BMPR-II in pulmonary endothelial cells promotes apoptosis and a release of factors that stimulate proliferation of pulmonary arterial smooth muscle cells. *Pulm. Circ.* 1, 103–110. doi: 10.4103/2045-8932.78100

Yu, A. Y., Shimoda, L. A., Iyer, N. V., Huso, D. L., Sun, X., Mcwilliams, R., et al. (1999). Impaired physiological responses to chronic hypoxia in mice partially deficient for hypoxia-inducible factor 1α. *J. Clin. Invest.* 103, 691–696. doi: 10.1172/JCI5912

Yu, Y., Kovacevic, Z., and Richardson, D. R. (2007). Tuning cell cycle regulation with an iron key. *Cell Cycle* 6, 1982–1994. doi: 10.4161/cc.6.16.4603

6

Pulmonary Artery Size in Interstitial Lung Disease and Pulmonary Hypertension: Association with Interstitial Lung Disease Severity and Diagnostic Utility

Matthew Chin[1], *Christopher Johns*[1], *Benjamin J. Currie*[1], *Nicholas Weatherley*[1], *Catherine Hill*[2], *Charlie Elliot*[2], *Smitha Rajaram*[2], *Jim M. Wild*[1], *Robin Condliffe*[2], *Stephen Bianchi*[2], *David G. Kiely*[2] *and Andrew J. Swift*[1,3]*

[1] *Department of Infection, Immunity and Cardiovascular Disease, University of Sheffield, Royal Hallamshire Hospital, Sheffield, United Kingdom,* [2] *Sheffield Teaching Hospitals NHS Foundation Trust, Sheffield, United Kingdom,* [3] *Institute for in silico Medicine, Sheffield, United Kingdom*

Correspondence:
Andrew J. Swift
a.j.swift@sheffield.ac.uk

Purpose: It is postulated that ILD causes PA dilatation independent of the presence of pulmonary hypertension (PH), so the use of PA size to screen for PH is not recommended. The aims of this study were to investigate the association of PA size with the presence and severity of ILD and to assess the diagnostic accuracy of PA size for detecting PH.

Methods: Incident patients referred to a tertiary PH centre underwent baseline thoracic CT, MRI and right heart catheterisation (RHC). Pulmonary artery diameter was measured on CT pulmonary angiography and pulmonary arterial areas on MRI. A thoracic radiologist scored the severity of ILD on CT from 0 to 4, 0 = absent, 1 = 1–25%, 2 = 26–50%, 3 = 51–75%, and 4 = 76–100% extent of involvement. Receiver operating characteristic analysis and linear regression were employed to assess diagnostic accuracy and independent associations of PA size.

Results: 110 had suspected PH due to ILD (age 65 years (SD 13), M:F 37:73) and 379 had suspected PH without ILD (age 64 years (SD 13), M:F 161:218). CT derived main PA diameter was accurate for detection of PH in patients both with and without ILD - AUC 0.873, $p =< 0.001$, and AUC 0.835, $p =< 0.001$, respectively, as was MRI diastolic PA area, AUC 0.897, $p =< 0.001$, and AUC 0.857, $p =< 0.001$, respectively Significant correlations were identified between mean pulmonary arterial pressure (mPAP) and PA diameter in ILD (r = 0.608, $p < 0.001$), and non-ILD cohort (r = 0.426, $p < 0.001$). PA size was independently associated with mPAP ($p < 0.001$) and BSA ($p = 0.001$), but not with forced vital capacity % predicted ($p = 0.597$), Transfer factor of the lungs for carbon monoxide (T_{LCO}) % predicted ($p = 0.321$) or the presence of ILD on CT ($p = 0.905$). The severity of ILD was not associated with pulmonary artery dilatation (r = 0.071, $p = 0.459$).

Conclusions: Pulmonary arterial pressure elevation leads to pulmonary arterial dilation, which is not independently influenced by the presence or severity of ILD measured by FVC, T_{LCO}'

Abbreviations: AA, Ascending Aorta; ILD, Interstitial Lung Disease; mPAP, mean Pulmonary Artery Pressure; NSIP, Non-specific Interstitial Pneumonia; PA, Pulmonary Artery; UIP, Usual Interstitial Pneumonia.

or disease severity on CT. Pulmonary arterial diameter has diagnostic value in patients with or without ILD and suspected PH.

Keywords: interstitial lung disease, computed tomography (CT) scanning, right heart catheterisation, pulmonary artery diameter, pulmonary hypertension

INTRODUCTION

Pulmonary hypertension (PH) is defined on right heart catheterisation (RHC), as a resting mean pulmonary artery pressure (mPAP) greater than or equal to 25 mmHg (1, 2). PH commonly complicates lung disease and chronic hypoxia, such as interstitial lung disease (ILD). When present in lung disease, PH is associated with a poor outcome (3).

CT is used to diagnose and phenotype suspected ILD, and is often part of the workup of patients with unexplained breathlessness and suspected PH (4). Dilatation of the main pulmonary artery (PA) or major branch vessels has been identified as markers of the presence of PH and is often the first imaging finding to suggest the diagnosis (5–9). As CT is commonly used in the investigation of patients with ILD, it would be useful to use the pulmonary arterial size to screen for the presence of pulmonary hypertension. Routine CT pulmonary angiography is performed without ECG gating. Pulmonary arterial size changes during the cardiac cycle. MRI is typically gated to the cardiac cycle and allows assessment of pulmonary arterial size at both systole and diastole. Some authors have suggested that in the presence of established lung fibrosis, the main PA diameter is not accurate for estimation of mean pulmonary arterial pressure as dilatation of the main PA develops in patients with pulmonary fibrosis in the absence of PH (5, 10).

The aim of this study was to investigate the role of main pulmonary arterial size in patients with ILD and suspected pulmonary hypertension. Firstly, by investigating the factors associated with main pulmonary arterial dilatation, including markers of disease severity in interstitial lung disease. Secondly, to compare the diagnostic accuracy of PA size in patients with suspected pulmonary hypertension with and without ILD.

METHODS

Patients

Consecutive patients who were referred to a pulmonary hypertension centre from 24 April 2012 to 30 March 2016 were identified from the ASPIRE registry (3). Patients with a CT scan within 90 days of MRI and RHC were included. In order to meet inclusion criteria, a diagnostic quality CT pulmonary angiogram (CTPA) with a slice thickness of less than 5 mm was required. Patients underwent systemic evaluation as part of their routine clinical workup, which included clinical review, multi-modality imaging and lung function testing.

The aetiology of pulmonary hypertension was decided at a multi-disciplinary team meeting, based upon review of radiological, RHC and clinical information. The North Sheffield Ethics Committee approved this study and institutional review board approval was attained.

All patients with ILD were assessed for radiological disease pattern on CT. The most common pathological patterns of fibrosis referred to our PH centre are usual interstitial pneumonia (UIP) and non-specific interstitial pneumonia (NSIP). These groups were prospectively separated to examine for differences between these groups.

CT Acquisition

The majority of CTPA scans (76.8%) were conducted at Sheffield's Pulmonary Vascular Disease Unit with a further 114 cases performed at the referring hospitals in Wales or the North of England. All Sheffield CTPA cases were performed on a 64-slice MDCT scanner (light-speed General Electric Medical Systems, Milwaukee, WI), with standard acquisition parameters: 100 mA with automated dose reduction, 120 kV, pitch 1, rotation time 0.5 s and 0.625 mm slice thickness. A 400 × 400 mm field of view was used with an acquisition matrix of 512 × 512. 100 ml of intravenous contrast agent (Ultravist, Bayer, Berlin, Germany) was administered at a rate of 5 ml/sec through a wide bore cannula, into a large central vein, typically in the ante-cubital fossa. The scan was then timed using a bolus tracking technique. HRCT was reconstructed using the contrast-enhanced acquisitions with 1.25 mm collimation from the apex of the lung to the diaphragm. In order to be included, any CTPA from an outside Trust had to be of diagnostic quality, as decided by a radiologist and slice thickness ≤5 mm. In the 23.2% (114) CTPAs performed outside of Sheffield, CT scanner and detailed acquisition parameters were not available for reporting.

MR Acquisition

Cardiac magnetic resonance (CMR) imaging was performed on a 1.5T whole body scanner GE HDx (GE Healthcare, Milwaukee, USA), using an 8-channel cardiac coil. Patients were in the supine position with a surface coil and with retrospective ECG gating. A retrospective cardiac gated multi-slice balanced steady state free precession (bSSFP) sequence was performed orthogonal to the main pulmonary artery. The bSSFP sequence parameters were: TR 2.8 ms, TE 1.0 ms, Flip angle of 50°, FOV = 48 × 43.2, 256 × 256 matrix, 125 kHz bandwidth and slice thickness of 10 mm (11).

Pulmonary Function Testing

All patients underwent lung function testing. Percent of predicted values for forced vital capacity (FVC), and transfer factor of the lungs for carbon monoxide (T_{LCO}) were calculated. The gender, age and physiology (GAP) score is a simple tool for estimating mortality in ILD from demographic and pulmonary function metrics and was calculated as previously described (12).

CT Image Analysis

Image analysis was carried out on picture archive and communication system (PACS) imaging on CE stamped Barco

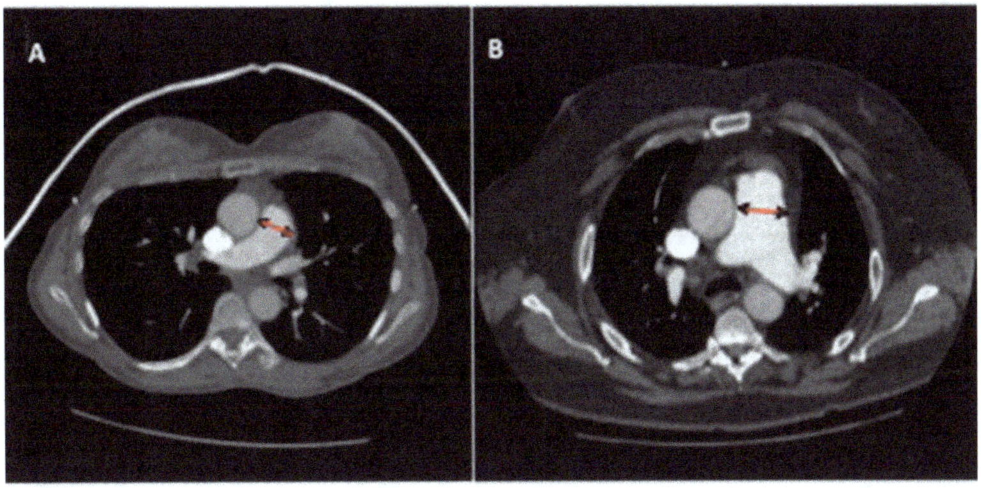

FIGURE 1 | CT images of pulmonary artery diameter measurements in patients with **(A)** a patient without PH (mean pulmonary arterial pressure of 20 mmHg), **(B)** a patient with PH with moderate elevation in pulmonary arterial pressure (mPAP 54 mmHg). Diameter measured where largest and most consistent - proximal to bifurcation, perpendicular to direction of vessel.

diagnostic monitors. The observer was blinded to the all other clinical and imaging data.

The main pulmonary artery was measured proximal to bifurcation, perpendicular to the direction of the vessel at the point where largest diameter is most consistent. The ascending aorta diameter was also measured on the same CT slice, see **Figure 1** Right and left pulmonary artery diameters were recorded 1 cm from the bifurcation, at their most consistent value. A thoracic radiologist scored the severity of ILD on CT, using the Likert semi-quantitative score, ranging from 0 to 4, 0 = absent, 1 = 1–25%, 2 = 26–50%, 3 = 51–75%, and 4 = 76–100% involvement (13). The imaging subtype of ILD was also recorded (UIP or NSIP).

MR Image Analysis

Image analysis was performed on a GE Advantage Workstation 4.4 and GE Advantage Workstation Report Card. Scans were defined as non-diagnostic when image quality significantly affected cardiac measurements or volumetric analysis could not be accurately performed. From the magnitude phase imaging images, the maximal (systolic) and minimal (diastolic) PA areas were measured, and relative area change (RAC) was defined by the following equation: RAC = (maximum area-minimum area)/ minimum area (14, 15).

Statistics

The differences in CT and MRI pulmonary arterial size between the patients with and without ILD were analysed using an independent *t*-test for continuous data and the chi-square for categorical data. ANOVA with Bonferroni correction was used for multiple group comparison. Pearson's correlation coefficient was used to assess the correlation between CT and MRI pulmonary arterial measurements and mPAP. Pearson correlations were conducted for cohorts of ILD, non-ILD and radiological subtypes against CT and MRI derived metric variables. Receiver operating characteristic (ROC) analysis was performed to determine diagnostic accuracy of CT and MRI pulmonary arterial size measurements with area under the ROC curve (AUC) results presented. Multiple t-tests were used to assess intergroup variance of PA diameter, PA to Aorta (PA:AA) ratio and PA relative to body mass index (PA index). The relationship between PA diameter with candidate predictors mPAP, ILD severity of CT, FVC T_{LCO}, and age, sex and body surface area (BSA) was assessed using multivariate linear regression analysis.

Statistical analysis was performed in IBM SPSS Statistics 22 (SPSS, Chicago) and graphed in GraphPad Prism (GraphPad, San Diego). A two-tailed *p*-value of <0.05 was considered statically significant.

RESULTS

Patients

From the ASPIRE database 489 patients with suspected PH were identified, including 198 males and 291 females. 420 patients had pulmonary hypertension. The mean age for the whole cohort was 65 (SD - SD 13). One hundred and ten patients had CT features of ILD (101 patients with pulmonary hypertension and 9 patents without), of which 46 patients had UIP and 43 had NSIP radiological subtypes. Chronic EAA (*n* = 1), asbestosis (*n* = 1), desquamative interstitial pneumonia (*n* = 1), chronic extrinsic allergic, alveolitis (*n* = 1), silicosis (*n* = 1), Langerhans cell histiocytosis (*n* = 1), radiotherapy (*n* = 1) and post infective interstitial disease and scarring (*n* = 4). 379 patients with suspected PH had no CT evidence of ILD (319 patients with pulmonary hypertension and 60 patients without) as shown in **Figure 2. Table 1** provides the baseline demographic data, lung function, CT and MRI derived variables for the study cohort as a whole and split into the ILD and not ILD cohorts. The mean (SD) interval between CT and RHC was 17.6 days (46.1), the interval between MRI and RHC was 0.2 days (4.2).

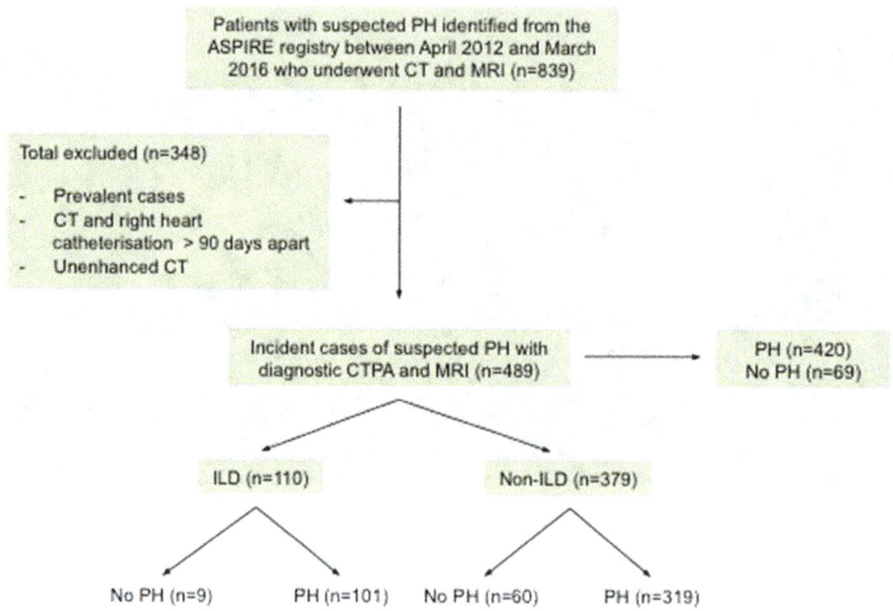

FIGURE 2 | The Study Cohort. PH, pulmonary hypertension; CT, computed tomography scan; MRI, magnetic resonance imaging; MPA, main pulmonary artery; CTPA, computed tomography pulmonary angiogram; ILD, interstitial.

TABLE 1 | Demographic table.

		Whole Cohort	ILD	Non-ILD	*p* Value*
		Mean (SD) *N* = 489	Mean (SD) *N* = 110	Mean (SD) *N* = 379	
Demographics					
Age		65 (13)	66 (11)	64 (13)	0.656
Sex	M/F	198/291	37/73	161/218	
	PH/No PH	420/69	101/9	319/60	0.003
WHO Functional Class	I/II/III/IV	1/59/378/42	0/9/80/18	1/50/298/24	<0.001
ILD Sub-Types	UIP/NSIP/Sarcoid/Chronic EAA, Other		46/43/11/1/20		
Right Heart Catheter					
	mRAP (mmHg)	10 (6)	9 (6)	10 (5)	0.017
	mPAP (mmHg)	41 (15)	41 (13)	42 (15)	0.856
	PAWP (mmHg)	13 (5)	12 (5)	13 (5)	0.014
	CI (L/min/m2)	2.7 (0.8)	2.7 (0.8)	2.7 (0.8)	0.981
	PVR (dyn.s.m-5)	529.2 (394.3)	539.7 (348.7)	526.1 (408.1)	0.267
Pulmonary function tests					
	Predicted FVC %	81.6	72.7	85.0	<0.001
	FVC (l)	2.9 (1.1)	2.4 (0.9)	3.1 (1.1)	<0.001
	Predicted T_{LCO} %	47.9	33.7	52.3	<0.001
	T_{LCO} (l)	3.9 (2.0)	2.5 (1.6)	4.3 (2.0)	<0.001
CT					
	Main PA diameter (mm)	32 (6)	31 (4.9)	32 (5.8)	0.092
	PA/AA	1 (0.2)	1 (0.2)	1 (0.2)	0.453
	PA/BSA	17.6 (3.5)	18 (3.0)	18 (3.6)	0.434
	Right PA diameter (mm)	26 (5)	25 (4.4)	26 (4.7)	0.234
	Left PA diameter (mm)	24 (4)	24 (3.4)	25 (4.0)	0.309
MRI					
	Systolic PA area (mm^2)	920 (306)	887 (269)	930 (316)	0.607
	Diastolic PA area (mm^2)	833 (276)	807 (255)	814 (281)	0.809
	PA relative area (mm^2)	10.9 (9.5)	10.6 (7.2)	10.9 (9.3)	0.394

WHO, World Health Organisation; mRAP, mean Right Arterial Pressure; mPAP, mean Pulmonary Arterial Pressure; PAWP, Pulmonary Artery Wedge Pressure; CI, Cardiac Index; PVR, Pulmonary Vascular Resistance; TLCO, Transfer Factor of the lungs for Carbon Monoxide; FVC, Forced Volume Capacity.

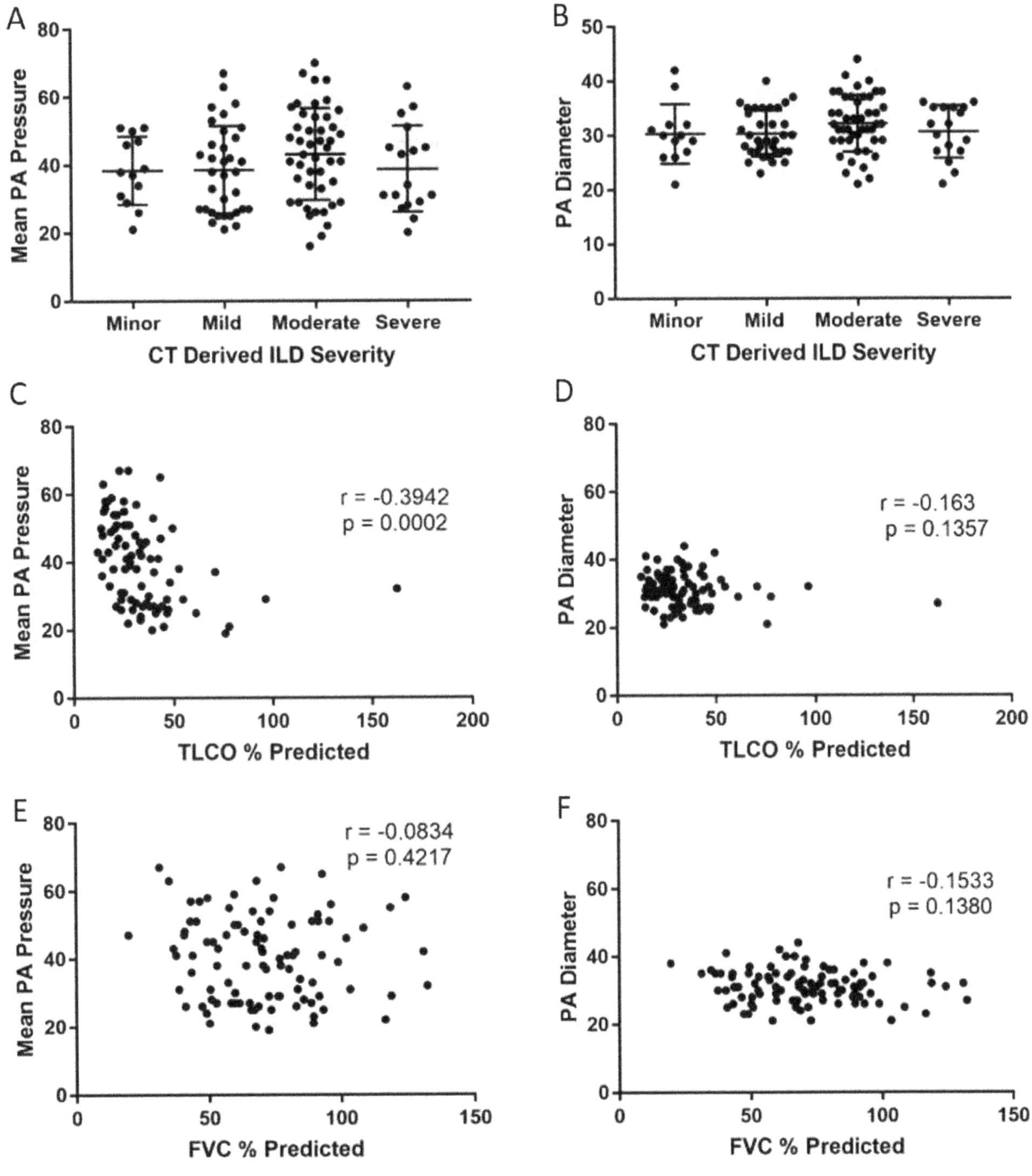

FIGURE 3 | Correlations between mean PA pressure and PA diameter with pulmonary function tests and CT-derived severity score. Graphs **(A)** and **(B)** represent the association with ILD severity on CT in ILD cohort. Graphs **(C)** and **(D)** scatter plot showing the association of PA pressure and diameter with TLCO %predicted and graphs **(E)** and **(F)** scatter plots showing the association of PA pressure and diameter with FVC %predicted.

Group Comparisons

Patients with PH had larger pulmonary arteries (33 mm) than patients without PH (27 mm) ($p < 0.001$) In the ILD cohort, there was no significance between PA size diameters in different semi-quantitative radiological severity scores of ILD, see (**Figure 3A**, mPAP and ILD severity). There was no

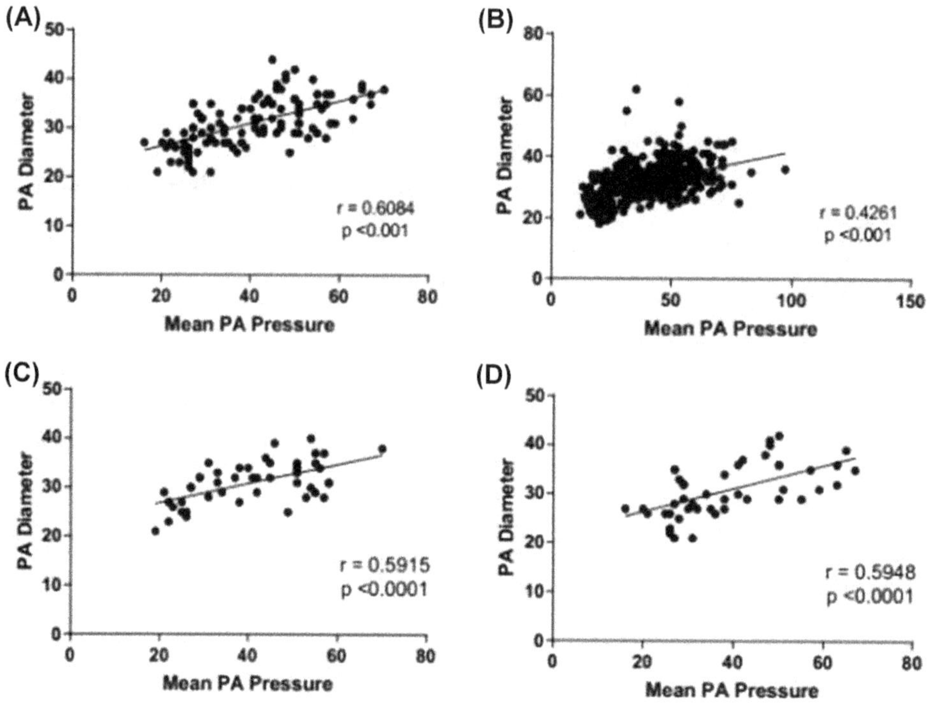

FIGURE 4 | Scatter distribution showing the relationship between mean PA pressure and PA diameter. Subgroups include ILD cohort **(A)**, non-ILD **(B)**, ILD with UIP pattern of disease **(C)** and ILD with NSIP pattern of disease **(D)**.

difference in mPAP between radiological severities of ILD scores (**Figure 3B**, PA diameter and ILD severity). Furthermore there were no significant differences in PA size or diameter between CT derived ILD severity within the pathological subgroups, UIP $p = 0.630$ and NSIP $p = 1.000$.

Correlations

CT derived main PA diameter correlated positively with mPAP in the ILD cohort (r = 0.608; $p < 0.001$), which improved when the pulmonary artery diameter was indexed to body surface area (r = 0.674 ; $p < 0.001$). MRI derived systolic and diastolic pulmonary artery area also correlated significantly with mPAP in the ILD cohort, (r = 0.423 and 0.479 respectively, $p < 0.001$). In the pathological subtypes, PA diameter correlated with mPAP for both UIP (r = 0.592; $p < 0.001$) and NSIP (r = 0.621; $p < 0.001$). Each are shown in **Figure 4.** In the non-ILD cohort, the correlation between mPAP and PA diameter was weaker but still significant, r = 0.426 ($p < 0.001$). **Table 2** presents Pearson correlations for ILD and non-ILD cohorts, with pathological UIP and NSIP subtype analysis. In the ILD cohort, there was

TABLE 2 | Correlations of CT and MRI measurements with mean pulmonary arterial pressure.

Pearson Correlations to mPAP	ILD		UIP		NSIP		Non ILD	
	R Value	*p Value*	*R Value*	*p Value*	*R Value*	*p Value*	*R Value*	*p Value*
CT								
PA Diameter	0.608	<0.001	0.592	<0.001	0.621	<0.001	0.426	<0.001
PA/AA Ratio	0.478	<0.001	0.515	<0.001	0.631	<0.001	0.431	<0.001
PA Index	0.498	<0.001	0.374	0.01	0.674	<0.001	0.402	<0.001
Right PA Diameter	0.466	<0.001	0.396	0.006	0.472	0.002	0.262	<0.001
Left PA Diameter	0.393	<0.001	0.406	0.005	0.656	0.029	0.332	<0.001
MRI								
Systolic PA area	0.423	<0.001	0.461	0.001	0.510	<0.001	0.353	<0.001
Diastolic PA area	0.479	<0.001	0.563	<0.001	0.558	<0.001	0.426	<0.001
PA relative area change	−0.397	<0.001	−0.457	0.001	−0.387	0.010	−0.310	<0.001

AA , Ascending Aorta; ILD , Interstitial Lung Disease; mPAP , mean Pulmonary Artery Pressure; NSIP , Non-specific Interstitial Pneumonia; PA , Pulmonary Artery; UIP , Usual Interstitial Pneumonia.

TABLE 3 | Area under the receiver operating characteristic curve for CT and MRI pulmonary arterial measurements in ILD and non-ILD cohorts.

CT and MRI Metrics	ILD		Non ILD	
	AUC	*p* value	AUC	*p* value
CT				
Main PA Diameter	0.873	<0.001	0.835	<0.001
PA/AA	0.799	0.003	0.794	<0.001
PA Index	0.595	0.347	0.836	<0.001
Right PA Diameter	0.753	0.012	0.757	<0.001
Left PA Diameter	0.729	0.023	0.754	<0.001
MRI				
Systolic PA area	0.887	<0.001	0.824	<0.001
Diastolic PA area	0.897	<0.001	0.857	<0.001
PA relative area change	0.388	0.266	0.365	<0.001

AA , Ascending Aorta; PA , Pulmonary Artery.

no significant correlation between PA diameter and FVC (r = −0.113; p = 0.301) or T_{LCO} (r = −0.041; p = 0.692) respectively, as shown in **Figure 3** shows the correlations between mean PA pressure and PA diameter for ILD (r = 0.608; $p < 0.001$), non-ILD (r = 0.461; $p < 0.001$), UIP (r = 0.592; $p < 0.001$), NSIP (r = 0.595; $p < 0.001$).

Diagnostic Accuracy

Table 3 provides the ROC area under the curve (AUC) values for CT and MRI metrics in both ILD and non-ILD cohorts for the diagnosis of PH. In the ILD cohort, main PA diameter on CT had strong diagnostic accuracy, AUC = 0.873 as did systolic and diastolic PA area on MRI (AUC = 0.887 and AUC = 0.897, respectively). In addition, high diagnostic accuracy of PA diameter on CT, AUC 0.835 and PA systolic and diastolic areas (AUC 0.824 and 0.857, respectively) on MRI were found in the non-ILD cohort. The relative area change of the pulmonary artery during the cardiac cycle was a weaker diagnostic marker than pulmonary arterial size.

TABLE 4 | Linear regression analysis, identifying covariates with independent association with pulmonary arterial diameter.

Model	Regression Co-efficient	SE	R	T Statistic	*p* value
(Constant)	11.060	3.471		3.187	0.002
PA Mean	0.205	0.033	0.525	6.168	<0.001
BSA	6.738	1.914	0.300	3.520	0.001

BSA, Body Surface Area; PA, Pulmonary Artery.

A previous threshold of 29mm tested in the ILD cohort resulted in 75.2% sensitivity, 88.9% specificity, 98.7% positive predictive values and 24.0% negative predictive value. In the non-ILD cohort, pulmonary arterial diameter was also accurate for the diagnosis of PH, with AUC=0.835 (p<0.001). The optimal threshold identified was 30mm, providing 76.3% sensitivity and 73.3% specificity. **Figure 5** shows the ROC curves for the CTPA measured pulmonary arterial diameter metrics (PA diameter, PA:AA ratio and PA index) in both ILD and non-ILD cohorts.

The highest AUC values for MRI derived variables in the ILD cohort (**Table 2**) were diastolic pulmonary arterial area (0.897) and systolic pulmonary arterial area (0.887). MRI variables have shown a similar diagnostic accuracy within this study cohort compared to CT derived parameters of PA size.

Factors Associated with Pulmonary Arterial Size in ILD

At multivariate linear regression analysis, mPAP and body surface area were independent predictors of pulmonary arterial size, [11.1 + (0.2 × mean pulmonary arterial pressure) + (6.7 × BSA)]. Age, sex, GAP score, ILD severity on CT, FVC %predicted and T_{LCO} %predicted were not multivariate predictors of pulmonary artery diameter (10). **Table 4** shows linear regression analysis.

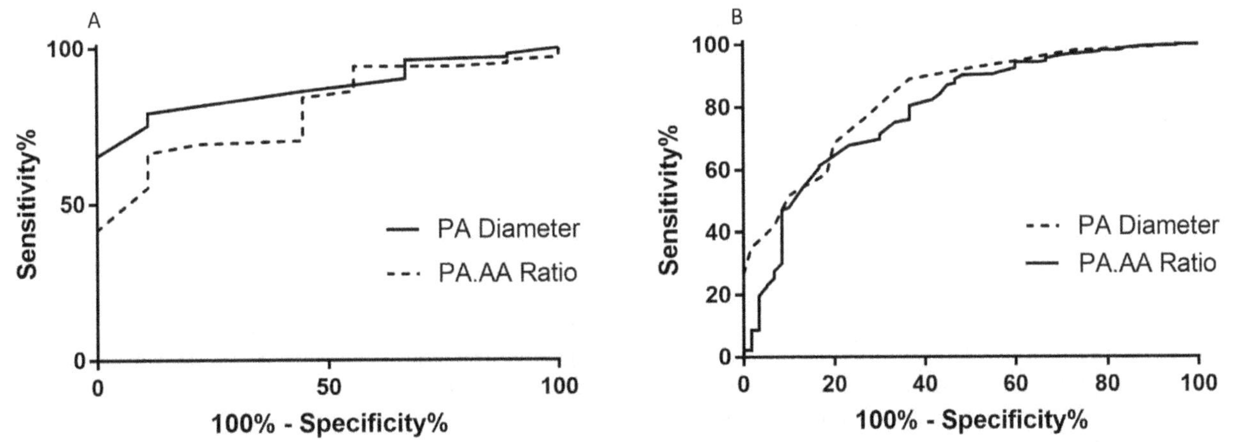

FIGURE 5 | ROC analysis showing the area under the curve for both ILD **(A)** and non-ILD **(B)** cohorts for the CT measured main pulmonary artery size (PA diameter and PA:AA Ratio)

Mean pulmonary arterial diameter had an adjusted correlation coefficient of 0.575 ($p < 0.001$) and BSA of 0.249 ($p = 0.001$).

DISCUSSION

In this retrospective study of 491 patients with suspected pulmonary hypertension referred to a tertiary referral centre, we show that main pulmonary arterial diameter has similar diagnostic utility in patients with and without ILD. In our cohort, pulmonary arterial diameter is independently associated with mean pulmonary arterial pressure and body size. The size of the pulmonary artery was not independently influenced by semi-quantitative radiological severity score of ILD, FVC, T_{LCO}, or GAP score.

It has been postulated that in patients with pulmonary fibrosis the pulmonary artery dilates in the absence of elevated pulmonary arterial pressure, as consequence of architectural distortion of the lung parenchyma. In contrast, in this cohort of patients, we have found that pulmonary arterial diameter is diagnostic of pulmonary hypertension in ILD, to a similar accuracy as seen in patients with pulmonary hypertension who do not have ILD (AUC 0.874 for ILD cohort and AUC 0.835 for non-ILD cohort), irrespective of the underlying radiological ILD pattern. UIP is typified by significant parenchymal distortion, including honeycombing, traction bronchiectasis and volume loss (16), therefore if PA size is driven by architectural destruction in ILD, it should be apparent in this group. However, PA size remains more closely associated with PH metrics than quantitative metrics of ILD severity in patients with UIP. In addition, the optimal pulmonary arterial diameter threshold for prediction of elevated mean pulmonary artery pressure was relatively low in patients with ILD at 29 mm, similar to 30 mm for patients in the non-ILD cohort. Mean pulmonary arterial diameter in our ILD cohort with pulmonary hypertension was 32 mm, compared to a mean of 25 mm in patients with ILD without pulmonary hypertension.

As expected, T_{LCO} and FVC were lower in the patients with ILD than those without. However, the ILD and non-ILD cohorts were well-matched in terms of PH severity, as defined by their RHC metrics. The clinical and radiological markers of ILD severity (T_{LCO}, FVC and CT semi-quantitative severity score) had weak correlations with pulmonary arterial diameter ($r = -0.148$, $p = 0.174$/$r = -0.153$, $p = 0.138$/$r = 0.082$, $p = 0.393$ respectively). Furthermore, there is a strong correlation between PA diameter and mean PA pressure within the ILD cohort ($r = 0.608$). On multivariate linear regression, the clinical and radiological markers of disease severity were not independent predictors of pulmonary arterial size. In fact, the independent predictors were body surface area and pulmonary arterial pressure.

Both CT and MRI derived pulmonary arterial size metrics were assessed. MRI variables showed high diagnostic accuracy with both systolic and diastolic pulmonary arterial area having diagnostic utility in both ILD and non-ILD cohorts. MRI derived diastolic pulmonary arterial area, was the most accurate diagnostic variable across the whole study cohort, regardless of the presence of ILD. Diastolic pulmonary arterial size was of systematically marginally higher diagnostic accuracy than systolic. We postulate that this is because of greater pulsatility of the pulmonary artery of a patient without pulmonary hypertension, allowing the pulmonary artery to reduce in size in diastole to a greater extent relative to a patient with pulmonary hypertension.

PA size measured on MRI also correlated well with RHC derived mean pulmonary arterial pressure and showed similar diagnostic accuracy to CT derived PA diameter. This trend was similar in both patients with and without interstitial lung disease. A limitation of routine CT pulmonary angiography is lack of cardiac gating; MRI with cardiac gating has provided additional proof of the equivalent utility of PA diameter in interstitial lung disease and non- interstitial lung disease

The pulmonary artery can dilate over time in a patient with elevated pulmonary arterial pressure (17). Hence the absolute instantaneous measure of pulmonary arterial pressure in a patient with pulmonary hypertension will be dependent not only on the pressure but also the duration of the disease, which explain the variable correlation observed between pulmonary arterial size and pressure in patients with suspected PH (5–7, 11, 18–20). All patients were referred with suspected pulmonary hypertension, however it is unknown how long the pressure has been elevated, given the insidious onset of the disease, absolute quantification of duration of disease is challenging.

LIMITATIONS

This study is limited by its retrospective design at a single tertiary referral centre, although in order to reduce bias from the retrospective analysis, the cohort is made up of consecutive patients. As this was performed in a pulmonary hypertension referral centre, there is a bias towards the presence of PH and as such there are only a few patients with no PH, so these results are only valid in the setting of a PH referral centre. It is expected, however that the strong correlation between mPAP and PA size in this cohort of patients would be similar in a non-selected patient cohort. A study in a non-PH centre, in a cohort with more even distribution of patients with and without pulmonary hypertension would be of benefit.

Interstitial lung diseases are a heterogeneous group of diseases with idiopathic and known-cause aetiologies. We have grouped the largest cohorts of fibrotic ILDs here to explore if the architectural destruction of UIP had a greater influence on PA dilatation than NSIP, but in practice these are not clinical diagnoses. However, in practice these are the patterns most likely to lead to fibrotic-driven architectural distortion and so we have taken a pragmatic approach in separating these. Further work evaluating the impact of varying forms of ILD, such as scleroderma related and drug induced ILD on the pulmonary vasculature, in terms of PA size and haemodynamic changes would be of value.

CONCLUSION

Pulmonary arterial pressure elevation leads to pulmonary arterial dilation, which is not independently influenced by the presence or severity of ILD measured by FVC, T_{LCO}, or disease severity on CT.

Pulmonary arterial diameter has diagnostic value in patients with or without ILD, key for the screening of suspected PH.

AUTHOR CONTRIBUTIONS

AS and DK conceived the idea for the study. AS, MC, NW, SB, BC and CJ participated in the study design. AS, DC acquired the MRI data. Image analysis was performed by AS, MC, BC, CJ. AS, MC, SR, CE, CJ, RC, DK, NW, JMW analysed and interpreted the MR data. AS, MC, SR, CE, CJ, NW, RC, DK, JMW, SB drafted the manuscript. All authors read and approved the final manuscript.

REFERENCES

1. Kiely DG, Elliot CA, Sabroe I, Condliffe R. Pulmonary hypertension: diagnosis and management. *BMJ* (2013) 346:f2028. doi: 10.1136/bmj.f2028
2. Galiè N, Humbert M, Vachiery JL, Gibbs S, Lang I, Torbicki A, et al. 2015 ESC/ERS Guidelines for the diagnosis and treatment of pulmonary hypertension: The Joint Task Force for the Diagnosis and Treatment of Pulmonary Hypertension of the European Society of Cardiology (ESC) and the European Respiratory Society (ERS): Endorsed by: Association for European Paediatric and Congenital Cardiology (AEPC), International Society for Heart and Lung Transplantation (ISHLT). *Eur Heart J* (2016) 37(1):67–119. doi: 10.1093/eurheartj/ehv317
3. Hurdman J, Condliffe R, Elliot CA, Davies C, Hill C, Wild JM, et al. ASPIRE registry: assessing the Spectrum of Pulmonary hypertension Identified at a REferral centre. *Eur Respir J* (2012) 39(4):945–55. doi: 10.1183/09031936.00078411
4. Rajaram S, Swift AJ, Condliffe R, Johns C, Elliot CA, Hill C, et al. CT features of pulmonary arterial hypertension and its major subtypes: a systematic CT evaluation of 292 patients from the ASPIRE Registry. *Thorax* (2015) 70(4):382–7. doi: 10.1136/thoraxjnl-2014-206088
5. Devaraj A, Wells AU, Meister MG, Corte TJ, Hansell DM. The effect of diffuse pulmonary fibrosis on the reliability of CT signs of pulmonary hypertension. *Radiology* (2008) 249(3):1042–9. doi: 10.1148/radiol.2492080269
6. Edwards PD, Bull RK, Coulden R. CT measurement of main pulmonary artery diameter. *Br J Radiol* (1998) 71(850):1018–20. doi: 10.1259/bjr.71.850.10211060
7. Shen Y, Wan C, Tian P, Wu Y, Li X, Yang T, et al. CT-base pulmonary artery measurement in the detection of pulmonary hypertension: a meta-analysis and systematic review. *Medicine* (2014) 93(27):e256. doi: 10.1097/MD.0000000000000256
8. Ng CS, Wells AU, Padley SP. A CT sign of chronic pulmonary arterial hypertension: the ratio of main pulmonary artery to aortic diameter. *J Thorac Imaging* (1999) 14(4):270–8.
9. Kuriyama K, Gamsu G, Stern RG, Cann CE, Herfkens RJ, Brundage BH. CT-determined pulmonary artery diameters in predicting pulmonary hypertension. *Invest Radiol* (1984) 19(1):16–22. doi: 10.1097/00004424-198401000-00005
10. Alhamad EH, Al-Boukai AA, Al-Kassimi FA, Alfaleh HF, Alshamiri MQ, Alzeer AH, et al. Prediction of pulmonary hypertension in patients with or without interstitial lung disease: reliability of CT findings. *Radiology* (2011) 260(3):875–83. doi: 10.1148/radiol.11103532
11. Swift AJ, Rajaram S, Condliffe R, Capener D, Hurdman J, Elliot CA, et al. Diagnostic accuracy of cardiovascular magnetic resonance imaging of right ventricular morphology and function in the assessment of suspected pulmonary hypertension results from the ASPIRE registry. *J Cardiovasc Magn Reson* (2012) 14:40. doi: 10.1186/1532-429X-14-40
12. Ley B, Ryerson CJ, Vittinghoff E, Ryu JH, Tomassetti S, Lee JS, et al. A multidimensional index and staging system for idiopathic pulmonary fibrosis. *Ann Intern Med* (2012) 156(10):684–91. doi: 10.7326/0003-4819-156-10-201205150-00004
13. Kazerooni EA, Martinez FJ, Flint A, Jamadar DA, Gross BH, Spizarny DL, et al. Thin-section CT obtained at 10-mm increments versus limited three-level thin-section CT for idiopathic pulmonary fibrosis: correlation with pathologic scoring. *AJR Am J Roentgenol* (1997) 169(4):977–83. doi: 10.2214/ajr.169.4.9308447
14. Sanz J, Kariisa M, Dellegrottaglie S, Prat-González S, Garcia MJ, Fuster V, et al. Evaluation of pulmonary artery stiffness in pulmonary hypertension with cardiac magnetic resonance. *JACC Cardiovasc Imaging* (2009) 2(3):286–95. doi: 10.1016/j.jcmg.2008.08.007
15. Toshner MR, Gopalan D, Suntharalingam J, Treacy C, Soon E, Sheares KK, et al. Pulmonary arterial size and response to sildenafil in chronic thromboembolic pulmonary hypertension. *J Heart Lung Transplant* (2010) 29(6):610–5. doi: 10.1016/j.healun.2009.12.014
16. Raghu G, Collard HR, Egan JJ, Martinez FJ, Behr J, Brown KK, et al. An official ATS/ERS/JRS/ALAT statement: idiopathic pulmonary fibrosis: evidence-based guidelines for diagnosis and management. *Am J Respir Crit Care Med* (2011) 183(6):788–824. doi: 10.1164/rccm.2009-040GL
17. Boerrigter B, Mauritz GJ, Marcus JT, Helderman F, Postmus PE, Westerhof N, et al. Progressive dilatation of the main pulmonary artery is a characteristic of pulmonary arterial hypertension and is not related to changes in pressure. *Chest* (2010) 138(6):1395–401. doi: 10.1378/chest.10-0363
18. Devaraj A, Hansell DM. Computed tomography signs of pulmonary hypertension: old and new observations. *Clin Radiol* (2009) 64(8):751–60. doi: 10.1016/j.crad.2008.12.005
19. Zisman DA, Karlamangla AS, Ross DJ, Keane MP, Belperio JA, Saggar R, et al. High-resolution chest CT findings do not predict the presence of pulmonary hypertension in advanced idiopathic pulmonary fibrosis. *Chest* (2007) 132(3):773–9. doi: 10.1378/chest.07-0116
20. Devaraj A, Wells AU, Meister MG, Corte TJ, Wort SJ, Hansell DM. Detection of pulmonary hypertension with multidetector CT and echocardiography alone and in combination. *Radiology* (2010) 254(2):609–16. doi: 10.1148/radiol.09090548

7

Nanotherapeutics for Treatment of Pulmonary Arterial Hypertension

*Victor Segura-Ibarra[1,2], Suhong Wu[1], Nida Hassan[1,3], Jose A. Moran-Guerrero[1,2], Mauro Ferrari[1,4], Ashrith Guha[5,6], Harry Karmouty-Quintana[7] and Elvin Blanco[1,5]**

[1] Department of Nanomedicine, Houston Methodist Research Institute, Houston, TX, United States, [2] Escuela de Ingeniería y Ciencias, Tecnológico de Monterrey, Monterrey, Mexico, [3] McGovern Medical School, The University of Texas Health Science Center at Houston, Houston, TX, United States, [4] Department of Medicine, Weill Cornell Medicine, New York, NY, United States, [5] Department of Cardiology, Houston Methodist DeBakey Heart and Vascular Center, Houston Methodist Hospital, Houston, TX, United States, [6] Houston Methodist J.C. Walter Jr. Transplant Center, Houston Methodist Hospital, Houston, TX, United States, [7] Department of Biochemistry and Molecular Biology, McGovern Medical School, The University of Texas Health Science Center at Houston, Houston, TX, United States

***Correspondence:**
Elvin Blanco
eblanco@houstonmethodist.org

Pulmonary arterial hypertension (PAH) is a devastating and fatal chronic lung disease. While current pharmacotherapies have improved patient quality of life, PAH drugs suffer from limitations in the form of short-term pharmacokinetics, instability, and poor organ specificity. Traditionally, nanotechnology-based delivery strategies have proven advantageous at increasing both circulation lifetimes of chemotherapeutics and accumulation in tumors due to enhanced permeability through fenestrated vasculature. Importantly, increased nanoparticle (NP) accumulation in diseased tissues has been observed pre-clinically in pathologies characterized by endothelial dysfunction and remodeled vasculature, including myocardial infarction and heart failure. Recently, this phenomenon has also been observed in preclinical models of PAH, leading to the exploration of NP-based drug delivery as a therapeutic modality in PAH. Herein, we discussed the advantages of NPs for efficacious treatment of PAH, including heightened therapeutic delivery to diseased lungs for increased drug bioavailability, as well as highlighted innovative nanotherapeutic approaches for PAH.

Keywords: pulmonary arterial hypertension, chronic lung disease, nanomedicine, nanoparticles, drug delivery

INTRODUCTION

Pulmonary arterial hypertension (PAH) is a progressive and fatal disease arising from restricted blood flow through pulmonary arterial circulation. Defined as having mean pulmonary artery pressures (mPAP) greater than 25 mm Hg (Pauwaa et al., 2011), the increased flow resistance in PAH causes an overload in the right ventricle (RV), leading to hypertrophy, hyperplasia, and fibrosis (Ryan and Archer, 2014). These ultimately lead to right heart failure, the major cause of death in PAH patients (Shah, 2012). PAH pertains to the Group I subset of PH, which encompasses idiopathic and heritable disease affecting pulmonary vasculature (Collum et al., 2017). Pathophysiologically, PAH is characterized by remodeling of the pulmonary vasculature that leads to vessel occlusion, muscularization of previously non-muscular vessels, and formation of complex vascular lesions (Stenmark et al., 2009), with pulmonary arteriole smooth muscle cells (PASMCs) and endothelial cells (PAECs) lying at the crux of these processes (Morrell et al., 2009).

Pulmonary arterial hypertension drug therapies have traditionally relied on regulation of vascular tone (Sahni et al., 2016), principally targeting the prostacyclin (PGI_2), endothelin (ET), and nitric oxide signaling pathways (Lang and Gaine, 2015). While pharmacotherapies have resulted in improvements in hemodynamics and quality of life (Lau et al., 2017), they are not without considerable shortcomings, including short drug half-lives and instability (Delcroix and Howard, 2015), as well as adverse side effects (Galie et al., 2009). Moreover, despite combination drug regimens, PAH undoubtedly progresses despite pharmacotherapy. Thus, there are currently no curative treatments available for PAH patients save for lung transplantation (Gottlieb, 2013), highlighting the pressing need to develop innovative treatments that can attenuate or even reverse vascular remodeling.

Nanotechnology-based drug delivery platforms prove effective vectors for packaging of drug and genetic material (Ferrari, 2005). Nanoparticles (NPs) are defined as possessing diameters between 0.1 and 100 nm, which can be composed of either naturally occurring or synthetic, man-made materials (Riehemann et al., 2009). These nanoconstructs can be precisely designed with regards to size and geometry, with versatile chemistry enabling tailorability of properties such as enhanced cellular entry and controlled release (Blanco et al., 2015). NP platforms prolong circulation lifetimes of drugs when administered intravenously (IV), proving pharmacokinetically advantageous when compared to conventional drug formulations (Blanco et al., 2011). Importantly, the myriad of pathophysiological alterations involved in PAH progression, particularly endothelial injury, provides a potential avenue for systemically administered nanotherapies in PAH. NP-based drug delivery has been extensively used in cancer primarily because of the ability of long-circulating NPs to accumulate passively in tumors by extravasating through leaky vasculature (Maeda et al., 2013). This phenomenon is commonly referred to as the enhanced permeability and retention (EPR) effect. Herein, we will discuss conventional pharmacotherapies in PAH. We will also describe the established NP platforms commonly used for drug delivery, and highlight the role that vascular remodeling in PAH can play in enhancing accumulation in lungs. Lastly, we will showcase several nanotherapeutic strategies that prove promising for the treatment of PAH.

CONVENTIONAL DRUG THERAPY IN PAH

Prostacyclin Agonists

Produced in vascular endothelial cells, the arachidonic acid metabolite PGI_2 plays an important role in vasodilation, and inhibits smooth muscle cell (SMC) proliferation and platelet aggregation (Del Pozo et al., 2017). By binding and activating the PGI_2 (IP) receptor on SMCs, PGI_2 activation increases cyclic adenosine monophosphate (cAMP) levels, which in turn results in vasodilation (Ricciotti and FitzGerald, 2011). In PAH, endogenous PGI_2 levels are decreased (Tuder et al., 1999), making PGI_2 and prostaglandin analogs attractive therapeutic options for treatment. Prostanoids have been used clinically over the past three decades for PAH therapy, with the synthetic PGI_2, epoprostenol sodium (Flolan®), being the first pharmacological agent to gain FDA approval for the treatment of PAH (Safdar, 2011), based on improvements in exercise capacity and hemodynamics in patients (Barst et al., 1996).

Endothelin Receptor Antagonists

Produced by endothelial cells, endothelin-1 (ET-1) promotes SMC vasoconstriction, proliferation, migration, and survival. ET-1 also promotes collagen synthesis by fibroblasts (Rosano et al., 2013). Binding of ET-1 to endothelin receptors (ET_A and ET_B) on SMCs activates phospholipase C, which in turn increases intracellular calcium, resulting in sustained vasoconstriction (Seo et al., 1994). Patients diagnosed with PAH have increased activation of ET-1 in both plasma and lung tissues (Galié et al., 2004) and elevated plasma levels of ET-1 can be correlated with severity of disease and prognosis (McLaughlin et al., 2009), leading to the exploration of various compounds capable of blocking either ET_A or ET_A and ET_B receptors. Three orally administered ET receptor antagonists (ERAs), ambrisentan (Letairis®, an ET_A receptor inhibitor), bosentan (Tracleer®, a dual ET_A and ET_B receptor inhibitor), and macitentan (Opsumit®, a dual ET_A and ET_B receptor inhibitor), have been clinically approved by the FDA based on randomized clinical trials where increases in 6-min walk distance (6MWD), improved hemodynamic parameters, and overall quality of life were observed (Raja, 2010).

Nitric Oxide Promoters

Nitric oxide (NO) is a product of endothelial cells and a potent vasodilator. By binding to and subsequent activation of soluble guanylate cyclase (sGC), NO increases levels of cyclic guanosine monophosphate (cGMP) (Russwurm and Koesling, 2004), resulting in reduced intracellular calcium levels and SMC relaxation (Carvajal et al., 2000). NO has also been shown to inhibit SMC proliferation and platelet activation (Tonelli et al., 2013). Levels of NO and NO-products in lungs and bronchoalveolar lavage fluid (BALF) of PAH patients have been shown to be significantly lower compared to control subjects (Kaneko et al., 1998). Therapies targeting the NO pathway in PAH consist of sGC agonists and phosphodiesterase type 5 (PDE5) inhibitors. While NO signaling in PAH patients is aberrant, sGC is expressed in PASMCs of PAH patients (Schermuly et al., 2008), making sGC stimulators attractive agents for increasing cGMP levels in these patients. One such oral sGC agonist, riociguat (Adempas®), was the first drug approved targeting the NO pathway for the treatment of PAH, and activates sGC directly despite the absence of NO (Klinger and Kadowitz, 2017). Findings also demonstrate that PDE5 is overexpressed in PASMCs of PAH patients (Murray et al., 2002). PDE5 inhibitors function by hindering the degradation of cGMP (Giovannoni et al., 2010). Administered orally, PDE5 inhibitors currently approved for the treatment of PAH are sildenafil (Viagra®) and tadalafil (Cialis®). sGC stimulators and PDE5 inhibitors have led to improved 6MWD in patients, as well as lessened time to clinical worsening (Humbert et al., 2014).

Pitfalls of Conventional Pharmacotherapies

Pharmacotherapies in PAH have improved patient hemodynamics and quality of life, but are not without significant shortcomings. Chief among these are drug half-life, stability, and formulation limitations, resulting in deleterious side effects. As an example, epoprostenol has a short half-life of 3–5 min, and instability at low pH values (Mubarak, 2010). As a result, the drug must be continuously infused IV by means of an implanted catheter and infusion pump, and the drug must be constantly maintained under refrigeration and prepared daily. Consequently, patients are at risk of infections, sepsis, and thrombosis (McLaughlin and Palevsky, 2013). Moreover, permanently implanted catheters may malfunction (Ruan et al., 2010). In the case of drugs such as PDE5 inhibitors, a high and continuous dosage is required to achieve beneficial effects, necessitating oral administration of 80 mg up to 3 times a day (Galie et al., 2005).

An additional pitfall is the non-specific distribution of pharmacotherapies, resulting in adverse systemic side effects. Prostanoid therapy is associated with flushing, headaches, and gastrointestinal symptoms, such as nausea and vomiting (Lang and Gaine, 2015). Traditional ET inhibitors result in peripheral edema, anemia, and hepatotoxicity (Aversa et al., 2015). And while the precise mechanism of liver toxicity has not been fully established, abnormal liver function is an indication for treatment discontinuation (McGoon et al., 2006). Lastly, targeting the NO pathway by either PDE5 inhibitors or sGC stimulators causes side effects such as headache, dyspepsia, peripheral edema, nausea, and dizziness (Ishikura et al., 2000; Ghofrani et al., 2013), in addition to retinal vascular disease and myocardial infarction (Duarte et al., 2013).

Novel drug formulations address limitations related to formulation and delivery. As an example, epoprostenol AS (Veletri®), contains arginine and sucrose, and can be stable at room temperature for up to 72 h depending on the concentration of the solution (Sitbon and Vonk Noordegraaf, 2017). More stable prostanoids such as inhaled iloprost (Ventavis®) showed improvements in exercise capacity and beneficial hemodynamic effects (LeVarge, 2015). Recently, a non-prostanoid PGI_2 receptor analog, selexipag (Uptravi®) was developed and approved for oral administration in PAH (Duggan et al., 2017). In the case of ERAs, the aforementioned macitentan reduced morbidity and mortality in PAH patients (Sitbon et al., 2014), lowering the incidence of liver toxicity. Despite these improvements, strategies capable of increasing the bioavailability of PAH pharmacotherapies in the lung have the potential to improve patient outcomes and reduce systemic adverse events.

NP PLATFORMS FOR DRUG AND GENE DELIVERY

Liposomes

Liposomes are composed of phospholipids with polar heads and hydrophobic tails, forming bilayered constructs with an aqueous core, typically on the order of 100 nm in size (**Figure 1A**) (Pattni et al., 2015). The aqueous compartment is ideal for accommodation of water-soluble drugs. Hydrophobic drugs can be incorporated within the bi-phospholipid membrane, albeit at the risk of membrane destabilization (Liu et al., 2006). Functionalization of liposomes with polyethylene glycol (PEG) on the surface led to significant enhancement of circulation lifetimes, best demonstrated by DOXIL®, a PEGylated liposomal formulation of doxorubicin (Hamilton et al., 2002). The increase in circulating half-life was a direct result of incorporating PEG onto the surface of liposomes, with the hydrating layer provided by PEG deterring protein adsorption and NP clearance by the mononuclear phagocyte system (MPS) (Harris and Chess, 2003). Importantly, liposomal doxorubicin was shown to reduce doxorubicin-associated cardiotoxicity compared to the conventional, clinically used formulation of doxorubicin (Berry et al., 1998). These advantages led to DOXIL® being the first NP platform approved by the FDA for the treatment of Kaposi's sarcoma in 1995 (Barenholz, 2012). Liposomes also prove advantageous for efficient delivery of genetic material through incorporation of cationic lipids such as [1,2-bis(oleoyloxy)-3-(trimethylammonio)propane] (DOTAP) (Zhang et al., 2012). Functionalization of liposomes with the thermoresponsive polymer N-isopropylacrylamide (NIPAAm) can be used to induce membrane disruption at high temperatures, resulting in increased local release of drug at specific sites (Ta and Porter, 2013).

Polymer Micelles

Polymer micelles are NPs formed from the self-assembly of amphiphilic-block copolymers in aqueous environments (Blanco et al., 2009). The core-shell morphology of polymer micelles consists of a hydrophobic core and a hydrophilic shell (**Figure 1B**), wherein the hydrophilic block of the constituent polymer is typically PEG. On the order of 10–100 nm in diameter, polymer micelles have traditionally been used as delivery vehicles for hydrophobic drugs. Of significant note, the tailorability of polymer chemistries makes micelles highly versatile carriers with a myriad of advantages for drug delivery. Cationic polymers such as polyethylenimine (PEI) (Dai et al., 2011b) or poly(L-lysine) (Christie et al., 2012) can be either grafted onto block copolymers or used as the core-forming block for loading of genetic material. Stimuli-responsive, tailored drug release can also be obtained based on the composition of the core forming polymer block. As an example, Bae et al. (2005) used PEG-b-poly(aspartate) (PEG-PAsp) for pH-sensitive release of doxorubicin by conjugating it to PAsp through a hydrazine linkage. Lastly, targeting moieties including antibodies, aptamers, and peptides fashioned onto polymer micelles can be used for active targeting to diseased tissues and cells (Jhaveri and Torchilin, 2014). As an example, the cyclic(Arg-Gly-Asp-DPhe-Lys) (cRGDfK) peptide has been used for polymer micelle targeting to the a_vb_3 integrin found overexpressed on tumor vasculature (Nasongkla et al., 2004; Song et al., 2014). Despite their numerous advantages, polymer micelles are limited by fast release of drug and long-term stability, with strategies such as interlayer-crosslinked cores (Dai et al., 2011a) shown to prevent premature drug release.

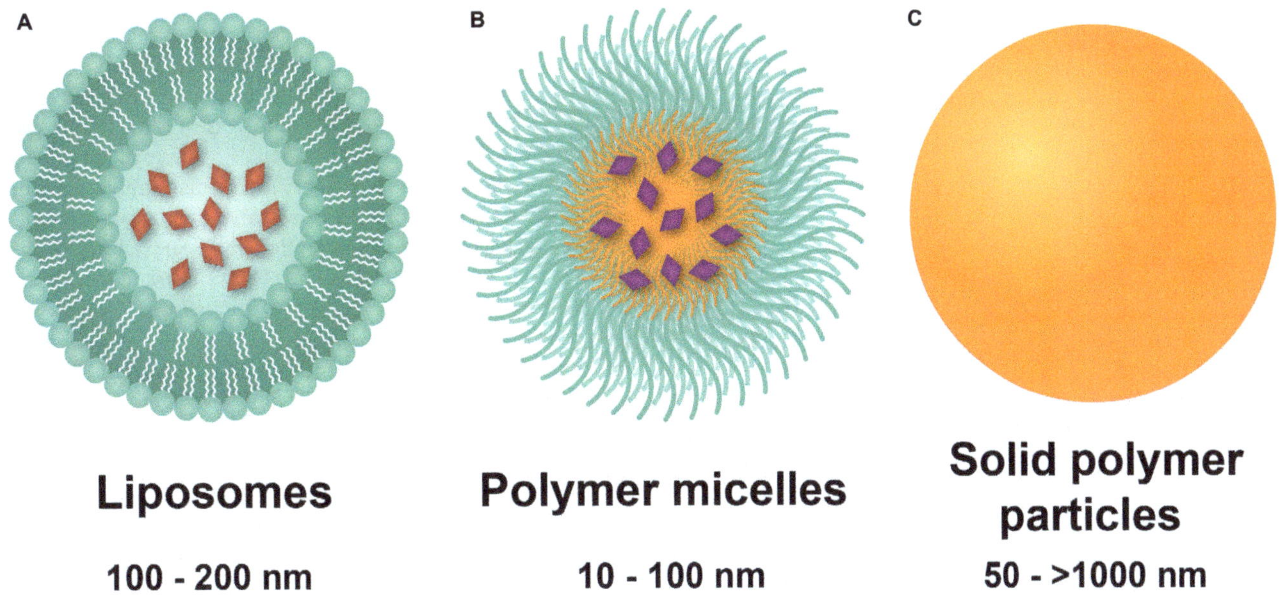

FIGURE 1 | Nanoparticle platforms explored in PAH drug and gene delivery. **(A)** Liposomes are comprised of a lipid bilayer, with an aqueous core ideal for encapsulation of water-soluble drugs (red). **(B)** Polymer micelles are comprised of amphiphilic block copolymers that self-assemble in water to form a hydrophilic corona and a hydrophobic core for encapsulation of lipophilic drugs (violet). **(C)** Solid polymer particles have drug dissolved or embedded within a polymer matrix.

Solid Polymer Particles

Solid polymer particles, typically comprised of the polyester polylactide-co-glycolide (PLGA), have long been employed in controlled drug release applications. These particles are spherical in morphology, can range from the nano- to micro-meter dimensions, and can be used for delivery of water soluble and insoluble drugs (Makadia and Siegel, 2011), with agents dissolved or encapsulated within the polymer matrix (**Figure 1C**; Danhier et al., 2012). PLGA remains the constituent polymer of choice for these NPs due to several advantages. Chief among these is the relative ease of fabrication, as well as the biocompatibility and biodegradability of the PLGA, a material approved by the FDA for a wide range of biomedical applications. In aqueous environments, ester linkages of PLGA undergo hydrolysis, producing the monomers lactic acid and glycolic acid, which are readily metabolized and removed from the body (Acharya and Sahoo, 2011). Moreover, drug release from PLGA NPs occurs through initial diffusion followed by degradation of the polymer matrix, which in turn is affected by crystallinity, composition, molecular weight, and size and shape of the matrix (Makadia and Siegel, 2011). Thus, highly controllable and sustained release profiles can be achieved by employing PLGA copolymers with the more hydrophobic polylactic acid (PLA) than polyglycolic acid (PGA), which give rise to NPs with less water absorption and slower degradation kinetics (Dinarvand et al., 2011). In addition to drugs, PLGA particles can incorporate cationic polymers (e.g., PEI) for delivery of genetic material (Bivas-Benita et al., 2004). PLGA NP drug delivery is limited by rapid initial release of payload due to hydration of the polymer (Kapoor et al., 2015), as well as dose dumping effects at longer timepoints (Khanal et al., 2016). Moreover, peptides and proteins may undergo chemical degradation within polymer matrices (Houchin and Topp, 2008).

Nanoparticle Size Considerations

The relative size of the different NPs influences *in vivo* fate following intravenous delivery. It is now well known that NPs with diameters < 5 nm are cleared rapidly by the kidneys (Choi et al., 2007). NPs that measure > 100 nm accumulate non-specifically in livers (Braet et al., 2007), those measuring > 200 nm accumulate in the spleen (Chen and Weiss, 1973), and particles > 2 μm accumulate in lung capillaries. Resident macrophages of the liver, spleen, and lungs rapidly internalize opsonized NPs in a size-dependent manner. Taken together, smaller sized NPs, measuring 100 nm or less, have been shown to be long circulating following intravenous administration (Blanco et al., 2010).

These size considerations play an important role in the design of nanotherapeutic constructs for purposes of targeting specific tissues. As an example, Xu et al. (2016) used particles with a diameter of 2.5 μm to specifically target breast cancer metastasis in the lung. Long-circulating NPs have a heightened propensity to passively accumulate in tissues with remodeled vasculature by extravasating through submicron sized pores in the endothelium (Hobbs et al., 1998). And while smaller sized NPs are able to extravasate from circulation into these diseased sites, the extent of NP penetration into the tissue depends on the size of the carrier. Cabral et al. (2011) were able to demonstrate that sub-100 nm NPs were able to penetrate into permeable tumors. However, in more fibrotic tumors, only NPs measuring < 50 nm were capable of penetrating into the tissue.

Inhalational delivery of NPs represents an attractive strategy for specifically targeting pulmonary tissues. However, particle size also dictates regional lung deposition after inhalation (Paranjpe and Muller-Goymann, 2014). When administered as a dry powder, large particles in the size range of 1–5 μm deposit in bronchioles and smaller airways, particles in the size range of 0.5–1 μm accumulate in alveolar regions, and smaller NPs (< 0.5 μm) can undergo exhalation.

ENHANCED NP ACCUMULATION IN LUNGS UNDERGOING PAH

Nanoparticle platforms such as liposomes and polymer micelles have been extensively explored in chemotherapy. While advantageous at increasing the circulation lifetimes of chemotherapeutics, it was the observation by Maeda et al. (2013) regarding the ability of IV-administered macromolecules to accumulate to a large extent in tumors that led to the excitement of NP-based drug delivery strategies in cancer (Matsumura and Maeda, 1986). Passive targeting of macromolecules and NPs to tumors is owed to the high degree of fenestrations (e.g., openings) present in tumor vasculature (McDonald and Choyke, 2003), a direct result of chaotic and ongoing angiogenic processes in tumors (Fang et al., 2011). This enhanced NP accumulation in tumors, combined with NP persistence due to impaired lymphatic drainage (Banerjee et al., 2011) is known as the EPR effect (Maeda et al., 2013).

While passive accumulation of NPs in disease sites is primarily associated with cancer, vascular permeability is prevalent in other diseases characterized by abnormal angiogenesis and vascular remodeling as a consequence of inflammation (Durymanov et al., 2017). As an example, in rheumatoid arthritis, where a combination of angiogenic and inflammatory processes promote vessel leakiness, several groups have reported passive targeting to the synovium (Metselaar et al., 2004; Anderson et al., 2010). Similarly, formation of new blood vessels in atherosclerotic plaques leads to enhanced NP uptake in these lesions (Chono et al., 2005; Stigliano et al., 2017). Vascular injury stemming from local inflammatory processes and hypoxia is present in diseases such as myocardial infarction and heart failure, resulting in enhanced vascular permeability to the heart. Nagaoka et al. (2015) and Nakano et al. (2016) demonstrated increased NP uptake in myocardial infarct areas following IV administration in a model of ischemia-reperfusion (IR) injury in the heart, mirroring previously published findings (Dvir et al., 2011; Paulis et al., 2012). Our laboratory recently demonstrated enhanced accumulation of micron-sized particles in failing hearts compared to healthy hearts (Ruiz-Esparza et al., 2016). It is important to note that the prevalence of immune-related cells in areas of inflammation can also contribute to increased uptake at these sites through macrophage phagocytosis (Ulbrich and Lamprecht, 2010).

Vascular permeability in PAH arises from injurious events such as inflammation and hypoxia, resulting in focal disruptions in endothelial cell basement membranes (McLaughlin and McGoon, 2006; Stenmark et al., 2006; Montani et al., 2014), as well as increased vascular pressure, which leads to fenestrations as a result of greater mechanical and shear stress (**Figure 2**) (Zhou et al., 2016). Moreover, mutations in bone morphogenetic protein receptor 2 (BMPR2), highly prevalent in heritable PAH, have been shown to contribute to increased vascular permeability through dysregulation of the TGF-β signaling pathway (Morrell, 2006). Our laboratory recently demonstrated

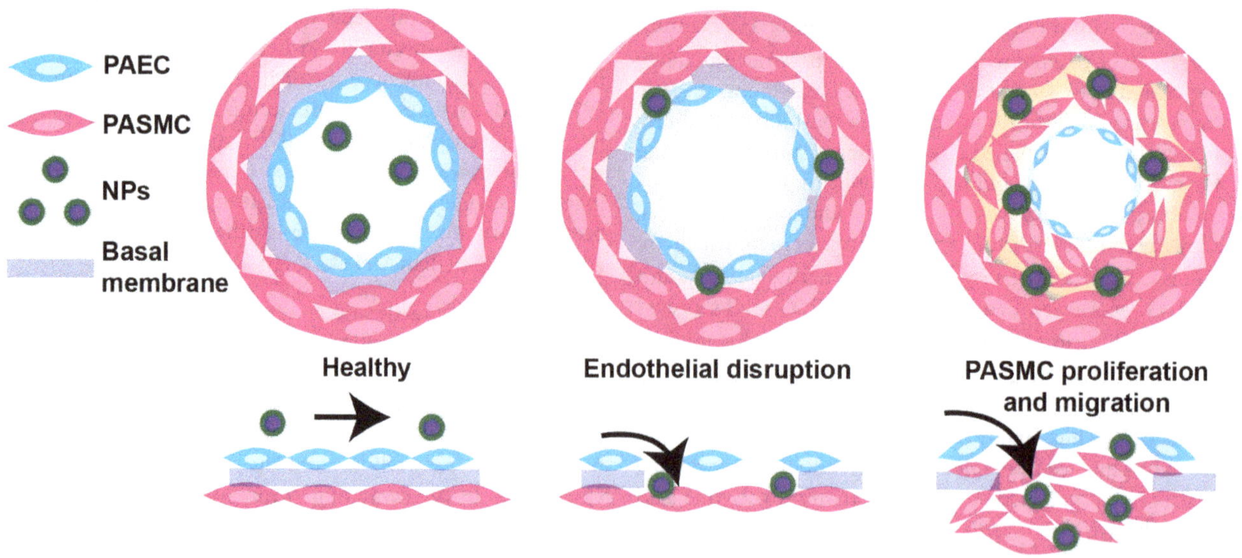

FIGURE 2 | Schematic representation of endothelial dysfunction in PAH and a proposed mechanism of NP extravasation into pulmonary vasculature. While healthy pulmonary vasculature is a semipermeable membrane barrier, the vasculature in lungs undergoing PAH exhibits endothelial dysfunction arising from a chronic inflammatory state and hypoxia, leading to fenestrations (openings) in the endothelium and a hyperpermeable state. Such permeability may be exploited by NPs to passively extravasate and accumulate in lungs undergoing PAH. Figure adapted from Segura-Ibarra et al. (2017), reproduced with permission courtesy of Elsevier.

that vascular permeability in PAH contributes to enhanced NP accumulation in diseased lungs (Segura-Ibarra et al., 2017), agreeing well with previous findings by Ishihara et al. (2015). In a monocrotaline (MCT)-induced model of PAH, poly(ethylene glycol)-*block*-poly(ε-caprolactone) (PEG-PCL) micelles containing rapamycin (RAP) resulted in increased drug accumulation in diseased lungs compared to healthy lungs 2 h after IV administration (**Figure 3A**). Moreover, LC/MS analysis comparing RAP-containing micelles and a free drug formulation of RAP showed a significantly higher increase in RAP accumulation in diseased lungs when packaged within NPs (**Figure 3A**). Upon closer examination of remodeled vasculature using confocal microscopy, heightened accumulation of PEG-PCL NPs was observed within the perivascular region (**Figures 3B,C**).

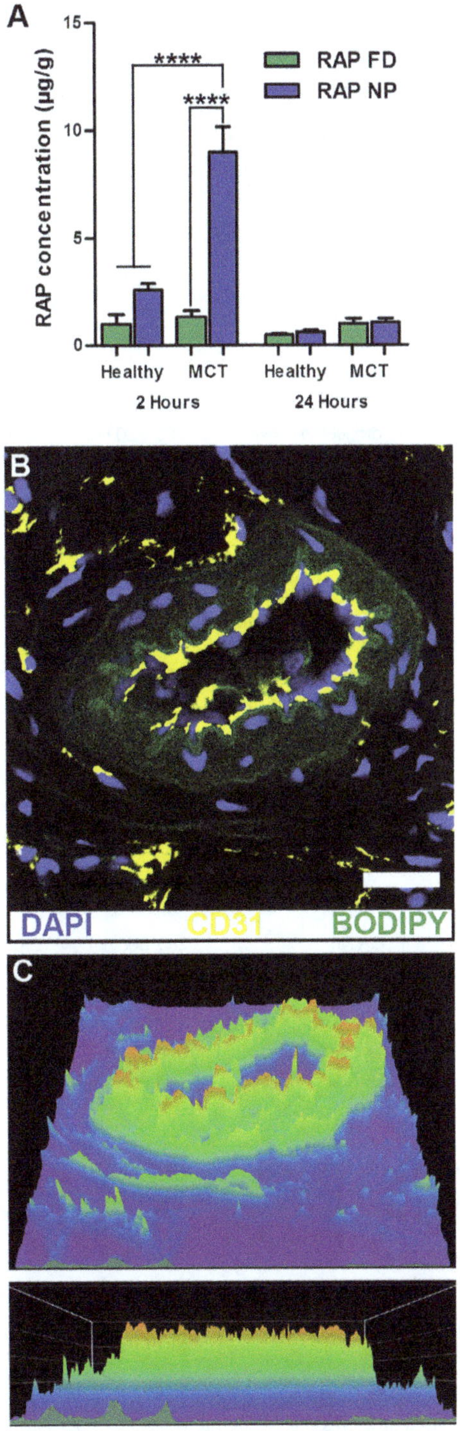

FIGURE 3 | NP accumulation in PAH lung vasculature. **(A)** LC/MS analysis of rapamycin (RAP) concentration in lung tissues 2 and 24 h after a single administration of 15 mg/kg of RAP, either as a free drug formulation (RAP FD) or nanoparticle form (RAP NP) in healthy and MCT-induced model of PH in rats (PH). Results represent mean ± SEM (*****P* < 0.0001). **(B)** Confocal imaging depicting fluorescently loaded NPs in diseased lungs. CD31 positive endothelial cells appear in yellow, NPs are green, while DAPI appears as blue. The scale bar represents 25 μm. **(C)** Surface intensity plot of the image from panel B representing NP signal. Figure adapted from Segura-Ibarra et al. (2017), reproduced with permission courtesy of Elsevier.

NANOTHERAPEUTICS IN PAH

Conventional pharmacotherapies for PAH treatment suffer from short half-lives, drug instability, and adverse side effects. NP-based strategies for the treatment of PAH offer advantages of improving short-term pharmacokinetics associated with drugs and increased localization of therapy to diseased tissues, in turn decreasing adverse effects. Herein, we highlight nanotherapeutic approaches aimed at delivering clinically approved PAH drugs, as well as nanoplatforms for delivery of novel agents, including genetic material (**Table 1**).

Prostanoid-Containing NPs

The clinically approved drug inhaled iloprost has an extremely short half-life, requiring at most 12 inhalations per day (Olschewski et al., 2000), largely impacting patient compliance. In hopes of increasing drug bioavailability, Kleemann et al. (2007) developed a liposomal formulation for sustained release of iloprost for aerosolized PAH therapy. Liposomes consisted of di-palmitoyl-phosphatidyl-choline (DPPC), cholesterol to enhance sustained delivery, and poly(ethylene glycol)-di-palmitoyl-phosphatidyl-ethanolamine (PEG-DPPE) to prevent clearance by alveolar macrophages, which would limit their bioavailability. Resulting liposomes ranged in size from 200 to 400 nm, and contained 11 μg iloprost/ml, which would significantly reduce the number of inhalations required.

Jain et al. (2014) fabricated iloprost-containing liposomes with cationic lipids in hopes of increasing drug loading efficiency and examined their efficacy based on changes in vascular tone of pulmonary arteries isolated from mice by means of a wire myograph. NPs averaged 168–178 nm in diameter and had drug loading efficiencies of ~50%. Pulmonary arteries were constricted by application of the thromboxane analog, U-46619, and treated either with free or liposomal iloprost. Liposomal iloprost resulted in significant enhancement of vasodilation (29% compared to 16% for free iloprost), with a much lower concentration of liposomal iloprost required to bring about efficacies similar to that of free drug.

The oral PGI_2 analog beraprost has proven vasodilatory and anti-platelet activity, but much like other prostanoids, has a

TABLE 1 | Nanotherapeutics explored pre-clinically in PAH.

Therapeutic agent	NP formulation	Size	Control	Advantage over control	Model	Reference
Iloprost	Liposomes (various formulations combining POPC, DOTAP, PVP, SA, DPPE-PEG2000, CH)	168–178 nm	Free iloprost	~1-fold ↑ vasodilation	BALB/c isolated intrapulmonary arteries	Jain et al., 2014
Beraprost	PEG-PLA NP	~128 nm	Free beraprost	↓ effective dose (20 μg/kg for NP vs. 100 μg/kg for control)	Rat MCT-induced PAH	Ishihara et al., 2015
Beraprost	PLGA NP	280–300 nm	Drug-free vehicle	1.3-fold ↑ survival rate in MCT model, ↓ RV hypertrophy, ↓ RVSP, ↓ muscularized pulmonary arteries in MCT and sugen/hypoxia models	Rat MCT-induced PAH, Rat sugen/ hypoxia-induced PAH	Akagi et al., 2016
NO	Liposomes (EDPPC, DOPC, CH, Ar)	–	NO in Ar saturated mannitol solution	7-fold ↑ NO uptake by VSMC	Cultured VSMC	Huang et al., 2009
NO	Hydrogel-like polymer NP (Methyl silicate, oligochitosan, PVP, PEG)	200–230 nm	Same formulation applied to healthy mice	Concentration-dependent ↑ vasodilation	Mice hypoxia-induced PAH	Mohamed et al., 2016
Pitavastatin	PLGA NP	~196	Free pitavastatin	↓ RVSP, ↓ arteriolar remodeling, ↓ macrophage infiltration, > 50% ↓ NF-κB positive cells, ↑ survival, ↑ NOS expression	Rat MCT-induced PAH	Chen et al., 2011
Fasudil	Aerosolized Liposomes (DPPC, CH)	~180 nm	Free fasudil	10-fold ↑ drug half-life, ↑ duration of vasodilation	Rat MCT-induced PAH	Gupta et al., 2013
Fasudil	Liposomes (DPPC, CH, DSPE-PEG, CAR peptide)	206–216 nm	Free fasudil	34-fold ↑ drug half-life in healthy rats; ↓ mPAP (40% reduction for NP vs. 35% for control in MCT model)	Healthy rats, Rat MCT-induced PAH	Nahar et al., 2014
Fasudil, SOD	Liposomes (DPPC, CH, DSPE-PEG-MAL, CAR peptide)	~150 nm	Fusudil + SOD	↓ mPAP, ↓ arterial medial wall thickness, ↑ vasodilatory effects duration	Rat MCT-induced PAH	Gupta et al., 2017
Ethyl pyruvate	PEG-LG NP	~286 nm	Free ethyl pyruvate	56% ↓ mPAP, > 50% ↓ arterial medial wall thickness, ~50% ↓ IL-6, ↓ T N F α, > 50% ↓ ROS, > 6 0 % ↓ HMGB 1	Rat Shunt flow-induced PAH	Liu et al., 2016
Imatinib	PLGA NP	280–300 nm	Drug-free vehicles	~40% ↓ RVSP, prevented ↑ in RV hypertrophy, ~50% ↓ small pulmonary vessel muscularization	Rat MCT-induced PAH	Akagi et al., 2015
Rapamycin	PEG-PCL NP	~17 nm	Free rapamycin	~50% ↓ Inflammatory cytokines levels, 10% ↓ in weight loss	Rat MCT-induced PAH	Segura-Ibarra et al., 2017
NF-κB decoy oligodeoxy-nucleotide	PEG-PLGA NP	~44 nm	Free NF-κB decoy	↓ RVSP, ↓ RV hypertrophy, ↓ small pulmonary vessel muscularization, > 50% ↓ inflammatory cytokine mRNA, > 50% ↓ NF-κB positive cells	Rat MCT-induced PAH	Kimura et al., 2009
Anti-sense oligonucleotide against miR-145	Liposomes (Star:Star-mPEG-550)	80–100 nm	Non-silencing oligonucleotide	~25% ↓ RVSP, ↓ in RV hypertrophy, ↓ arterial medial wall thickness, > 50% ↓ in miR-145 expression	Rat Sugen/ Hypoxia-induced PAH	McLendon et al., 2015

POPC, 1-palmitoyl-2oleoyl-sn-glycero-3-phosphocholine; DOTAP, 1,2-di-(9Z-octadecenoyl)-3-trimethylammonium-propane; PVP, polyvinylpyrrolidone; SA, stearylamine; DPPE-PEG2000, [methoxy (polyethyleneglycol)-2000]-dipalmitoyl-phosphatidylethanolamine; PEG, polyethylene glycol; PLA, polylactic acid; NP, nanoparticle; MCT, monocrotaline; PAH, pulmonary arterial hypertension; PLGA, poly(lactic-co-glycolic acid); RV, right ventricle; RVSP, right venticular systolic pressure; NO, nitric oxide; EDPPC, 1,2-dipalmitoyl-sn-glycero-3-ethylphosphocholine; DOPC, 1,2-dioleoyl-sn-glycero-3-phosphocholine; CH, cholesterol; Ar, argon; VSMC, vascular smooth muscle cells; SP, systolic pressure; NF-κB, nuclear factor kappa-light-chain-enhancer of activated B cells; NOS, nitric oxide synthase; DPPC, 1,2-dipalmitoyl-sn-glycero-3-phosphocholine; DSPE-PEG-MAL, 1,2-distearoyl-sn-glycero-3-phosphoethanolamineN-[maleimide(polyethylene glycol)-2000]; CAR peptide, peptide with amino acid sequence CARSKNKDC; mPAP, mean pulmonary arterial pressure; PEG-LG, poly(ethylene glycol)-block-lactide/glycolide copolymer; TNFα, tumor necrosis factor alpha; HMGB1, high mobility group box 1 protein; ROS, reactive oxygen species; IL-6, Interleukin 6; PEG-PCL, poly(ethylene glycol)-block-poly(ε-caprolactone); Star, staramine; mPEG, methoxypolyethylene glycol.

very short half-life (~1 h) (Barst et al., 2003). In attempts to overcome pharmacokinetic limitations of the drug, Ishihara et al. (2015), who previously formulated NPs containing prostaglandin E1 (PGE1) (Takeda et al., 2009), encapsulated beraprost within poly(ethyleneglycol)-*block*- poly(lactide) (PEG-PLA) micelles and examined their efficacy in an MCT-induced PAH rat model and hypoxia-induced mouse model of PAH. Resulting NPs possessed average diameters of 128 nm and exhibited slow drug release kinetics (~20% over 1 week). Beraprost NPs showed significantly reduced drug clearance from plasma compared to free beraprost, the former present in circulation at timepoints of 24 h, while the latter was cleared within 6 h. Upon IV administration in an MCT-induced model of PAH in rats, NPs accumulated more in MCT-damaged lungs compared to healthy control lungs, and were found associated with pulmonary peripheral arteries. Importantly, once a week IV administration of beraprost NPs at a dose of 20 μg/kg in an MCT-induced PAH rat model reduced pulmonary arterial remodeling and right ventricular hypertrophy; the efficacy proving similar to that of a daily oral administration of the drug at a much higher dose (100 μg/kg). A similar improvement in pulmonary arterial remodeling was observed in the hypoxia-induced model in mice. This study effectively highlights the advantages afforded by NP-based drug delivery, mainly the need for lower doses and less frequent administrations to achieve similar efficacious responses.

In another study, Akagi et al. (2016) fabricated PLGA NPs containing beraprost and examined the efficacy of the platform in MCT- and Sugen/Hypoxia-induced models of PAH. After a single intratracheal administration of beraprost-containing NPs, RV systolic pressure (RVSP), RV hypertrophy, and the percentage of fully muscularized small pulmonary arteries were significantly reduced compared to disease controls in both PAH models. Moreover, the survival rate increased to 65% following administration of NP-based beraprost, compared to 27.8% in disease controls. Of note, NPs administered intratracheally in the Sugen/Hypoxia-induced model of PAH were found associated with the media of pulmonary arteries and interstitium at timepoints of up to 3 days, whereas no NPs were evident in healthy control lungs.

NP-Based Targeting of the NO Pathway

Nitric oxide plays an important role in healthy pulmonary physiology, driving SMC relaxation (Perez-Zoghbi et al., 2010), with added anti-inflammatory and proliferative properties (Tonelli et al., 2013). Huang et al. (2009) developed a liposomal formulation of NO consisting of 1,2-dipalmitoyl-sn-glycero-3-ethylphosphocholine (EDPPC), 1,2-dioleoyl-sn-glycero-3-phosphocholine (DOPC), and cholesterol. These liposomes encapsulated 10 μL of NO per mg of lipids and Argon (Ar) was used as an excipient for NO. Upon examination of release kinetics *in vitro*, release of NO from liposomes was slower in the presence of Ar, resulting in a sustained release profile. No significant toxicity was observed *in vitro* in cultured rat vascular smooth muscle cells (VSMCs), and based on a colorimetric NO assay kit, a sevenfold increase in uptake of NO was observed with liposomal NO than NO formulated in Ar saturated mannitol solution. Moreover, liposomes protected NO from microenvironmental scavengers such as hemoglobin. To evaluate *in vivo* efficacy, a balloon injury was induced in the common carotid arteries of rabbits and liposomes containing NO were administered locally. After 2 weeks, a significant decrease in intimal hyperplasia was observed in rabbits treated with liposomal NO compared to vehicle controls (empty liposomes), demonstrating the feasibility of delivery of bio-active gases NPs.

Recently, Mohamed et al. (2016) developed a novel hydrogel-like polymer composite NP formulation for delivery of NO. NPs released NO in a sustained fashion over time, and showed concentration-dependent vasodilation of U-46619-induced preconstricted pulmonary arteries, with a more pronounced effect observed in arteries from hypoxia-induced PAH mice compared to healthy mice.

Beck-Broichsitter et al. (2012) have explored novel spray-drying techniques to fabricate PLGA microparticles for deposition in the lungs and release of sildenafil. Using a vibrational spray drying procedure, resulting microparticles measured 4–8 μm in size and had a high sildenafil encapsulation efficiency of > 90% (Beck-Broichsitter et al., 2017). Moreover, the formulation resulted in a sustained release of sildenafil over time, making these microparticles potentially beneficial for controlled pulmonary drug delivery in PAH and chronic lung diseases.

Nanotherapeutic Delivery of Novel Agents Targeting PAH

Currently, statins are one of the first-line medications given to patients with elevated cholesterol levels to prevent cardiovascular disease. The mechanism of action involves inhibiting the rate-limiting step of cholesterol biosynthesis by competitive inhibition of HMG-CoA reductase (Istvan, 2003). Statins also improve endothelial function (Beckman and Creager, 2006), displaying anti-tumoral (Crescencio et al., 2009), anti-proliferative (Kamigaki et al., 2011), and anti-inflammatory (Ridker et al., 1999; Lefer, 2002) effects.

Given that inflammation, endothelial injury, and cellular proliferation play a crucial role in PAH progression, Chen et al. (2011) explored the use of statin nanotherapeutics for treatment of PAH. The anti-proliferative effects of different statins (pravastatin, losuvastatin, simvastatin, atorvastatin, fluvastatin, and pitavastatin) were evaluated in human PASMCs, and pitavastatin was selected for PLGA NP encapsulation based on its potent effects. Distribution of PLGA NPs following intratracheal instillation were examined, and FITC-containing NPs were found in lungs of rats undergoing MCT-induced PAH 3 days after administration, specifically in small arteries, bronchi, alveoli, and alveolar macrophages. Of significant note, FITC was detected in lungs at timepoints of up to 14 days after a single administration. A single administration of pitavastatin-containing NPs was performed at the time of PAH induction of rats, and 21 days after administration, right ventricular catheterization revealed a significant decrease in RV systolic pressure compared to rats treated with free pitavastatin or vehicle controls. A significant decrease in systolic pressure in pulmonary arterioles was also observed. Of note, lower levels of macrophages and monocytes were found in rats treated with pitavastatin-containing NPs. Moreover, compared to free pitavastatin, the NP formulation resulted in a > 50% decrease of cells positive for nuclear factor kappa-light-chain-enhancer of activated B (NF-κB), which plays an important role in cell proliferation and survival (Hoesel and Schmid, 2013). The NP formulation increased expression of endothelial NO synthase (eNOS), which can potentially promote endothelial healing. Following NP administration in rats 21 days after MCT induction of PAH, pitavastatin-containing NPs significantly increased survival by 64% compared to control groups (**Figure 4A**) and significantly decreased RVSP compared to disease controls (**Figure 4B**). It is important to note that a Phase I clinical trial involving pitavastatin PLGA NP-based delivery for PAH has recently been completed (Nakamura et al., 2017).

Activation of the Ras homolog gene family, member A (RhoA) GTPase and it downstream effector, the Rho-associated kinase (ROCK), have been implicated in several processes driving PAH pathogenesis, including SMC vasoconstriction and proliferation, and endothelial cell contraction (Oka et al., 2008). Thus, inhibitors of RhoA/ROCK signaling such as Fasudil can potentially prove efficacious in the treatment of PAH. However, Fasudil has a short half-life of ~45 min (Shibuya et al., 2005). In light of these limitations, Gupta et al. (2013) developed a liposomal formulation of fasudil for purposes of aerosolized delivery to lungs undergoing PAH. Resulting liposomes measured ~180 nm following nebulization, had loading efficiencies > 60%, and released ~70% of the drug over the course of 35 h. Pulmonary delivery of liposomes via intratracheal administration increased the half-life by more than 10-fold, as well as the bioavailability of the drug, compared to a free drug formulation administered IV. Upon efficacy examination in an MCT-induced PAH model in rats, an intratracheally administered liposomal formulation of fasudil was compared to a free formulation of fasudil administered intratracheally and by IV. Liposomal fasudil resulted in an increase in the duration of vasodilatory effects compared to controls, with a maximal reduction in mPAP of ~40%.

In an attempt to enhance site-specific accumulation of NPs to the lungs, Nahar et al. (2014) subsequently developed fasudil liposomes with the cyclic peptide CARSKNKDC, which binds to cell surface heparan sulfate found overexpressed in pulmonary vasculature in PAH. Liposomes were in the range of 206–216 nm and had a sustained release of fasudil over the course of 120 h. Peptide-coated liposomes resulted in ~34-fold increase in half-life of the drug compared to an IV-administered formulation of free drug. As a result, the mPAP in an MCT-induced model and a Sugen/Hypoxia model of PAH in rats was greatly reduced compared to controls. In a recent study, Gupta et al. (2017) incorporated superoxide dismutase (SOD) into their peptide-targeted fasudil liposomes, with the hypothesis that inclusion of a reactive oxygen species (ROS) scavenger would further enhance efficacy, given the role that increased ROS levels play in vascular remodeling in PAH. In an MCT-model of PAH, wherein the liposomal formulation was administered every 72 h for 21 days, the duration of vasodilatory effects was significantly increased in rats receiving targeted liposomes containing both fasudil and SOD compared to free drug controls. In a Sugen/Hypoxia model of PAH, mPAP, RV hypertrophy, fractions of occluded blood vessels, and arterial medial wall thickness were all reduced in rats receiving targeted liposomes containing both fasudil and SOD compared to free drug controls.

Liu et al. (2016) also examined the potential of ROS scavenging nanotherapeutics for the treatment of PAH. In their study, ethyl pyruvate, a derivative of pyruvic acid and an inhibitor of nuclear protein HMGB1, which in turn activates pro-inflammatory cytokines, was incorporated within poly(ethylene glycol)-*block*-lactide/glycolide (PEG-LG) NPs and examined their efficacy in a hyperkinetic model of PAH induced by shunt flow. At a timepoint of 24 h after intratracheal instillation, NPs were evident in lungs, predominantly in bronchi, alveoli, alveolar macrophages, and small arteries, with evidence of NPs present up to timepoints of 7 days. Following weekly administration of ethyl pyruvate NPs immediately after model induction for a time period of 12 weeks, medial wall thickness index (TI) and medial wall area index (AI) of small pulmonary arteries was significantly reduced by >50% compared to free ethyl pyruvate controls. Moreover, IL-6 and

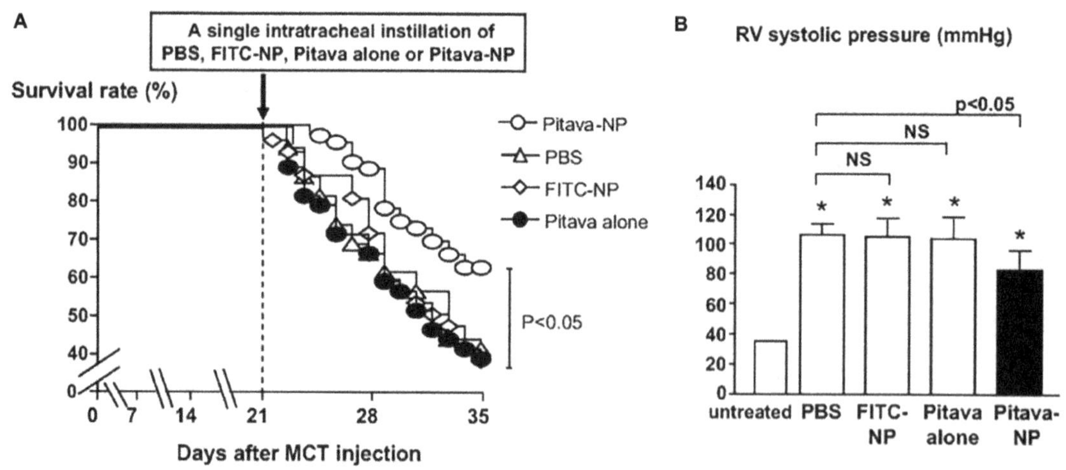

FIGURE 4 | Effects on survival and RV systolic pressures following pitavastatin-NP delivery. **(A)** Kaplan–Meier curve depicting survival of MCT-induced PAH rats following a single intratracheal administration of Pitavastatin-NP compared to controls consisting of intratracheal delivery of PBS, free pitavastatin, and fluorescein isothiocyanate (FITC)-NPs. **(B)** Effects of pitavastatin-NPs on RV systolic pressure (expressed as mmHg). **P* < 0.01 vs. untreated control. Figure adapted from Chen et al. (2011), reproduced with permission courtesy of Wolters Kluwer Health, Inc.

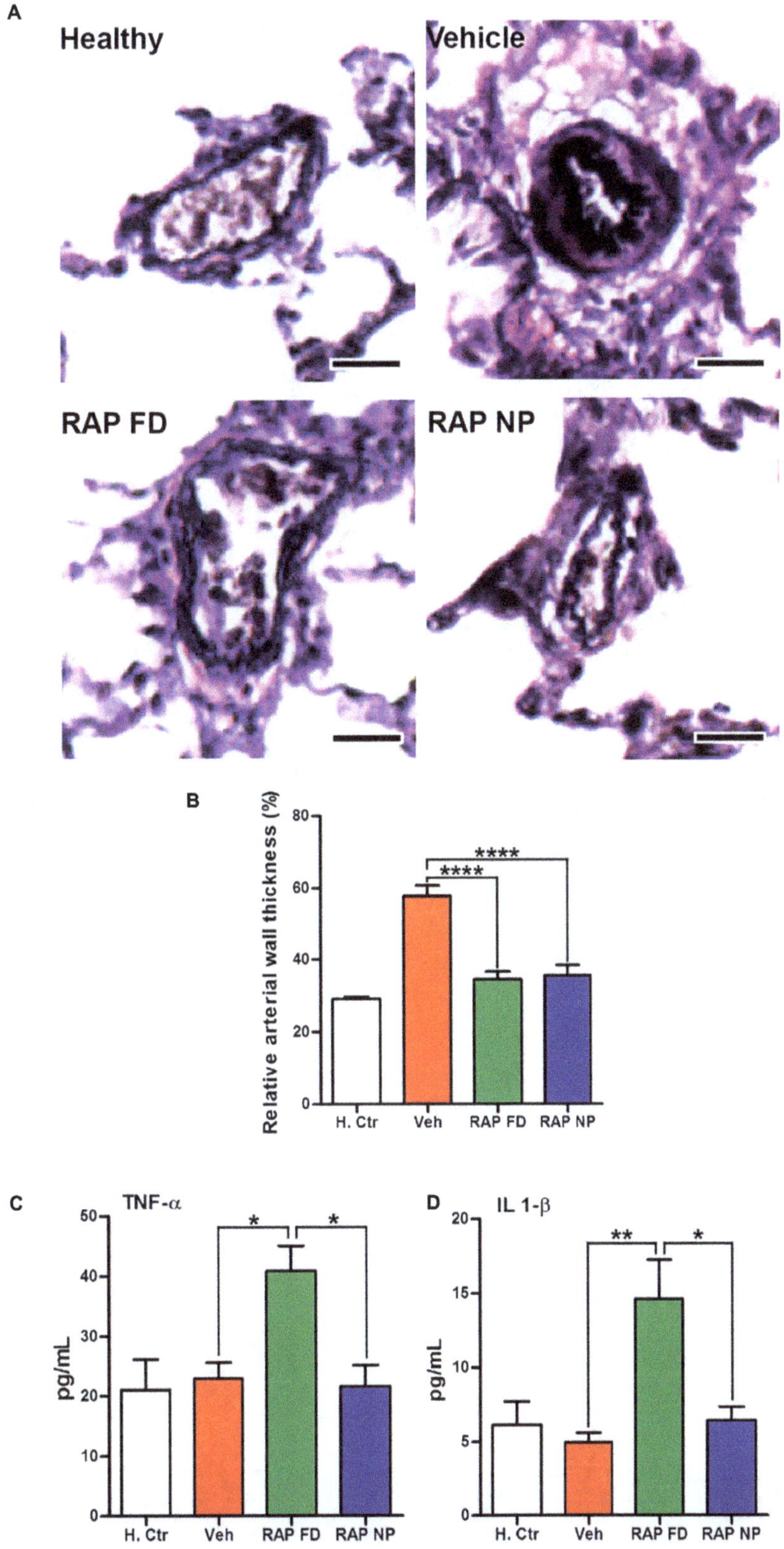

FIGURE 5 | Rapamycin NPs prevented pulmonary arteriole hypertrophy in PAH and did not lead to an increase in inflammatory cytokines. **(A)** Verhoeff–Van Gieson (VVG) stain of pulmonary arterioles from MCT-induced model of PAH in rats treated with free rapamycin (RAP FD), NP vehicle (Vehicle), and RAP NPs. Scale bars represent 50 μm. **(B)** Quantification of the relative wall thickness among treated groups in **(A)**. Results shown as mean ± SEM (****$P < 0.0001$). Serum levels of inflammatory cytokines TNF-α **(C)** and IL-1β **(D)** measured after the course of treatment. Results represent mean ± SEM values (**$P < 0.01$, *$P < 0.05$). Figure adapted from Segura-Ibarra et al. (2017), reproduced with permission courtesy of Elsevier.

TNFα levels were significantly reduced (~50%), as were levels of HMGB1 and ROS by more than 50 and 60%, respectively.

PASMC abnormal proliferation is vital to pathogenesis of PAH, with platelet–derived growth factor (PDGF) stimulation resulting in increased growth rate of PASMCs (Ikeda et al., 2010). Akagi et al. (2015) incorporated the PDGF-receptor tyrosine kinase inhibitor imatinib in PLGA NPs and examined their efficacy in an MCT-induced model of PAH. Imatinib is used for the treatment of chronic myelogenous leukemia (CML) and acute lymphocytic leukemia (ALL), and has resulted in 10-year progression-free survivals of 82% in CML (Kalmanti et al., 2015). It is important to note that a limitation of imatinib is patient resistance due to BCR-ABL1 amplification and multidrug-resistant P-glycoprotein (MDR-1) overexpression (Milojkovic and Apperley, 2009). Following a single intratracheal administration immediately after model induction, imatinib-containing NPs significantly reduced RV systolic pressure (~40% reduction) and RV hypertrophy, as well as muscularization of pulmonary small vessels (~50% reduction) compared to vehicle controls.

Aberrant activation of the mammalian target of rapamycin (mTOR) plays an important role in diseases such as cancer (Blanco et al., 2014), leading to the therapeutic exploration of mTOR inhibitors such as RAP. mTOR is also a key player in PAH progression due to its effects on PASMC growth and survival (Goncharova, 2013). Rapamycin has been shown to prevent PAH progression pre-clinically (Houssaini et al., 2013) while clinical exploration of everolimus, a rapalog, led to improvements in pulmonary vascular resistance and 6MWD (Seyfarth et al., 2013). Similar to the aforementioned imatinib, resistance to RAP is a limitation of the drug, stemming from mutations in mTOR or mutations in downstream effectors of mTOR (S6K1 or 4E-BP1) (Huang and Houghton, 2001). Our laboratory recently examined the potential of RAP NPs for the treatment of PAH (Segura-Ibarra et al., 2017). RAP was encapsulated within PEG-PCL polymer micelles measuring ~17 nm in diameter. In an MCT-induced rat model of PAH, RAP NPs led to a significant increase in RAP in diseased lungs compared to healthy lungs. Similarly, RAP NPs led to an increase in RAP in diseased lungs compared to a free drug formulation. Moreover, NPs were localized primarily in pulmonary vasculature. Following twice a week administration of RAP NPs at the time of PAH induction for a duration of 4 weeks, RAP NPs significantly reduced pulmonary arteriole hypertrophy (**Figures 5A,B**) and RV ventricular remodeling compared to vehicle controls, and prevented increases in right ventricular systolic pressures and phosphorylation of S6, a downstream effector of mTOR. Importantly, compared to a free drug formulation of RAP, a 10% decrease in weight loss associated with RAP was observed in rats receiving RAP NPs, accompanied as well by a decrease (~50%) in levels of pro-inflammatory cytokines (**Figures 5C,D**).

NP Delivery of Genetic Material in PAH

Enhanced insights into molecular machinery driving PAH progression, including those involved in inflammation, have resulted in the identification of several viable therapeutic targets, with NP-based delivery platforms enabling gene therapy. As an example, NF-κB is a transcription factor that regulates numerous inflammatory cytokines, including IL-6 and TNF-α, which are involved in PAH (Hoesel and Schmid, 2013).

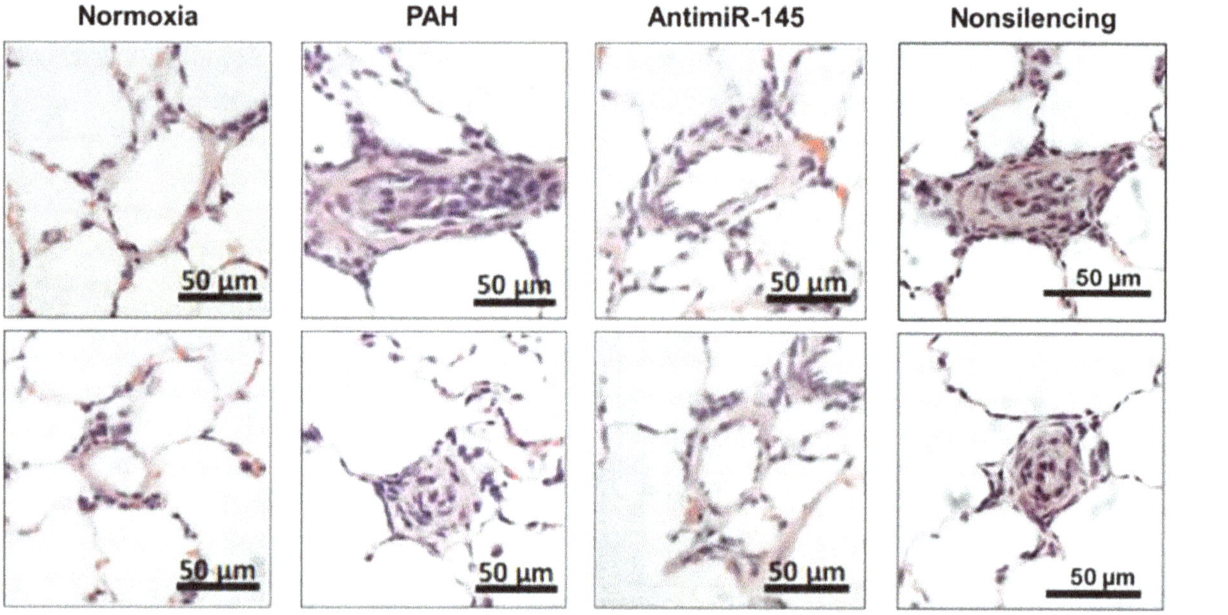

FIGURE 6 | Effects of anti-miR-145 loaded liposomes on arteriole hyperplasia in an MCT-induced model of PAH. Hematoxylin and Eosin (H&E) stained histological sections depicting pulmonary arterioles following anti-miR-145 liposome treatment of rats with Sugen/Hypoxia induced PAH. Results highlight anti-miR-145 liposome treatment compared to controls consisting of healthy controls (normoxia), rats undergoing PAH (PAH), and liposomes containing non-silencing control oligonucleotide (non-silencing). Scale bar represents 50 μm. Figure adapted from McLendon et al. (2015), reproduced with permission courtesy of Elsevier.

Kimura et al. (2009) examined the role of NF-κB in PAH, as well as the potential for NP-based therapeutics targeting NF-κB as a treatment strategy. An NF-κB decoy oligodeoxynucleotide meant to inhibit binding of NF-κB to the promoter region was encapsulated within poly(ethylene glycol)-*block*-lactide/glycolide (PEG-PLGA) polymer micelles. Resulting NPs measured 44 nm in diameter, and displayed release of ~40% of NF-κB decoy over 24 h and sustained release over the course of 28 days. Efficacy of NF-κB NPs were examined in preventive (NP intratracheal administration at the time of model induction) and treatment (NP intratracheal administration 21 days after model induction) protocols in an MCT-induced model of PAH. Using FITC-labeled NF-κB for visualization of NPs, FITC signal was found in small arteries, arterioles, small bronchi, and alveoli of diseased lungs at timepoints of 7 and 14 days after administration. In the preventive study, NF-κB positive cells were significantly reduced (> 50%) compared to free NF-κB decoy controls 7 days after model induction. In the treatment study, NF-κB NPs resulted in a significant decrease in RV systolic pressure, RV hypertrophy, and percentage of muscularized pulmonary arteries compared to PBS controls. Moreover, mRNA levels of inflammatory factors such as monocyte chemoattractant protein (MCP) 1, TNF-α, IL-6, and ICAM-1, were reduced by more than 50% following treatment with NF-κB NPs compared to free NF-κB decoy controls, and animal survival rate was increased compared to vehicle controls.

In a study by McLendon et al. (2015), NPs were used to deliver anti-sense oligonucleotide against microRNA-145 (miR-145) in hopes of exploiting RNA interference (RNAi) as a viable treatment strategy in PAH. Increased expression of miR-145 has been shown in lungs undergoing PAH, playing a vital role in vascular remodeling and pulmonary artery muscularization (Zhou et al., 2015). Moreover, downregulation of miR-145 prevents the onset of PAH in preclinical models (Caruso et al., 2012). Anti-miR-145 oligonucleotides were encapsulated within cationic lipid nanoconstructs in the range of 80–100 nm in size. Efficacy was examined in a Sugen/Hypoxia model of PAH in rats, wherein NPs were administered IV every 2 weeks starting on week 8 after model induction. Liposomes delivered anti-miR-145 to diseased lungs, and decreased the expression of miR-145 by more than 50%. The median wall thickness of pulmonary arteries was reduced following treatment with anti-miR-145 liposomes (**Figure 6**), with results suggesting that the therapy was capable of repairing vascular remodeling. Moreover, RV systolic pressure decreased by ~25% and RV hypertrophy was reduced following treatment with anti-miR-145 liposomes compared to non-silencing oligonucleotide controls.

CONCLUSION

Pulmonary arterial hypertension results in considerable patient morbidity, proving irreversible and fatal. Present-day pharmacotherapies suffer from considerable limitations. Short-term drug pharmacokinetics, where half-lives are on the order of minutes, contribute to low bioavailability in diseased tissues and adverse side effects. Nanoplatforms have improved the pharmacokinetic profiles of chemotherapeutics, with increased accumulation of NPs in tumors through the EPR effect. Importantly, enhanced accumulation and persistence of NPs has been observed in lungs undergoing PAH following both intravenous and inhalational routes of delivery. Endothelial dysfunction present in diseased lung vasculature results in NP accumulation in pulmonary arterioles, and NPs are found largely associated with vascular cells such as PAECs and PASMCs. Given the vital role these cells play in PAH progression, NPs stand to significantly impact PAH treatment strategies and patient outcomes.

Herein, we have provided an overview of NP-based drug delivery strategies in PAH, with particular emphasis on improvements in vascular remodeling and hemodynamics. Several nanotherapies involved the use of clinically approved drugs for PAH, while others exploited novel signaling pathways and molecular targets. The future of NP-based drug delivery in PAH will surely involve advancements on two fronts. On the one hand, innovations in materials science will lead to sophisticated nanotechnology platforms highly capable of delivering drugs to target cells in diseased lungs. These nanoconstructs will incorporate moieties for successful navigation of barriers to transport to the lungs, facilitate sustained delivery of therapeutics over time, and enable combined delivery of drugs and genetic material for synergistic treatment. Additionally, nanotherapies in PAH will benefit from enhanced understanding of molecular drivers of the disease. Insights into processes of PAH pathogenesis can potentially provide overexpressed surface receptors for active targeting to target cells and provide novel targets for gene therapy. Thus, rational design of NPs that can effectively target diseased lungs combined with molecular-targeted therapeutics will lead to more efficacious treatment outcomes in PAH.

AUTHOR CONTRIBUTIONS

All authors listed have made a substantial, direct and intellectual contribution to the work, and approved it for publication.

FUNDING

This work was supported by the George and Angelina Kostas Research Center for Cardiovascular Nanomedicine. VS-I is grateful for support from the Instituto Tecnológico y de Estudios Superiores de Monterrey and the Consejo Nacional de Ciencia y Tecnología (CONACyT, 490202/278979). MF is grateful for the Ernest Cockrell Jr. Presidential Distinguished Endowed Chair in the Department of Nanomedicine at the Houston Methodist Research Institute. AG is grateful for funding from the Vaughan Foundation. HK-Q is grateful for funding from the National Institutes of Health (NIH 1R01 HL138510-01) and the UTHealth Pulmonary Center of Excellence Discovery Award Program.

ACKNOWLEDGMENTS

We thank Matthew G. Landry for assistance with schematics.

REFERENCES

Acharya, S., and Sahoo, S. K. (2011). PLGA nanoparticles containing various anticancer agents and tumour delivery by EPR effect. *Adv. Drug Deliv. Rev.* 63, 170–183. doi: 10.1016/j.addr.2010.10.008

Akagi, S., Nakamura, K., Matsubara, H., Kondo, M., Miura, D., Matoba, T., et al. (2016). Intratracheal administration of prostacyclin analogue-incorporated nanoparticles ameliorates the development of monocrotaline and sugen-hypoxia-induced pulmonary arterial hypertension. *J. Cardiovasc. Pharmacol.* 67, 290–298. doi: 10.1097/FJC.0000000000000352

Akagi, S., Nakamura, K., Miura, D., Saito, Y., Matsubara, H., Ogawa, A., et al. (2015). Delivery of imatinib-incorporated nanoparticles into lungs suppresses the development of monocrotaline-induced pulmonary arterial hypertension. *Int. Heart J.* 56, 354–359. doi: 10.1536/ihj.14-338

Anderson, R., Franch, A., Castell, M., Perez-Cano, F. J., Brauer, R., Pohlers, D., et al. (2010). Liposomal encapsulation enhances and prolongs the anti-inflammatory effects of water-soluble dexamethasone phosphate in experimental adjuvant arthritis. *Arthritis Res. Ther.* 12:R147. doi: 10.1186/ar3089

Aversa, M., Porter, S., and Granton, J. (2015). Comparative safety and tolerability of endothelin receptor antagonists in pulmonary arterial hypertension. *Drug Saf.* 38, 419–435. doi: 10.1007/s40264-015-0275-y

Bae, Y., Nishiyama, N., Fukushima, S., Koyama, H., Yasuhiro, M., and Kataoka, K. (2005). Preparation and biological characterization of polymeric micelle drug carriers with intracellular pH-triggered drug release property: tumor permeability, controlled subcellular drug distribution, and enhanced in vivo antitumor efficacy. *Bioconjug. Chem.* 16, 122–130. doi: 10.1021/bc0498166

Banerjee, D., Harfouche, R., and Sengupta, S. (2011). Nanotechnology-mediated targeting of tumor angiogenesis. *Vasc. Cell* 3:3. doi: 10.1186/2045-824X-3-3

Barenholz, Y. (2012). Doxil®–the first FDA-approved nano-drug: lessons learned. *J. Control. Release* 160, 117–134. doi: 10.1016/j.jconrel.2012.03.020

Barst, R. J., McGoon, M., McLaughlin, V., Tapson, V., Rich, S., Rubin, L., et al. (2003). Beraprost therapy for pulmonary arterial hypertension. *J. Am. Coll. Cardiol.* 41, 2119–2125. doi: 10.1016/S0735-1097(03)00463-7

Barst, R. J., Rubin, L. J., Long, W. A., McGoon, M. D., Rich, S., Badesch, D. B., et al. (1996). A comparison of continuous intravenous epoprostenol (prostacyclin) with conventional therapy for primary pulmonary hypertension. *N. Engl. J. Med.* 334, 296–301. doi: 10.1056/NEJM199602013340504

Beck-Broichsitter, M., Bohr, A., Aragao-Santiago, L., Klingl, A., and Kissel, T. (2017). Formulation and process considerations for the design of sildenafil-loaded polymeric microparticles by vibrational spray-drying. *Pharm. Dev. Technol.* 22, 691–698. doi: 10.3109/10837450.2015.1098661

Beck-Broichsitter, M., Schweiger, C., Schmehl, T., Gessler, T., Seeger, W., and Kissel, T. (2012). Characterization of novel spray-dried polymeric particles for controlled pulmonary drug delivery. *J. Control. Release* 158, 329–335. doi: 10.1016/j.jconrel.2011.10.030

Beckman, J. A., and Creager, M. A. (2006). The nonlipid effects of statins on endothelial function. *Trends Cardiovasc. Med.* 16, 156–162. doi: 10.1016/j.tcm.2006.03.003

Berry, G., Billingham, M., Alderman, E., Richardson, P., Torti, F., Lum, B., et al. (1998). The use of cardiac biopsy to demonstrate reduced cardiotoxicity in AIDS Kaposi's sarcoma patients treated with pegylated liposomal doxorubicin. *Ann. Oncol.* 9, 711–716. doi: 10.1023/A:1008216430806

Bivas-Benita, M., Romeijn, S., Junginger, H. E., and Borchard, G. (2004). PLGA-PEI nanoparticles for gene delivery to pulmonary epithelium. *Eur. J. Pharm. Biopharm.* 58, 1–6. doi: 10.1016/j.ejpb.2004.03.008

Blanco, E., Bey, E. A., Khemtong, C., Yang, S. G., Setti-Guthi, J., Chen, H., et al. (2010). Beta-lapachone micellar nanotherapeutics for non-small cell lung cancer therapy. *Cancer Res.* 70, 3896–3904. doi: 10.1158/0008-5472.CAN-09-3995

Blanco, E., Hsiao, A., Mann, A. P., Landry, M. G., Meric-Bernstam, F., and Ferrari, M. (2011). Nanomedicine in cancer therapy: innovative trends and prospects. *Cancer Sci.* 102, 1247–1252. doi: 10.1111/j.1349-7006.2011.01941.x

Blanco, E., Kessinger, C. W., Sumer, B. D., and Gao, J. (2009). Multifunctional micellar nanomedicine for cancer therapy. *Exp. Biol. Med.* 234, 123–131. doi: 10.3181/0808-MR-250

Blanco, E., Sangai, T., Wu, S., Hsiao, A., Ruiz-Esparza, G. U., Gonzalez-Delgado, C. A., et al. (2014). Colocalized delivery of rapamycin and paclitaxel to tumors enhances synergistic targeting of the PI3K/Akt/mTOR pathway. *Mol. Ther.* 22, 1310–1319. doi: 10.1038/mt.2014.27

Blanco, E., Shen, H., and Ferrari, M. (2015). Principles of nanoparticle design for overcoming biological barriers to drug delivery. *Nat. Biotechnol.* 33, 941–951. doi: 10.1038/nbt.3330

Braet, F., Wisse, E., Bomans, P., Frederik, P., Geerts, W., Koster, A., et al. (2007). Contribution of high-resolution correlative imaging techniques in the study of the liver sieve in three-dimensions. *Microsc. Res. Tech.* 70, 230–242. doi: 10.1002/jemt.20408

Cabral, H., Matsumoto, Y., Mizuno, K., Chen, Q., Murakami, M., Kimura, M., et al. (2011). Accumulation of sub-100 nm polymeric micelles in poorly permeable tumours depends on size. *Nat. Nanotechnol.* 6, 815–823. doi: 10.1038/nnano.2011.166

Caruso, P., Dempsie, Y., Stevens, H. C., McDonald, R. A., Long, L., Lu, R., et al. (2012). A role for miR-145 in pulmonary arterial hypertension: evidence from mouse models and patient samples. *Circ. Res.* 111, 290–300. doi: 10.1161/CIRCRESAHA.112.267591

Carvajal, J. A., Germain, A. M., Huidobro-Toro, J. P., and Weiner, C. P. (2000). Molecular mechanism of cGMP-mediated smooth muscle relaxation. *J. Cell. Physiol.* 184, 409–420. doi: 10.1002/1097-4652(200009)184:3<409::AID-JCP16>3.0.CO;2-K

Chen, L., Nakano, K., Kimura, S., Matoba, T., Iwata, E., Miyagawa, M., et al. (2011). Nanoparticle-mediated delivery of pitavastatin into lungs ameliorates the development and induces regression of monocrotaline-induced pulmonary artery hypertension. *Hypertension* 57, 343–350. doi: 10.1161/HYPERTENSIONAHA.110.157032

Chen, L. T., and Weiss, L. (1973). The role of the sinus wall in the passage of erythrocytes through the spleen. *Blood* 41, 529–537.

Choi, H. S., Liu, W., Misra, P., Tanaka, E., Zimmer, J. P., Itty Ipe, B., et al. (2007). Renal clearance of quantum dots. *Nat. Biotechnol.* 25, 1165–1170. doi: 10.1038/nbt1340

Chono, S., Tauchi, Y., Deguchi, Y., and Morimoto, K. (2005). Efficient drug delivery to atherosclerotic lesions and the antiatherosclerotic effect by dexamethasone incorporated into liposomes in atherogenic mice. *J. Drug Target.* 13, 267–276. doi: 10.1080/10611860500159030

Christie, R. J., Matsumoto, Y., Miyata, K., Nomoto, T., Fukushima, S., Osada, K., et al. (2012). Targeted polymeric micelles for siRNA treatment of experimental cancer by intravenous injection. *ACS Nano* 6, 5174–5189. doi: 10.1021/nn300942b

Collum, S. D., Amione-Guerra, J., Cruz-Solbes, A. S., DiFrancesco, A., Hernandez, A. M., Hanmandlu, A., et al. (2017). Pulmonary hypertension associated with Idiopathic pulmonary fibrosis: current and future perspectives. *Can. Respir. J.* 2017:1430350. doi: 10.1155/2017/1430350

Crescencio, M. E., Rodríguez, E., Páez, A., Masso, F. A., Montaño, L. F., and López-Marure, R. (2009). Statins inhibit the proliferation and induce cell death of human papilloma virus positive and negative cervical cancer cells. *Int. J. Biomed. Sci.* 5, 411–420.

Dai, J., Lin, S., Cheng, D., Zou, S., and Shuai, X. (2011a). Interlayer-crosslinked micelle with partially hydrated core showing reduction and pH dual sensitivity for pinpointed intracellular drug release. *Angew. Chem. Int. Ed. Engl.* 50, 9404–9408. doi: 10.1002/anie.201103806

Dai, J., Zou, S., Pei, Y., Cheng, D., Ai, H., and Shuai, X. (2011b). Polyethylenimine-grafted copolymer of poly(L-lysine) and poly(ethylene glycol) for gene delivery. *Biomaterials* 32, 1694–1705. doi: 10.1016/j.biomaterials.2010.10.044

Danhier, F., Ansorena, E., Silva, J. M., Coco, R., Le Breton, A., and Preat, V. (2012). PLGA-based nanoparticles: an overview of biomedical applications. *J. Control. Release* 161, 505–522. doi: 10.1016/j.jconrel.2012.01.043

Del Pozo, R., Hernandez Gonzalez, I., and Escribano-Subias, P. (2017). The prostacyclin pathway in pulmonary arterial hypertension: a clinical review. *Expert Rev. Respir. Med.* 11, 491–503. doi: 10.1080/17476348.2017.1317599

Delcroix, M., and Howard, L. (2015). Pulmonary arterial hypertension: the burden of disease and impact on quality of life. *Eur. Respir. Rev.* 24, 621–629. doi: 10.1183/16000617.0063-2015

Dinarvand, R., Sepehri, N., Manoochehri, S., Rouhani, H., and Atyabi, F. (2011). Polylactide-co-glycolide nanoparticles for controlled delivery of anticancer agents. *Int. J. Nanomedicine* 6, 877–895. doi: 10.2147/IJN.S18905

Duarte, J. D., Hanson, R. L., and Machado, R. F. (2013). Pharmacologic treatments for pulmonary hypertension: exploring pharmacogenomics. *Future Cardiol.* 9, 335–349. doi: 10.2217/fca.13.6

Duggan, S. T., Keam, S. J., and Burness, C. B. (2017). Selexipag: a review in pulmonary arterial hypertension. *Am. J. Cardiovasc. Drugs* 17, 73–80. doi: 10.1007/s40256-016-0209-9

Durymanov, M., Kamaletdinova, T., Lehmann, S. E., and Reineke, J. (2017). Exploiting passive nanomedicine accumulation at sites of enhanced vascular permeability for non-cancerous applications. *J. Control. Release* 261, 10–22. doi: 10.1016/j.jconrel.2017.06.013

Dvir, T., Bauer, M., Schroeder, A., Tsui, J. H., Anderson, D. G., Langer, R., et al. (2011). Nanoparticles targeting the infarcted heart. *Nano Lett.* 11, 4411–4414. doi: 10.1021/nl2025882

Fang, J., Nakamura, H., and Maeda, H. (2011). The EPR effect: unique features of tumor blood vessels for drug delivery, factors involved, and limitations and augmentation of the effect. *Adv. Drug Deliv. Rev.* 63, 136–151. doi: 10.1016/j.addr.2010.04.009

Ferrari, M. (2005). Cancer nanotechnology: opportunities and challenges. *Nat. Rev. Cancer* 5, 161–171. doi: 10.1038/nrc1566

Galie, N., Ghofrani, H. A., Torbicki, A., Barst, R. J., Rubin, L. J., Badesch, D., et al. (2005). Sildenafil citrate therapy for pulmonary arterial hypertension. *N. Engl. J. Med.* 353, 2148–2157. doi: 10.1056/NEJMoa050010

Galie, N., Hoeper, M. M., Humbert, M., Torbicki, A., Vachiery, J. L., Barbera, J. A., et al. (2009). Guidelines for the diagnosis and treatment of pulmonary hypertension: the task force for the diagnosis and treatment of pulmonary hypertension of the European Society of Cardiology (ESC) and the European Respiratory Society (ERS), endorsed by the International Society of Heart and Lung Transplantation (ISHLT). *Eur. Heart J.* 30, 2493–2537. doi: 10.1093/eurheartj/ehp297

Galié, N., Manes, A., and Branzi, A. (2004). The endothelin system in pulmonary arterial hypertension. *Cardiovasc. Res.* 61, 227–237. doi: 10.1016/j.cardiores.2003.11.026

Ghofrani, H. A., Galie, N., Grimminger, F., Grunig, E., Humbert, M., Jing, Z. C., et al. (2013). Riociguat for the treatment of pulmonary arterial hypertension. *N. Engl. J. Med.* 369, 330–340. doi: 10.1056/NEJMoa1209655

Giovannoni, M. P., Vergelli, C., Graziano, A., and Dal Piaz, V. (2010). PDE5 inhibitors and their applications. *Curr. Med. Chem.* 17, 2564–2587. doi: 10.2174/092986710791859360

Goncharova, E. A. (2013). mTOR and vascular remodeling in lung diseases: current challenges and therapeutic prospects. *FASEB J.* 27, 1796–1807. doi: 10.1096/fj.12-222224

Gottlieb, J. (2013). Lung transplantation for interstitial lung diseases and pulmonary hypertension. *Semin. Respir. Crit. Care Med.* 34, 281–287. doi: 10.1055/s-0033-1348462

Gupta, N., Rashid, J., Nozik-Grayck, E., McMurtry, I. F., Stenmark, K. R., and Ahsan, F. (2017). Cocktail of superoxide dismutase and fasudil encapsulated in targeted liposomes slows PAH progression at a reduced dosing frequency. *Mol. Pharm.* 14, 830–841. doi: 10.1021/acs.molpharmaceut.6b01061

Gupta, V., Gupta, N., Shaik, I. H., Mehvar, R., McMurtry, I. F., Oka, M., et al. (2013). Liposomal fasudil, a rho-kinase inhibitor, for prolonged pulmonary preferential vasodilation in pulmonary arterial hypertension. *J. Control. Release* 167, 189–199. doi: 10.1016/j.jconrel.2013.01.011

Hamilton, A., Biganzoli, L., Coleman, R., Mauriac, L., Hennebert, P., Awada, A., et al. (2002). EORTC 10968: a phase I clinical and pharmacokinetic study of polyethylene glycol liposomal doxorubicin (Caelyx, Doxil) at a 6-week interval in patients with metastatic breast cancer. European organization for research and treatment of cancer. *Ann. Oncol.* 13, 910–918. doi: 10.1093/annonc/mdf157

Harris, J. M., and Chess, R. B. (2003). Effect of pegylation on pharmaceuticals. *Nat. Rev. Drug Discov.* 2, 214–221. doi: 10.1038/nrd1033

Hobbs, S. K., Monsky, W. L., Yuan, F., Roberts, W. G., Griffith, L., Torchilin, V. P., et al. (1998). Regulation of transport pathways in tumor vessels: role of tumor type and microenvironment. *Proc. Natl. Acad. Sci. U.S.A.* 95, 4607–4612. doi: 10.1073/pnas.95.8.4607

Hoesel, B., and Schmid, J. A. (2013). The complexity of NF-kappaB signaling in inflammation and cancer. *Mol. Cancer* 12:86. doi: 10.1186/1476-4598-12-86

Houchin, M. L., and Topp, E. M. (2008). Chemical degradation of peptides and proteins in PLGA: a review of reactions and mechanisms. *J. Pharm. Sci.* 97, 2395–2404. doi: 10.1002/jps.21176

Houssaini, A., Abid, S., Mouraret, N., Wan, F., Rideau, D., Saker, M., et al. (2013). Rapamycin reverses pulmonary artery smooth muscle cell proliferation in pulmonary hypertension. *Am. J. Respir. Cell Mol. Biol.* 48, 568–577. doi: 10.1165/rcmb.2012-0429OC

Huang, S., and Houghton, P. J. (2001). Mechanisms of resistance to rapamycins. *Drug Resist. Updat.* 4, 378–391. doi: 10.1054/drup.2002.0227

Huang, S. L., Kee, P. H., Kim, H., Moody, M. R., Chrzanowski, S. M., Macdonald, R. C., et al. (2009). Nitric oxide-loaded echogenic liposomes for nitric oxide delivery and inhibition of intimal hyperplasia. *J. Am. Coll. Cardiol.* 54, 652–659. doi: 10.1016/j.jacc.2009.04.039

Humbert, M., Lau, E. M., Montani, D., Jais, X., Sitbon, O., and Simonneau, G. (2014). Advances in therapeutic interventions for patients with pulmonary arterial hypertension. *Circulation* 130, 2189–2208. doi: 10.1161/CIRCULATIONAHA.114.006974

Ikeda, T., Nakamura, K., Akagi, S., Kusano, K. F., Matsubara, H., Fujio, H., et al. (2010). Inhibitory effects of simvastatin on platelet-derived growth factor signaling in pulmonary artery smooth muscle cells from patients with idiopathic pulmonary arterial hypertension. *J. Cardiovasc. Pharmacol.* 55, 39–48. doi: 10.1097/FJC.0b013e3181c0419c

Ishihara, T., Hayashi, E., Yamamoto, S., Kobayashi, C., Tamura, Y., Sawazaki, R., et al. (2015). Encapsulation of beraprost sodium in nanoparticles: analysis of sustained release properties, targeting abilities and pharmacological activities in animal models of pulmonary arterial hypertension. *J. Control. Release* 197, 97–104. doi: 10.1016/j.jconrel.2014.10.029

Ishikura, F., Beppu, S., Hamada, T., Khandheria, B. K., Seward, J. B., and Nehra, A. (2000). Effects of sildenafil citrate (Viagra) combined with nitrate on the heart. *Circulation* 102, 2516–2521. doi: 10.1161/01.CIR.102.20.2516

Istvan, E. (2003). Statin inhibition of HMG-CoA reductase: a 3-dimensional view. *Atheroscler. Suppl.* 4, 3–8. doi: 10.1016/S1567-5688(03)00003-5

Jain, P. P., Leber, R., Nagaraj, C., Leitinger, G., Lehofer, B., Olschewski, H., et al. (2014). Liposomal nanoparticles encapsulating iloprost exhibit enhanced vasodilation in pulmonary arteries. *Int. J. Nanomedicine* 9, 3249–3261. doi: 10.2147/IJN.S63190

Jhaveri, A. M., and Torchilin, V. P. (2014). Multifunctional polymeric micelles for delivery of drugs and siRNA. *Front. Pharmacol.* 5:77. doi: 10.3389/fphar.2014.00077 doi: 10.3389/fphar.2014.00077

Kalmanti, L., Saussele, S., Lauseker, M., Muller, M. C., Dietz, C. T., Heinrich, L., et al. (2015). Safety and efficacy of imatinib in CML over a period of 10 years: data from the randomized CML-study IV. *Leukemia* 29, 1123–1132. doi: 10.1038/leu.2015.36

Kamigaki, M., Sasaki, T., Serikawa, M., Inoue, M., Kobayashi, K., Itsuki, H., et al. (2011). Statins induce apoptosis and inhibit proliferation in cholangiocarcinoma cells. *Int. J. Oncol.* 39, 561–568. doi: 10.3892/ijo.2011.1087

Kaneko, F. T., Arroliga, A. C., Dweik, R. A., Comhair, S. A., Laskowski, D., Oppedisano, R., et al. (1998). Biochemical reaction products of nitric oxide as quantitative markers of primary pulmonary hypertension. *Am. J. Respir. Crit. Care Med.* 158, 917–923. doi: 10.1164/ajrccm.158.3.9802066

Kapoor, D. N., Bhatia, A., Kaur, R., Sharma, R., Kaur, G., and Dhawan, S. (2015). PLGA: a unique polymer for drug delivery. *Ther. Deliv.* 6, 41–58. doi: 10.4155/tde.14.91

Khanal, S., Adhikari, U., Rijal, N. P., Bhattarai, S. R., Sankar, J., and Bhattarai, N. (2016). pH-responsive PLGA nanoparticle for controlled payload delivery of diclofenac sodium. *J. Funct. Biomater.* 7:E21. doi: 10.3390/jfb7030021

Kimura, S., Egashira, K., Chen, L., Nakano, K., Iwata, E., Miyagawa, M., et al. (2009). Nanoparticle-mediated delivery of nuclear factor kappaB decoy into lungs ameliorates monocrotaline-induced pulmonary arterial hypertension. *Hypertension* 53, 877–883. doi: 10.1161/HYPERTENSIONAHA.108.121418

Kleemann, E., Schmehl, T., Gessler, T., Bakowsky, U., Kissel, T., and Seeger, W. (2007). Iloprost-containing liposomes for aerosol application in pulmonary arterial hypertension: formulation aspects and stability. *Pharm. Res.* 24, 277–287. doi: 10.1007/PL00022055

Klinger, J. R., and Kadowitz, P. J. (2017). The nitric oxide pathway in pulmonary vascular disease. *Am. J. Cardiol.* 120, S71–S79. doi: 10.1016/j.amjcard.2017.06.012

Lang, I. M., and Gaine, S. P. (2015). Recent advances in targeting the prostacyclin pathway in pulmonary arterial hypertension. *Eur. Respir. Rev.* 24, 630–641. doi: 10.1183/16000617.0067-2015

Lau, E. M. T., Giannoulatou, E., Celermajer, D. S., and Humbert, M. (2017). Epidemiology and treatment of pulmonary arterial hypertension. *Nat. Rev. Cardiol.* 14, 603–614. doi: 10.1038/nrcardio.2017.84

Lefer, D. J. (2002). Statins as potent antiinflammatory drugs. *Circulation* 106, 2041–2042. doi: 10.1161/01.CIR.0000033635.42612.88

LeVarge, B. L. (2015). Prostanoid therapies in the management of pulmonary arterial hypertension. *Ther. Clin. Risk Manag.* 11, 535–547. doi: 10.2147/TCRM.S75122

Liu, J. B., Lee, H., Huesca, M., Young, A. P., and Allen, C. (2006). Liposome formulation of a novel hydrophobic aryl-imidazole compound for anti-cancer therapy. *Cancer Chemother. Pharmacol.* 58, 306–318. doi: 10.1007/s00280-005-0161-x

Liu, K., Zhang, X., Cao, G., Liu, Y., Liu, C., Sun, H., et al. (2016). Intratracheal instillation of ethyl pyruvate nanoparticles prevents the development of shunt-flow-induced pulmonary arterial hypertension in a rat model. *Int. J. Nanomedicine* 11, 2587–2599. doi: 10.2147/IJN.S103183

Maeda, H., Nakamura, H., and Fang, J. (2013). The EPR effect for macromolecular drug delivery to solid tumors: improvement of tumor uptake, lowering of systemic toxicity, and distinct tumor imaging in vivo. *Adv. Drug Deliv. Rev.* 65, 71–79. doi: 10.1016/j.addr.2012.10.002

Makadia, H. K., and Siegel, S. J. (2011). Poly Lactic-co-Glycolic Acid (PLGA) as biodegradable controlled drug delivery carrier. *Polymers* 3, 1377–1397. doi: 10.3390/polym3031377

Matsumura, Y., and Maeda, H. (1986). A new concept for macromolecular therapeutics in cancer chemotherapy: mechanism of tumoritropic accumulation of proteins and the antitumor agent smancs. *Cancer Res.* 46(12 Pt 1), 6387–6392.

McDonald, D. M., and Choyke, P. L. (2003). Imaging of angiogenesis: from microscope to clinic. *Nat. Med.* 9, 713–725. doi: 10.1038/nm0603-713

McGoon, M. D., Frost, A. E., Oudiz, R. J., Badesch, D. B., Galie, N., Olschewski, H., et al. (2006). Ambrisentan rescue therapy in patients with pulmonary arterial hypertension who discontinued bosentan or sitaxsentan due to liver function abnormalities. *Chest* 130:254S. doi: 10.1378/chest.130.4_MeetingAbstracts.254S-a

McLaughlin, V. V., Archer, S. L., Badesch, D. B., Barst, R. J., Farber, H. W., Lindner, J. R., et al. (2009). ACCF/AHA 2009 expert consensus document on pulmonary hypertension: a report of the American College of Cardiology Foundation task force on expert consensus documents and the American Heart Association: developed in collaboration with the American College of Chest Physicians, American Thoracic Society, Inc., and the Pulmonary Hypertension Association. *Circulation* 119, 2250–2294. doi: 10.1161/CIRCULATIONAHA.109.192230

McLaughlin, V. V., and McGoon, M. D. (2006). Pulmonary arterial hypertension. *Circulation* 114, 1417–1431. doi: 10.1161/CIRCULATIONAHA.104.503540

McLaughlin, V. V., and Palevsky, H. I. (2013). Parenteral and inhaled prostanoid therapy in the treatment of pulmonary arterial hypertension. *Clin. Chest Med.* 34, 825–840. doi: 10.1016/j.ccm.2013.09.003

McLendon, J. M., Joshi, S. R., Sparks, J., Matar, M., Fewell, J. G., Abe, K., et al. (2015). Lipid nanoparticle delivery of a microRNA-145 inhibitor improves experimental pulmonary hypertension. *J. Control. Release* 210, 67–75. doi: 10.1016/j.jconrel.2015.05.261

Metselaar, J. M., van den Berg, W. B., Holthuysen, A. E., Wauben, M. H., Storm, G., and van Lent, P. L. (2004). Liposomal targeting of glucocorticoids to synovial lining cells strongly increases therapeutic benefit in collagen type II arthritis. *Ann. Rheum. Dis.* 63, 348–353. doi: 10.1136/ard.2003.009944

Milojkovic, D., and Apperley, J. (2009). Mechanisms of resistance to imatinib and second-generation tyrosine inhibitors in chronic myeloid leukemia. *Clin. Cancer Res.* 15, 7519–7527. doi: 10.1158/1078-0432.CCR-09-1068

Mohamed, N. A., Ahmetaj-Shala, B., Duluc, L., Mackenzie, L. S., Kirkby, N. S., Reed, D. M., et al. (2016). A new NO-releasing nanoformulation for the treatment of pulmonary arterial hypertension. *J. Cardiovasc. Transl. Res.* 9, 162–164. doi: 10.1007/s12265-016-9684-2

Montani, D., Chaumais, M. C., Guignabert, C., Gunther, S., Girerd, B., Jais, X., et al. (2014). Targeted therapies in pulmonary arterial hypertension. *Pharmacol. Ther.* 141, 172–191. doi: 10.1016/j.pharmthera.2013.10.002

Morrell, N. W. (2006). Pulmonary hypertension due to BMPR2 mutation: a new paradigm for tissue remodeling? *Proc. Am. Thorac. Soc.* 3, 680–686. doi: 10.1513/pats.200605-118SF

Morrell, N. W., Adnot, S., Archer, S. L., Dupuis, J., Jones, P. L., MacLean, M. R., et al. (2009). Cellular and molecular basis of pulmonary arterial hypertension. *J. Am. Coll. Cardiol.* 54(Suppl. 1), S20–S31. doi: 10.1016/j.jacc.2009.04.018

Mubarak, K. K. (2010). A review of prostaglandin analogs in the management of patients with pulmonary arterial hypertension. *Respir. Med.* 104, 9–21. doi: 10.1016/j.rmed.2009.07.015

Murray, F., MacLean, M. R., and Pyne, N. J. (2002). Increased expression of the cGMP-inhibited cAMP-specific (PDE3) and cGMP binding cGMP-specific (PDE5) phosphodiesterases in models of pulmonary hypertension. *Br. J. Pharmacol.* 137, 1187–1194. doi: 10.1038/sj.bjp.0704984

Nagaoka, K., Matoba, T., Mao, Y., Nakano, Y., Ikeda, G., Egusa, S., et al. (2015). A new therapeutic modality for acute myocardial infarction: nanoparticle-mediated delivery of pitavastatin induces cardioprotection from ischemia-reperfusion injury via activation of pi3k/akt pathway and anti-inflammation in a rat model. *PLoS One* 10:e0132451. doi: 10.1371/journal.pone.0132451

Nahar, K., Absar, S., Gupta, N., Kotamraju, V. R., McMurtry, I. F., Oka, M., et al. (2014). Peptide-coated liposomal fasudil enhances site specific vasodilation in pulmonary arterial hypertension. *Mol. Pharm.* 11, 4374–4384. doi: 10.1021/mp500456k

Nakamura, K., Matsubara, H., Akagi, S., Sarashina, T., Ejiri, K., Kawakita, N., et al. (2017). Nanoparticle-mediated drug delivery system for pulmonary arterial hypertension. *J. Clin. Med.* 6:E48. doi: 10.3390/jcm6050048

Nakano, Y., Matoba, T., Tokutome, M., Funamoto, D., Katsuki, S., Ikeda, G., et al. (2016). Nanoparticle-mediated delivery of irbesartan induces cardioprotection from myocardial ischemia-reperfusion injury by antagonizing monocyte-mediated inflammation. *Sci. Rep.* 6:29601. doi: 10.1038/srep29601

Nasongkla, N., Shuai, X., Ai, H., Weinberg, B. D., Pink, J., Boothman, D. A., et al. (2004). cRGD-functionalized polymer micelles for targeted doxorubicin delivery. *Angew. Chem. Int. Ed. Engl.* 43, 6323–6327. doi: 10.1002/anie.200460800

Oka, M., Fagan, K. A., Jones, P. L., and McMurtry, I. F. (2008). Therapeutic potential of RhoA/Rho kinase inhibitors in pulmonary hypertension. *Br. J. Pharmacol.* 155, 444–454. doi: 10.1038/bjp.2008.239

Olschewski, H., Ghofrani, H. A., Schmehl, T., Winkler, J., Wilkens, H., Hoper, M. M., et al. (2000). Inhaled iloprost to treat severe pulmonary hypertension. an uncontrolled trial. German PPH study group. *Ann. Intern. Med.* 132, 435–443. doi: 10.7326/0003-4819-132-6-200003210-00003

Paranjpe, M., and Muller-Goymann, C. C. (2014). Nanoparticle-mediated pulmonary drug delivery: a review. *Int. J. Mol. Sci.* 15, 5852–5873. doi: 10.3390/ijms15045852

Pattni, B. S., Chupin, V. V., and Torchilin, V. P. (2015). New developments in liposomal drug delivery. *Chem. Rev.* 115, 10938–10966. doi: 10.1021/acs.chemrev.5b00046

Paulis, L. E., Geelen, T., Kuhlmann, M. T., Coolen, B. F., Schafers, M., Nicolay, K., et al. (2012). Distribution of lipid-based nanoparticles to infarcted myocardium with potential application for MRI-monitored drug delivery. *J. Control. Release* 162, 276–285. doi: 10.1016/j.jconrel.2012.06.035

Pauwaa, S., Machado, R. F., and Desai, A. A. (2011). Survival in pulmonary arterial hypertension: a brief review of registry data. *Pulm. Circ.* 1, 430–431. doi: 10.4103/2045-8932.87314

Perez-Zoghbi, J. F., Bai, Y., and Sanderson, M. J. (2010). Nitric oxide induces airway smooth muscle cell relaxation by decreasing the frequency of agonist-induced Ca^{2+} oscillations. *J. Gen. Physiol.* 135, 247–259. doi: 10.1085/jgp.200910365

Raja, S. G. (2010). Endothelin receptor antagonists for pulmonary arterial hypertension: an overview. *Cardiovasc. Ther.* 28, e65–e71. doi: 10.1111/j.1755-5922.2010.00158.x

Ricciotti, E., and FitzGerald, G. A. (2011). Prostaglandins and inflammation. *Arterioscler. Thromb. Vasc. Biol.* 31, 986–1000. doi: 10.1161/ATVBAHA.110.207449

Ridker, P. M., Rifai, N., Pfeffer, M. A., Sacks, F., and Braunwald, E. (1999). Long-term effects of pravastatin on plasma concentration of c-reactive protein. The cholesterol and recurrent events (CARE) investigators. *Circulation* 100, 230–235. doi: 10.1161/01.CIR.100.3.230

Riehemann, K., Schneider, S. W., Luger, T. A., Godin, B., Ferrari, M., and Fuchs, H. (2009). Nanomedicine–challenge and perspectives. *Angew. Chem. Int. Ed. Engl.* 48, 872–897. doi: 10.1002/anie.200802585

Rosano, L., Spinella, F., and Bagnato, A. (2013). Endothelin 1 in cancer: biological implications and therapeutic opportunities. *Nat. Rev. Cancer* 13, 637–651. doi: 10.1038/nrc3546

Ruan, C. H., Dixon, R. A., Willerson, J. T., and Ruan, K. H. (2010). Prostacyclin therapy for pulmonary arterial hypertension. *Tex. Heart Inst. J.* 37, 391–399.

Ruiz-Esparza, G. U., Segura-Ibarra, V., Cordero-Reyes, A. M., Youker, K. A., Serda, R. E., Cruz-Solbes, A. S., et al. (2016). A specifically designed nanoconstruct associates, internalizes, traffics in cardiovascular cells, and accumulates in failing myocardium: a new strategy for heart failure diagnostics and therapeutics. *Eur. J. Heart Fail.* 18, 169–178. doi: 10.1002/ejhf.463

Russwurm, M., and Koesling, D. (2004). NO activation of guanylyl cyclase. *EMBO J.* 23, 4443–4450. doi: 10.1038/sj.emboj.7600422

Ryan, J. J., and Archer, S. L. (2014). The right ventricle in pulmonary arterial hypertension: disorders of metabolism, angiogenesis and adrenergic signaling in right ventricular failure. *Circ. Res.* 115, 176–188. doi: 10.1161/CIRCRESAHA.113.301129

Safdar, Z. (2011). Treatment of pulmonary arterial hypertension: the role of prostacyclin and prostaglandin analogs. *Respir. Med.* 105, 818–827. doi: 10.1016/j.rmed.2010.12.018

Sahni, S., Ojrzanowski, M., Majewski, S., and Talwar, A. (2016). Pulmonary arterial hypertension: a current review of pharmacological management. *Pneumonol. Alergol. Pol.* 84, 47–61. doi: 10.5603/PiAP.a2015.0084

Schermuly, R. T., Stasch, J. P., Pullamsetti, S. S., Middendorff, R., Muller, D., Schluter, K. D., et al. (2008). Expression and function of soluble guanylate cyclase in pulmonary arterial hypertension. *Eur. Respir. J.* 32, 881–891. doi: 10.1183/09031936.00114407

Segura-Ibarra, V., Amione-Guerra, J., Cruz-Solbes, A. S., Cara, F. E., Iruegas-Nunez, D. A., Wu, S., et al. (2017). Rapamycin nanoparticles localize in diseased lung vasculature and prevent pulmonary arterial hypertension. *Int. J. Pharm.* 524, 257–267. doi: 10.1016/j.ijpharm.2017.03.069

Seo, B., Oemar, B. S., Siebenmann, R., von Segesser, L., and Luscher, T. F. (1994). Both ETA and ETB receptors mediate contraction to endothelin-1 in human blood vessels. *Circulation* 89, 1203–1208. doi: 10.1161/01.CIR.89.3.1203

Seyfarth, H. J., Hammerschmidt, S., Halank, M., Neuhaus, P., and Wirtz, H. R. (2013). Everolimus in patients with severe pulmonary hypertension: a safety and efficacy pilot trial. *Pulm. Circ.* 3, 632–638. doi: 10.1086/674311

Shah, S. J. (2012). Pulmonary hypertension. *JAMA* 308, 1366–1374. doi: 10.1001/jama.2012.12347

Shibuya, M., Hirai, S., Seto, M., Satoh, S., Ohtomo, E., and Fasudil Ischemic Stroke Study Group (2005). Effects of fasudil in acute ischemic stroke: results of a prospective placebo-controlled double-blind trial. *J. Neurol. Sci.* 238, 31–39. doi: 10.1016/j.jns.2005.06.003

Sitbon, O., Channick, R. N., Delcroix, M., Ghofrani, H.-A., Jansa, P., Le Brun, F.-O., et al. (2014). Macitentan reduces the risk of morbidity and mortality irrespective of the presence or absence of right ventricular (RV) impairment: results from the randomised SERAPHIN trial in pulmonary arterial hypertension (PAH). *Eur. Respir. J.* 44:3419.

Sitbon, O., and Vonk Noordegraaf, A. (2017). Epoprostenol and pulmonary arterial hypertension: 20 years of clinical experience. *Eur. Respir. Rev.* 26:160055. doi: 10.1183/16000617.0055-2016

Song, W., Tang, Z., Zhang, D., Zhang, Y., Yu, H., Li, M., et al. (2014). Anti-tumor efficacy of c(RGDfK)-decorated polypeptide-based micelles co-loaded with docetaxel and cisplatin. *Biomaterials* 35, 3005–3014. doi: 10.1016/j.biomaterials.2013.12.018

Stenmark, K. R., Fagan, K. A., and Frid, M. G. (2006). Hypoxia-induced pulmonary vascular remodeling: cellular and molecular mechanisms. *Circ. Res.* 99 675–691. doi: 10.1161/01.RES.0000243584.45145.3f

Stenmark, K. R., Meyrick, B., Galie, N., Mooi, W. J., and McMurtry, I. F. (2009). Animal models of pulmonary arterial hypertension: the hope for etiological discovery and pharmacological cure. *Am. J. Physiol. Lung Cell. Mol. Physiol.* 297, L1013–L1032. doi: 10.1152/ajplung.00217.2009

Stigliano, C., Ramirez, M. R., Singh, J. V., Aryal, S., Key, J., Blanco, E., et al. (2017). Methotraxate-loaded hybrid nanoconstructs target vascular lesions and inhibit atherosclerosis progression in ApoE(-/-) mice. *Adv. Healthc. Mater.* 6:1601286. doi: 10.1002/adhm.201601286

Ta, T., and Porter, T. M. (2013). Thermosensitive liposomes for localized delivery and triggered release of chemotherapy. *J. Control. Release* 169, 112–125. doi: 10.1016/j.jconrel.2013.03.036

Takeda, M., Maeda, T., Ishihara, T., Sakamoto, H., Yuki, K., Takasaki, N., et al. (2009). Synthesis of prostaglandin E-1 phosphate derivatives and their encapsulation in biodegradable nanoparticles. *Pharm. Res.* 26, 1792–1800. doi: 10.1007/s11095-009-9891-5

Tonelli, A. R., Haserodt, S., Aytekin, M., and Dweik, R. A. (2013). Nitric oxide deficiency in pulmonary hypertension: pathobiology and implications for therapy. *Pulm. Circ.* 3, 20–30. doi: 10.4103/2045-8932.109911

Tuder, R. M., Cool, C. D., Geraci, M. W., Wang, J., Abman, S. H., Wright, L., et al. (1999). Prostacyclin synthase expression is decreased in lungs front patients with severe pulmonary hypertension. *Am. J. Respir. Crit. Care Med.* 159, 1925–1932. doi: 10.1164/ajrccm.159.6.9804054

Ulbrich, W., and Lamprecht, A. (2010). Targeted drug-delivery approaches by nanoparticulate carriers in the therapy of inflammatory diseases. *J. R. Soc. Interface* 7(Suppl. 1), S55–S66. doi: 10.1098/rsif.2009.0285.focus

Xu, R., Zhang, G., Mai, J., Deng, X., Segura-Ibarra, V., Wu, S., et al. (2016). An injectable nanoparticle generator enhances delivery of cancer therapeutics. *Nat. Biotechnol.* 34, 414–418. doi: 10.1038/nbt.3506

Zhang, X. X., McIntosh, T. J., and Grinstaff, M. W. (2012). Functional lipids and lipoplexes for improved gene delivery. *Biochimie* 94, 42–58. doi: 10.1016/j.biochi.2011.05.005

Zhou, C., Townsley, M. I., Alexeyev, M., Voelkel, N. F., and Stevens, T. (2016). Endothelial hyperpermeability in severe pulmonary arterial hypertension: role of store-operated calcium entry. *Am. J. Physiol. Lung Cell. Mol. Physiol.* 311, L560–L569. doi: 10.1152/ajplung.00057.2016

Zhou, G., Chen, T., and Raj, J. U. (2015). MicroRNAs in pulmonary arterial hypertension. *Am. J. Respir. Cell Mol. Biol.* 52, 139–151. doi: 10.1165/rcmb.2014-0166TR

8

Thin Air, Thick Vessels: Historical and Current Perspectives on Hypoxic Pulmonary Hypertension

Jason M. Young[1,2], *David R. Williams*[2] *and A. A. Roger Thompson*[2,3*]

[1] *Edinburgh Medical School, University of Edinburgh, Edinburgh, United Kingdom,* [2] *Apex (Altitude Physiology Expeditions), Edinburgh, United Kingdom,* [3] *Department of Infection, Immunity and Cardiovascular Disease, University of Sheffield, Sheffield, United Kingdom*

***Correspondence:**
A. A. Roger Thompson
r.thompson@sheffield.ac.uk

The association between pulmonary hypertension (PH) and hypoxia is well-established, with two key mechanistic processes, hypoxic pulmonary vasoconstriction and hypoxia-induced vascular remodeling, driving changes in pulmonary arterial pressure. In contrast to other forms of pulmonary hypertension, the vascular changes induced by hypoxia are reversible, both in humans returning to sea-level from high altitude and in animal models. This raises the intriguing possibility that the molecular drivers of these hypoxic processes could be targeted to modify pulmonary vascular remodeling in other contexts. In this review, we outline the history of research into PH and hypoxia, before discussing recent advances in our understanding of this relationship at the molecular level, focussing on the role of the oxygen-sensing transcription factors, hypoxia inducible factors (HIFs). Emerging links between HIF and vascular remodeling highlight the potential utility in inhibiting this pathway in pulmonary hypertension and raise possible risks of activating this pathway using HIF-stabilizing medications.

Keywords: hypoxia, pulmonary hypertension, altitude, vascular remodeling, hypoxic pulmonary vasoconstriction (HPV)

INTRODUCTION

Pulmonary hypertension (PH) is a feature of several distinct clinical phenotypes which, by differing means, result in increased pressure within the pulmonary vasculature. Despite some advancements in treatment over recent years (1), most forms of PH are progressive and life-limiting. In the current classification of PH etiology, Group III (PH due to lung diseases and/or hypoxia) is the second commonest cause of elevated pulmonary artery pressure, behind heart disease (2). Group III encompasses a broad range of conditions such as chronic obstructive pulmonary disease (COPD), interstitial lung disease (ILD) and sleep apnoea (3). Alongside parenchymal changes, two key pathological process, pulmonary vascular remodeling and vasoconstriction, contribute to PH in this group of patients but treatment with pulmonary vasodilators has, to date, been disappointing. New approaches to the management of these patients are thus urgently required to improve outcomes as 3 year survival remains as low as 33% for COPD patients with mean pulmonary artery pressures >40 mmHg (1, 2, 4). While pathologic mechanisms might vary depending on the underlying disease or phenotype, a better understanding of the defining component of Group III disorders, hypoxia, may help provide new targets for therapies.

A causal relationship between hypoxia and PH is well established; hypoxia is frequently used to both precipitate PH in animal models (5) and to induce aberrant cell phenotypes *in vitro* (6). These approaches have greatly improved our understanding of the underlying physiological mechanisms that drive the pathology. In humans, compelling evidence of the effects of hypoxia on pulmonary vascular tone and remodeling derives from studies performed at altitude, where the inherent reduction in barometric pressure results in hypobaric hypoxia. This approach is advantageous for evaluation of the effects of hypoxia on the pulmonary vasculature in relative isolation, without the complicating factors of disease. In this review, we outline the historical context of research into PH and hypoxia and discuss emerging molecular mechanisms for this relationship. We focus on the role of the oxygen-sensing transcription factors, hypoxia inducible factors (HIFs), and links between HIFs and vascular remodeling.

IMPORTANT DEFINITIONS

Before embarking on this review, it is important to consider the definitions of PH used within this manuscript and others. The term PH is used to describe elevation in mean pulmonary artery pressure (mPAP) from any cause. PH was first classified as a mPAP exceeding 25 mmHg at the 1st World Symposium on Pulmonary Hypertension (WSPH) in 1973 (7). Notably, at the recent 6th WSPH, the upper limit of normal for mPAP was set at 20 mmHg, argued in part due to emerging evidence of poorer survival in patients with mPAPs of 21–24 mmHg and in part based on the distribution of values in healthy population data (8). For a diagnosis of pre-capillary pulmonary hypertension, of any cause, an increased pulmonary vascular resistance (PVR > 3 WU) is also required (8). Pre-capillary hemodynamics that meet the above definition, are not uncommon in patients with lung disease (4, 9), but the prevalence of increased PVR in healthy individuals who are hypoxic without lung disease, for example altitude residents and those with sleep apnoea, is less clear and will be discussed later (10). To avoid confusion we have, where possible, included values (±SD) from the cited literature indicating recorded pulmonary artery pressures and/or PVR.

PULMONARY HYPERTENSION: A HISTORY

Pathological changes in the pulmonary arteries co-existing with right ventricular hypertrophy (RVH) were first observed by the German physician Ernst von Romberg toward the end of the nineteenth century, which he coined "pulmonary vascular sclerosis" (11). However, the etiology of PH remained elusive at this time and was wrongly attributed to syphilis for many years (12, 13). Whilst the British cardiologist Oscar Brenner eventually disproved this link in 1935, he could not provide an explanation for pulmonary vascular changes coinciding with RVH (14). It was only with the advent of right heart catheterization in the mid-twentieth century that these observations were intrinsically linked by raised pulmonary artery pressure (PAP). Despite extensive use in animals in the early twentieth century, cardiac catheterization in humans was widely considered unsafe until Werner Forssman's gallant self-catheterization of his right heart in 1929 (15, 16). Whilst this act of bravery was initially poorly received and widely ignored by the medical community, American physicians Dickinson Richards and Andrew Cournard would recognize the importance of Forssman's work in the 1940s. Their pioneering research characterized mPAP in cardiac and pulmonary diseases for the first time, a feat for which they were awarded a Nobel Prize, together with Forssman, in 1956 (17, 18).

Further work in the 1950s began to establish the clinical and pathological features of PH. In 1951, one of the first detailed descriptions of the haemodynamic profiles of the disease was provided by David Dresdale who also observed cyanosis, orthopnoea and haemoptysis amongst patients with idiopathic PH. Dresdale and others termed their findings "primary pulmonary hypertension" (19, 20); this terminology provided important nomenclature for the emerging research community. Additionally, an extensive characterization of histological changes in PH was described by Donald Heath who, in collaboration with William Whitaker, first detailed extensive thickening of the pulmonary arterial wall associated with fibrosis in 1953, amongst individuals with congenital heart disease, mitral stenosis and idiopathic PH (21, 22). Heath and Jesse Edwards subsequently produced a detailed histological classification system correlated to PH severity in Eisenmenger's syndrome, which ranged from early vascular medial hypertrophy in mild PH to late intimal fibrosis in severe disease (23).

EARLY LINKS BETWEEN ACUTE HYPOXIA AND PULMONARY HYPERTENSION

Despite elevated PAP being first associated with ventilatory failure in 1852 (24), a causal relationship between hypoxia and PH only became established in 1946 when von Euler and colleagues demonstrated increased mPAP on exposing cats to both hypoxia and hypercapnia (25); in 1947, Dresdale reported similar findings in humans (26). These reports constituted the first measurements of pulmonary arteriole constriction to hypoxia, or hypoxic pulmonary vasoconstriction (HPV), a phenotype which contrasts the vasodilating properties of hypoxia on the systemic circulation (27). At the time, von Euler correctly hypothesized that this physiological response is beneficial in order to shunt blood from areas of regional lung hypoxia that stems from reduced ventilation, thus maintaining blood oxygenation (a concept now termed ventilation-perfusion matching).

However, the adverse effects of this response in the context of more global alveolar hypoxia soon became apparent, particularly in relation to high-altitude pulmonary oedema (HAPE). Whilst a syndrome of cough, blood-stained sputum and severe breathlessness was previously recognized in high altitude sojourners, Hurtado was the first to attribute this to pulmonary oedema in 1937 (28). PH was first identified as co-existing with HAPE in 1962 by Fred et al. (29) in one patient with a mPAP of 46 mmHg, although Hultgren and Spickard had proposed this association in 1960, providing clinical descriptions of a loud second heart sound and electrographic changes consistent with PH in 41 cases of HAPE in Peru (30). Hultgren et al. subsequently confirmed this in seven individuals following acute exposure to high altitude in 1964, in whom mPAP ranged from 33 to 117 mmHg (PVR reported in 2 patients; 8 and 36 WU). Importantly, the authors could also demonstrate a degree of reversibility of pulmonary oedema and elevated mPAP on administration of 100% oxygen (31). Further work from this group, along with others (32), identified a predisposition to pulmonary oedema amongst five individuals with mPAPs of 38.8 ± 10.3 mmHg on ascent to 3,100 m (33).

Despite the early identification of PH as a factor in the pathogenesis of HAPE, how this results in oedema formation remains unclear. Hultgren proposed that because HPV is heterogeneous, areas of the lung are over-perfused leading to pulmonary capillary stress failure in HAPE (34). Indeed, subsequent studies in HAPE-susceptible individuals have provided evidence of exaggerated heterogeneity of perfusion (35), whilst haemodynamic studies have also demonstrated elevated pulmonary capillary pressures (19 ± 1 mmHg vs. 13 ± 1 mmHg in controls) and arterial pressures (mPAP 37 ± 2 mmHg vs. 26 ± 1 mmHg in controls) amongst such individuals at high altitude (36). Other factors in HAPE pathogenesis include impaired nitric oxide (NO) biosynthesis and reduced alveolar fluid reabsorption, as reviewed here (37, 38).

CHRONIC HYPOXIA AND REMODELING OF THE PULMONARY VASCULATURE

Concurrently, research began to investigate the effects of chronic hypoxia on the pulmonary vasculature of high-altitude populations. This initially began in cattle which often developed significant oedema around the lower chest at high altitude, dubbed "brisket disease," a condition that caused significant mortality upon ascent. In the 1940s, Rue Jensen first identified right ventricular dilatation and failure co-existing with brisket disease amongst the high-altitude cattle populations in Colorado (39), with further work with Grover, Reeves and Will identifying a positive correlation between the severity of RVH and the degree of raised PAP (40). Further breeding experiments led by Grover and Reeves suggested an autosomal dominant inheritance of HAPH among these cattle (41, 42). In contrast to Hultgren's later findings amongst patients with HAPE (31), 100% oxygen did not fully reverse PH in cattle (40), indicating a lesser role of HPV in PH pathogenesis in the setting of chronic hypoxia. Interestingly, similar findings were documented by Anand et al. amongst a human population, detailing evidence of peripheral oedema and shortness of breath amongst Indian soldiers who had sojourned at altitudes above 5,800 m for 18 weeks. While no measurements were made at altitude, shortly after return to sea level right heart catheter studies on these patients provided evidence of mild pre-capillary pulmonary hypertension, with mPAP and PVR measured as 26.1 ± 4.5 mmHg and 3.41 ± 2.46 WU, respectively (43).

Elevated PAP in human populations at high altitude was first reported in 1956 by Canepa in one of the first reports of human right heart catheterization in Peruvians from Morochoca (4,540 m), recorded as 25 (range 18–29) mmHg amongst 7 highlanders and 34 and 35 mmHg amongst two chronic mountain sickness patients; however, these findings were initially attributed to polycythaemia, abnormal ventilation and increased cardiac output (44). It would take the work of fellow Peruvians Dante Peñaloza and Javier Arias-Stella in the 1960s to demonstrate that PH amongst high altitude populations was associated with remodeling of the pulmonary vasculature (45–47). Earlier work from Peñaloza confirmed elevated mPAP (23 ± 5.1 mmHg) associated with RVH in Peruvians at high altitude (48, 49) and interestingly, also identified PH amongst new born children both at sea level and altitude, with a swift resolution at sea level that was not recognized amongst Peruvian infants (50). Importantly, the authors found no difference in PAWP and CO between residents at sea level and altitude, with PVR elevated at 4.15 ± 2.66 WU in high altitude dwellers (46, 49). Oxygen administration to Peruvian adults resulted in minor reductions in mPAP of 15–20% (45, 47), mirroring prior results in brisket disease (40) and indicating that pulmonary vascular remodeling was primarily responsible for PH in chronic hypoxia. Further weight to this hypothesis was added by Jensen and Alexander, who later demonstrated a linear relationship between medial hypertrophy of the pulmonary arteries and PAP amongst cattle (51). Notably, despite a failure of immediate resolution with oxygen, Peñaloza identified a normalization of mPAP (12 ± 1.9 mmHg) and PVR (1.81 ± 0.44 WU) amongst high altitude populations following 2 years spent at sea level, demonstrating that changes as a result of chronic hypoxic exposure are not permanent (52). Complementing this finding, the Indian soldiers studied by Anand et al., who had developed signs of right heart failure during their altitude sojourn, made a full recovery, with reversal of cardiomegaly and normalization of mPAP (16.3 ± 2.9 mmHg) and PVR pulmonary vascular resistance (1.34 ± 0.48 WU) 12–16 weeks after descent from high altitude (43).

While the above studies in healthy individuals imply that elevated pulmonary artery pressures are found ubiquitously at altitude, whether the magnitude of elevation in healthy altitude residents reaches that which would define pre-capillary PH remains unclear. A recent meta-analysis by Soria et al. revealed an average systolic PAP of 25.3 mmHg across high altitude populations with a wider distribution than amongst lowlanders implying a low prevalence of PH even by the new WHO criteria (8, 10). Furthermore, PVR is seldom reported and a notable limitation of reported PVRs among historical catheterization studies at altitude, is the lack of correction for hematocrit. Resistance to blood flow is dependent upon viscosity as well as vessel dimensions [reviewed by Vanderpool and Naeije (53)], with equations describing the relationship derived from isolated perfused lung experiments involving alterations in haematocrit (54). Thus, reporting of haematocrit is important in determining true PVR (53, 55) and may lead to false assumptions regarding the extent of vascular remodeling in healthy individuals following hypoxic exposure.

Nonetheless, similar to observations in patients with lung disease, there is a sub-population of altitude residents who develop more severe PH. A consensus definition for high altitude PH (HAPH) was reported in 2005, to encompass those at altitude with exaggerated elevation in PAP and signs of RVH and right heart failure (56). HAPH was defined as a mean PAP of >30 mmHg (or systolic PAP > 50 mmHg) in the absence of excessive erythrocytosis (hemoglobin concentration > 19 g/dl for women, > 21 g/dl for men). This definition allowed discrimination between HAPH and chronic mountain sickness (CMS), in which there is excessive erythrocytosis (57, 58). Despite aforementioned epidemiological studies indicating the rarity of HAPH by the above definition amongst high altitude dwellers (10), the study of such individuals may provide important insights into molecular pathways that drive vasoconstrictive and remodeling processes in both hypoxic PH and, potentially, other forms of PAH. However, it could be argued that a revision of the current definition of HAPH, to include haematocrit-corrected PVR, would facilitate this research.

INTER-SPECIES VARIATION AT HIGH ALTITUDE

Following these results in both humans and cattle, Donald Heath became interested in inter-species variability in the pulmonary vasculature of high-altitude populations. Heath traveled to Cerro de Pasco, Peru (4,330 m) alongside Peter Harris in 1965, in what became the first of many high-altitude research expeditions dedicated to PH research. A descriptive overview of this work is provided by one of this article's authors in **Box 1**. In 1974, Heath published their research in llamas (*Lama glama*) demonstrating a lack of pulmonary arteriole muscularisation or RVH at altitude, contrasting previous findings in humans and cattle (*Bos taurus*) (59). A similarly thin walled pulmonary vasculature was also identified in the Himalayan yak (*Bos grunniens*) (60), indicating a role of natural selection in the loss of the thick-walled, reactive pulmonary arteries typically characteristic of the Bos genus.

An interesting biological issue arises when species from within the same genus interbreed; one such example is the interbreeding of cattle giving rise to species such as the dzo (cow x yak) and stol (dzo x bull) (61). In 1986, work from Peter Harris' group identified that protection from PH correlated with the degree of yak heritage; whilst dzos and yaks demonstrated minimal PH, half of the stols had significantly raised PAPs similar to that of cattle (62), indicating a degree of inheritance. These observations lend support to the concept that animals indigenous to high altitude have become genetically adapted to their hypoxic environment, vs. acclimatization as seen in other species.

Box 1 | Adaptation to chronic hypoxia in the andes.

The recognition of the different biological classes of man and mammals at high altitude is best illustrated by taking a mental stroll around the streets and surrounding countryside of any small town in the high Andes. The studies undertaken demonstrated that there was no single stereotypical man or mammal at high altitude.

Cerro de Pasco is a mining community with a population of 70,000 people, situated at an attitude of 4330 m in the central Andes of Peru. In the streets will be a number of lowlanders who may have arrived at high altitude in a matter of hours from Lima on the coast. Approximately 50% will suffer from benign acute mountain sickness mainly characterized by headache, insomnia, anorexia, nausea and dizziness. These symptoms are the consequence of hypobaric hypoxia and may be regarded as the physiological components of early acclimatization.

In contrast, most people are native Quechua Indians born and bred in the high Andes. These descendants of the Inca people have very characteristic physical features of skin color with deeply polycythaemic and suffused conjunctiva and lips. Many will have a capacious chest which looks prominent and out of proportion to their short and stocky physique. These native highlanders lead normal busy lives at high altitude. They participate in vigorous games of football at altitudes exceeding the summit of the Matterhorn in the Swiss Alps.

Living on the pastures surrounding Cerro de Pasco are examples of indigenous mountain animals such as the llama, alpaca, vicuna and guanaco. These animals have been living on the Andean altiplano for many thousands of years. One cannot help but be impressed by the vigor and activity of these animals in an atmosphere characterized by severe hypobaric hypoxia.

MOLECULAR MECHANISMS OF PH IN ACUTE AND CHRONIC HYPOXIC EXPOSURE

While the evidence above clearly illustrates connections between hypoxic exposure and pulmonary hypertension, the underlying genetic, molecular and cellular mechanisms that regulate these phenotypes remain unclear and in part, controversial. Nonetheless, basic science work over the last 25 years has advanced our understanding of common pathways that govern both adaptation to altitude and hypoxia-induced PH. Reviewed extensively elsewhere (63–65), pulmonary vasoconstriction in acute hypoxia comprises at least two phases involving distinct mechanisms. Initially, changes in redox status within smooth muscle cell mitochondria mediate alterations in potassium and voltage-gated calcium channel flux, promoting contraction (63). Subsequently, vasoconstriction is maintained by mechanisms that include reduced bioavailability of NO (66), release of endothelial-derived vasoconstrictors (67) and increases in myofilament calcium sensitivity (68). The focus of this article will be on the role of the hypoxia-inducible factors (HIFs) in vascular remodeling due to chronic hypoxic exposure.

HYPOXIA-INDUCIBLE FACTORS (HIFs) AND PULMONARY VASCULAR REMODELING

HIFs are a family of heterodimeric transcription factors, discovered in 1995 (69), whose alpha subunits are stabilized in hypoxia by the inhibition of oxygen-dependent prolyl hydroxylase (PHD) enzyme activity (70); under normoxic conditions, hydroxylation of HIF-alpha by PHDs targets them for ubiquitination by the VHL complex, resulting in subsequent proteasomal degradation (**Figure 1**) (71). Whilst HIF-1α is expressed ubiquitously throughout body tissues (72), HIF-2α expression is tissue specific with an endothelial bias (73, 74). In hypoxia, stabilization of HIF-α subunits induces transcription of targets with a wide range of functions.

Perhaps unsurprisingly, genetic variation in the HIF pathway has been identified amongst indigenous altitude dwellers. Notably, genome wide association studies in the Tibetan

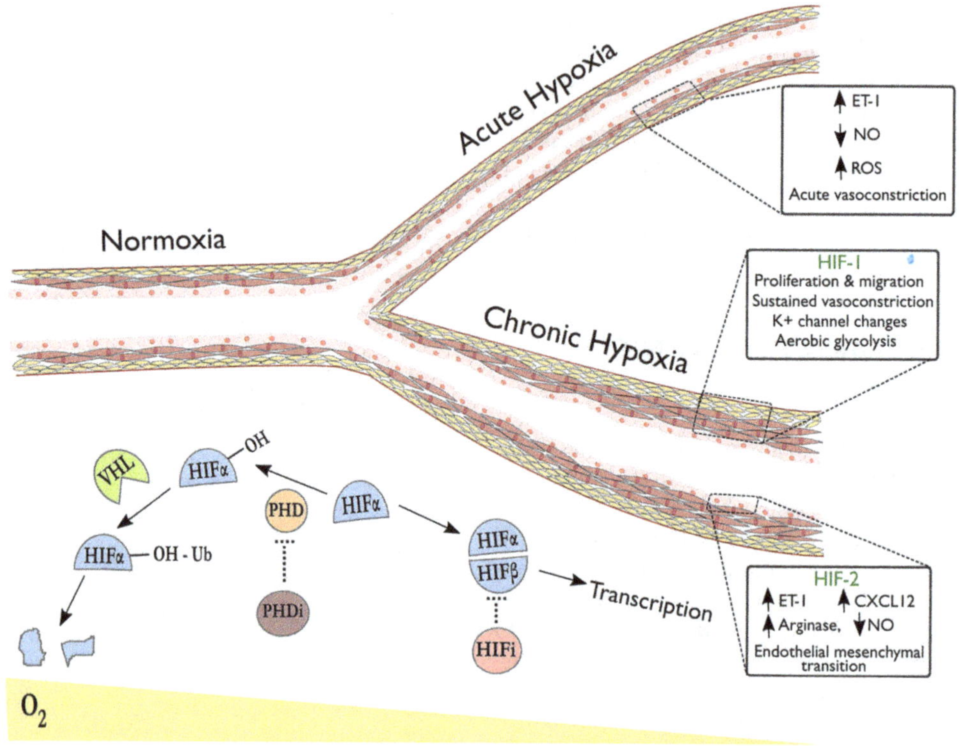

FIGURE 1 | Pulmonary vascular responses to hypoxia with emphasis on the role of HIF isoforms in remodeling. The right upper branch of this vessel depicts vasoconstriction in acute hypoxia, occurring due to alterations in redox and NO signaling and release of vasoactive mediators. The lower branch indicates remodeling in the context of sustained hypoxic exposure and illustrates HIF-dependent processes revealed by tissue-specific deletion of HIF-isoforms in endothelial cells (HIF-2α) or smooth muscle cells (HIF-1α). Below the vessel, a schematic shows degradation of hydroxylated HIF-α subunits in normoxia via the von-Hippel Lindau (VHL) pathway. In hypoxia or following treatment with prolyl hydroxylase inhibitors (PHDi), HIF-α stabilization and dimerization with HIF-β occurs, leading to transcription of target genes. HIF inhibitors (HIFi) with specific activity against HIF-2α are in clinical development.

population have identified single nucleotide polymorphisms (SNPs) in *EPAS1* (encoding HIF-2α) and *ELGN1* (encoding PHD2) that were not enriched in lowlanders (75–77). *EPAS1* variants were associated with lower PAP (78) and a high frequency *ELGN1* mutation has been linked to reduced proliferation of erythroid progenitors in response to EPO, thus dampening hypoxia-induced erythrocytosis (79). These findings demonstrate a selection pressure for specific HIF pathway polymorphisms over 25,000 years at altitude that has aided adaptation for the Tibetan population. Interestingly, such variation is not observed in Andean counterparts, a population that has resided at altitude for 15,000 years and who are more susceptible to PH (80, 81) and erythrocytosis (82).

However, the evidence for HIF pathway polymorphisms influencing remodeling processes is weakened by the observation that correction for erythrocytosis reduces mPAP amongst Andean populations to values near those of Tibetans (57). Thus, correcting for erythrocytosis argues against a susceptibility of Andean populations to HIF-mediated remodeling processes. In light of the new PH definition (8), however, Andean corrected mPAP remains consistently above 20 mmHg at rest and the slope of rise in mPAP with cardiac output is steeper than that of lowlanders (57).

Furthermore, evidence from murine models strongly implicates the HIF pathway in hypoxia-induced vascular remodeling. Soon after the discovery of the pathway, early work in both *Hif1a* and *Hif2a* heterozygotes revealed a marked reduction in PH and vascular remodeling following chronic exposure to 10% oxygen (83, 84). Conversely, *HIF2A* (*EPAS1*) gain-of-function mutations can predispose to PH; a *Hif2a* variant in high altitude cattle increases susceptibility to brisket disease (85), whilst a *HIF2A* mutation causing familial erythrocytosis is also associated with elevated systolic PAP in humans (86). A mouse generated to have the same G536W gain-of-function mutation in the *Hif2a* gene also developed erythrocytosis and PH, providing further evidence of cross-species conservation of this HIF-2α role (87). Additionally, both animal models and patients with Chuvash polycythaemia (CP), characterized by a VHL mutation, exhibit marked erythrocytosis and elevated PAP that could be rescued in mice by *Hif2a* but not *Hif1a* deletion (88–90). While the descriptions of elevated PAP in humans with CP did not include right heart catheter data or haematocrit-corrected PVR, it is worth noting that elevations in systolic PAP and vessel muscularisation in young mice with homozygous VHL mutations, preceded the onset of polycythaemia (90).

TISSUE-SPECIFIC MANIPULATION OF HIF EXPRESSION REVEALS DISTINCT ROLES FOR HIF ISOFORMS IN PULMONARY VASCULAR REMODELING

Evidence is now emerging as to how the HIF isoforms regulate pulmonary vascular cell function, with advances gained through use of murine tissue-specific deletion models, see **Figure 1**. For example, HIF-1α has been implicated in both vasoconstriction and vascular cell proliferation, the two key components of hypoxic pulmonary hypertension. Ball et al. demonstrated that inducible *Hif1a* deletion in PASMCs reduced right ventricular systolic pressure, arterial wall thickness and vessel muscularisation in chronic hypoxia (91), whilst Shiekh et al. reported a dependence on *Hif1a* in PASMC progenitors in order to drive distal migration and expansion (92). Proposed mechanisms that could explain these findings include enhanced intracellular calcium via *Hif1a* dependent downregulation of K^+ channels (93) and upregulation of transient receptor potential calcium channels (94), recognized to enhance vasoconstriction, PASMC proliferation and migration (95). HIF-1α also mediates pro-proliferative metabolic changes in PASMCs and fibroblasts that could contribute to hypoxia-induced remodeling. One widely recognized consequence of HIF signaling amongst cancer cells is the favoring of glycolysis over oxidative phosphorylation in aerobic conditions, known as the "Warburg effect," inducing glycolytic enzymes to enhance ATP production and promote tumor growth (96, 97). Interestingly, HIF signaling amongst pulmonary arterial smooth muscle cells (PASMCs) and fibroblasts results in a similar shift to aerobic glycolysis as seen in tumors (98–100), with increased glucose uptake observed in the lungs of rats with hypoxia-induced PH and in PAH patients (101, 102). This metabolic reprogramming of pulmonary vascular cells has proven stable *ex vivo* with evidence of underlying epigenetic regulation (103, 104). Targeting these mechanisms may limit hypoxia-induced PASMC proliferation in the pulmonary vasculature.

Consistent with its predominantly endothelial expression profile, a growing body of evidence implicates endothelial cell (EC) HIF-2α expression as essential for pulmonary vascular remodeling through varied biological mechanisms, see **Figure 1** Two studies have demonstrated severe and spontaneous PH following *Phd2* knockdown in murine ECs (105, 106). Double knockouts of *Phd2* and either HIF isoform revealed that this was a *Hif2a*-mediated phenotype (105, 106) but the studies highlighted different mechanisms: one associating HIF-2α expression with reduced expression of the potent vasoconstrictor endothelin-1 (ET-1) (106) and the other demonstrating HIF-2α involvement in CXCL12-mediated PASMC proliferation (105). Reduced EC *Phd2* expression was also observed amongst occlusive vessels in IPAH (105), implying relevance to human pathology. Notably, these *Phd2* knockout mice did not develop polycythaemia prior to the development of PH.

The NO synthesis pathway has also been implicated in EC HIF-2α-mediated remodeling. Cowburn et al. observed a similar level of protection from hypoxia-induced PH as *Hif2a* knockdown following EC-specific deletion of arginase-1 (*Arg1*), a downstream HIF-2α target and negative regulator of NO synthesis (107). Additionally, ECs from PH patients demonstrated impaired NO production *in vitro*, restored on arginase inhibition (107). A further mechanism by which HIF-2α could contribute to remodeling is through regulation of endothelial-mesenchymal transition (EMT), a process implicated in pathogenic remodeling (108). Tang et al. showed that markers of EMT were regulated by HIF-2α in ECs and that while endothelial-specific deletion of *Hif2a* protected mice from hypoxia-induced PH, deletion of *Hif2a* in vascular smooth muscle cells did not (109).

There remain notable controversies in the literature surrounding HIF-mediated regulation of remodeling. Whilst Ball et al. demonstrated a role for PASMC *Hif1a* in chronic hypoxic remodeling using a tamoxifen-inducible conditional deletion (91), Kim et al. reported enhanced pulmonary arterial tone in the absence of arterial muscularisation following constitutive PASMC-specific *Hif1a* deletion (110). Similarly, constitutive EC *Hif1a* deletion was found to confer no protection to PH by three authors (105–107), whilst Shiekh et al. could ameliorate PH following tamoxifen-inducible conditional EC *Hif1a* deletion, which prevented PASMC expansion and distal migration (92). Alongside evidence detailing the importance of embryonic HIF signaling for the developing vasculature (111), these observed differences imply a role of early HIF-1α signaling in pulmonary vessel development.

The crucial role of HIF isoforms in hypoxia-induced PH has identified the inhibition of these molecules as an important strategy for targeting remodeling processes. Whilst efforts to develop HIF pathway inhibitors have previously proven challenging due to poor efficacy, HIF isoform specificity and adverse effects (112, 113), a specific HIF-2α small molecule inhibitor developed to treat renal cancer has demonstrated a favorable safety profile in a recent Phase I trial (114). Encouragingly, the use of another HIF-2α inhibitor, C76, has recently been demonstrated to attenuate remodeling in three murine models of PH, with no notable inhibition of HIF-1α (115).

The pleiotropic nature of HIF signaling has identified several other pathways as possible therapeutic targets. Using congenic linkage analysis, Zhao et al. discovered a dependence on intracellular zinc in hypoxia-induced remodeling. Homozygous deletion of the zinc transporter ZIP12, a target of both HIF-1α and HIF-2α, was found to attenuate PAP, RVH and vascular remodeling in chronic hypoxia (116). Additionally, induction of ZIP12 was also reported in the pulmonary tissue in Brisket disease and highland human populations (116). How intracellular zinc influences hypoxia-induced remodeling remains unclear; however, targeting intracellular zinc homeostasis may represent a further therapeutic strategy.

CONCLUSIONS

This article has reviewed historical observations connecting hypoxia and pulmonary hypertension and described more recent insights into the molecular mechanisms involved in hypoxia-induced remodeling. Notably, the evidence linking HIF expression to processes involved in vascular remodeling strongly raises the prospect of HIF inhibition, and in particular HIF-2α inhibition, as a strategy in order to ameliorate vascular pathology in the context of chronic hypoxia. The recent success of a HIF-2α inhibitor in several murine models is supportive of such a strategy and may lead to the consideration of clinical trials amongst PH patients in the future. However, the mechanistic links between HIF-pathway activation and PH, notably the development of spontaneous PH following *Phd2* deletion, should also raise a note of caution for use of PHD inhibitors which are currently undergoing Phase II/III clinical trials in renal anemia (117).

Genetic insights gained through study of high-altitude populations suggests that a greater appreciation of factors underlying altitude adaptation may highlight further mechanisms involved in the regulation of vascular remodeling. However, while similarities exist between the pathological features of hypoxia-induced PH and other forms of the disease, the extent of overlap in the pathological mechanisms, even for patients with chronic respiratory disease, remains unclear. Furthermore, the notable lack of correction for haematocrit in previous work reporting PVR at altitude casts some doubt over some of the apparent differences between altitude populations, which may in fact be due to differences in haematocrit. Nonetheless, a reversal of PH on return to sea level provides the tantalizing possibility that exploiting endogenous mechanisms might provide agents that reverse vascular remodeling in hypoxic disease. Therefore, there is still hope that lessons learned from studying hypoxia-induced disease could impact on the search for agents that target pervasive vascular remodeling in other forms of PH.

AUTHOR CONTRIBUTIONS

JY wrote the manuscript. DW and AART drafted additional text and edited the manuscript. All authors approved the final version.

REFERENCES

1. Gall H, Felix JF, Schneck FK, Milger K, Sommer N, Voswinckel R, et al. The giessen pulmonary hypertension registry: survival in pulmonary hypertension subgroups. *J Hear Lung Transplant.* (2017) 36:957–67. doi: 10.1016/j.healun.2017.02.016
2. Strange G, Playford D, Stewart S, Deague JA, Nelson H, Kent A, et al. Pulmonary hypertension: prevalence and mortality in the Armadale echocardiography cohort. *Heart.* (2012) 98:1805–11. doi: 10.1136/heartjnl-2012-301992
3. Simonneau G, Gatzoulis MA, Adatia I, Celermajer D, Denton C, Ghofrani A, et al. Updated clinical classification of pulmonary hypertension. *J Am Coll Cardiol.* (2013) 62:D34–41. doi: 10.1016/j.jacc.2013.10.029
4. Hurdman J, Condliffe R, Elliot CA, Swift A, Rajaram S, Davies C, et al. Pulmonary hypertension in COPD: results from the ASPIRE registry. *Eur Respir J.* (2013) 41:1292–301. doi: 10.1183/09031936.00079512
5. Maarman G, Lecour S, Butrous G, Thienemann F, Sliwa K. A comprehensive review: the evolution of animal models in pulmonary hypertension research; are we there yet? *Pulm Circ.* (2013) 3:739–56. doi: 10.1086/674770
6. Pugliese SC, Poth JM, Fini MA, Olschewski A, El Kasmi KC, Stenmark KR. The role of inflammation in hypoxic pulmonary hypertension: from cellular mechanisms to clinical phenotypes. *Am J Physiol Lung Cell Mol Physiol.* (2015) 308:L229–52. doi: 10.1152/ajplung.00238.2014
7. Hatano S, Strasser T, World Health Organization. *Primary Pulmonary Hypertension: Report on a WHO Meeting, Geneva, 15-17 October 1973.* Geneva: World Health Organization (1975).
8. Galiè N, McLaughlin V V, Rubin LJ, Simonneau G. An overview of the 6th World Symposium on Pulmonary Hypertension. *Eur Respir J.* (2019) 53:1802148. doi: 10.1183/13993003.02148-2018
9. Seeger W, Adir Y, Barberà JA, Champion H, Coghlan JG, Cottin V, et al. Pulmonary hypertension in chronic lung diseases. *J Am Coll Cardiol.* (2013) 62:D109–16. doi: 10.1016/j.jacc.2013.10.036
10. Soria R, Egger M, Scherrer U, Bender N, Rimoldi SF, Rimoldi SF. Pulmonary artery pressure and arterial oxygen saturation in people living at high or low altitude: systematic review and meta-analysis. *J Appl Physiol.* (2016) 121:1151–9. doi: 10.1152/japplphysiol.00394.2016.-More
11. Park MH. Historical perspective on the classification and nomenclature of pulmonary hypertension. In: Maron B, Zamanian R, Waxman A, editors. *Pulmonary Hypertension.* Cham: Springer International Publishing (2016). p. 3–15.
12. Escudero P. The Black Cardiacs and the Ayerza's disease. *Rev Crit.* (1911).
13. Mazzei JA, Mazzei ME. A tribute: Abel Ayerza and pulmonary hypertension. *Eur Respir Rev.* (2011) 20:220–1. doi: 10.1183/09059180.000 06811
14. Brenner O. Pathology of the vessels of the pulmonary circulation. *Arch Intern Med.* (1935) 56:211. doi: 10.1001/archinte.1935.03920020003001
15. Forssmann W. Die Sondierung des Rechten Herzens. *Klin Wochenschr.* (1929) 8:2085–7. doi: 10.1007/BF01875120
16. van Wolferen SA, Grünberg K, Vonk Noordegraaf A. Diagnosis and management of pulmonary hypertension over the past 100 years. *Respir Med.* (2007) 101:389–98. doi: 10.1016/J.RMED.2006.11.022
17. Cournand A. Control of the pulmonary circulation in man with some remarks on methodology. In: *Nobel Lectures: Physiology or Medicine.* Amsterdam: Elsevier Publishing (1964). p. 529–42.
18. Richards DW. The contributions of right heart catheterization to physiology and medicine, with some observations on the physiopathology of pulmonary heart disease. *Am Heart J.* (1957) 54:161–71. doi: 10.1016/0002-8703(57)90143-6
19. Dresdale DT, Schultz M, Michtom RJ. Primary pulmonary hypertension. *Am J Med.* (1951) 11:686–705. doi: 10.1016/0002-9343(51)90020-4
20. Gilmour JR, Evans W. Primary pulmonary hypertension. *J Pathol Bacteriol.* (1946) 58:687–97. doi: 10.1002/path.1700580410
21. Heath D, Whitaker W. Hypertensive pulmonary vascular disease. *Circulation.* (1956) 14:323–43. doi: 10.1161/circ.14.3.323
22. Whitaker W. The initiation of an interest in the pulmonary circulation. *Thorax.* (1994) 49:S2–4. doi: 10.1136/thx.49.Suppl.S2
23. Heath D, Edwards J. The pathology of hypertensive pulmonary vascular disease. *Circulation.* (1958) 18:533–47. doi: 10.1161/circ.18.4.533
24. Beutner CA. Ueber die Strom-und Druckkrafte des Blutes in der Arteria pulmonalis. *Z Ration Med.* (1852) 2:97–138.
25. Euler USV, Liljestrand G. Observations on the pulmonary arterial blood pressure in the cat. *Acta Physiol Scand.* (1946) 12:301–20. doi: 10.1111/j.1748-1716.1946.tb00389.x
26. Motley HL, Cournand A, Werko L, Himmelstein A, Dresdale D. The influence of short periods of induced acute anoxia upon pulmonary artery pressures in man. *Am J Physiol Content.* (1947) 150:315–20. doi: 10.1152/ajplegacy.1947.150.2.315
27. Kulandavelu S, Balkan W, Hare JM. Regulation of oxygen delivery to the body via hypoxic vasodilation. *Proc Natl Acad Sci USA.* (2015) 112:6254–5. doi: 10.1073/pnas.1506523112
28. Hurtado A. Aspectos Fisiologicos y Patologicos de la Vida en la Altura. *Rev Med Peru.* (1937) 9:3–52.
29. Fred HL, Schmidt AM, Bates T, Hecht HH. Acute pulmonary edema of altitude: clinical and physiologic observations. *Circulation.* (1962) 25:929–37. doi: 10.1161/01.CIR.25.6.929
30. West JB. *High Life : A History of High-Altitude Physiology and Medicine.* New York: Springer (1998).
31. Hultgren HN, Lopez CE, Lundberg E, Miller H. Physiologic studies of pulmonary edema at high altitude. *Circulation.* (1964) 29:393–408. doi: 10.1161/01.CIR.29.3.393
32. Viswanathan R, Jain SK, Subramanian S, Subramanian TAV, Dua GL, Giri J. Pulmonary Edema of High Altitude. *Am Rev Respir Dis.* (1969) 100:334–41. doi: 10.1164/arrd.1969.100.3.334

33. Hultgren HN, Grover RF, Hartley LH. Abnormal circulatory responses to high altitude in subjects with a previous history of high-altitude pulmonary edema. *Circulation.* (1971) 44:759–70. doi: 10.1161/01.CIR.44.5.759
34. Hultgren HN. High-altitude pulmonary edema: current concepts. *Annu Rev Med.* (1996) 47:267–84. doi: 10.1146/annurev.med.47.1.267
35. Dehnert C, Risse F, Ley S, Kuder TA, Buhmann R, Puderbach M, et al. Magnetic resonance imaging of uneven pulmonary perfusion in hypoxia in humans. *Am J Respir Crit Care Med.* (2006) 174:1132–8. doi: 10.1164/rccm.200606-780OC
36. Maggiorini M, Mélot C, Pierre S, Pfeiffer F, Greve I, Sartori C, et al. High-altitude pulmonary edema is initially caused by an increase in capillary pressure. *Circulation.* (2001) 103:2078–83. doi: 10.1161/01.CIR.103.16.2078
37. Scherrer U, Rexhaj E, Jayet PY, Allemann Y, Sartori C. New insights in the pathogenesis of high-altitude pulmonary edema. *Prog Cardiovasc Dis.* (2010) 52:485–92. doi: 10.1016/j.pcad.2010.02.004
38. Swenson ER, Bärtsch P. High-altitude pulmonary edema. *Comprehen Physiol.* (2012) 2: 2753–73. doi: 10.1002/cphy.c100029
39. Rhodes J. Comparative physiology of hypoxic pulmonary hypertension: historical clues from brisket disease. *J Appl Physiol.* (2005) 98:1092–100. doi: 10.1152/japplphysiol.01017.2004
40. Alexander AF, Will DH, Grover RF, Reeves JT. Pulmonary hypertention and right ventricular hypertrophy in catle at high altitude. *Am J Vet Res* (1960) 21:199–204.
41. Will DH, Hicks JL, Card CS, Alexander AF. Inherited susceptibility of cattle to high-altitude pulmonary hypertension. *J Appl Physiol.* (1975) 38:491–4. doi: 10.1152/jappl.1975.38.3.491
42. Weir EK, Tucker A, Reeves JT, Will DH, Grover RF. The genetic factor influencing pulmonary hypertension in cattle at high altitude. *Cardiovasc Res.* (1974) 8:745–9.
43. Anand IS, Chandrashekhar Y, Bali HK, Wahi PL, Jindal SK, Malhotra RM, et al. Adult subacute mountain sickness—a syndrome of congestive heart failure in man at very high altitude. *Lancet.* (1990) 335:561–5. doi: 10.1016/0140-6736(90)90348-9
44. Rotta A, Cánepa A, Hurtado A, Velásquez T, Chávez R. Pulmonary circulation at sea level and at high altitudes. *J Appl Physiol.* (1956) 9:328–36. doi: 10.1152/jappl.1956.9.3.328
45. Arias-Stella J, Saldana M. The terminal portion of the pulmonary arterial tree in people native to high altitudes. *Circulation.* (1963) 28:915–25. doi: 10.1161/01.CIR.28.5.915
46. Penaloza D, Arias-Stella J. The heart and pulmonary circulation at high altitudes: healthy highlanders and chronic mountain sickness. *Circulation* (2007) 115:1132–46. doi: 10.1161/CIRCULATIONAHA.106.624544
47. Arias-Stella J, Castillo Y. The muscular pulmonary arterial branches in stillborn natives of high altitude. *Lab Invest.* (1966) 15:1951–9.
48. Peñaloza D, Gamboa R, Marticorena E, Echevarría M, Dyer J, Gutierrez E. The influence of high altitudes on the electrical activity of the heart. *Am Heart J.* (1961) 61:101–15. doi: 10.1016/0002-8703(61)90522-1
49. Peñaloza D, Sime F, Banchero N, Gamboa R, Cruz J, Marticorena E. Pulmonary hypertension in healthy men born and living at high altitudes. *Am J Cardiol.* (1963) 11:150–7. doi: 10.1016/0002-9149(63)90055-9
50. Peñaloza D, Gamboa R, Dyer J, Echevarría M, Marticorena E. The influence of high altitudes on the electrical activity of the heart. I. Electrocardiographic and vectocardiographic observations in the newborn, infants, and children. *Am Heart J.* (1960) 59:111–28. doi: 10.1016/0002-8703(60)90390-2
51. Alexander AF, Jensen R. Pulmonary vascular pathology of high-altitude induced pulmonary hypertension in cattle. *Am J Vet Res.* (1963) 24:1112–22.
52. Sime F, Peñaloza D, Ruiz L. Bradycardia, increased cardiac output, and reversal of pulmonary hypertension in altitude natives living at sea level. *Br Heart J.* (1971) 33:647–57. doi: 10.1136/hrt.33.5.647
53. Vanderpool RR, Naeije R. Hematocrit-corrected pulmonary vascular resistance. *Am J Respir Crit Care Med.* (2018) 198:305–9. doi: 10.1164/rccm.201801-0081PP
54. Linehan JH, Haworth ST, Nelin LD, Krenz GS, Dawson CA. A simple distensible vessel model for interpreting pulmonary vascular pressure-flow curves. *J Appl Physiol.* (1992) 73:987–94. doi: 10.1152/jappl.1992.73.3.987
55. Hoffman JIE. Pulmonary vascular resistance and viscosity: the forgotten factor. *Pediatr Cardiol.* (2011) 32:557–61. doi: 10.1007/s00246-011-9954-3
56. León-Velarde F, Maggiorini M, Reeves JT, Aldashev A, Asmus I, Bernardi L, et al. Consensus statement on chronic and subacute high altitude diseases. *High Alt Med Biol.* (2005) 6:147–57. doi: 10.1089/ham.2005.6.147
57. Naeije R, Vanderpool R. Pulmonary hypertension and chronic mountain sickness. *High Alt Med Biol.* (2013) 14:117–25. doi: 10.1089/ham.2012.1124
58. Villafuerte FC, Corante N. Chronic mountain sickness: clinical aspects, etiology, management, and treatment. *High Alt Med Biol.* (2016) 17:61–9. doi: 10.1089/ham.2016.0031
59. Heath D, Smith P, Williams D, Harris P, Arias-Stella J, Krüger H. The heart and pulmonary vasculature of the llama (Lama glama). *Thorax.* (1974) 29:463–71. doi: 10.1136/thx.29.4.463
60. Heath D, Williams D, Dickinson J. The pulmonary arteries of the yak. *Cardiovasc Res.* (1984) 18:133–139. doi: 10.1093/cvr/18.3.133
61. Porter V, Alderson L, Hall S, Sponenberg P. *Mason's World Encyclopedia of Livestock Breeds and Breeding: 2 Volume Pack.* Wallington: CAB International (2016).
62. Anand IS, Harris E, Ferrari R, Pearce P, Harris P. Pulmonary haemodynamics of the yak, cattle, and cross breeds at high altitude. *Thorax.* (1986) 41:696–700. doi: 10.1136/thx.41.9.696
63. Dunham-Snary KJ, Wu D, Sykes EA, Thakrar A, Parlow LRG, Mewburn JD, et al. Hypoxic pulmonary vasoconstriction: from molecular mechanisms to medicine. *Chest.* (2017) 151:181–92 doi: 10.1016/j.chest.2016.09.001
64. Wilkins MR, Ghofrani H-A, Weissmann N, Aldashev A, Zhao L. Pathophysiology and treatment of high-altitude pulmonary vascular disease. *Circulation.* (2015) 131:582–90. doi: 10.1161/CIRCULATIONAHA.114.006977
65. Siques P, Brito J, Pena E. Reactive oxygen species and pulmonary vasculature during hypobaric hypoxia. *Front Physiol.* (2018) 9:865. doi: 10.3389/fphys.2018.00865
66. Bailey DM, Dehnert C, Luks AM, Menold E, Castell C, Schendler G, et al. High-altitude pulmonary hypertension is associated with a free radical-mediated reduction in pulmonary nitric oxide bioavailability. *J Physiol.* (2010) 588:4837–47. doi: 10.1113/jphysiol.2010.194704
67. Kourembanas S, Marsden PA, McQuillan LP, Faller DV. Hypoxia induces endothelin gene expression and secretion in cultured human endothelium. *J Clin Invest.* (1991) 88:1054–7. doi: 10.1172/JCI115367
68. Weigand L, Shimoda LA, Sylvester JT. Enhancement of myofilament calcium sensitivity by acute hypoxia in rat distal pulmonary arteries. *Am J Physiol Lung Cell Mol Physiol.* (2011) 301:L380–7. doi: 10.1152/ajplung.00068.2011
69. Wang GL, Jiang BH, Rue EA, Semenza GL. Hypoxia-inducible factor 1 is a basic-helix-loop-helix-PAS heterodimer regulated by cellular O2 tension. *Proc Natl Acad Sci USA.* (1995) 92:5510–4. doi: 10.1073/pnas.92.12.5510
70. Jaakkola P, Mole DR, Tian YM, Wilson MI, Gielbert J, Gaskell SJ, et al. Targeting of HIF-alpha to the von Hippel-Lindau ubiquitylation complex by O2-regulated prolyl hydroxylation. *Science.* (2001) 292:468–72. doi: 10.1126/science.1059796
71. Maxwell PH, Wiesener MS, Chang G-W, Clifford SC, Vaux EC, Cockman ME, et al. The tumour suppressor protein VHL targets hypoxia-inducible factors for oxygen-dependent proteolysis. *Nature.* (1999) 399:271–5. doi: 10.1038/20459
72. Semenza GL. Hypoxia-inducible factor 1: master regulator of O2 homeostasis. *Curr Opin Genet Dev.* (1998) 8:588–94.
73. Patel SA, Simon MC. Biology of hypoxia-inducible factor-2alpha in development and disease. *Cell Death Differ.* (2008) 15:628–34. doi: 10.1038/cdd.2008.17
74. Tian H, McKnight SL, Russell DW. Endothelial PAS domain protein 1 (EPAS1), a transcription factor selectively expressed in endothelial cells. *Genes Dev.* (1997) 11:72–82. doi: 10.1101/gad.11.1.72
75. Beall CM, Cavalleri GL, Deng L, Elston RC, Gao Y, Knight J, et al. Natural selection on EPAS1 (HIF2) associated with low hemoglobin concentration in Tibetan highlanders. *Proc Natl Acad Sci USA.* (2010) 107:11459–64. doi: 10.1073/pnas.1002443107
76. Yi X, Liang Y, Huerta-Sanchez E, Jin X, Cuo ZXP, Pool JE, et al. Sequencing of 50 human exomes reveals adaptation to high altitude. *Science.* (2010) 329:75–8. doi: 10.1126/science.1190371
77. Xiang K, Ouzhuluobu, Peng Y, Yang Z, Zhang X, Cui C, et al. Identification of a Tibetan-specific mutation in the hypoxic gene EGLN1 and its contribution to high-altitude adaptation. *Mol Biol Evol.* (2013) 30:1889–98. doi: 10.1093/molbev/mst090
78. Peng Y, Cui C, He Y, Ouzhuluobu, Zhang H, Yang D, et al. Down-regulation of EPAS1 transcription and genetic adaptation of tibetans to high-altitude hypoxia. *Mol Biol Evol.* (2017) 34:818–30. doi: 10.1093/molbev/msw280
79. Lorenzo FR, Huff C, Myllymäki M, Olenchock B, Swierczek S, Tashi T, et al. A genetic mechanism for Tibetan high-altitude adaptation. *Nat Genet.* (2014)

46:951–6. doi: 10.1038/ng.3067

80. Groves BM, Sutton J, Droma T, McCullough RG, McCullough RE, Zhuang J, et al. Minimal hypoxic pulmonary hypertension in normal Tibetans at 3,658 m. *J Appl Physiol.* (1993) 74:312–8. doi: 10.1152/jappl.1993.74.1.312
81. Gupta ML, Rao KS, Anand IS, Banerjee AK, Boparai MS. Lack of smooth muscle in the small pulmonary arteries of the native Ladakhi: is the Himalayan highlander adapted? *Am Rev Respir Dis.* (1992) 145:1201–4. doi: 10.1164/ajrccm/145.5.1201
82. Beall CM. Two routes to functional adaptation: Tibetan and Andean high-altitude natives. *Proc Natl Acad Sci USA.* (2007) 104:8655–60. doi: 10.1073/pnas.0701985104
83. Yu AY, Shimoda LA, Iyer N V, Huso DL, Sun X, McWilliams R, et al. Impaired physiological responses to chronic hypoxia in mice partially deficient for hypoxia-inducible factor 1alpha. *J Clin Invest.* (1999) 103:691–6. doi: 10.1172/JCI5912
84. Brusselmans K, Compernolle V, Tjwa M, Wiesener MS, Maxwell PH, Collen D, et al. Heterozygous deficiency of hypoxia-inducible factor−2α protects mice against pulmonary hypertension and right ventricular dysfunction during prolonged hypoxia. *J Clin Invest.* (2003) 111:1519–27. doi: 10.1172/JCI200315496
85. Newman JH, Holt TN, Cogan JD, Womack B, Phillips JA, Li C, et al. Increased prevalence of EPAS1 variant in cattle with high-altitude pulmonary hypertension. *Nat Commun.* (2015) 6:6863. doi: 10.1038/ncomms7863
86. Tan Q, Kerestes H, Percy MJ, Pietrofesa R, Chen L, Khurana TS, et al. Erythrocytosis and pulmonary hypertension in a mouse model of human HIF2A gain of function mutation. *J Biol Chem.* (2013) 288:17134–44. doi: 10.1074/jbc.M112.444059
87. Gale DP, Harten SK, Reid CDL, Tuddenham EGD, Maxwell PH. Autosomal dominant erythrocytosis and pulmonary arterial hypertension associated with an activating HIF2 alpha mutation. *Blood.* (2008) 112:919–21. doi: 10.1182/blood-2008-04-153718
88. Bushuev VI, Miasnikova GY, Sergueeva AI, Polyakova LA, Okhotin D, Gaskin PR, et al. Endothelin-1, vascular endothelial growth factor and systolic pulmonary artery pressure in patients with Chuvash polycythemia. *Haematologica.* (2006) 91:744–9. Available online at: http://www.haematologica.org/content/91/6/744.full.pdf+html
89. Bond J, Gale DP, Connor T, Adams S, de Boer J, Gascoyne DM, et al. Dysregulation of the HIF pathway due to VHL mutation causing severe erythrocytosis and pulmonary arterial hypertension. *Blood.* (2011) 117:3699–701. doi: 10.1182/blood-2010-12-327569
90. Hickey MM, Richardson T, Wang T, Mosqueira M, Arguiri E, Yu H, et al. The von Hippel–Lindau Chuvash mutation promotes pulmonary hypertension and fibrosis in mice. *J Clin Invest.* (2010) 120:827–39. doi: 10.1172/JCI36362
91. Ball MK, Waypa GB, Mungai PT, Nielsen JM, Czech L, Dudley VJ, et al. Regulation of hypoxia-induced pulmonary hypertension by vascular smooth muscle hypoxia-inducible factor-1alpha. *Am J Respir Crit Care Med.* (2014) 189:314–24. doi: 10.1164/rccm.201302-0302OC
92. Sheikh AQ, Saddouk FZ, Ntokou A, Mazurek R, Greif DM. Cell autonomous and non-cell autonomous regulation of SMC progenitors in pulmonary hypertension. *Cell Rep.* (2018) 23:1152–65. doi: 10.1016/j.celrep.2018.03.043
93. Shimoda LA, Manalo DJ, Sham JS, Semenza GL, Sylvester JT. Partial HIF-1alpha deficiency impairs pulmonary arterial myocyte electrophysiological responses to hypoxia. *Am J Physiol Lung Cell Mol Physiol.* (2001) 281:L202–8. doi: 10.1152/ajplung.2001.281.1.L202
94. Wang J, Weigand L, Lu W, Sylvester JT, Semenza GL, Shimoda LA. Hypoxia inducible factor 1 mediates hypoxia-induced TRPC expression and elevated intracellular Ca2+ in pulmonary arterial smooth muscle cells. *Circ Res.* (2006) 98:1528–37. doi: 10.1161/01.RES.0000227551.68124.98
95. Martin E, Dahan D, Cardouat G, Gillibert-Duplantier J, Marthan R, Savineau JP, et al. Involvement of TRPV1 and TRPV4 channels in migration of rat pulmonary arterial smooth muscle cells. *Pflugers Arch Eur J Physiol.* (2012) 464:261–72. doi: 10.1007/s00424-012-1136-5
96. Vander Heiden MG, Cantley LC, Thompson CB. Understanding the Warburg effect: the metabolic requirements of cell proliferation. *Science.* (2009) 324:1029–33. doi: 10.1126/science.1160809
97. Liberti MV, Locasale JW. The Warburg effect: how does it benefit cancer cells? *Trends Biochem Sci.* (2016) 41:211–8. doi: 10.1016/j.tibs.2015.12.001
98. Fijalkowska I, Xu W, Comhair SAA, Janocha AJ, Mavrakis LA, Krishnamachary B, et al. Hypoxia inducible-factor1α regulates the metabolic shift of pulmonary hypertensive endothelial cells. *Am J Pathol.* (2010) 176:1130–8. doi: 10.2353/ajpath.2010.090832
99. Plecitá-Hlavatá L, Tauber J, Li M, Zhang H, Flockton AR, Pullamsetti SS, et al. Constitutive reprogramming of fibroblast mitochondrial metabolism in pulmonary hypertension. *Am J Respir Cell Mol Biol.* (2016) 55:47–57. doi: 10.1165/rcmb.2015-0142OC
100. Stenmark KR, Tuder RM, El Kasmi KC. Metabolic reprogramming and inflammation act in concert to control vascular remodeling in hypoxic pulmonary hypertension. *J Appl Physiol.* (2015) 119:1164–72. doi: 10.1152/japplphysiol.00283.2015
101. Marsboom G, Wietholt C, Haney CR, Toth PT, Ryan JJ, Morrow E, et al. Lung ^{18}F-fluorodeoxyglucose positron emission tomography for diagnosis and monitoring of pulmonary arterial hypertension. *Am J Respir Crit Care Med.* (2012) 185:670–9. doi: 10.1164/rccm.201108-1562OC
102. Zhao L, Ashek A, Wang L, Fang W, Dabral S, Dubois O, et al. Heterogeneity in lung 18FDG uptake in PAH: potential of dynamic 18FDG-PET with kinetic analysis as a bridging biomarker for pulmonary remodeling targeted treatments. *Circulation.* (2013) 128:1214–24. doi: 10.1161/CIRCULATIONAHA.113.004136
103. Li M, Riddle SR, Frid MG, El Kasmi KC, McKinsey TA, Sokol RJ, et al. Emergence of fibroblasts with a proinflammatory epigenetically altered phenotype in severe hypoxic pulmonary hypertension. *J Immunol.* (2011) 187:2711–22. doi: 10.4049/jimmunol.1100479
104. Zhao L, Chen C-N, Hajji N, Oliver E, Cotroneo E, Wharton J, et al. Histone deacetylation inhibition in pulmonary hypertension: therapeutic potential of valproic acid and suberoylanilide hydroxamic acid. *Circulation.* (2012) 126:455–67. doi: 10.1161/CIRCULATIONAHA.112.103176
105. Dai Z, Li M, Wharton J, Zhu MM, Zhao YY. Prolyl-4 Hydroxylase 2 (PHD2) deficiency in endothelial cells and hematopoietic cells induces obliterative vascular remodeling and severe pulmonary arterial hypertension in mice and humans through hypoxia-inducible factor-2α. *Circulation.* (2016) 133:2447–58. doi: 10.1161/CIRCULATIONAHA.116.021494
106. Kapitsinou PP, Rajendran G, Astleford L, Michael M, Schonfeld MP, Fields T, et al. The endothelial prolyl-4-hydroxylase domain 2/hypoxia-inducible factor 2 axis regulates pulmonary artery pressure in mice. *Mol Cell Biol.* (2016) 36:1584–94. doi: 10.1128/MCB.01055-15
107. Cowburn AS, Crosby A, Macias D, Branco C, Colaço RDDR, Southwood M, et al. HIF2α-arginase axis is essential for the development of pulmonary hypertension. *Proc Natl Acad Sci USA.* (2016) 113:8801–6. doi: 10.1073/pnas.1602978113
108. Good RB, Gilbane AJ, Trinder SL, Denton CP, Coghlan G, Abraham DJ, et al. Endothelial to mesenchymal transition contributes to endothelial dysfunction in pulmonary arterial hypertension. *Am J Pathol.* (2015) 185:1850–8. doi: 10.1016/j.ajpath.2015.03.019
109. Tang H, Babicheva A, McDermott KM, Gu Y, Ayon RJ, Song S, et al. Endothelial HIF-2α contributes to severe pulmonary hypertension by inducing endothelial-to-mesenchymal transition. *Am J Physiol Cell Mol Physiol.* (2017) 314:ajplung.00096.2017. doi: 10.1152/ajplung.00096.2017
110. Kim Y-M, Barnes EA, Alvira CM, Ying L, Reddy S, Cornfield DN. Hypoxia-inducible factor-1 in pulmonary artery smooth muscle cells lowers vascular tone by decreasing myosin light chain phosphorylation. *Circ Res.* (2013) 112:1230–3. doi: 10.1161/CIRCRESAHA.112.300646
111. Iyer NV, Kotch LE, Agani F, Leung SW, Laughner E, Wenger RH, et al. Cellular and developmental control of O2 homeostasis by hypoxia- inducible factor 1α. *Genes Dev.* (1998) 12:149–62. doi: 10.1101/gad.12.2.149
112. Wigerup C, Påhlman S, Bexell D. Therapeutic targeting of hypoxia and hypoxia-inducible factors in cancer. *Pharmacol Ther.* (2016) 164:152–69. doi: 10.1016/j.pharmthera.2016.04.009
113. Yu T, Tang B, Sun X. Development of inhibitors targeting hypoxia-inducible factor 1 and 2 for cancer therapy. *Yonsei Med J.* (2017) 58:489–96. doi: 10.3349/ymj.2017.58.3.489
114. Courtney KD, Infante JR, Lam ET, Figlin RA, Rini BI, Brugarolas J, et al. Phase I dose-escalation trial of PT2385, a first-in-class hypoxia-inducible factor-2α antagonist in patients with previously treated advanced clear cell renal cell carcinoma. *J Clin Oncol.* (2017) 36:JCO.2017.74.2627. doi: 10.1200/JCO.2017.74.2627
115. Dai Z, Zhu MM, Peng Y, Machireddy N, Evans CE, Machado R, et al. Therapeutic targeting of vascular remodeling and right heart failure in PAH with HIF-2α inhibitor. *Am J Respir Crit Care Med.* (2018) 198:1423–34. doi: 10.1164/rccm.201710-2079OC

116. Zhao L, Oliver E, Maratou K, Atanur SS, Dubois OD, Cotroneo E, et al. The zinc transporter ZIP12 regulates the pulmonary vascular response to chronic hypoxia. *Nature*. (2015) 524:356–60. doi: 10.1038/nature14620
117. Gupta N, Wish JB. Hypoxia-inducible factor prolyl hydroxylase inhibitors: a potential new treatment for anemia in patients with CKD. *Am J Kidney Dis*. (2017) 69:815–26. doi: 10.1053/j.ajkd.2016.12.011

9

Vascular Endothelial Cell-Specific Connective Tissue Growth Factor (CTGF) is Necessary for Development of Chronic Hypoxia-Induced Pulmonary Hypertension

Liya Pi[1], Chunhua Fu[2], Yuanquing Lu[2], Junmei Zhou[1], Marda Jorgensen[2], Vinayak Shenoy[3], Kenneth E. Lipson[4], Edward W. Scott[5] and Andrew J. Bryant[2]*

[1] Department of Pediatrics, University of Florida, Gainesville, FL, United States, [2] Division of Pulmonary, Critical Care, and Sleep Medicine, Department of Medicine, College of Medicine, University of Florida, Gainesville, FL, United States, [3] Department of Pharmaceutical and Biomedical Sciences, California Health Sciences University, Clovis, CA, United States, [4] FibroGen, Inc., San Francisco, CA, United States, [5] Department of Molecular Genetics and Microbiology, University of Florida, Gainesville, FL, United States

***Correspondence:**
Andrew J. Bryant
andrew.bryant@medicine.ufl.edu

Chronic hypoxia frequently complicates the care of patients with interstitial lung disease, contributing to the development of pulmonary hypertension (PH), and premature death. Connective tissue growth factor (CTGF), a matricellular protein of the Cyr61/CTGF/Nov (CCN) family, is known to exacerbate vascular remodeling within the lung. We have previously demonstrated that vascular endothelial-cell specific down-regulation of CTGF is associated with protection against the development of PH associated with hypoxia, though the mechanism for this effect is unknown. In this study, we generated a transgenic mouse line in which the *Ctgf* gene was floxed and deleted in vascular endothelial cells that expressed Cre recombinase under the control of VE-Cadherin promoter (eCTGF KO mice). Lack of vascular endothelial-derived CTGF protected against the development of PH secondary to chronic hypoxia, as well as in another model of bleomycin-induced pulmonary hypertension. Importantly, attenuation of PH was associated with a decrease in infiltrating inflammatory cells expressing CD11b or integrin α_M (ITGAM), a known adhesion receptor for CTGF, in the lungs of hypoxia-exposed eCTGF KO mice. Moreover, these pathological changes were associated with activation of—Rho GTPase family member—cell division control protein 42 homolog (Cdc42) signaling, known to be associated with alteration in endothelial barrier function. These data indicate that endothelial-specific deletion of CTGF results in protection against development of chronic-hypoxia induced PH. This protection is conferred by both a decrease in inflammatory cell recruitment to the lung, and a reduction in lung Cdc42 activity. Based on our studies, CTGF inhibitor treatment should be investigated in patients with PH associated with chronic hypoxia secondary to chronic lung disease.

Keywords: pulmonary hypertension, hypoxia, connective tissue growth factor (CTGF), CD11b/integrin α_M (ITGAM), cell division control protein 42 homolog (Cdc42)

INTRODUCTION

Hypoxia is traditionally held to be a necessary factor in the pathogenesis of pulmonary hypertension (PH) secondary to chronic lung disease, classified as World Health Organization (WHO) Group III PH (Klinger, 2016). This contribution is clinically important, as Group III PH patients have at least a four-fold increased risk of death compared to disease controls without pulmonary vascular disease (Lettieri et al., 2006), and no proven treatments exist. Thus, studies of novel molecular pathways contributing to disease are needed in order to identify therapeutic targets.

To this end, the tissue response to low oxygen mediated by hypoxia-inducible factor (HIF)—a tightly conserved and regulated transcription factor across species—is known to be integral in the development of PH (Yu et al., 1999; Brusselmans et al., 2003). Building on these data, our group has recently uncovered a necessary role for tissue-specific—vascular endothelium derived—HIF in several models of PH (Bryant et al., 2015, 2016). Specifically, we found that deletion of endothelial HIF leads to improved vascular barrier integrity in response to injury, and is associated with protection against pulmonary vessel "leakiness" leading to PH. These findings echo previously reported results that described normalization of pulmonary pressures, in a genetic model of PH, associated with a decrease in endothelial layer permeability (Burton et al., 2011a). Of note, protection against these lung vasculopathic changes was in part due to reduced extravasation of circulating myeloid cell mediators into the pulmonary vascular bed (Burton et al., 2011b), although an exact mechanism is a topic of ongoing debate.

Therefore, a primary objective was to find a candidate targetable hypoxia-response element gene that is both (1) a protein involved in cell-cell adhesion and remodeling, and (2) a chemoattractant for circulating myeloid cells. Significantly, we discovered that connective tissue growth factor (CTGF)—a matricellular protein of the CCN family important for cell-cell and cell-matrix crosstalk (Lipson et al., 2012)—is upregulated in an endothelial cell autonomous fashion during hypoxia exposure (Bryant et al., 2016). Notably, CTGF is an identified coordinator of vascular repair (Pi et al., 2011), and a known ligand for the integrin α_M (ITGAM)—also known as CD11b—adhesion receptor expressed by peripheral blood leukocytes (Schober et al., 2002). Based on these findings, we asked the question: what is the mechanistic role of CTGF in pulmonary vascular remodeling? Our central hypothesis, based upon this query, is that endothelial CTGF is necessary for recruitment of CD11b expressing leukocytes to the lung, and development of PH. In this study, we demonstrate in two models of PH, that endothelial CTGF is necessary for development of disease, through accumulation of CD11b$^+$ cells and downstream factors promoting aberrant vascular repair.

MATERIALS AND METHODS

Reagents, Antibodies, and Primers

FG-3019 (10 mg/kg) and control IgG (10 mg/kg)—both administered intraperitoneal every week at initiation of hypoxia exposure (Wang et al., 2011)—were the kind gift of FibroGen Inc. (San Francisco, CA). Bleomycin Sulfate, ML141, and dichloromethylenediphosphonic acid disodium salt (clodronate) was purchased through MilliporeSigma. Lipids and cholesterol for liposome production were bought from Avanti Polar Lipids. EBM-2 culture media (Lonza), with EGM-2 bulletkit, was utilized for all *in vitro* experiments. Primer sequences are as follows: CTGF forward primer GGGAGAACTGTGTACGGAGC; CTGF reverse primer AGTGCACACTCCGATCTTGC; CD11b forward primer ATGGACGCTGATGGCAATACC; CD11b reverse primer TCCCCATTCACGTCTCCCA; 18S forward primer ACCTGGTTGATCCTGCCAGTAG; and, 18S reverse primer TTAATGAGCCATTCGCAGTTTC. Antibodies used in this study were: anti-GFP (Aves), MECA-32 (BD Biosciences), CTGF (BD Biosciences), CD11b (Abcam), F4/80 (BD Biosciences), CD31 (Santa Cruz Biotechnology), and GAPDH (Abcam). Antibodies for flow cytometry used in this study were: CD45 (FITC; BioLegend), CD11b (APC-Cy7; BioLegend), and IgG2 (isotype control; BioLegend). Active Cdc42 detection kit was purchased through Cell Signaling Technology. Secondary fluorescent antibodies were from Jackson Immunoresearch. Refer to **Supplementary Table 1** for full details of antibody catalog number and dilutions.

Animals

All wild-type (Jackson Laboratory) and transgenic mice generated for this study were on the C57BL/6J background, were greater than 8 weeks of age at the study onset, included both males and females, and ranged in weight from 20 to 30 g. Transgenic mice expressing Cre-recombinase under control of the mouse VE-Cadherin promoter (VECad.Cre) (Alva et al., 2006) were crossed with mice in which exon 4 was flanked by two loxP sites (*Ctgf*^{fl}) to create Cre mediated deletion the *Ctgf* gene within vascular endothelium (*Ctgf*$^{fl/fl}$, VECad-Cre). Breeding pairs were set up such that *floxed* Ctgf allele was maintained in homozygous state while VECad-Cre was in the heterozygous state, yielding Cre-positive mice with endothelial deletion of CTGF while *Ctgf*$^{fl/fl}$ mice served as littermate controls. To control for potential Cre-positive effects, in some experiments, VECad.Cre mice were used as part of the control cohort. Experiments to identify CTGF-expressing cells used CTGF-GFP mice, in which transgenic expression of green fluorescent protein (GFP) is driven by the *Ctgf* promoter (Pi et al., 2011). Mice were housed in the central animal care facility at University of Florida College of Medicine (Gainesville, FL) and were given food and water *ad libitum*. The experimental protocol was reviewed and approved by the institutional animal care and utilization committee at University of Florida.

Chronic Hypoxia and Bleomycin Models

Mice exposed to chronic hypoxia were placed in a normobaric chamber (Coy Laboratory Products) with continuous monitoring of oxygen and carbon dioxide concentration, ensuring that ventilation was maintained such that carbon dioxide levels remain <0.1%. Mice were housed in the same room under normoxia (room air, FiO_2 21%) or hypoxia

(FiO_2 10%) for a period of 4 weeks. At the completion of the chronic hypoxia protocol, mice underwent harvest for histology and hemodynamic measurement (Bryant et al., 2016). In indicated experiments, a separate group of mice underwent intraperitoneal injection with 0.018 U/g bleomycin (Thermo Fisher Scientific) or vehicle twice weekly for 28 days (Baran et al., 2007; Bryant et al., 2015). A group of vehicle- or bleomycin-treated mice were concomitantly dosed with 100 μL intraperitoneal liposomal clodronate (CL_2MDP) 1 week prior to either bleomycin or chronic hypoxia exposure, and every 3 days thereafter, in order to induce lung macrophage apoptosis. Clodronate liposomes, and control PBS liposomes, were generated as previously described (Murray et al., 2011; Zaynagetdinov et al., 2013). One week after the last injection, mice were then harvested for histology and hemodynamic measurements, similar to hypoxia-treated groups. ML141 (5 mg per kg body weight), a Cdc42 inhibitor, was dissolved in dimethyl sulfoxide (DMSO), and was intraperitoneally injected daily throughout bleomycin administration protocol (Chen et al., 2015), in described experiments.

PH Assessment

Invasive hemodynamic measurement was conducted, as described previously (West et al., 2008). In brief, upon induction of a surgical plane of anesthesia with avertin (500 mg/kg, intraperitoneal) the right internal jugular vein was exposed. The distal portion of the vein was completely occluded, while the proximal end of the jugular was loosely tied. A small incision was made in the exposed vein, and a Millar 1.4 French pressure-volume microtip catheter transducer (SPR-839; Millar Instruments, Houston, TX) connected to a PowerLab/8s (ADInstruments) was inserted through the incision and threaded down into the right ventricle. Data were collected using Chart 5 (ADInstruments). The heart was then excised with removal of the atria, and the RV and left ventricle (LV) plus septum were isolated for measurement of the RV:LV+S as previously described (Hemnes et al., 2014).

Isolation of Pulmonary Microvascular Endothelial Cells (PMVECs)

Primary isolates of PMVECs were obtained from transgenic mice and littermate controls, as previously described (West et al., 2014). In brief, cells were prepared from uninjured mice using collagenase type 2 and red blood cell lysis buffer. Endothelium was then isolated by fluorescence-activated cells sorting (FACS) based on CD31-PECAM-1 expression. To induce endothelial differentiation, sorted cells were plate on gelatin-coated plastic and were cultured in endothelial growth medium (Lonza, Walkersville, MD), until cells were confluent. Cells were then incubated with Alexa 488-labeled AcDiLDL (Life Technologies, Grand Island, NY) as previously described (Irwin et al., 2007), and positively stained cells were enriched by flow cytometry. Cells were then expanded and phenotyped as described.

Flow Cytometry

Flow cytometry analyses were performed on a BD LSR II or on FACSCalibur upgraded at three lasers and 8 colors (Cytek). Cell populations were identified using sequential gating strategy characterized within body of manuscript (excluding debris and doublets). Fluorescence minus one (FMO) and isotype controls were used when necessary. The expression of markers is presented as median fluorescence intensity (MFI). Data were analyzed using FlowJo software (Tree Star).

Immunohistochemical, RNA, and Protein Analyses

Upon harvest, the left lobe of the lung was inflated and placed in either 10% formalin or 4% PFA followed by sucrose for histological processing as previously described (Degryse et al., 2011; Tanjore et al., 2013), and the right lobes were snap frozen in liquid nitrogen for RNA and protein processing. Sections were prepared and processed for immunohistochemistry and immuno-fluorescence staining as previously described (Tanjore et al., 2009). Semiquantitative lung fibrosis scoring (10) and hydroxyproline microplate assay were performed, as previously described (11). For morphometric measurement, CTGF expression was analyzed quantitatively based on green fluorescence intensity from CTGF-GFP transgenic animals and CD11b expression was based on red fluorescence intensity from eCTGF KO lungs. At least 10 images (20x magnification)/lung sections were analyzed using ImageJ software (http://rsb.info.nih.gov/ij/). Relative expression was calculated as a percentage of total pixel intensity in each image. Western blots were performed on tissue and cell lysates as previously described (Tanjore et al., 2011). Total RNA was isolated from frozen whole-lung tissue and human cell lysate using a RNEasy kit (Qiagen) per manufacturer recommendations, DNase treated and prepared for quantitative RT-PCR according to previous report (Pi et al., 2015). Specific transcript levels for target genes were then determined by normalization to 18s. Values are presented as mean normalized transcript level using the comparative C_t method ($2^{-\Delta\Delta C_t}$).

Statistical Analyses

Statistical analysis was performed using GraphPad Prism 6.0 (GraphPad Software). Data are expressed as means ± SEM. As appropriate, groups were compared by ANOVA; follow-up comparisons between groups were conducted using Student's t-test. A $P \leq 0.05$ was considered to be significant.

RESULTS

Blockade of CTGF in Hypoxia Model Rescues PH Phenotype

In order to investigate the therapeutic targeting of CTGF in chronic hypoxia induced PH, we determined whether the pulmonary vascular response could be suppressed by systemic administration of a CTGF inhibitory monoclonal antibody, FG-3019. FG-3019 was therefore administered by intraperitoneal injection three times weekly starting the day prior to the onset of hypoxia exposure, in a preventive regimen. The extent of PH, as measured by right-ventricular systolic pressure (RVSP; mmHg), was significantly reduced in those mice treated with FG-3019, as compared to control IgG treated mice (**Figure 1A**). Additionally, the extent of protection against PH development by FG-3019 was also quantified by assessing the ratio of right ventricle to left ventricle plus septal mass (RV:LV+S; %), a surrogate marker of right ventricular remodeling in response to PH. Though there was a trend toward a decrease in RV remodeling, there was no statistically significant difference between hypoxia-exposed groups. Collectively, these findings suggested that an intrinsic lung vascular change accounted for differences in pressures (**Figure 1B**). In order to evaluate this vascular specific effect further we performed co-immunofluorescent staining for MECA32 (highlighting the vascular endothelium) in CTGF-GFP reporter mice—in which GFP expression is driven by the *Ctgf* promoter—exposed to normoxia vs. hypoxia. We found that the vascular endothelium significantly increased expression of CTGF in lung sections from hypoxia vs. normoxia animals (**Figures 1C,D**). Taken together, these data indicate that CTGF importantly contributes to the development of PH, and that FG-3019 can suppress PH—in the described murine models—through CTGF-inhibition.

CTGF Expression Is Enhanced in Hypoxia Model in Lung CD11b$^+$ Cells

The induction of CTGF under hypoxic conditions has been recognized as a key contributor to conditions of aberrant tissue remodeling (Higgins et al., 2004). Likewise, CTGF-expression is known to contribute to perivascular myeloid cell accumulation in the pathology of atherosclerotic arterial changes in cardiac disease (Schober et al., 2002). Therefore, we hypothesized that CTGF expressed during chronic hypoxia exposure critically influences accumulation of CD11b$^+$ cells in the lung. To investigate the contribution of CTGF to CD11b$^+$ cell accrual during the development of PH, we first confirmed global lung increase in CTGF expression in response to chronic hypoxia (**Figure 2A**). In CTGF-GFP mice, lung-sections co-stained for CD11b exhibited co-localization with CTGF that was qualitatively increased in hypoxia compared to normoxia exposed mice (**Figure 2B**). This is consistent with either increased binding of CTGF to CD11b$^+$ cells, or

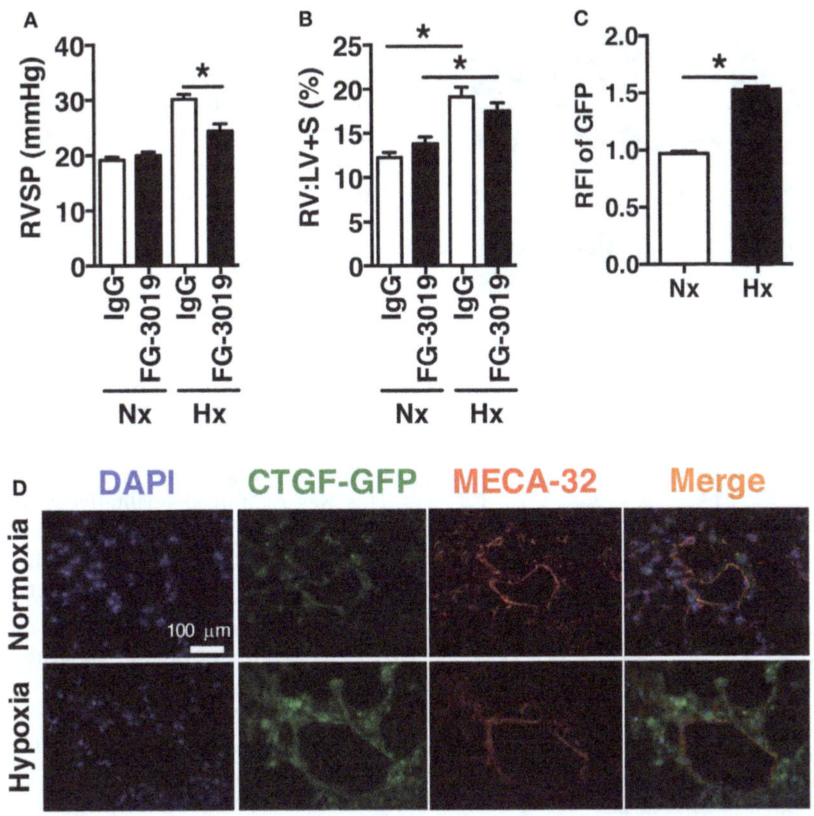

FIGURE 1 | Pharmacological inhibition of CTGF protects mice from hypoxia-induced PH. **(A)** Right ventricular systolic pressure (RVSP) and **(B)** Right ventricle to left ventricle plus septal mass ratio (RV:LV+S) in control IgG- or FG-3019-treated mice, exposed to normoxia (FiO_2 21%) or chronic hypoxia (FiO_2 10%; day 28, $n = 8$ mice/group). Dose for both FG-3019 and IgG was 10 mg/kg, injected intraperitoneally, once weekly. **(C)** Quantification of GFP relative fluorescent intensity (RFI) and **(D)** representative immunofluorescent images (40x magnification; scale bar 100 μm) from CTGF-GFP mice exposed to normoxia or hypoxia, also co-stained for vascular endothelial cell marker, MECA-32. *$P < 0.05$; data are presented as mean ± SEM.

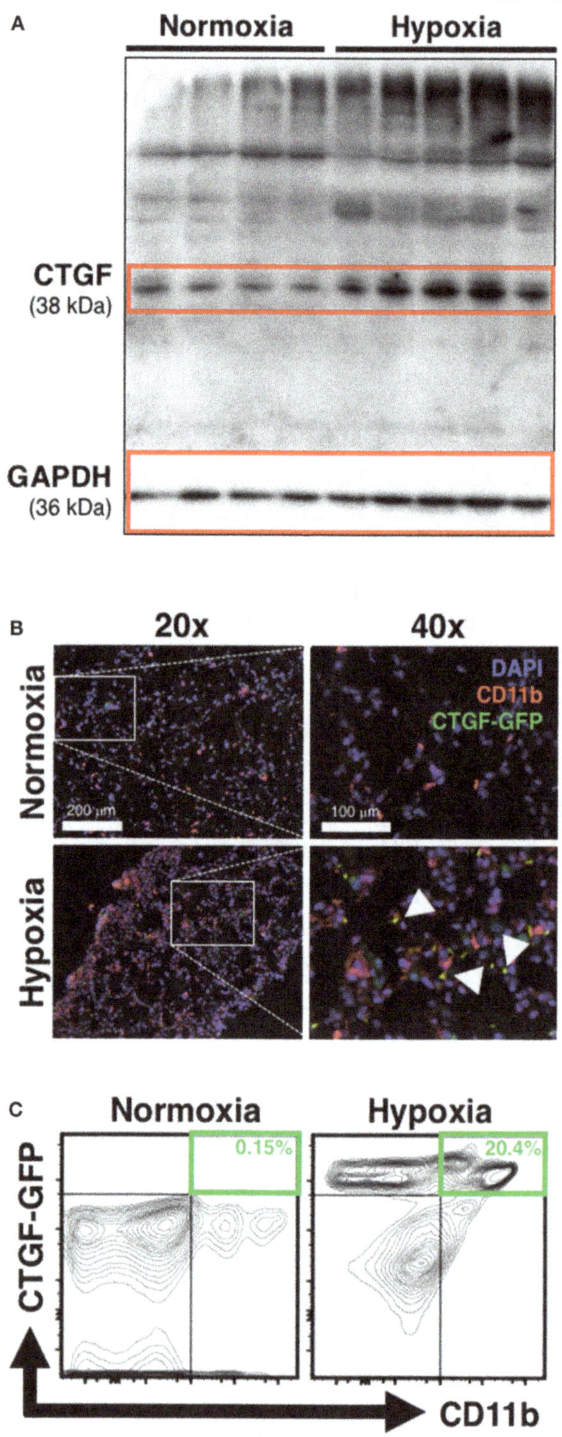

FIGURE 2 | Chronic hypoxia-induced PH is associated with CTGF- and CD11b-expression within the lung. **(A)** Western blot on whole lung of mice exposed to normoxia vs. chronic hypoxia ($n = 4$ and 5 mice/group, respectively). **(B)** Representative CD11b (white arrowheads) immunofluorescent staining of lung section from CTGF-GFP reporter mice exposed to either normoxia or hypoxia (20x and 40x magnification; scale bars 100 and 200 μm, respectively). **(C)** Representative flow cytometry contour plots detailing GFP and CD11b co-expression of whole lung $CD45^+$ cells, after normoxia or hypoxia treatment for 28 days, with percentages listed ($n = 8$–10 mice/group).

to increased expression of CTGF in the CD11b-expressing cells, though the latter is less likely since CD11b-expressing leukocytes are known to produce little CTGF intrinsically (Cicha et al., 2005). Flow cytometric assessment confirmed that the percentage of dual positive CTGF and CD11b cells in the lungs was increased in hypoxia (20.4% of $CD45^+$ cells) vs. normoxic (0.15% of $CD45^+$ cells; **Figure 2C**) controls. These data suggest that CTGF contributes to the expansion of the $CD11b^+$ myeloid cell pool within the lung, possibly through direct interaction with CD11b upon exposure to hypoxia, since CTGF is a ligand for this adhesion receptor that is encoded by the *ITGAM* gene on leukocytes (Schober et al., 2002).

Vascular Endothelial CTGF Is Necessary for Development of PH Secondary to Hypoxia

Based on our lab's previous work demonstrating alteration in vascular endothelial cell CTGF as associated with PH pathophysiology (Bryant et al., 2015, 2016), we next sought to evaluate the impact that endothelial cell CTGF deletion would have on disease progression. In order to test our central hypothesis, we developed a genetic mouse model in which $Ctgf^{fl/fl}$ alleles were deleted by the Cre recombinase under the control of the VECadherin-promoter, creating endothelial specific knockouts (eCTGF KO). Immunohistochemical staining for CTGF expression corroborated that in eCTGF KO mice, CTGF was not expressed in the thin vascular endothelial cells lining blood vessels within the lung after hypoxia exposure (**Figure 3A**). In addition, we examined isolated pulmonary microvascular endothelial cells (PMVECs) from our genetic model, for RNA (**Figure 3B**) expression level confirmation that CTGF was not present in cells compared to controls. We also found little to no CTGF staining in isolated PMVECs by immunofluorescence, co-stained with CD31 (**Figure 3C**). Next, we exposed our eCTGF KO mice to chronic hypoxia, and found that they were protected against development of PH (**Figure 4A**), with an associated decrease in RV remodeling (**Figure 4B**). The decrease in RVSP was associated with a decrease in leukocyte CD11b expression within the lung, as assessed by flow cytometry (**Figure 4C**). This was reinforced qualitatively, and semi-quantitatively, by examining CD11b immunofluorescent staining of lung sections, demonstrating fewer $CD11b^+$ cells in the lungs of eCTGF KO mice after hypoxia (**Figures 4D,E**). RNA level expression of CD11b in whole lung was likewise decreased in eCTGF KO mice after hypoxic exposure, compared to controls (**Figures 4F,G**). Taken together, these data demonstrate the critical role of endothelial CTGF to the pulmonary vascular response to chronic hypoxia, associated with increased CD11b-expression.

Endothelial CTGF Expression Is Necessary in a Bleomycin Model of PH

In order to establish rationale for the following series of experiments, we must consider possible cell sources of CTGF. CTGF is known to be increased in whole lung of patients

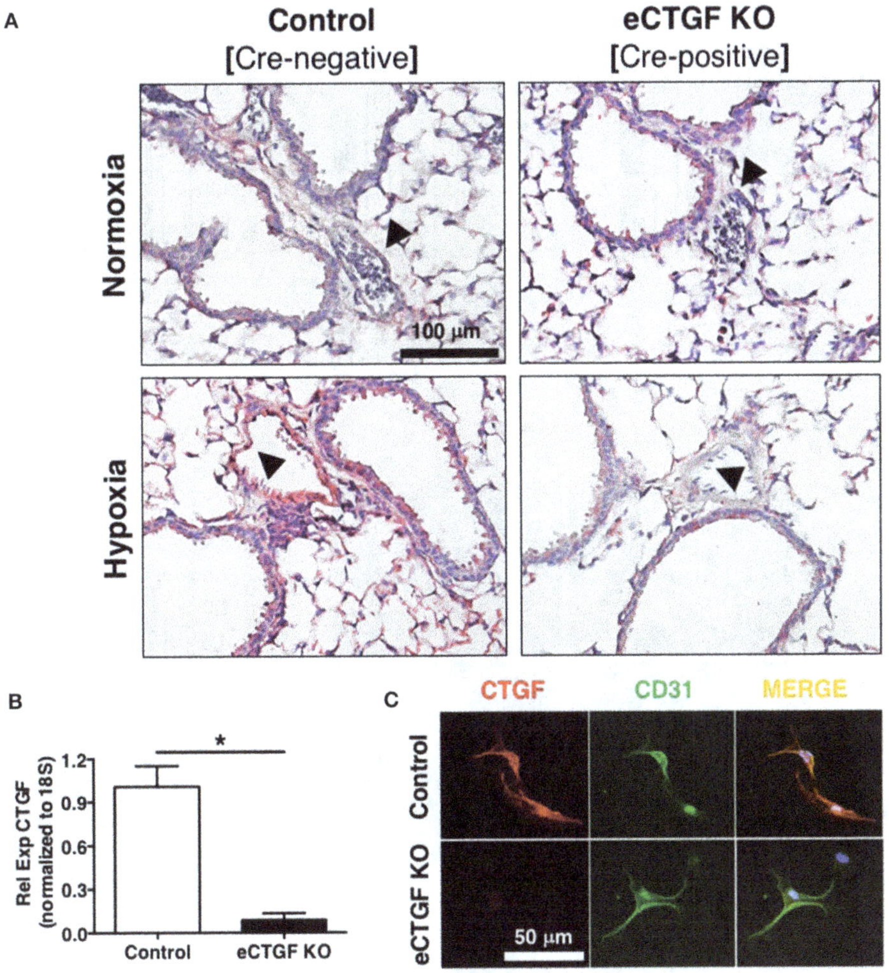

FIGURE 3 | Mice designated eCTGF KO (VECadherin.Cre-CTGF$^{fl/fl}$) have no CTGF expression in pulmonary vascular endothelial cells. **(A)** Representative immunohistochemical stain for CTGF (red) in whole lung sections from Control and eCTGF KO mice, upon exposure to normoxia or hypoxia. **(B)** qPCR for CTGF mRNA ($n = 4$ mice/group) and **(C)** immunofluorescent double staining for CD31 and CTGF proteins, in pulmonary microvascular endothelial cells isolated from wild type (WT) and eCTGF KO mice (200x magnification, scale bar 50 μm). $^{*}P < 0.05$; data are presented as mean ± SEM.

with chronic lung disease (Noguchi et al., 2017). In pulmonary fibrosis, CTGF is expressed in interstitial fibroblasts and type 2 alveolar epithelial cells (Pan et al., 2001). In addition to endothelial cells, other vascular cells can express CTGF, including pericytes (Suzuma et al., 2000) and vascular smooth muscle cells (Lee et al., 2005). Likewise, in hepatic fibrosis models, production of CTGF has been shown to be a necessary factor in progression of scarring of chronic fibrosis, and co-localization of CTGF was observed with liver macrophages/Kuppfer cells in a biliary fibrosis model (Pi et al., 2015). Importantly, modest expression of CTGF in myeloid cells has also been observed in other models. For example, *in vitro* CTGF expression in monocyte-derived macrophages can be induced (Ikezumi et al., 2015), and modest CTGF expression was observed in THP-1 cells polarized to M1, M2a or M2c macrophage phenotypes, with much more robust expression if the polarized macrophages were co-cultured with a mesenchymal cell population (Finlin et al., 2013). Similarly, we found in the intraperitoneal bleomycin model of pulmonary fibrosis an increase in CTGF expression by F4/80^{+} macrophages within the lung (**Figure 5A**). The fact that these non-endothelial cells express CTGF may explain, in part, our findings that after chronic intraperitoneal bleomycin exposure alone (twice weekly for 33 days), eCTGF KO mice were not protected against development of PH (**Figure 5B**), or pulmonary fibrosis (**Supplementary Figure 1**). Intriguingly, our group has recently described a novel model for PH, administering bleomycin in combination with clodronate (CL_2MDP, in figures) liposomes, resulting in depletion of macrophages and robust PH, with nearly no evidence of pulmonary fibrosis (Bryant et al., 2017). In light of these findings, we hypothesized that depletion of lung phagocytes with clodronate liposome administration

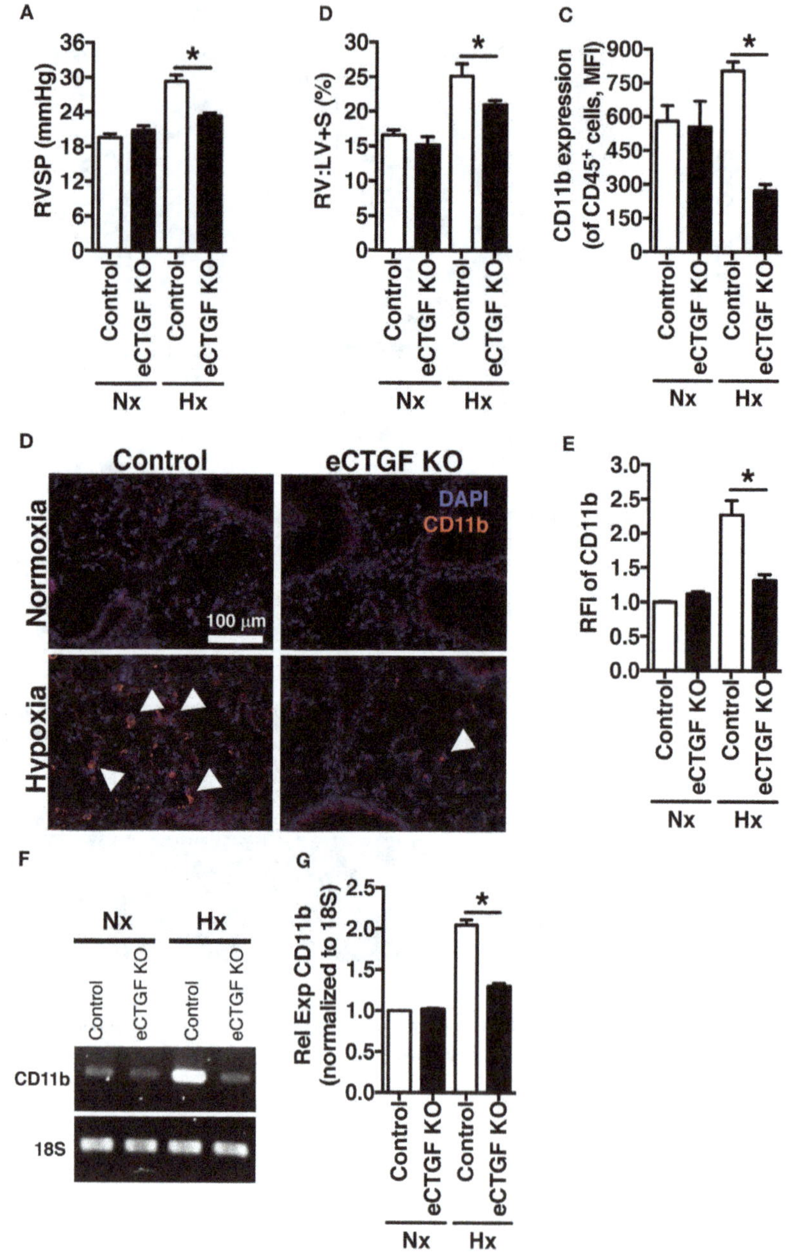

FIGURE 4 | The development of chronic-hypoxia induced PH is dependent upon pulmonary vascular endothelial cell expression of CTGF, and CD11b$^+$ cell accumulation within the lung. **(A)** RVSP and **(B)** RV:LV+S in Control and eCTGF KO mice, exposed to normoxia or chronic hypoxia (n = 10 mice/group). **(C)** CD11b-expression (MFI) as determined by flow cytometric analysis of CD45$^+$ cells from lungs of mice treated with either normoxia or hypoxia (n = 8 mice/group); **(D)** Representative immunofluorescent images of lung sections from described groups, staining for CD11b (40x magnification; scale bar 100 μm), and **(E)** quantification of CD11b relative fluorescent intensity (RFI). **(F,G)** PCR for CD11b-expression in whole lung of mice in indicated groups. $^*P < 0.05$; data are presented as mean ± SEM.

would lead to decreased whole lung CTGF-expression, with a greater dependence on CTGF from the vascular/endothelial compartment in maintaining the wound regulatory balance. Given this rationale, we found an appreciable decrease in CTGF in lungs of mice treated with clodronate, compared to PBS liposome controls (**Figures 5C,D**). Using this model, we were next able to confirm the main findings of the chronic hypoxia experiments, validating that eCTGF KO mice were protected against development of PH (**Figure 5E**). The normalization of pulmonary pressures was also shown to correlate with a decrease in CD45$^+$ cell CD11b expression (**Figure 5F**). These results suggest that endothelial CTGF is integral in recruited myeloid-cell associated pulmonary vascular remodeling in multiple models of PH.

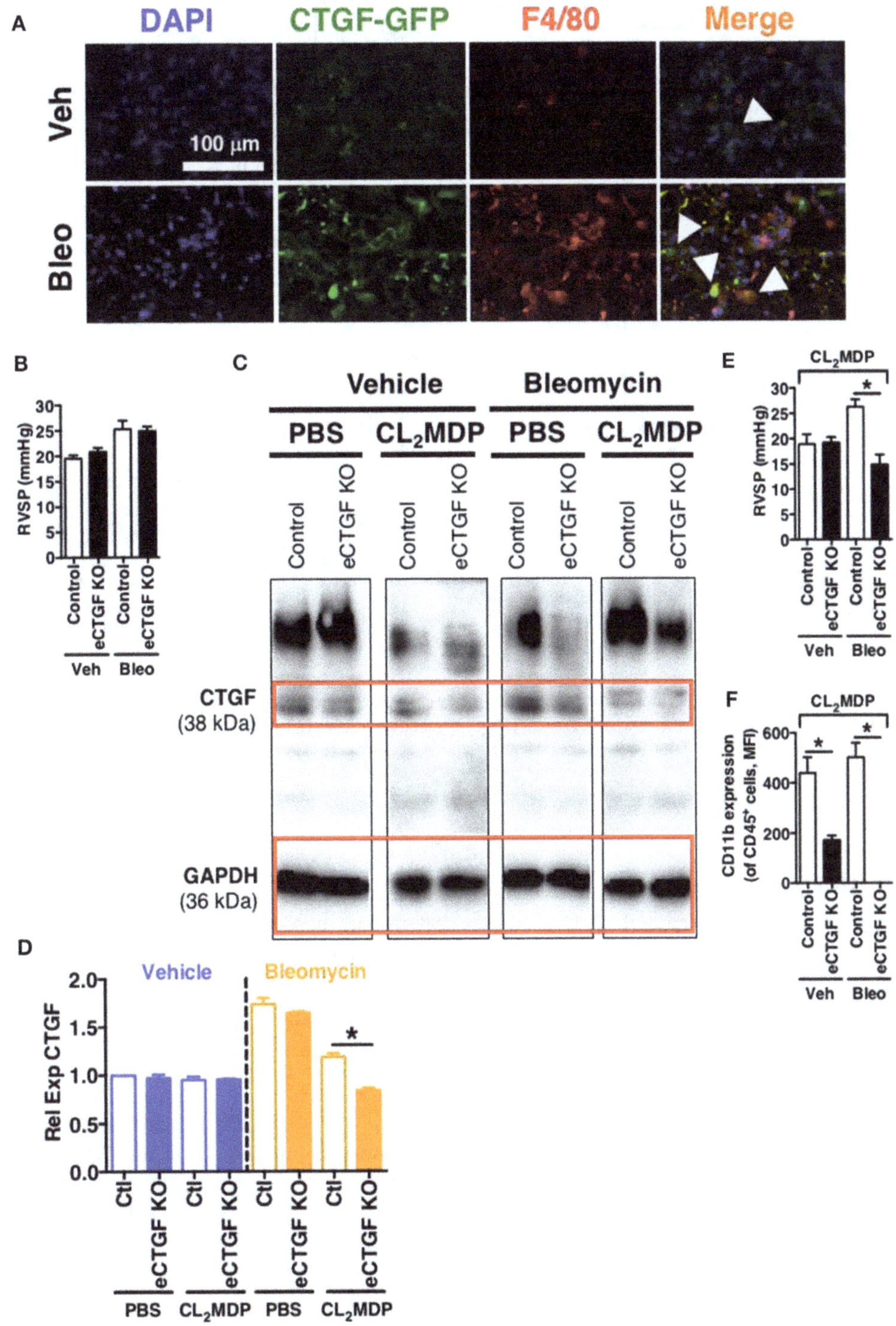

FIGURE 5 | Vascular endothelial cell CTGF production induced in a bleomycin model of PH is necessary for development of elevated pulmonary pressures. **(A)** Representative immunofluorescent images (40x magnification; scale bar 100 μm) from CTGF-GFP mice exposed to normoxia or hypoxia, co-stained for macrophage marker, F4/80. **(B)** RVSP measurement in Control and eCTGF KO mice, exposed to vehicle (PBS) or intraperitoneal bleomycin (day 33; $n = 8$ mice/group). **(C)** Western blot and **(D)** densitometry analysis on whole lung of Control and eCTGF KO mice detailing CTGF expression upon exposure to bleomycin and either PBS- or clodronate (CL_2MDP) liposomes. **(E)** RVSP in Control and eCTGF KO mice, exposed to CL_2MDP liposomes and either vehicle (PBS) or intraperitoneal bleomycin (day 33; $n = 8$–10 mice/group). **(F)** CD11b-expression, by flow cytometry, of CD45+ cells from lungs of treated mice ($n = 8$ mice/group). $^*P < 0.05$; data are presented as mean ± SEM.

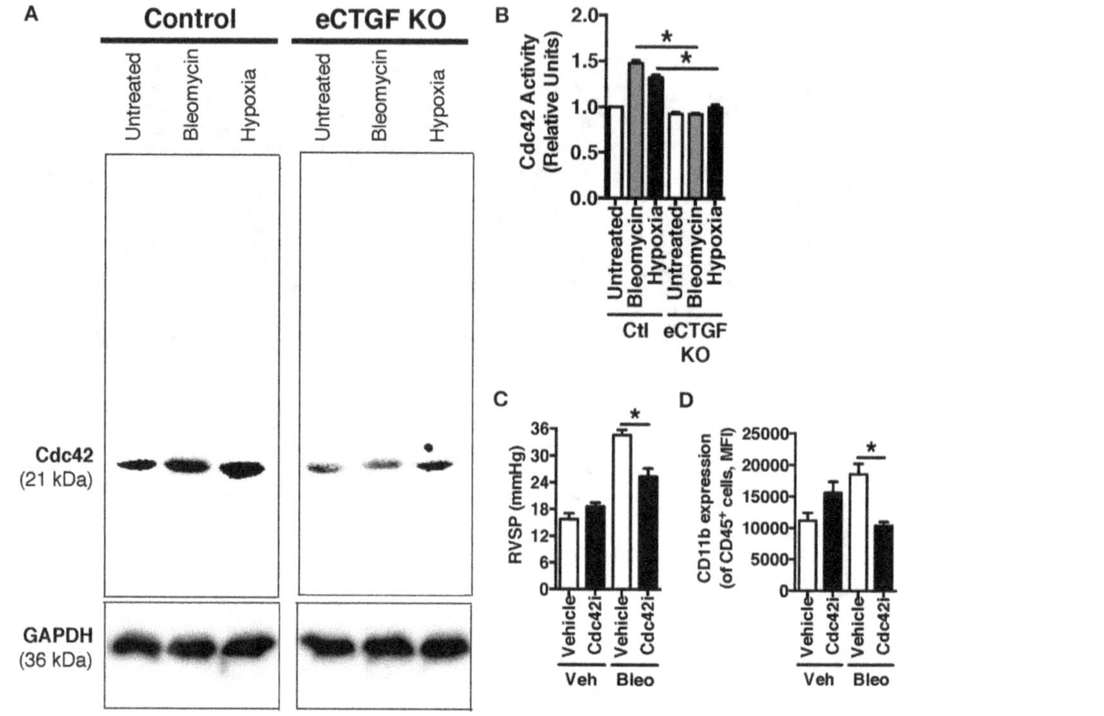

FIGURE 6 | Inhibition of Cdc42 suppressed PH in response to chronic hypoxia. **(A,B)** Cdc42 activation under normoxic/vehicle-, bleomycin-treated, and hypoxic conditions in lungs of Control and eCTGF KO mice. **(C)** RVSP in vehicle or Cdc42 inhibitor-treated (ML141; indicated as "Cdc42i") mice exposed to either vehicle or intraperitoneal bleomycin ($n = 8$ mice/group). **(D)** CD11b-expression, by flow cytometry, of CD45+ cells from lungs of treated mice ($n = 8$ mice/group). $^*P < 0.05$; data are presented as mean ± SEM.

Endothelial CTGF Expression Activates Cdc42 in Lungs of Mice Exposed to Hypoxia and Bleomycin, While Cdc42 Inhibition Protects against Development of PH

Vascular permeability is a consistent change observed in PH development (Burton et al., 2011a,b). Previous studies have shown that inhibition of vascular endothelial cell hypoxia signaling resulted in improvement in pulmonary vascular leak, associated with a decrease in CTGF production (Bryant et al., 2016). As a next step, to further investigate a potential mechanism of CTGF contribution to a known potentiator of vascular permeability and PH, we chose to examine the Rho GTPase proteins in a model of PH. This group is known to contribute to microvascular permeability (Spindler et al., 2010)—with candidate family member Cdc42 being mediated by CTGF—integrating cell polarization and migration in response to injury (Crean et al., 2004; Black and Trackman, 2008). As demonstrated in **Figures 6A,B**, Cdc42 activity is increased in response to both bleomycin and hypoxia treatment, and is nearly absent in whole lung samples from our eCTGF KO mice. Given difficulties with feasibility in the experimental approach of administering a daily Cdc42 inhibitor (ML141; referred to as "Cdc42i," in figure) to mice undergoing either hypoxia exposure (frequently interrupting the development of the phenotype), or multiple injections (with bleomycin and clodronate liposome administration), and—finally—given the robust upregulation in the bleomycin model alone, we chose to test whether Cdc42 inhibition would be protective against development of bleomycin-induced PH. The administration of a Cdc42 inhibitor prevented development of PH in response to bleomycin treatment, though not to completely normal pressure measurements (**Figure 6C**). Importantly, pulmonary pressures were lowered in association with decreased CD11b expression (**Figure 6D**). Taken together, these results suggest that endothelial CTGF plays a pivotal role in inducing PH through coordinating CD11b$^+$-cell trafficking to the lung due to change in induction of Cdc42 activity, which is known to influence cell polarization and motility (Summary, **Figure 7**).

DISCUSSION

Balanced regulation of wound-healing response through CTGF is a necessity for survival of an organism. Too little CTGF can impair efficiency of tissue regeneration after injury (Gibson et al., 2014), but too much can result in fibrosis and eventual organ dysfunction (Wang et al., 2011). While numerous cell-types have been found to secrete CTGF in response to chronic inflammation or injury, the tissue-specific contribution to development of aberrant vascular remodeling continues to be actively scrutinized.

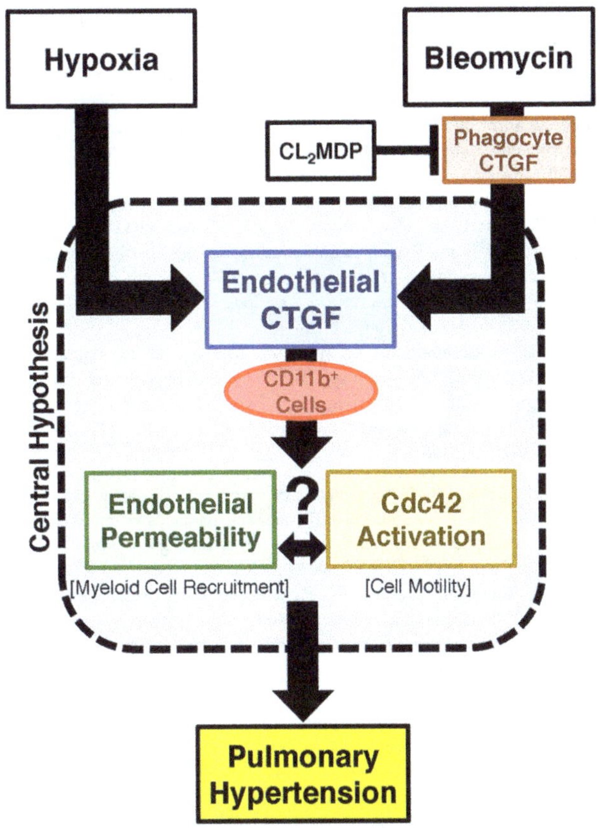

FIGURE 7 | Proposed schema for development of PH regulated by endothelial cell CTGF. Endothelial CTGF contributes to recruitment of CD11b-expressing leukocytes to the lung. Cd11b^{+} cells feasibly traffic to the lung through alteration in vascular endothelial barrier function, in combination with changes in cell motility factors, such as Cdc42. Together, these factors contribute to the development of PH.

To this end, proper and coordinated release of CTGF by specific cells within the vascular niche, and the subsequent downstream orchestration of cell motility and proliferation, is necessary for normal vascular repair. Among the factors known to facilitate cell migration is Cdc42, which dynamically mediates actin cytoskeleton rearrangement and is directly regulated by a CTGF-integrated mechanism (Crean et al., 2004). However, the contribution of vascular endothelial CTGF to Cdc42-mediated actin polymerization and cell-cell adhesion is complex, depending on the coordinated reaction of multiple cell types within the lung. In this study, we have shown that endothelial cell expression of CTGF is necessary for development of PH secondary to chronic hypoxia, implicating a potential mechanism in the regulation of Rho family GTPase, Cdc42.

While other members of the Rho family of GTPases—such as RhoA and Rac1—have been confirmed as important in endothelial cell permeability upon exposure to noxious stimuli, the role of Cdc42 in this process remains disputed Wojciak-Stothard et al., 2001; Fediuk et al., 2014). However, changes in endothelial cytoskeleton, adherens junctions, and permeability do correlate with Cdc42 activity in a model of hypoxia-induced neonatal pulmonary hypertension (Wojciak-Stothard et al., 2006). Importantly, CTGF works in concert with other protein mediators to increase the angiogenic response to injury, including downstream Cdc42 activation (Pi et al., 2012; Kiwanuka et al., 2016). Thus, it is interesting to speculate—based on our findings—that the spatiotemporal integration of signals that regulate cytoskeletal dynamics through CTGF, specifically Cdc42, are necessary for PH development. Future studies examining vascular endothelial models of Cdc42 up- or down-regulation upon exposure to hypoxia will help to elucidate this mechanism.

Moreover, as described above, CTGF may be directly responsible for binding to CD11b in promoting the adhesion and diapedesis of myeloid cells within inflamed vasculature (Schober et al., 2002). This finding is consistent with another report detailing that, in a model of renal fibrosis, while CTGF is expressed by myeloid cells to a slight degree, the predominant expression is in other surrounding kidney cells (Tateishi et al., 2015). Furthermore, CTGF expression is sufficient to induce bone marrow mesenchymal stem cells/stromal cells to differentiate into collagen-producing fibroblasts, contributing to fibrogenesis and pathological fibrosis (Lee et al., 2010). Interestingly, our group has recently described a contributory role of a similarly immature CD11b^{+} myeloid cell population in vascular remodeling necessary for development of chronic hypoxia-induced PH (Bryant et al., 2017). A next step in parsing out the mechanistic pathway leading to disease, will involve exploring the CTGF/CD11b interaction in *in vitro* and *in vivo* models, to understand the true molecular effect on pathophysiology of pulmonary vascular remodeling.

Though the central hypothesis is strongly supported by our experimental design—including use of our novel genetic knock out model—there are several limitations in this study worth noting. First, these data do not address a central question: what is the role of pulmonary macrophage CTGF-expression in development of pulmonary vasculopathy? As mentioned above, many different cells can express CTGF, and they often express it more strongly than macrophages. Therefore, it remains to be determined what is the relative contribution of CTGF from each of the cells toward development of PH. Though one hypothesis is that protection conferred in the bleomycin and clodronate liposome model is due to depletion of phagocyte produced CTGF, the role of those cells in the model, and the source of CTGF that drives their accumulation, requires further exploration. The contribution of other cells is also reinforced by recent studies detailing the necessary function of CTGF in bone marrow development and myeloid precursor-cell release by the stroma (Battula et al., 2013; Wang et al., 2015). Similarly, though the VECadherin Cre-recombinase is expressed primarily within vascular endothelial cells, there is slight, but potentially contributory, expression within bone marrow cells. Thus, a second caveat to the reported study is that CTGF expression may be decreased within the bone marrow stromal microenvironment in our model, resulting in inhibition of myeloid cells discharge from the developmental niche (Istvánffy et al., 2015). Such a finding would result in decreased numbers of CD11b-expressing cells in the circulation of these animals.

However, contrary to this concern, we detected no gross decrease in global hematopoiesis in our murine models. Nevertheless, such a concern does emphasize the need to search for bone marrow contribution to the PH phenotype, through either generation of bone marrow chimera mice or by knocking out CTGF expression in bone marrow stromal cell populations (Cheung et al., 2014).

Overall, regulation of CTGF expression in response to injury is poorly understood on a broad spectrum encompassing potential deficits of wound repair and chronic scarring leading to fibrosis. The current study demonstrates that tissue-specific expression of CTGF by the vascular endothelium significantly influences the delicate balance between extremes of aberrant vascular wound repair, leading to development of PH. As well, we observed that inhibition of CTGF-regulated Cdc42 results in near normalization of pulmonary artery pressures. Given that vasodilator therapy use—clinically applied based primarily upon the treatment of familial/genetic pulmonary arterial hypertension—has to date failed in application to patients with Group III PH, there is a significant clinical need for evaluation of novel drug targets that meaningfully impact disease pathogenesis. We believe that endothelial cell CTGF-dependent interaction with Cdc42 in the recruitment of circulating CD11b+ myeloid cells is a singular example of a relevant protective pathway, possibly contributing to observed benefit in human clinical trials of anti-CTGF drugs related to pulmonary disease. Ultimately, cell-specific targeting may improve the clinical benefit of such therapies (Liu H. et al., 2006; Liu L. et al., 2006; Jung et al., 2017), with an ancillary decrease in off-target effects.

AUTHOR CONTRIBUTIONS

LP: designed and performed experiments, analyzed data, and wrote the manuscript; CF, YL, JZ, MJ, and VS: performed experiments; KL and ES: designed experiments and edited the manuscript; AB: designed experiments, analyzed data, and edited the manuscript.

SUPPLEMENTARY MATERIAL

Supplementary Figure 1 | Mice without vascular endothelial cell expression of CTGF are not protected against development of pulmonary fibrosis. **(A)** Fibrosis score and **(B)** collagen content of lungs from Control and eCTGF KO mice exposed to bleomycin ($n = 8$ mice/group).

Supplementary Table 1 | Antibodies used for immunostaining and flow cytometry.

REFERENCES

Alva, J. A., Zovein, A. C., Monvoisin, A., Murphy, T., Salazar, A., Harvey, N. L., et al. (2006). VE-Cadherin-Cre-recombinase transgenic mouse: a tool for lineage analysis and gene deletion in endothelial cells. *Dev. Dyn.* 235, 759–767. doi: 10.1002/dvdy.20643

Baran, C. P., Opalek, J. M., McMaken, S., Newland, C. A., O'Brien, J. M. Jr., Hunter, M. G., et al. (2007). Important roles for macrophage colony-stimulating factor, CC chemokine ligand 2, and mononuclear phagocytes in the pathogenesis of pulmonary fibrosis. *Am. J. Respir. Crit. Care Med.* 176, 78–89. doi: 10.1164/rccm.200609-1279OC

Battula, V. L., Chen, Y., Cabreira Mda, G., Ruvolo, V., Wang, Z., Ma, W., et al. (2013). Connective tissue growth factor regulates adipocyte differentiation of mesenchymal stromal cells and facilitates leukemia bone marrow engraftment. *Blood* 122, 357–366. doi: 10.1182/blood-2012-06-437988

Black, S. A. Jr., and Trackman, P. C. (2008). Transforming growth factor-beta1 (TGFbeta1) stimulates connective tissue growth factor (CCN2/CTGF) expression in human gingival fibroblasts through a RhoA-independent, Rac1/Cdc42-dependent mechanism: statins with forskolin block TGFbeta1-induced CCN2/CTGF expression. *J. Biol. Chem.* 283, 10835–10847. doi: 10.1074/jbc.M710363200

Brusselmans, K., Compernolle, V., Tjwa, M., Wiesener, M. S., Maxwell, P. H., Collen, D., et al. (2003). Heterozygous deficiency of hypoxia-inducible factor-2alpha protects mice against pulmonary hypertension and right ventricular dysfunction during prolonged hypoxia. *J. Clin. Invest.* 111, 1519–1527. doi: 10.1172/JCI15496

Bryant, A. J., Carrick, R. P., McConaha, M. E., Jones, B. R., Shay, S. D., Moore, C. S., et al. (2016). Endothelial HIF signaling regulates pulmonary fibrosis-associated pulmonary hypertension. *Am. J. Physiol. Lung Cell. Mol. Physiol.* 310, L249–L262. doi: 10.1152/ajplung.00258.2015

Bryant, A. J., Robinson, L. J., Moore, C. S., Blackwell, T. R., Gladson, S., Penner, N. L., et al. (2015). Expression of mutant bone morphogenetic protein receptor II worsens pulmonary hypertension secondary to pulmonary fibrosis. *Pulm. Circ.* 5, 681–690. doi: 10.1086/683811

Bryant, A. J., Shenoy, V., Fu, C., Marek, G., Lorentsen, K. J., Herzog, E. L., et al. (2017). Myeloid-derived suppressor cells are necessary for development of pulmonary hypertension. *Am. J. Respir. Cell Mol. Biol.* 58, 170–180. doi: 10.1165/rcmb.2017-0214OC

Burton, V. J., Ciuclan, L. I., Holmes, A. M., Rodman, D. M., Walker, C., and Budd, D. C. (2011a). Bone morphogenetic protein receptor II regulates pulmonary artery endothelial cell barrier function. *Blood* 117, 333–341. doi: 10.1182/blood-2010-05-285973

Burton, V. J., Holmes, A. M., Ciuclan, L. I., Robinson, A., Roger, J. S., Jarai, G., et al. (2011b). Attenuation of leukocyte recruitment via CXCR1/2 inhibition stops the progression of PAH in mice with genetic ablation of endothelial BMPR-II. *Blood* 118, 4750–4758. doi: 10.1182/blood-2011-05-347393

Chen, C., Song, X., Ma, S., Wang, X., Xu, J., Zhang, H., et al. (2015). Cdc42 inhibitor ML141 enhances G-CSF-induced hematopoietic stem and progenitor cell mobilization. *Int. J. Hematol.* 101, 5–12. doi: 10.1007/s12185-014-1690-z

Cheung, L. C., Strickland, D. H., Howlett, M., Ford, J., Charles, A. K., Lyons, K. M., et al. (2014). Connective tissue growth factor is expressed in bone marrow stromal cells and promotes interleukin-7-dependent B lymphopoiesis. *Haematologica* 99, 1149–1156. doi: 10.3324/haematol.2013.102327

Cicha, I., Yilmaz, A., Klein, M., Raithel, D., Brigstock, D. R., Daniel, W. G., et al. (2005). Connective tissue growth factor is overexpressed in complicated atherosclerotic plaques and induces mononuclear cell chemotaxis *in vitro*. *Arterioscler. Thromb. Vasc. Biol.* 25, 1008–1013. doi: 10.1161/01.ATV.0000162173.27682.7b

Crean, J. K., Furlong, F., Finlay, D., Mitchell, D., Murphy, M., Conway, B., et al. (2004). Connective tissue growth factor [CTGF]/CCN2 stimulates mesangial cell migration through integrated dissolution of focal adhesion complexes and activation of cell polarization. *FASEB J.* 18, 1541–1543. doi: 10.1096/fj.04-1546fje

Degryse, A. L., Tanjore, H., Xu, X. C., Polosukhin, V. V., Jones, B. R., Boomershine, C. S., et al. (2011). TGFbeta signaling in lung epithelium regulates bleomycin-induced alveolar injury and fibroblast recruitment. *Am. J. Physiol. Lung Cell. Mol. Physiol.* 300, L887–L897. doi: 10.1152/ajplung.00397.2010

Fediuk, J., Sikarwar, A. S., Nolette, N., and Dakshinamurti, S. (2014). Thromboxane-induced actin polymerization in hypoxic neonatal pulmonary arterial myocytes involves Cdc42 signaling. *Am. J. Physiol. Lung Cell. Mol. Physiol.* 307, L877–L887. doi: 10.1152/ajplung.00036.2014

Finlin, B. S., Zhu, B., Starnes, C. P., McGehee, R. E. Jr., Peterson, C. A., and Kern, P. A. (2013). Regulation of thrombospondin-1 expression in alternatively activated macrophages and adipocytes: role of cellular cross talk and omega-3 fatty acids. *J. Nutr. Biochem.* 24, 1571–1579. doi: 10.1016/j.jnutbio.2013.01.007

Gibson, D. J., Pi, L., Sriram, S., Mao, C., Petersen, B. E., Scott, E. W., et al.

(2014). Conditional knockout of CTGF affects corneal wound healing. *Invest. Ophthalmol. Vis. Sci.* 55, 2062–2070. doi: 10.1167/iovs.13-12735

Hemnes, A. R., Brittain, E. L., Trammell, A. W., Fessel, J. P., Austin, E. D., Penner, N., et al. (2014). Evidence for right ventricular lipotoxicity in heritable pulmonary arterial hypertension. *Am. J. Respir. Crit. Care Med.* 189, 325–334. doi: 10.1164/rccm.201306-1086OC

Higgins, D. F., Biju, M. P., Akai, Y., Wutz, A., Johnson, R. S., and Haase, V. H. (2004). Hypoxic induction of Ctgf is directly mediated by Hif-1. *Am. J. Physiol. Renal Physiol.* 287, F1223–F1232. doi: 10.1152/ajprenal.00245.2004

Ikezumi, Y., Suzuki, T., Yamada, T., Hasegawa, H., Kaneko, U., Hara, M., et al. (2015). Alternatively activated macrophages in the pathogenesis of chronic kidney allograft injury. *Pediatr. Nephrol.* 30, 1007–1017. doi: 10.1007/s00467-014-3023-0

Irwin, D., Helm, K., Campbell, N., Imamura, M., Fagan, K., Harral, J., et al. (2007). Neonatal lung side population cells demonstrate endothelial potential and are altered in response to hyperoxia-induced lung simplification. *Am. J. Physiol. Lung Cell. Mol. Physiol.* 293, L941–L951. doi: 10.1152/ajplung.00054.2007

Istvánffy, R., Vilne, B., Schreck, C., Ruf, F., Pagel, C., Grziwok, S., et al. (2015). Stroma-derived connective tissue growth factor maintains cell cycle progression and repopulation activity of hematopoietic stem cells *in vitro*. *Stem Cell Reports* 5, 702–715. doi: 10.1016/j.stemcr.2015.09.018

Jung, K., Heishi, T., Khan, O. F., Kowalski, P. S., Incio, J., Rahbari, N. N., et al. (2017). Ly6Clo monocytes drive immunosuppression and confer resistance to anti-VEGFR2 cancer therapy. *J. Clin. Invest.* 127, 3039–3051. doi: 10.1172/JCI93182

Kiwanuka, E., Lee, C. C., Hackl, F., Caterson, E. J., Junker, J. P., Gerdin, B., et al. (2016). Cdc42 and p190RhoGAP activation by CCN2 regulates cell spreading and polarity and induces actin disassembly in migrating keratinocytes. *Int. Wound J.* 13, 372–381. doi: 10.1111/iwj.12315

Klinger, J. R. (2016). Group III pulmonary hypertension: pulmonary hypertension associated with lung disease: epidemiology, pathophysiology, and treatments. *Cardiol. Clin.* 34, 413–433. doi: 10.1016/j.ccl.2016.04.003

Lee, C. H., Shah, B., Moioli, E. K., and Mao, J. J. (2010). CTGF directs fibroblast differentiation from human mesenchymal stem/stromal cells and defines connective tissue healing in a rodent injury model. *J. Clin. Invest.* 120, 3340–3349. doi: 10.1172/JCI43230

Lee, Y. S., Byun, J., Kim, J. A., Lee, J. S., Kim, K. L., Suh, Y. L., et al. (2005). Monocrotaline-induced pulmonary hypertension correlates with upregulation of connective tissue growth factor expression in the lung. *Exp. Mol. Med.* 37, 27–35. doi: 10.1038/emm.2005.4

Lettieri, C. J., Nathan, S. D., Barnett, S. D., Ahmad, S., and Shorr, A. F. (2006). Prevalence and outcomes of pulmonary arterial hypertension in advanced idiopathic pulmonary fibrosis. *Chest* 129, 746–752. doi: 10.1378/chest.129.3.746

Lipson, K. E., Wong, C., Teng, Y., and Spong, S. (2012). CTGF is a central mediator of tissue remodeling and fibrosis and its inhibition can reverse the process of fibrosis. *Fibrogenesis Tissue Repair* 5(Suppl. 1):S24. doi: 10.1186/1755-1536-5-S1-S24

Liu, H., Liu, L., Fletcher, B. S., and Visner, G. A. (2006). Sleeping Beauty-based gene therapy with indoleamine 2,3-dioxygenase inhibits lung allograft fibrosis. *FASEB J.* 20, 2384–2386. doi: 10.1096/fj.06-6228fje

Liu, L., Liu, H., Visner, G., and Fletcher, B. S. (2006). Sleeping Beauty-mediated eNOS gene therapy attenuates monocrotaline-induced pulmonary hypertension in rats. *FASEB J.* 20, 2594–2596. doi: 10.1096/fj.06-6254fje

Murray, L. A., Chen, Q., Kramer, M. S., Hesson, D. P., Argentieri, R. L., Peng, X., et al. (2011). TGF-beta driven lung fibrosis is macrophage dependent and blocked by Serum amyloid P. *Int. J. Biochem. Cell Biol.* 43, 154–162. doi: 10.1016/j.biocel.2010.10.013

Noguchi, S., Saito, A., Mikami, Y., Urushiyama, H., Horie, M., Matsuzaki, H., et al. (2017). TAZ contributes to pulmonary fibrosis by activating profibrotic functions of lung fibroblasts. *Sci. Rep.* 7:42595. doi: 10.1038/srep42595

Pan, L. H., Yamauchi, K., Uzuki, M., Nakanishi, T., Takigawa, M., Inoue, H., et al. (2001). Type II alveolar epithelial cells and interstitial fibroblasts express connective tissue growth factor in IPF. *Eur. Respir. J.* 17, 1220–1227. doi: 10.1183/09031936.01.00074101

Pi, L., Robinson, P. M., Jorgensen, M., Oh, S. H., Brown, A. R., Weinreb, P. H., et al. (2015). Connective tissue growth factor and integrin alphavbeta6: a new pair of regulators critical for ductular reaction and biliary fibrosis in mice. *Hepatology* 61, 678–691. doi: 10.1002/hep.27425

Pi, L., Shenoy, A. K., Liu, J., Kim, S., Nelson, N., Xia, H., et al. (2012). CCN2/CTGF regulates neovessel formation via targeting structurally conserved cystine knot motifs in multiple angiogenic regulators. *FASEB J.* 26, 3365–3379. doi: 10.1096/fj.11-200154

Pi, L., Xia, H., Liu, J., Shenoy, A. K., Hauswirth, W. W., and Scott, E. W. (2011). Role of connective tissue growth factor in the retinal vasculature during development and ischemia. *Invest. Ophthalmol. Vis. Sci.* 52, 8701–8710. doi: 10.1167/iovs.11-7870

Schober, J. M., Chen, N., Grzeszkiewicz, T. M., Jovanovic, I., Emeson, E. E., Ugarova, T. P., et al. (2002). Identification of integrin alpha(M)beta(2) as an adhesion receptor on peripheral blood monocytes for Cyr61 (CCN1) and connective tissue growth factor (CCN2): immediate-early gene products expressed in atherosclerotic lesions. *Blood* 99, 4457–4465. doi: 10.1182/blood.V99.12.4457

Spindler, V., Schlegel, N., and Waschke, J. (2010). Role of GTPases in control of microvascular permeability. *Cardiovasc. Res.* 87, 243–253. doi: 10.1093/cvr/cvq086

Suzuma, K., Naruse, K., Suzuma, I., Takahara, N., Ueki, K., Aiello, L. P., et al. (2000). Vascular endothelial growth factor induces expression of connective tissue growth factor via KDR, Flt1, and phosphatidylinositol 3-kinase-akt-dependent pathways in retinal vascular cells. *J. Biol. Chem.* 275, 40725–40731. doi: 10.1074/jbc.M006509200

Tanjore, H., Cheng, D. S., Degryse, A. L., Zoz, D. F., Abdolrasulnia, R., Lawson, W. E., et al. (2011). Alveolar epithelial cells undergo epithelial-to-mesenchymal transition in response to endoplasmic reticulum stress. *J. Biol. Chem.* 286, 30972–30980. doi: 10.1074/jbc.M110.181164

Tanjore, H., Degryse, A. L., Crossno, P. F., Xu, X. C., McConaha, M. E., Jones, B. R., et al. (2013). Beta-catenin in the alveolar epithelium protects from lung fibrosis after intratracheal bleomycin. *Am. J. Respir. Crit. Care Med.* 187, 630–639. doi: 10.1164/rccm.201205-0972OC

Tanjore, H., Xu, X. C., Polosukhin, V. V., Degryse, A. L., Li, B., Han, W., et al. (2009). Contribution of epithelial-derived fibroblasts to bleomycin-induced lung fibrosis. *Am. J. Respir. Crit. Care Med.* 180, 657–665. doi: 10.1164/rccm.200903-0322OC

Tateishi, Y., Osada-Oka, M., Tanaka, M., Shiota, M., Izumi, Y., Ishimura, E., et al. (2015). Myeloid HIF-1 attenuates the progression of renal fibrosis in murine obstructive nephropathy. *J. Pharmacol. Sci.* 127, 181–189. doi: 10.1016/j.jphs.2014.12.011

Wang, Q., Usinger, W., Nichols, B., Gray, J., Xu, L., Seeley, T. W., et al. (2011). Cooperative interaction of CTGF and TGF-beta in animal models of fibrotic disease. *Fibrogenesis Tissue Repair* 4:4. doi: 10.1186/1755-1536-4-4

Wang, W., Strecker, S., Liu, Y., Wang, L., Assanah, F., Smith, S., et al. (2015). Connective tissue growth factor reporter mice label a subpopulation of mesenchymal progenitor cells that reside in the trabecular bone region. *Bone* 71, 76–88. doi: 10.1016/j.bone.2014.10.005

West, J., Harral, J., Lane, K., Deng, Y., Ickes, B., Crona, D., et al. (2008). Mi expressing BMPR2R899X transgene in smooth muscle develop pulmonary vascular lesions. *Am. J. Physiol. Lung Cell. Mol. Physiol.* 295, L744–L755. doi: 10.1152/ajplung.90255.2008

West, J. D., Austin, E. D., Gaskill, C., Marriott, S., Baskir, R., Bilousova, G., et al. (2014). Identification of a common wnt associated genetic signature across multiple cell types in pulmonary arterial hypertension. *Am. J. Physiol. Cell Physiol.* 307, C415–430. doi: 10.1152/ajpcell.00057.2014

Wojciak-Stothard, B., Potempa, S., Eichholtz, T., and Ridley, A. J. (2001). Rho and Rac but not Cdc42 regulate endothelial cell permeability. *J. Cell Sci.* 114(Pt 7), 1343–1355.

Wojciak-Stothard, B., Tsang, L. Y., Paleolog, E., Hall, S. M., and Haworth, S. G. (2006). Rac1 and RhoA as regulators of endothelial phenotype and barrier function in hypoxia-induced neonatal pulmonary hypertension. *Am. J. Physiol. Lung Cell. Mol. Physiol.* 290, L1173–L1182. doi: 10.1152/ajplung.00309.2005

Yu, A. Y., Shimoda, L. A., Iyer, N. V., Huso, D. L., Sun, X., McWilliams, R., et al. (1999). Impaired physiological responses to chronic hypoxia in mice partially deficient for hypoxia-inducible factor 1alpha. *J. Clin. Invest.* 103, 691–696. doi: 10.1172/JCI5912

Zaynagetdinov, R., Sherrill, T. P., Kendall, P. L., Segal, B. H., Weller, K. P., Tighe, R. M., et al. (2013). Identification of myeloid cell subsets in murine lungs using flow cytometry. *Am. J. Respir. Cell Mol. Biol.* 49, 180–189. doi: 10.1165/rcmb.2012-0366MA

10

Using Omics to Understand and Treat Pulmonary Vascular Disease

*Anna R. Hemnes**

Division of Allergy, Pulmonary and Critical Care Medicine, Vanderbilt University Medical Center, Nashville, TN, United States

***Correspondence:**
Anna R. Hemnes
anna.r.hemnes@vanderbilt.edu

Pulmonary arterial hypertension (PAH) is a devastating disease for which there is no cure. Presently this condition is differentiated from other diseases of the pulmonary vasculature by a practitioner's history, physical examination, and clinical studies with clinical markers of disease severity primarily guiding therapeutic choices. New technologies such as next generation DNA sequencing, high throughput RNA sequencing, metabolomics and proteomics have greatly enhanced the amount of data that can be studied efficiently in patients with PAH and other rare diseases. There is emerging data on the use of these "Omics" for pulmonary vascular disease classification and diagnosis and also new work that suggests molecular markers, including Omics, may be used to more efficiently match patients to their own most effective therapies. This review focuses on the state of knowledge on molecular classification and treatment of PAH. Strengths and weaknesses of current Omic technologies are discussed and how these new technologies can be used in the future to improve diagnosis of pulmonary vascular disease, more effectively treat patients with existing and future drugs, and generate new understanding of disease pathogenesis and mechanisms underlying treatment success or failure. Bioinformatic methods to analyze the large volumes of data are developing rapidly, but still present major challenges to interpretation of potential Omic findings in pulmonary vascular disease, with low numbers of patients studied and a potentially high false discovery rate. With more experience, precise and established drug response definitions, this field with move forward and will likely be a major component of the clinical care of PH patients in the future.

Keywords: pulmonary hypertension, omics-technologies, precision medicine, right ventricle, OMICS data

INTRODUCTION

Despite major advances in the last several decades, pulmonary vascular disease is a major source of morbidity and mortality. Primarily manifest as elevated pulmonary arterial pressure or pulmonary hypertension (PH), pulmonary vascular disease also includes pulmonary embolism and vascular malformations. PH has been subdivided in the current classification scheme into conditions that have a primary pulmonary vasculopathy, e.g., pulmonary arterial hypertension (PAH) and chronic thromboembolic PH (CTEPH) and conditions in which PH is considered to be a secondary phenomenon (1). For instance, left atrial hypertension raises pulmonary venous pressure and subsequently pulmonary arterial pressure, but if the left atrial pressure were removed, the PH would regress, theoretically. Similarly, parenchymal lung disease such as chronic obstructive pulmonary disease is associated with PH occasionally, but pathologic specimens do not uniformly demonstrate pulmonary arterial vasculopathy. Many of these conditions predispose to right ventricular failure and ultimately result in death, despite new treatments, making improved diagnostic and therapeutic options potentially highly clinically impactful.

Some forms of PH, e.g., PAH and chronic thromboembolic pulmonary hypertension (CTEPH), have specific medical or surgical therapies (2, 3), however the majority of PH and pulmonary vascular disease in general have no therapy aside from supportive care. Further complicating this group of diseases is the lack of specific diagnostic material. Lung biopsy is generally considered high risk in patients with PH or other forms of pulmonary vascular disease (4, 5), making diagnosis reliant on clinical factors, radiographic findings and invasive hemodynamics. This leaves clinicians with a major challenge of potentially missing a treatable condition such as PAH or CTEPH when they diagnose other forms of PH. Alternatively, PAH-directed therapy has been shown to potentially harm patients with non-PAH PH (6, 7), thus a practice pattern of simply treating all PH as PAH is potentially dangerous. In short, the field is in need of improved diagnostic modalities and more efficient mechanisms through which to identify patients who respond to a specific treatment.

Recent advances in biomedical research and bioinformatics approaches are now available to apply to pulmonary vascular disease and hold tremendous promise to improve diagnostic accuracy and improve treatments of all forms of pulmonary vascular disease. The term "Omics," hereafter referred to Omics, refers to the field of study generally ending in "-omics" such as genomics, proteomics, and transcriptomics. Broadly speaking, Omics suggests study of the entire field of proteins, metabolites or genes that may contribute to a disease state or phenomenon. Although early work in Omics included studies of genomics, transcriptomics, metabolomics, and proteomics, more recent work has added other fields such as radiology (radiomics) and cell biology (cell biomics). The use of transcriptomics and genomics in pulmonary vascular disease is most established, but recent work has drawn attention to how other Omics may be used to understand and optimally treat pulmonary vascular disease. This review will focus on these two key areas: First, use of Omics to classify PH and, second, use of Omics to optimize therapy in PAH and PH more broadly.

OMICS TO CLASSIFY PH

Originally developed in the second World Symposium on Pulmonary Hypertension in 1998, the classification of PH attempts to categorize patients by similar clinical and hemodynamic patters that correlate with specific pathologic findings and response to therapies (8). Although modifications have been made, the classification of PH continues to rely on clinical metrics (1). One notable exception to this is heritable PAH in which genetic mutations such as those in bone morphogenetic protein receptor type 2 (BMPR2) and other mutations are well-described (9–13) and may be used to assist in classification of patients.

Although the classification is generally quite useful in predicting response to PAH-directed therapies, many patients have features of multiple forms of PH, so-called "mixed" or "combined" PH. An example of a patient with combined group 1 and 2 PH is the 75 year old woman, an aunt in the blood line of a patient with heritable PAH who has normal lungs by chest imaging and spirometry, no evidence of chronic thromboembolic PH by ventilation perfusion lung scan, and a right heart catheterization demonstrating a pulmonary arterial wedge pressure of 20 mmHg and pulmonary arterial pressure of 95/50 mmHg with a normal cardiac output. Her elevated pulmonary arterial wedge pressure suggests group 2 PH, however she has a wide diastolic pressure gradient, suggesting underling pulmonary vasculopathy. Further, she likely carries a BMPR2 mutation, making PAH possible. After the 2012 World Symposium on PH, this patient would be called combined pre- and post-capillary PH (Cpc-PH) (14) and her case demonstrates a common clinical scenario of a patient with multiple potential etiologies of PH. As lung biopsies are not routinely obtained due to risk of bleeding and increased surgical risk in PH patients (3, 4), precise classification of many patients' pulmonary vascular disease may not be possible. Further, since most medical therapy is reserved for patients with exclusively PAH (2, 3, 15), patients with indicators they may have other forms of PH in addition to PAH may not be recommended for life-saving therapies. Thus, there are significant limitations to the current clinical classification of PH.

Although specific gene sequencing for mutations in BMPR2, ALK1, and other genes can, in the right clinical context, confirm a diagnosis of heritable PAH, these are specific, targeted tests and only applicable to small number of even patients with PAH, and a minute fraction of PH in general (9, 16, 17). Recently there has been interest in using Omic technologies to enhance the current classification of PH, thus moving beyond tests of single gene mutations. Early work in this field has used multiple Omic technologies to understand primarily how PAH patients are different from healthy controls. Given that PAH can be challenging to diagnose and is a relatively heterogeneous group of diseases including congenital heart disease and multiple different connective tissue diseases, some of the earliest Omic work focused on heritable PAH, in which the diagnosis is firm and the disease etiology less heterogeneous. West and colleagues used microarray analysis on cultured peripheral blood lymphocytes to define RNA transcript patterns in patients with heritable PAH compared with controls (18). Cultured lymphocytes offer the advantage of several weeks of *ex vivo* culture, thereby removing environmental influences on the cells. These data demonstrated alterations in estrogen metabolism, actin organization, growth, and apoptosis signaling with significant differences between heritable PAH and control patients. These early studies used a very well-defined disease phenotype to compare to controls and served as a prototype for future Omic analysis, focusing on tight phenotype and pathway or gene ontology analysis.

More recently, Rhodes and colleagues performed a comprehensive study of 1,416 plasma metabolites using ultraperformance liquid chromatography mass spectrometry in patients with PAH and healthy controls (19). They included only idiopathic and heritable PAH patients, again ensuring a relatively homogenous population and compared with both healthy and disease controls. Using an unbiased approach to analysis, they identified metabolites that discern PAH from controls and, after correcting for various factors, found 20 metabolites that distinguish PAH from healthy and disease controls. A network analysis of these metabolites highlights alterations in amino acid, nucleoside and glucose and lipid metabolism. They further developed a discriminant score using seven metabolites to separate PAH from healthy and disease controls. Taken together, these data demonstrate that metabolomics can be used to define detectable, metabolic differences between PAH and control patients and perhaps point to pathways key to development or maintenance of PAH.

Our own group has used genomics to understand whether patients with Cpc-PH have genetic variant patterns that are more similar to PAH than to group 2 PH with isolated post-capillary PH (Ipc-PH). Assad and colleagues first defined demographics in the three groups of patients and showed the Cpc-PH is distinct and characterized by younger age than Ipc-PH patients with more severe pulmonary hemodynamics (20). Using a DNA biorepository with pre-existing data on single nucleotide variants linked to de-identified clinical data, distinct gene variant patterns in Cpc-PH were identified that were more similar to PAH than to Ipc-PH patients and were in pathways known to be of relevance to PAH such as extracellular matrix and immune function. These data show that there may be genetic variant patterns that could be used to both understand etiology of pulmonary vascular disease, but also to define phenotypes and endophenotypes of pulmonary vascular disease.

Other groups have used similar methodologies to explore expression patterns in the lung, clearly a highly relevant tissue to pulmonary vascular disease. Geraci and colleagues demonstrated different expression patterns in PAH compared to controls in lung tissue (21). Others have used Omics in tissue and peripheral blood to study differences in RNA expression patterns in scleroderma-associated PAH (22, 23). Taken together, these data show the broad applicability of RNA expression pattern studies to pulmonary vascular disease, both in the peripheral blood and the affected tissues. Unfortunately, due to low numbers of patients undergoing lung transplantation or autopsy, studies of tissues are limited in number, thereby potentially limiting data generated and increasing false discovery rate. Nonetheless, when available, tissue can provide key insights into disease pathology and also critical confirmatory information of peripheral blood findings.

There is much enthusiasm that Omics will 1 day either augment or replace our current clinical classification of PH. With large numbers of patient enrollees, new molecular classifications discovered using Omics, may allow for more precise diagnoses, similar to progress made in cancer diagnostics. With homogenous diagnostic categories, discovery of molecular etiologies, identification of new therapeutics and more targeted clinical trials will all be possible (24). The National Institutes of Health/National Heart, Lung and Blood Institute (NHLBI) has funded a multi-center United States cohort study to use Omics, including genomics, transcriptomics, proteomics, and metabolomics, among other Omics, to advance understanding and classification of PH patients and is presently enrolling (NCT02980887) (25). Studies such as these potentially will change the classification and diagnosis of PH type to one that incorporates measurement of blood-based metrics into clinical parameters to define disease etiology and treatment recommendations.

OMICS TO IMPROVE THERAPY IN PH

PAH is a specific form of PH in which the distal pulmonary arterioles develop occlusive lesions, termed plexiform lesions, as well as other changes resulting in elevations in pulmonary vascular resistance generally with right heart failure and death within 3–5 years if untreated. While major progress has been made in therapy of PAH in the last several decades, it remains a highly mortal disease, with a recent publication showing that despite modern therapy, 40% of newly diagnosed patients die within 5 years (26), survival similar to early stage lung cancer. There are 10 FDA-approved therapies in three broad classes, however, clinicians have a very limited capacity to determine which patients are likely to respond to which drug class. This leads to costly prescription of multiple classes of medications, greater exposure to side effects of medications and greater burden of therapy, without clear therapeutic benefit. While the combination of tadalafil and ambrisentan has been shown to improve time to clinical worsening (27), there is very limited data on the efficacy of other combinations of medications. Additionally, PAH therapy is expensive, with annual costs ranging from \$20,000 to \$1,000,000 per patient. Use of costly and potentially ineffective drugs is untenable for healthcare systems. Thus, there is a pressing need to develop novel treatment strategies in PAH, ideally using drugs that are presently FDA-approved in the short term, and applying these strategies to future pivotal trials of drugs in all forms of PH.

Omics technologies have been used to improve patient care through identification of markers or patterns of markers that indicate positive responses to specific therapies, often drugs. While occasionally the same marker that defines a disease state can be used to predict treatment responses, e.g., the presence of cystic fibrosis with G551D mutation responds to treatment with ivacaftor (28), it is possible and perhaps likely that markers of drug responsiveness are different from those of disease diagnosis. Here we focus on Omic predictors of responses to PAH therapies, as there are presently no data for other forms of PH.

Some forms of PAH may provide clues as to how we can more effectively and efficiently treat PH. It has long been recognized that about 5–10% of patients with PAH have an acute pulmonary vasodilatory response when confronted with vasodilator therapy with normalization or near-normalization of pulmonary arterial pressures and preservation of cardiac output (29). Patients meeting these criteria can be treated safely with calcium channel blocker medications with substantially improved mortality and a much cheaper drug treatment cost (30). The identification of acute vasodilator response as a predictor of long term response

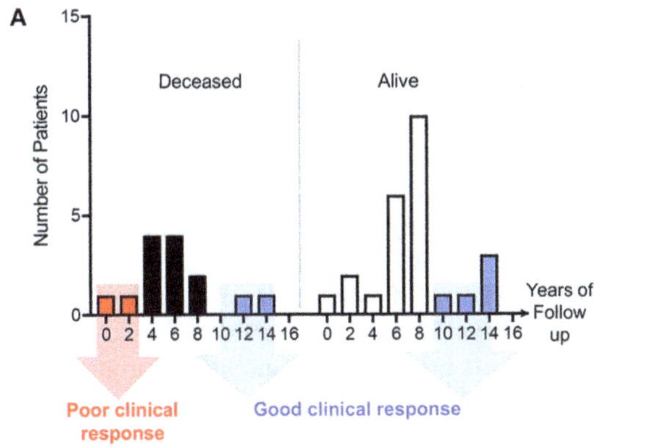

B

	Poor clinical response	Good clinical response
Change in 6MWD	<30m	>100m
RV function on Echo	Severe RV dysfunction	Normalizes
Change in FC	FC III or IV	FC I or II
Cardiac Index	<2	Normalizes
BNP	Persistently elevated	Normalizes
Survival	<3 years	>5 years
Transplant	Within 3 years	Never

6MWD = 6 minute walk distance; RV = right ventricle, BNP = brain natriuretic peptide, FC = functional class

FIGURE 1 | (A) Histograms of survival in ongoing survivors ($n = 25$) vs. deceased patients ($n = 14$). Y axis depicts years since initiation of IV epoprostenol. Patients with good response may be considered those still alive after 8 years of drug or those who are deceased but after 8 years of IV epoprostenol therapy. Eight years is the median survival in our cohort (31). **(B)** Table showing proposed single or combined metrics of response to parenteral prostacyclin therapy.

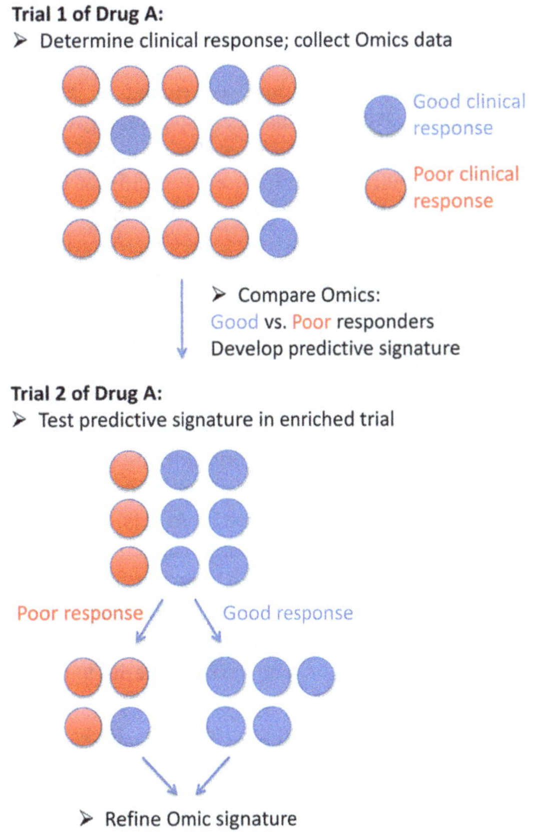

FIGURE 2 | Schematic of how Omic data could be used in a precision medicine trial of a drug in pulmonary arterial hypertension.

to calcium channel blocker therapy was a key development in the therapy of PAH as it (1) was the first foray into precision medicine in the field of pulmonary vascular disease and (2) defined a phenotypically homogenous group of drug responders that later could be studied to understand molecular etiology and markers of drug responsiveness in PAH.

Years after the discovery of this distinct phenotype, Omic technologies had advanced such that their use to find predictors of drug responsiveness now seemed plausible. Our group used transcriptomics to determine if the clinical response to calcium channel blocker therapies could be predicted using molecular markers (32). A major limitation to studying this condition is its extreme rarity making study of untreated patients infeasible. We overcame this limitation using cultured lymphocytes as above. Because the lymphocytes were cultured *ex vivo* for weeks, potential confounding by exposure to calcium channel blockers was minimized. We used microarray to measure mRNA expression levels and found that there were distinct patterns of RNA expression in the vasodilator-responsive PAH patients compared to those that were not. Since our primary goal was to define a simple RNA expression pattern to predict vasodilator responsive PAH, we confirmed the most differentially expressed genes using whole blood RNA. After doing this, we developed an algorithm of RNA expression patterns that predicted this drug-responsive PAH phenotype and validated it in an external cohort. The strengths of this approach are that the RNAs were selected agnostic of their biologic plausibility, allowing the selection of the strongest predictors and the use of cultured lymphocytes to remove environmental influences on RNA patterns. These data suggested that in a cohort of tightly phenotyped drug responders, with a clear definition of drug response, Omic predictors might potentially be used to predict drug responses.

The most appealing Omic field for predicting drug responses is genomics. Generally not impacted by external forces or intercurrent illness, DNA is also more stable facilitating transfer to different facilities and readily available through blood draws or buccal mucosa swab. In addition, DNA would not be expected to change if a patient is already started on PAH-directed therapy, whereas metabolomics, proteomics, and transcriptomics may be altered by the therapy itself. Given these appealing qualities, there have been a few recent attempts to predict drug responses using genomics. First, Benza and colleagues used targeted DNA sequencing to study gene variants in the endothelin signaling pathway (33). They identified several variants that predict clinical outcomes with endothelin receptor antagonist therapy in PAH. The authors approach was limited to only genes known to be in the endothelin pathway and it is possible that with a discovery-based approach they would have identified even stronger predictors of endothelin receptor antagonist therapy outcomes.

Our group used whole exome sequencing in PAH patients with and without acute vasodilatory response. Again using this distinct endophenotype as a proof of the concept that genomics can be used to predict drug responses. We did not identify one single gene or gene variant that predicts calcium channel blocker responses, however we did find over 1,500 DNA variants unique to PAH patients. Next generation DNA sequencing is well known to identify hundreds of variants of undetermined significance, a limitation we attempted to avoid using pathway analysis of identified variants, comparing patients with acute response to vasodilators and those without. After filtering out gene variants associated with the presence of idiopathic pulmonary fibrosis and those not predicted to be deleterious using online resources, we studied the variants based on their frequency and found that there were generally more gene variants in patients with vasodilator-responsive PAH and also these genes were enriched in pathways associated with smooth muscle cell contraction. In the case of vasodilator-responsive PAH, we learned that there likely is not a single gene that differentiates PAH from control, but more likely a pattern of gene variants. Perhaps with greater numbers, these data can be refined and a gene variant risk score for PAH may be developed. Presently, these drug Omic methodologies are not appropriate for clinical care, though hopefully their use is not far away.

Future areas in which Omics may be useful in PAH therapeutics include development of genetic or other markers of predictors of response to endothelin receptor antagonists, phosphodiesterase type 5 inhibitors, riociguat, and prostacyclin pathway therapeutics. Prostacyclins may be particularly appealing for this sort of analysis as excellent clinical response are well described, and endpoints such as death and transplant are unfortunately relatively common, making numbers of enrollees required to generate useful data relatively low (34). Examples of how groups may be defined, either singly or in combination, are shown in **Figure 1**, including a demonstration of how survival (**Figure 1A**) or clinical metrics (**Figure 1B**) could be used to define good or poor clinical response. **Figure 2** outlines a schema of how Omics could be used to refine future trials in pulmonary hypertension medications, both existing and future.

CHALLENGES IN THE USE OF OMICS IN PULMONARY VASCULAR DISEASE

In order to move this field forward, we need a commonly agreed upon definition of "good response" to drugs to allow segregation of groups. A key feature that made analysis of RNA expression patterns in PAH patients with and without acute vasodilator responses possible was the distinct acute drug responses and long term survival data. This clear endophenotype could be exploited on a molecular level. However, most clinical drug responses are less well-established, with perhaps the exception of the occasional exceptional prostacyclin response. Moreover, use of a single drug to treat PAH is becoming less common, making identification of molecular predictors of response to a single drug less likely. Further, while Omics may select one or several biomarkers of prognosis in PAH, they must be carefully tested in their predictive value against traditional, highly predictive clinical models of survival in PAH such as the REVEAL risk score (26, 35, 36).

Further, we need to refine our pipeline for analysis of Omics data. Each methodology generates at a minimum, hundreds and, more commonly, thousands of data points that have to be filtered and prioritized. The use of biologic plausibility may lose strongly predictive Omic metrics and alternatively a simple "strength of expression" analysis may miss biologically important molecules with low level expression. Finally, integration of data across Omic platforms is presently challenging and required advanced computational skills with different analytic techniques. This has the potential to bias the final data and its interpretation. Thus different methods for analyzing data may yield very different results, each with its own strengths and weaknesses. Recent developments such as predictive modeling and machine learning, reviewed here (37) and here (38), may be a powerful way forward to integrate and understand these large datasets. Detailed discussion of these methodologies and their applications are outside the scope of this manuscript.

CONCLUSION

In conclusion, Omic technologies hold tremendous promise to improve the diagnosis and treatment of PH. There are major limitations to their present use, however, including potentially high false discovery rate with low numbers of patients, imprecise phenotypes and bioinformatics challenges. With more experience, precise and established drug response definitions, this field with move forward and will likely be a major component of the clinical care of PH patients in the future.

AUTHOR CONTRIBUTIONS

The author confirms being the sole contributor of this work and approved it for publication.

REFERENCES

1. Simonneau G, Gatzoulis MA, Adatia I, Celermajer D, Denton C, Ghofrani A, et al. Updated clinical classification of pulmonary hypertension. *J Am Coll Cardiol.* (2013) **62**(25 Suppl.):D34–41. doi: 10.1016/j.jacc.2013.10.029
2. Galie N, Corris PA, Frost A, Girgis RE, Granton J, Jing ZC, et al. Updated treatment algorithm of pulmonary arterial hypertension. *J Am Coll Cardiol.* (2013) **62**(25 Suppl.):D60–72. doi: 10.1016/j.jacc.2013.10.031
3. Galie N, Humbert M, Vachiery JL, Gibbs S, Lang I, Torbicki A, et al. 2015 ESC/ERS guidelines for the diagnosis and treatment of pulmonary hypertension. *Rev Esp Cardiol.* (2016) **69**:177. doi: 10.1016/j.rec.2016.01.002
4. Castro M, Krowka MJ, Schroeder DR, Beck KC, Plevak DJ, Rettke SR, et al. Frequency and clinical implications of increased pulmonary artery pressures in liver transplant patients. *Mayo Clin Proc.* (1996) **71**:543–51.
5. Galie N, Hoeper MM, Humbert M, Torbicki A, Vachiery JL, Barbera JA, et al. Guidelines for the diagnosis and treatment of pulmonary hypertension. *Eur Respir J.* (2009) **34**:1219–63. doi: 10.1183/09031936.00139009

6. Kalra PR, Moon JC, Coats AJ. Do results of the ENABLE (Endothelin Antagonist Bosentan for Lowering Cardiac Events in Heart Failure) study spell the end for non-selective endothelin antagonism in heart failure? *Int J Cardiol.* (2002) **85**:195–7. doi: 10.1016/S0167-5273(02)00182-1
7. Montalescot G, Drobinski G, Meurin P, MacLouf J, Sotirov I, Philippe F, et al. Effects of prostacyclin on the pulmonary vascular tone and cardiac contractility of patients with pulmonary hypertension secondary to end-stage heart failure. *Am J Cardiol.* (1998) **82**:749–55.
8. Simonneau G, Galie N, Rubin LJ, Langleben D, Seeger W, Domenighetti G, et al. Clinical classification of pulmonary hypertension. *J Am Coll Cardiol.* (2004) **43**(12 Suppl. S):5S–12S. doi: 10.1016/j.jacc.2004.02.037
9. Newman JH, Wheeler L, Lane KB, Loyd E, Gaddipati R, Phillips JA, III, et al. Mutation in the gene for bone morphogenetic protein receptor II as a cause of primary pulmonary hypertension in a large kindred. *N Engl J Med.* (2001) **345**:319–24. doi: 10.1056/NEJM200108023450502
10. Best DH, Sumner KL, Austin ED, Chung WK, Brown LM, Borczuk AC, et al. EIF2AK4 mutations in pulmonary capillary hemangiomatosis. *Chest* (2013) **145**:231–6. doi: 10.1378/chest.13-2366
11. Germain M, Eyries M, Montani D, Poirier O, Girerd B, Dorfmuller P, et al. Genome-wide association analysis identifies a susceptibility locus for pulmonary arterial hypertension. *Nat Genet.* (2013) **45**:518–21. doi: 10.1038/ng.2581
12. Ma L, Roman-Campos D, Austin ED, Eyries M, Sampson KS, Soubrier F, et al. A novel channelopathy in pulmonary arterial hypertension. *N Engl J Med.* (2013) **369**:351–61. doi: 10.1056/NEJMoa1211097
13. Austin ED, Ma L, LeDuc C, Berman Rosenzweig E, Borczuk A, Phillips JA, III, et al. Whole exome sequencing to identify a novel gene (caveolin-1) associated with human pulmonary arterial hypertension. *Circ Cardiovasc Genet.* (2012) **5**:336–43. doi: 10.1161/CIRCGENETICS.111.961888
14. Vachiery JL, Adir Y, Barbera JA, Champion H, Coghlan JG, Cottin V, et al. Pulmonary hypertension due to left heart diseases. *J Am Coll Cardiol.* (2013) **62**(25 Suppl.):D100–8. doi: 10.1016/j.jacc.2013.10.033
15. McLaughlin VV, Archer SL, Badesch DB, Barst RJ, Farber HW, Lindner JR, et al. ACCF/AHA 2009 expert consensus document on pulmonary hypertension a report of the American College of Cardiology Foundation Task Force on Expert Consensus Documents and the American Heart Association developed in collaboration with the American College of Chest Physicians; American Thoracic Society, Inc.; and the Pulmonary Hypertension Association. *J Am Coll Cardiol.* (2009) **53**:1573–619. doi: 10.1016/j.jacc.2009.01.004
16. Machado RD, Pauciulo MW, Thomson JR, Lane KB, Morgan NV, Wheeler L, et al. BMPR2 haploinsufficiency as the inherited molecular mechanism for primary pulmonary hypertension. *Am J Hum Genet.* (2001) **68**:92–102. doi: 10.1086/316947
17. Thomson JR, Machado RD, Pauciulo MW, Morgan NV, Humbert M, Elliott GC, et al. Sporadic primary pulmonary hypertension is associated with germline mutations of the gene encoding BMPR-II, a receptor member of the TGF-beta family. *J Med Genet.* (2000) **37**:741–5. doi: 10.1136/jmg.37.10.741
18. West J, Cogan J, Geraci M, Robinson L, Newman J, Phillips JA, et al. Gene expression in BMPR2 mutation carriers with and without evidence of pulmonary arterial hypertension suggests pathways relevant to disease penetrance. *BMC Med Genomics* (2008) **1**:45. doi: 10.1186/1755-8794-1-45
19. Rhodes CJ, Ghataorhe P, Wharton J, Rue-Albrecht KC, Hadinnapola C, Watson G, et al. Plasma metabolomics implicates modified transfer RNAs and altered bioenergetics in the outcomes of pulmonary arterial hypertension. *Circulation* (2017) **135**:460–75. doi: 10.1161/CIRCULATIONAHA.116.024602
20. Assad TR, Hemnes AR, Larkin EK, Glazer AM, Xu M, Wells QS, et al. Clinical and biological insights into combined post- and pre-capillary pulmonary hypertension. *J Am Coll Cardiol.* (2016) **68**:2525–36. doi: 10.1016/j.jacc.2016.09.942
21. Geraci MW, Moore M, Gesell T, Yeager ME, Alger L, Golpon H, et al. Gene expression patterns in the lungs of patients with primary pulmonary hypertension: a gene microarray analysis. *Circ Res.* (2001) **88**:555–62. doi: 10.1161/01.RES.88.6.555
22. Hsu E, Shi H, Jordan RM, Lyons-Weiler J, Pilewski JM, Feghali-Bostwick CA. Lung tissues in patients with systemic sclerosis have gene expression patterns unique to pulmonary fibrosis and pulmonary hypertension. *Arthritis Rheum.* (2011) **63**:783–94. doi: 10.1002/art.30159
23. Bull TM, Coldren CD, Moore M, Sotto-Santiago SM, Pham DV, Nana-Sinkam SP, et al. Gene microarray analysis of peripheral blood cells in pulmonary arterial hypertension. *Am J Respir Crit Care Med.* (2004) **170**:911–9. doi: 10.1164/rccm.200312-1686OC
24. Newman JH, Rich S, Abman SH, Alexander JH, Barnard J, Beck GJ, et al. Enhancing insights into pulmonary vascular disease through a precision medicine approach. A joint NHLBI-cardiovascular medical research and education fund workshop report. *Am J Respir Crit Care Med.* (2017) **195**:1661–70. doi: 10.1164/rccm.201701-0150WS
25. Hemnes AR, Beck GJ, Newman JH, Abidov A, Aldred MA, Barnard J, et al. PVDOMICS: a multi-center study to improve understanding of pulmonary vascular disease through phenomics. *Circ Res* (2017) **121**:1136–9. doi: 10.1161/CIRCRESAHA.117.311737
26. Farber HW, Miller DP, Poms AD, Badesch DB, Frost AE, Muros-Le Rouzic E, et al. Five-Year outcomes of patients enrolled in the REVEAL Registry. *Chest* (2015) **148**:1043–54. doi: 10.1378/chest.15-0300
27. Galie N, Barbera JA, Frost AE, Ghofrani HA, Hoeper MM, McLaughlin VV, et al. Initial use of ambrisentan plus tadalafil in pulmonary arterial hypertension. *N Engl J Med.* (2015) **373**:834–44. doi: 10.1056/NEJMoa1413687
28. Whiting P, Al M, Burgers L, Westwood M, Ryder S, Hoogendoorn M, et al. Ivacaftor for the treatment of patients with cystic fibrosis and the G551D mutation: a systematic review and cost-effectiveness analysis. *Health Technol Assess.* (2014) **18**:1–106. doi: 10.3310/hta18180
29. Rich S, Brundage BH. High-dose calcium channel-blocking therapy for primary pulmonary hypertension: evidence for long-term reduction in pulmonary arterial pressure and regression of right ventricular hypertrophy. *Circulation* (1987) **76**:135–41. doi: 10.1161/01.CIR.76.1.135
30. Sitbon O, Humbert M, Jais X, Ioos V, Hamid AM, Provencher S, et al. Long-term response to calcium channel blockers in idiopathic pulmonary arterial hypertension. *Circulation* (2005) **111**:3105–11. doi: 10.1161/CIRCULATIONAHA.104.488486
31. Brittain EL, Pugh ME, Wheeler LA, Robbins IM, Loyd JE, Newman JH, et al. Shorter survival in familial versus idiopathic pulmonary arterial hypertension is associated with hemodynamic markers of impaired right ventricular function. *Pulm Circ.* (2013) 3:589–98. doi: 10.1086/674326
32. Hemnes AR, Trammell AW, Archer SL, Rich S, Yu C, Nian H, et al. Peripheral blood signature of vasodilator-responsive pulmonary arterial hypertension. *Circulation* (2015) **131**:401–9; discussion: 9. doi: 10.1161/CIRCULATIONAHA.114.013317
33. Benza RL, Gomberg-Maitland M, Demarco T, Frost AE, Torbicki A, Langleben D, et al. Endothelin-1 pathway polymorphisms and outcomes in pulmonary arterial hypertension. *Am J Respir Crit Care Med.* (2015) **192**:1345–54. doi: 10.1164/rccm.201501-0196OC
34. Halliday SJ, Hemnes AR. Identifying "super responders" in pulmonary arterial hypertension. *Pulm Circ.* (2017) 7:300–11. doi: 10.1177/2045893217697708
35. Benza RL, Miller DP, Barst RJ, Badesch DB, Frost AE, McGoon MD. An evaluation of long-term survival from time of diagnosis in pulmonary arterial hypertension from the REVEAL Registry. *Chest* (2012) **142**:448–56. doi: 10.1378/chest.11-1460
36. Benza RL, Miller DP, Gomberg-Maitland M, Frantz RP, Foreman AJ, Coffey CS, et al. Predicting survival in pulmonary arterial hypertension: insights from the Registry to Evaluate Early and Long-Term Pulmonary Arterial Hypertension Disease Management (REVEAL). *Circulation* (2010) **122**:164–72. doi: 10.1161/CIRCULATIONAHA.109.898122
37. Zeng ISL, Lumley T. Review of statistical learning methods in integrated omics studies (an integrated information science). *Bioinform Biol Insights* (2018) **12**:1177932218759292. doi: 10.1177/1177932218759292
38. Karczewski KJ, Snyder MP. Integrative omics for health and disease. *Nat Rev Genet.* (2018) **19**:299–310. doi: 10.1038/nrg.2018.4

11

Increased Drp1-Mediated Mitochondrial Fission Promotes Proliferation and Collagen Production by Right Ventricular Fibroblasts in Experimental Pulmonary Arterial Hypertension

*Lian Tian, Francois Potus, Danchen Wu, Asish Dasgupta, Kuang-Hueih Chen, Jeffrey Mewburn, Patricia Lima and Stephen L. Archer**

Department of Medicine, Queen's University, Kingston, ON, Canada

Correspondence:
Stephen L. Archer
stephen.archer@queensu.ca

Introduction: Right ventricular (RV) fibrosis contributes to RV failure in pulmonary arterial hypertension (PAH). The mechanisms underlying RV fibrosis in PAH and the role of RV fibroblasts (RVfib) are unknown. Activation of the mitochondrial fission mediator dynamin-related protein 1 (Drp1) contributes to dysfunction of RV myocytes in PAH through interaction with its binding partner, fission protein 1 (Fis1). However, the role of mitochondrial fission in RVfib and RV fibrosis in PAH is unknown.

Objective: We hypothesize that mitochondrial fission is increased in RVfib of rats with monocrotaline (MCT)-induced PAH. We evaluated the contribution of Drp1 and Drp1–Fis1 interaction to RVfib proliferation and collagen production in culture and to RV fibrosis *in vivo*.

Methods: Vimentin (+) RVfib were enzymatically isolated and cultured from the RVs of male Sprague–Dawley rats that received MCT (60 mg/kg) or saline. Mitochondrial morphology, proliferation, collagen production, and expression of Drp1, Drp1 binding partners and mitochondrial fusion mediators were measured. The Drp1 inhibitor mitochondrial division inhibitor 1 (Mdivi-1), P110, a competitive peptide inhibitor of Drp1–Fis1 interaction, and siRNA targeting Drp1 were assessed. Subsequently, prevention and regression studies tested the antifibrotic effects of P110 (0.5 mg/kg) *in vivo*. At week 4 post MCT, echocardiography and right heart catheterization were performed. The RV was stained for collagen.

Results: Mitochondrial fragmentation, proliferation rates and collagen production were increased in MCT-RVfib versus control-RVfib. MCT-RVfib had increased expression of activated Drp1 protein and a trend to decreased mitofusin-2 expression. Mdivi-1 and P110 inhibited mitochondrial fission, proliferation and collagen III expression in MCT-RVfib. However, P110 was only effective at high doses (1 mM). siDrp1 also reduced fission in MCT-RVfib. Despite promising results in cell therapy, *in vivo* therapy with P110 failed to prevent or regress RV fibrosis in MCT rats, perhaps due to failure to achieve adequate P110 levels or to the greater importance of interaction of Drp1 with other binding partners.

Conclusion: PAH RVfib have increased Drp1-mediated mitochondrial fission. Inhibiting Drp1 prevents mitochondrial fission and reduces RVfib proliferation and collagen production. This is the first description of disordered mitochondrial dynamics in RVfib and suggests that Drp1 is a potential new antifibrotic target.

Keywords: mitochondrial fission, mitochondrial dynamics, dynamin-related protein 1 (Drp1), fibrosis, mitochondrial division inhibitor 1 (Mdivi-1), P110

INTRODUCTION

Pulmonary arterial hypertension (PAH) is characterized by pulmonary vascular obstruction, vascular stiffening and vasoconstriction, leading to increased right ventricular (RV) afterload and, consequently, right ventricular hypertrophy (RVH). Ultimately, pulmonary vascular disease leads to death from RV failure. Despite the importance of pulmonary vascular hemodynamics in PAH, RV function is the major determinant of the long-term prognosis (D'Alonzo et al., 1991; Sandoval et al., 1994; Campo et al., 2010; Ghio et al., 2010; Humbert et al., 2010; Sachdev et al., 2011; Voelkel et al., 2015). Some PAH patients, such as those with Eisenmenger's syndrome, respond to increased afterload with an adaptive form of RVH, which is associated with a good prognosis; whereas, others, such as patients with scleroderma, have a maladaptive form of RVH. While the differences between adaptive and maladaptive RVH remain poorly defined, patients with maladaptive RVH have worse functional capacity. These patients have greater impairment of angiogenesis, adrenergic signaling and metabolism, and display impaired RV morphology characterized by RV dilatation and fibrosis (Archer et al., 2013; Ryan and Archer, 2014).

Disorders of mitochondrial metabolism, notably an increase in uncoupled glycolysis due to activation of pyruvate dehydrogenase kinase (the Warburg phenomenon), contribute to impaired RV myocyte function in RVH (Piao et al., 2010, 2013; Fang et al., 2012). The Warburg phenomenon also promotes an hyperproliferative, apoptosis-resistant phenotype in pulmonary artery smooth muscle cells (PASMC) in PAH (Michelakis et al., 2002; McMurtry et al., 2004; Bonnet et al., 2006). A similar Warburg shift in metabolism in pulmonary adventitial fibroblasts, mediated by epigenetic changes in pyruvate kinase muscle isoform 2/isoform 1 ratio, contributes to a hyperproliferative, profibrotic vascular fibroblast phenotype in PAH (Zhang et al., 2017).

In addition to metabolic changes (Sutendra and Michelakis, 2014), the mitochondria in PAH display structural changes due to disorders of mitochondrial dynamics that are linked to cell cycle regulation (Marsboom et al., 2012) and production of reactive oxygen species (Tian et al., 2017). Mitochondria undergo dynamic cycles of fission (division) and fusion (union) to form a highly plastic network. The mitochondrial network is regulated by various GTPase, including the fusion mediators mitofusin-1 (MFN1), mitofusin-2 (MFN2), and optic atrophy-1 (OPA1) and the fission mediator, dynamin-related protein 1 (Drp1) (Chen et al., 2003; Westermann, 2010). Inactivated Drp1 resides in the cytosol. Once activated by either dephosphorylation at Serine 637 (Cereghetti et al., 2008; Sharp et al., 2014, 2015), phosphorylation at Serine 616 (Taguchi et al., 2007; Marsboom et al., 2012), or both (Rehman et al., 2012), Drp1 translocates to the outer mitochondrial membrane where it associates with one or more of its binding partners, including fission protein 1 (Fis1), mitochondrial fission factor (MFF), and mitochondrial dynamics proteins of 49 and 51 kDa (MiD49 and MiD51) (Otera et al., 2010; Zhao et al., 2011; Loson et al., 2013; Chen et al., 2018). Activated Drp1 and its binding partners multimerize, forming a ring-like structure, which constricts and divides the mitochondrion, resulting in mitochondrial fission (Lee et al., 2004; Zhu et al., 2004; Chan, 2007; Youle and van der Bliek, 2012; Archer, 2013). Increased rates of mitochondrial fission are observed in PASMC in PAH, resulting in a fragmented mitochondrial network that promotes a hyperproliferative, apoptosis-resistant phenotype (Bonnet et al., 2007; Marsboom et al., 2012). This increase in mitotic fission is coordinated with cell cycle progression and reflects a shared reliance of fission and mitosis on certain kinases, including cyclin B1-CDK1 (Marsboom et al., 2012). However, the importance of increased fission is contextual and varies by cell type. For example, excessive mitochondrial fission in RV myocytes in PAH leads to increased production of mitochondrial-derived reactive oxygen species and impaired RV diastolic function (Tian et al., 2017), rather than changes in cell proliferation.

Inhibiting mitochondrial fission by targeting Drp1 has therapeutic potential in PAH. Mitochondrial division inhibitor 1 (Mdivi-1), a selective Drp1 GTPase activity inhibitor (Cassidy-Stone et al., 2008), inhibits mitochondrial fission and reduces proliferation in PASMC from PAH patients and improves hemodynamics *in vivo* in animal models of pulmonary hypertension (Marsboom et al., 2012). Mdivi-1 also inhibits mitochondrial fission in rat left ventricular (LV) myocytes and improves LV function both in *ex vivo* Langendorff ischemia-reperfusion injury model in rat and in *in vivo* cardiac arrest model in mouse (Sharp et al., 2014, 2015). P110, a relatively novel drug, is a 7-amino acid peptide representing a homology sequence between Drp1 and Fis1 (Guo et al., 2013; Qi et al., 2013). It is delivered across cell membranes and can cross the blood–brain barrier with the TAT_{47-57} carrier peptide (Guo et al., 2013). P110 selectively inhibits pathological, but not physiological mitochondrial fission (Guo et al., 2013; Qi et al., 2013). Blocking the interaction between Drp1 and Fis1 with P110 also preserves mitochondrial morphology and cellular function in rat cardiac myocytes under ischemia-reperfusion injury *in vitro* and *ex vivo* and improves LV function in an ischemia-reperfusion injury model *in vivo* (Disatnik et al., 2013). Our group has also demonstrated that P110 improves mitochondrial function and preserves RV diastolic function in both normal and monocrotaline (MCT)-induced PAH rat RVs in ischemia-reperfusion injury model using the Langendorff preparation (Tian et al., 2017). However, Fis1 is not important to the increased fission observed in PAH PASMC (Chen et al., 2018). The mitochondrial metabolic and mitochondrial dynamics profile of RV fibroblasts (RVfib) is unknown, as its potential relevance to RV fibrosis.

Here, we isolated RVfib from normal and pulmonary hypertensive rats and studied changes in mitochondrial dynamics. We focused on these cells as they are likely the major determinant of the RV fibrosis that occurs in maladaptive RVH. We compared RVfib from control versus monocrotaline (MCT)-induced PAH rats, using this well-established model because of the predisposition of the MCT RV to develop fibrosis and the MCT rat to die of RV failure. We characterized the mitochondrial dynamics in RVfib and examined the relationship between the observed increase in mitochondrial fission and increased rates of RVfib proliferation and collagen production. We then examined the effects of Mdivi-1 and P110 on mitochondrial morphology, cell proliferation and collagen production. We also evaluated the role of Drp1–Fis1 interaction in the regulation of mitochondrial fission in RVfib in PAH.

We demonstrate that MCT-RVfib have a fragmented mitochondrial phenotype due to excessive mitochondrial fission mediated by Drp1 activation. This phenotype persists in culture, suggesting it may be epigenetically mediated. This increase in fission promotes excess proliferation and collagen production. The Drp1 inhibitor Mdivi-1, small inhibitory RNA targeting Drp1 (siDrp1), and high doses of P110 each reverse mitochondrial fission. Both Mdivi-1 and high dose P110 reduce proliferation and collagen production in MCT-RVfib *in vitro* Despite promising results in cell culture, P110 was not effective *in vivo*, at the administered dose. This is the first description of increased mitochondrial fission as a mediator of cardiac fibroblast proliferation and collagen production. Drp1 is a potential new antifibrotic target in PAH.

MATERIALS AND METHODS

Experiments were conducted in accordance with the published guidelines of the Canadian Council on Animal Care and approved by the Queen's University Animal Care Committee.

Reagents

Monocrotaline (MCT; C2401), Mdivi-1 (M0199), dimethyl sulfoxide (DMSO; D2650), collagenase (C0130), Dulbecco's modified Eagle's medium (DMEM; D5796), 10% neutral buffered formalin (HT501128), and bovine serum albumin (A7906) were purchased from Sigma (St. Louis, MO, United States). Both P110 and the peptide control sequence, TAT, were purchased from United Peptide (Herndon, VA, United States). L-glutamine (25030081), fetal bovine serum (SH3039603), penicillin-streptomycin (15140163), trypsin-EDTA (25200056), Hanks' Balanced Salt Solution (SH3058802), phosphate-buffered saline (PBS; SH3025601), paraformaldehyde (AC416780250), Triton X-100 (BP151-100), and Tween-20 (BP337-100) were purchased from Thermo Fisher Scientific (Waltham, MA, United States). Fibroblast growth factor-basic was purchased from ProSpec (CYT-608; East Brunswick, NJ, United States).

Monocrotaline-Induced PAH Animal Model

Male Sprague–Dawley rats (~270 g) (Charles River, QC, Canada) received a single subcutaneous injection of monocrotaline (MCT; 60 mg/kg) (n = 45) or PBS (n = 5). We assessed the effects of P110 both as a prevention and as a regression intervention. In both protocols, P110 and TAT were administered at 0.5 mg/kg via intraperitoneal injection. In the prevention group (MCT-P3 group; n = 5), P110 was injected once at the time of injection of MCT.

There were two regression protocols. In one, P110 (MCT-P1 group; n = 14) or TAT (MCT-T1 group; n = 14) was injected on day 14 and 19 post MCT injection. In the other, P110 (MCT-P2 group; n = 7) or TAT (MCT-T2 group; n = 5) was injected on alternating days beginning day-10 post MCT injection.

Echocardiography

At week 4 after MCT injection, Doppler, 2-dimensional, and M-mode echocardiography was performed using a high-frequency ultrasound system (Vevo 2100; Visual Sonics, Toronto, ON, Canada), as described (Urboniene et al., 2010; Tian et al., 2017). The following variables were measured: pulmonary artery acceleration time (PAAT), main pulmonary artery (PA) inner diameter at the level of the pulmonary outflow tract during mid-systole, diastolic and systolic thickness of the RV free wall (RVFW), and tricuspid annular plane systolic excursion (TAPSE). RVFW systolic thickening was calculated as $(RVFW_{systole} - RVFW_{diastole})/RVFW_{diastole}$, and cardiac output (CO) was estimated as HR × VTI × $ID^2/4$, where HR is the heart rate, VTI is the systolic velocity time integral over the main PA flow obtained from pulsed-wave Doppler, and ID is the inner diameter of the main PA at mid-systole, as described previously (Piao et al., 2010; Urboniene et al., 2010; Prins et al., 2017; Tian et al., 2017).

Right Heart Catheterization (RHC)

At week 4, following cardiac ultrasound, invasive closed-chest RHC was performed to obtain RV pressure-volume loops. Briefly, rats were anesthetized with 5% isoflurane induction and maintained with 3% during procedures. A high-fidelity catheter (Scisense pressure-volume catheter; Transonic, London, ON, Canada) was advanced to RV through the right jugular vein and the right atria in closed-chest animals. During catheterization, animals were intubated and ventilated. RV pressure and volume were recorded continuously using Scisense ADV500 Pressure-Volume Measurement System (Transonic, London, ON, Canada) and LabScribe2 software (iWorx, Dover, NH, United States). RV systolic pressure and end-diastolic pressure (RVSP and RVEDP, respectively) were directly obtained from the pressure trace. Total pulmonary resistance (TPR) was then calculated as mPAP/CO, where CO is cardiac output calculated as (RV end-diastolic volume − RV end-systolic volume) × heart rate, and mPAP is the mean pulmonary artery pressure estimated as 0.61 × RVSP + 2 (Chemla et al., 2004).

Histological Analysis

After RHC, animals were sacrificed. RV and LV plus septum were then dissected for tissue weight measurement. Biopsies of RV free wall tissues were fixed in 10% buffered formalin. The fixed tissues were then embedded in paraffin and stained with picrosirius red, for measurement of collagen deposition.

Images of RV stained with picrosirius red were taken by a scientist who was blinded to the experimental groups, using a Leica digital color camera (Leica DFC310 FX, Leica Microsystems; Wetzlar, Germany) and Leica DM4000 B LED microscope with a 20X objective (Leica Microsystems; Wetzlar, Germany). For each sample, more than 4 areas were imaged and analyzed for the percentage of the collagen area using Leica software (LAS V4.7, Leica Microsystems; Wetzlar, Germany). Results are presented as the average percentage of all the sample areas stained with picrosirius red.

RV Fibroblasts Isolation

RVfib were isolated from control and monocrotaline rats (n = 8 each) using a modification of a previously described method (Agocha and Eghbali-Webb, 1997). Briefly, excised fresh RV free wall tissues were rinsed with ice-cold PBS twice and minced in ice-cold PBS into small pieces at ~0.5 mm. The minced tissues were then digested at 37°C in 2 mL Hanks' Balanced Salt Solution supplemented with 0.1% trypsin-EDTA and 200 U/mL collagenase in 15 mL conical tube by constant stirring at a speed of 1000 RPM via Eppendorf™ ThermoMixer temperature control device (05412503; Thermo Fisher Scientific, Waltham, MA, United States) for 5 min, and the supernatant was discarded. A total of 2 mL digestion solution was added to the 15 mL conical tube for the next digestion. The second to the sixth digestions underwent constant stirring for 15 min each, and at the end of each digestion period the supernatant was aspirated and centrifuged. The pellet was suspended in culture medium and placed on a 100-mm culture dish (12-556-02; Fisher Scientific, Waltham, MA, United States). After the supernatant was aspirated, 2 mL of fresh digestion solution was added for the next cycle. On the second and the third days after the cell isolation, the cell culture dish was washed with PBS and replaced with new culture medium. Starting from the fourth day, the culture medium was replaced every 2 or 3 days. The identity of fibroblasts was confirmed by immunofluorescence using previously published criteria (positive for vimentin and negative for α-smooth muscle actin, von Willebrand factor, and heavy chain cardiac myosin) (Neuss et al., 1996; Agocha and Eghbali-Webb, 1997).

Cell Culture

Isolated RVfib were cultured in DMEM containing glucose (4500 mg/L), supplemented with 2 mM L-glutamine, 10% fetal bovine serum, penicillin/streptomycin (100 U/mL), and 4.6 ng/L fibroblast growth factor basic. Cells were treated with P110 or control peptide TAT (10, 50, 100 μM or 1 mM) daily, with small interfering RNA of Drp1 (siDrp1) or its negative control (NC1), or with Mdivi-1 (25 μM) or DMSO once. Depending on the experiment they were studied 5, 24, 48, or 72 h post incubation with the study drug.

qRT-PCR

The mRNA was extracted from RVfib using the Invitrogen™ Ambion PureLink RNA Mini Kit (12183025; Thermo Fisher Scientific, Waltham, MA, United States), and then converted to cDNA with High-Capacity cDNA Reverse Transcription Kit (4368814; Thermo Fisher Scientific, Waltham, MA, United States). mRNA levels of Drp1, Fis1, MFF, MiD49, and MiD51 were assessed by Bio-Rad CFX96 qPCR instrument (Mississauga, ON, Canada). mRNA expression was normalized to GAPDH mRNA and the relative expression between groups was assessed using $2^{-\Delta\Delta Ct}$ equation. All the primers were purchased from IDT (San Jose, CA, United States).

Mitochondrial Networking

Mitochondrial fragmentation was evaluated with MitoTracker™ Green FM (M7514; Thermo Fisher Scientific, Waltham, MA, United States) or tetramethylrhodamine methyl ester (TMRM; Cat #T668, Lifetechnologies; Carlsbad, CA, United States). Briefly, RVfib were cultured in a 35-mm glass-bottom dish (P35G-1.5-14-C; MatTek Corporation, Ashland, MA, United States) and incubated in culture medium containing 400 nM MitoTracker™ Green FM or 25 nM TMRM at 37°C in the dark for 40 or 20 min, respectively. Images were then taken with a Leica SP8 confocal, laser-scanning microscope (Leica Microsystems; Wetzlar, Germany) with a 1.40 NA, 63X oil immersion objective with 3X digital zoom. Mitochondrial segments were identified using ImageJ (National Institutes of Health, Bethesda, MD, United States), and mitochondrial fragmentation count was calculated as the ratio of the number of individual mitochondria and the total area of these mitochondria, as described (Marsboom et al., 2012; Rehman et al., 2012).

In addition, mitochondrial morphology was also quantified via a machine-learning algorithm using the Leica LAS X software (Leica Microsystems; Wetzlar, Germany), as described (Chen et al., 2018). This algorithm automatically measures the percentage area of three morphology-based categories (punctate, intermediate, and filamentous) in an entire field of cells, independent of the operator. Briefly, an image that has mitochondria covering a large range of area, length, and aspect ratio was chosen, and more than 15 mitochondria from each category were manually selected from this image to inform the machine-leaning algorithm. Subsequently, the algorithm was applied to all the images to obtain the percentage area of each category in each image. Results are presented as the average distribution of the three categories.

Proliferation Assay

Cell proliferation was assessed using the Click-iT® EdU Flow Cytometry Assay Kit following the manufacturer's instructions (C10420; Thermo Fisher Scientific, Waltham, MA, United States), as described (Hong et al., 2017). Briefly, 10 μM EdU (5-ethynyl-2′-deoxyuridine) was added to the culture medium for incorporation into DNA during active DNA synthesis and the cell culture dish that did not have addition of EdU was taken as a negative staining control. A total of 24 h following the addition of EdU, cells were harvested, fixed, permeabilized, and labeled with Alexa Fluor® 488 azide. The analysis for proliferation was then performed using the analysis mode of the flow sorter SH800S (Sony Biotechnology Inc., San Jose, CA, United States). A total of 10,000 events were recorded, adjusted according forward and side scatter and the positive population was gated and analyzed using the 488 nm laser and FL2 filter (525 ± 50).

Immunoblotting

Proteins were extracted from RVfib with cell lysis buffer (#9803; Cell Signaling Technologies, Beverly, MA, United States) and 50 or 70 μg (for phosphorylated Drp1 at Serine 616) protein was loaded to SDS-PAGE gel for immunoblotting. Images were taken with Chemidoc MP Imaging System (Bio-Rad Laboratories; Mississauga, ON, Canada) and analyzed with ImageJ (National Institutes of Health, Bethesda, MD, United States). The following antibodies were used: anti-β-actin (A5441; Sigma, St. Louis, MO, United States), anti-MFN2 (ab56889; Abcam, Cambridge, MA, United States), anti-phospho-Drp1 (Ser616) (#3455; Cell Signaling Technology, Danvers, MA, United States), anti-Drp1 (611112; BD Transduction Laboratories™, San Jose, CA, United States). β-actin was used as loading control. Note that for the gels running for phosphorylated Drp1 at Serine 616, the cells were collected on ice and low temperature was carefully maintained throughout all steps of protein isolation and processing.

Immunofluorescence

Cells were fixed in 4% paraformaldehyde at room temperature for 10 min, permeabilized with 1% Triton X-100 in PBS, blocked in 2% bovine serum albumin plus 0.05% Tween-20 in PBS for 30 min, and incubated with primary antibodies at 4°C overnight. The following primary antibodies were used: anti-collagen III (ab6310; Abcam, Cambridge, MA, United States), anti-collagen I (ab34710; Abcam, Cambridge, MA, United States), anti-phospho-Drp1 (Ser616) (#3455; Cell Signaling Technology, Danvers, MA, United States), anti-vimentin (ab8069; Abcam, Cambridge, MA, United States), anti-α-smooth muscle actin (ab5694; Abcam, Cambridge, MA, United States), anti-von Willebrand factor (ab6994; Abcam, Cambridge, MA, United States), and anti-heavy chain cardiac myosin (ab15; Abcam, Cambridge, MA, United States). Slides were then washed with PBS for 5 min three times and then incubated with secondary antibodies (Alexa Fluor-conjugated secondary antibodies Alexa Fluor 488 goat anti-rabbit #A-11034 and Alexa Fluor goat anti-mouse #A-11031; Invitrogen, Carlsbad, CA, United States) for 60 min at room temperature. Finally, slides were washed with PBS three times in the dark and mounted in ProLong™ Gold Antifade Mountant with DAPI (P36935; Thermo Fisher Scientific, Waltham, MA, United States). Images on phospho-Drp1 (Ser616) and collagen were taken with a Leica SP8 confocal, laser-scanning microscope (Leica Microsystems; Wetzlar, Germany) with a 1.40 NA, 63X oil immersion objective with 3X digital zoom and with Leica DM4000 B LED microscope with a 20X objective (Leica Microsystems; Wetzlar, Germany). A microscopist blinded to treatment groups performed the analysis. Images for cell characterization were acquired with an EVOS image system (EVOS FL Color, Life Technologies; Carlsbad, CA, United States). The intensity of fluorescent signal for phospho-Drp1 (Ser616) and collagen I and III was measured using ImageJ software (National Institutes of Health; Bethesda, MD, United States).

Statistical Analysis

All of the data are reported as mean ± standard error of the mean (SEM). Two-tailed, Student's *t*-test, paired *t*-test, Chi-Square test, or analysis of variance (ANOVA) was performed as appropriate. Statistical analyses were performed using the GraphPad Prism version 7.04 for Windows (GraphPad[1] Software, La Jolla, CA, United States). A $P < 0.05$ was considered statistically significant.

RESULTS

Mdivi-1, siDrp1, and P110 at High Dose Inhibit Mitochondrial Fission in MCT-RV Fibroblasts

The identity of isolated fibroblasts from RV was confirmed with immunofluorescence positive for vimentin and negative for α-smooth muscle actin, von Willebrand factor, and heavy chain cardiac myosin staining (Supplementary Figure S1). Compared to control-RVfib, MCT-RVfib displayed excessive mitochondrial fission indicated by increased mitochondrial fragmentation count (MFC) and decreased percentage area of filamentous mitochondria (**Figure 1**). Both Mdivi-1 (25 μM) treatment for 5 or 24 h and siDrp1 for 48 h inhibited mitochondrial fission in MCT-RVfib, whereas P110 treatment for either 5, 24, or 48 h at a dose of 10, 50, or 100 μM did not significantly inhibited mitochondrial fission in MCT-RVfib (**Figure 1** and Supplementary Figure S2). Treatment with P110 at a high dose (1 mM) for 3 days significantly inhibited mitochondrial fission in MCT-RVfib with no effect on Control-RVfib (**Figures 1D,E**).

Mdivi-1 and P110 at High Dose Reduce Proliferation in MCT-RV Fibroblasts

Compared to Control-RVfib, MCT-RVfib had higher proliferation rates (**Figure 2**). Mdivi-1 (25 μM) treatment for 48 h significantly reduced proliferation rates in MCT-RVfib (**Figure 2**). Treatment with P110 for 48 h at a dose of 10, 50, or 100 μM had no significant effect on the proliferation of MCT-RVfib (**Figure 2**). Again, treatment with P110 at a high dose (1 mM) for 3 days significantly reduced proliferation rates in MCT-RVfib but also in Control-RVfib (**Figure 2**). Preliminary study found that treatment with P110 at low doses (0.5 mM or lower) for 3 days did not reduce proliferation rates on RV fibroblasts from two MCT rats (data not shown).

[1] www.graphpad.com

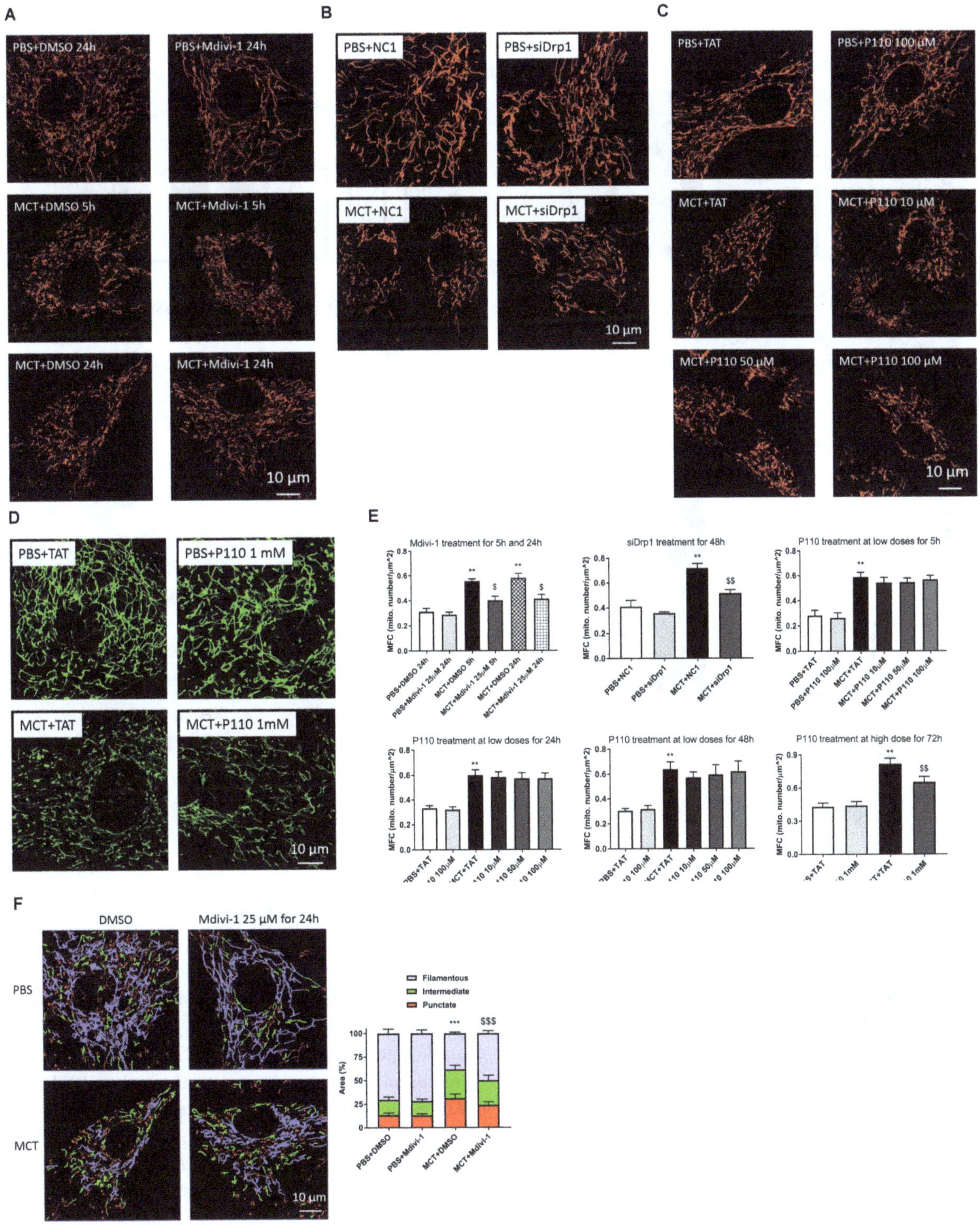

FIGURE 1 | Monocrotaline (MCT)-induced RVfib display mitochondrial fragmentation and mitochondrial division inhibitor 1 (Mdivi-1; 25 μM) for both 5 and 24 h, small interfering RNA targeting Drp1 (siDrp1) for 48 h, and P110 treatment at high dose (1 mM) for 3 days inhibited mitochondrial fission, whereas P110 at a dose up to 100 μM for 5, 24, and 48 h has no significant effect. Representative mitochondrial network stained with TMRM in RVfib with and without **(A)** Mdivi-1 for 5 and 24 h, **(B)** siDrp1 for 48 h, or **(C)** P110 (up to 100 μM) treatment for 5 h; **(D)** Representative mitochondrial network stained with MitoTracker^{TM} Green FM with P110 and its control TAT (1 mM) treatment for 3 days; **(E)** Summary of mitochondrial fragmentation count (MFC) in RVfib; **(F)** Representative mitochondrial network divided into three categories (punctate, red; intermediate, green; filamentous, purple) in RVfib treated with Mdivi-1 (25 μM) for 24 h and summary of area distribution of the three categories. $^{**}P < 0.01$ and $^{***}P < 0.001$ versus PBS+DMSO, PBS+NC1, or PBS+TAT group; $^{\$}P < 0.05$, $^{\$\$}P < 0.01$, and $^{\$\$\$}P < 0.001$ versus the corresponding vehicle control group (i.e., MCT+DMSO, MCT+NC1, or MCT+TAT). $n = 5$ per group except for the PBS+NC1 and PBS+siDrp1 groups ($n = 2$).

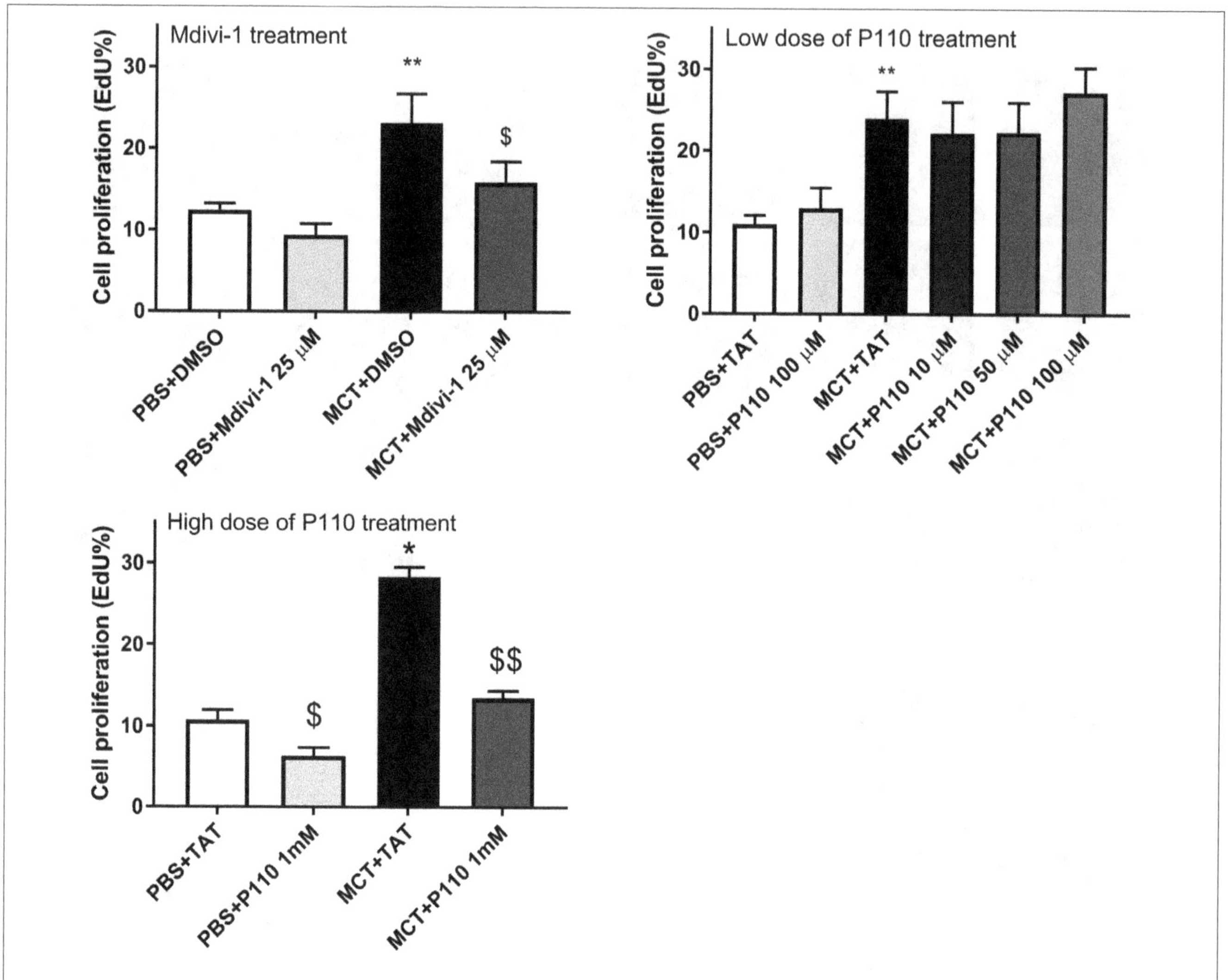

FIGURE 2 | Compared to control, monocrotaline (MCT)-induced RVfib are hyperproliferative as measured by Click-iT® EdU assay. Mitochondrial division inhibitor 1 (Mdivi-1; 25 μM) for 2 days and high dose of P110 (1 mM) for 3 days reduced proliferation in MCT-RVfib whereas lower doses of P110 had no effect. $^{*}P < 0.05$ and $^{**}P < 0.01$ versus PBS+DMSO or PBS+TAT group; $^{\$}P < 0.05$ and $^{\$\$}P < 0.01$ versus the corresponding vehicle control group. $n = 5$ per group.

Mdivi-1 Reduces Collagen Production in MCT-RV Fibroblasts

Compared to Control-RVfib, MCT-RVfib increased collagen production in both types I and III, though only statistically significantly in type III (**Figure 3**). Mdivi-1 (25 μM) for 3 days significantly reduced type III collagen production in MCT-RVfib, while P110 (1 mM) for 3 days showed a trend ($P = 0.14$) in reducing type III collagen production in MCT-RVfib (**Figure 3**).

MCT-RV Fibroblasts Have Increased Phosphorylated Drp1 at Serine 616

Activated Drp1 (phosphorylation at Serine 616) measured via immunofluorescence was significantly increased in MCT-RVfib versus Control-RVfib (**Figures 4A–C**), which is confirmed with immunoblotting (**Figure 4D**). qRT-PCR measurement showed that there was no significant difference between Control-RVfib and MCT-RVfib in the mRNA expression of total Drp1, Fis1, MFF, MiD49, or MiD51 (**Figure 4E**). Immunoblotting also did not find significant change in total Drp1 in MCT-RVfib versus the control (**Figure 4F**). In addition, qRT-PCR measurement found no significant difference between groups in the mRNA expression of fusion mediators (MFN1, MFN2 and OPA1) (Supplementary Figure S3). However, there was a trend toward reduction in the expression of MFN2 mRNA ($P = 0.32$) and protein ($P = 0.18$) in MCT-RVfib versus Control-RVfib (Supplementary Figures S3, S4).

P110 Does Not Improve RV Function in MCT Rats

At week 4 post-injection of MCT or PBS, the body weight of MCT rats was significantly less than PBS (i.e., control) rats and was not altered by P110 treatment (either prevention or regression) (Supplementary Figure S5). Compared to control (i.e., PBS), MCT rats had significantly increased total

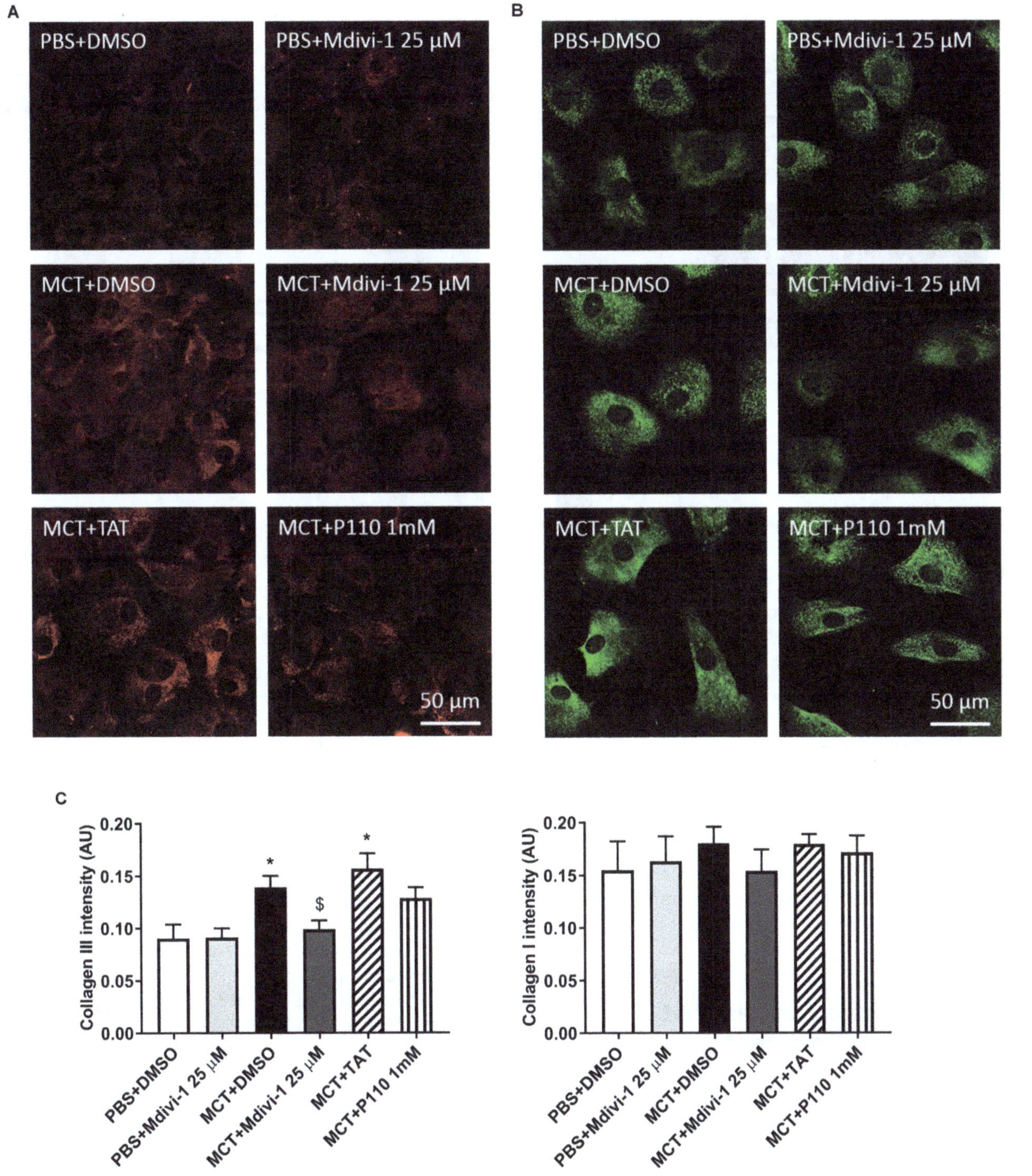

FIGURE 3 | Compared to control, monocrotaline (MCT)-induced RVfib have significantly greater production of collagen type III but not collagen type I. Mitochondrial division inhibitor 1 (Mdivi-1; 25 μM) significantly reduced type III collagen production and P110 (1 mM) for 3 days showed a trend in reducing type III collagen production ($P = 0.14$). Representatives of **(A)** type III (red) and **(B)** type I (green) collagen in RVfib characterized by immunofluorescence; **(C)** Summary of intensity of the fluorescent signal. $^{*}P < 0.05$ versus PBS+DMSO group; $^{\$}P < 0.05$ versus MCT+DMSO group. n = 5~6 per group.

pulmonary resistance (TPR, estimated from RHC; **Figure 5A**) and developed RV hypertrophy (RVH) (**Figure 5B**). MCT rats had higher pressure in both PA and RV as indicated by shorter pulmonary artery acceleration time (PAAT) (measured by echocardiography; **Figure 5B**) and higher RV systolic pressure (RVSP) and RV end-diastolic pressure (RVEDP)

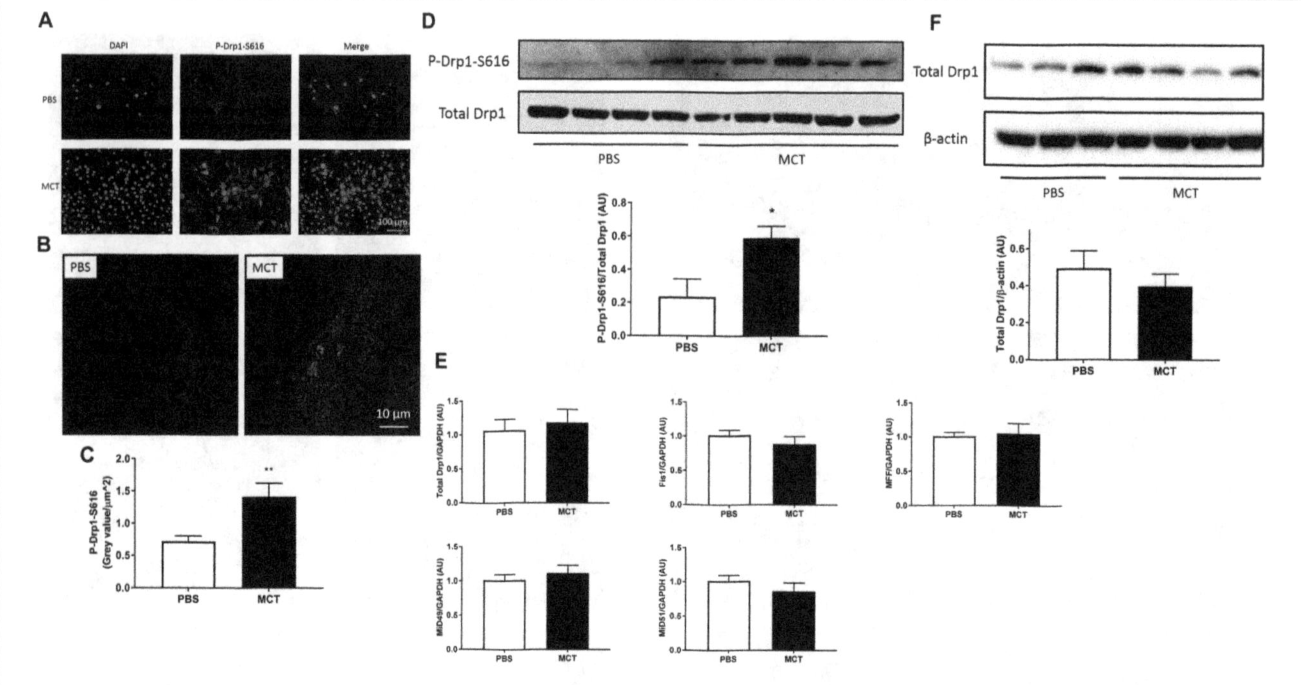

FIGURE 4 | Compared to control, monocrotaline (MCT)-induced RVfib have upregulation of phosphorylation of dynamin-related protein 1(Drp1) at Serine 616 but no significant changes in total Drp1 or Drp1 binding partners. Representative immunofluorescence images of phosphorylated Drp1 at Serine 616 (P-Drp1-S616; red) in RVfib **(A)** at 20X with DAPI at blue and **(B)** at 63X; **(C)** Summary of the intensity of phosphorylated Drp1 at Serine 616 (n = 5~6 per group); **(D)** Immunoblotting on P-Drp1-S616 and its ratio to total Drp1 (n = 4~5 per group); **(E)** mRNA expression of total Drp1, fission protein 1 (Fis1), mitochondrial fission factor (MFF), and mitochondrial dynamics proteins of 49 and 51 kDa (MiD49 and MiD51, respectively) in RVfib (n = 6~8 per group); **(F)** Immunoblotting on total Drp1 in RVfib (n = 4~6 per group). *$P < 0.05$ and **$P < 0.01$ versus PBS group.

(measured by RHC; **Figure 5A**). Also, MCT rats had reduced RV contractility manifest as reduced RVFW systolic thickening, reduced tricuspid annular plane systolic excursion (TAPSE), and reduced cardiac output (CO) (**Figure 5B**). P110 treatment did not improve RV function in MCT rats in either the prevention protocol (P110 was administered at the time of MCT injection) or the two regression protocols (P110 administered on day 14 and 19 or every other day from day 10) (**Figure 5**).

MCT RV Develops Fibrosis That Is Not Altered by P110 Treatment

Compared to control, MCT rats developed greater RV fibrosis, as observed from picrosirius red staining (**Figure 6**). *In vivo* P110 treatment did not prevent or regress RV fibrosis in MCT rats (**Figure 6**).

DISCUSSION

This study examined the role of disordered mitochondrial dynamics in the hyperproliferative, collagen-producing phenotype of RV fibroblasts derived from rats with MCT-induced PAH. The study revealed five significant findings. First, MCT-RVfib display excessive mitochondrial fission and this phenotype persists in culture. Second, MCT-RVfib are hyperproliferative. Third, MCT-RVfib have increased expression of activated Drp1 (phosphorylated at Serine 616). Fourth, the mitochondrial fission is crucial to the hyperproliferative, profibrotic phenotype, since Mdivi-1 treatment, which inhibits mitochondrial fission, also reduces proliferation and collagen production, indicating Drp1 is a potential antifibrotic target. Fifth, P110, a competitive peptide that antagonizes the interaction between Drp1 and Fis1 also reduces mitochondrial fission and RVfib proliferation *in vitro*; however, it only has these effects at very high doses. Moreover, P110 failed to prevent or regress RV fibrosis or improve RV function *in vivo*. These data suggest that Drp1-mediated fission is central to the RVfib hyperproliferative, profibrotic phenotype in MCT-PAH.

Changes in mitochondrial dynamics regulates vital cellular functions including metabolism, cell cycle progression, and apoptosis (Archer et al., 2008; Suen et al., 2008; Rehman et al., 2012). Excessive mitochondrial fission has been observed in PAH in RV myocytes (Tian et al., 2017), pulmonary artery smooth muscle cells (PASMC) (Marsboom et al., 2012; Chen et al., 2018), and pulmonary adventitial fibroblasts (Plecita-Hlavata et al., 2016). In PASMC, excessive mitotic fission is associated with increased proliferation and is thought to reflect coordination between division of the nucleus and mitochondria (Marsboom et al., 2012; Chen et al., 2018). In PAH PASMC, this fissogenic phenotype is mediated by both posttranslational modification of Drp1, leading to its activation, and increased interaction of Drp1 and upregulation of its recently discovered binding partners, MiD49 and MiD51 (Chen et al., 2018). Similar

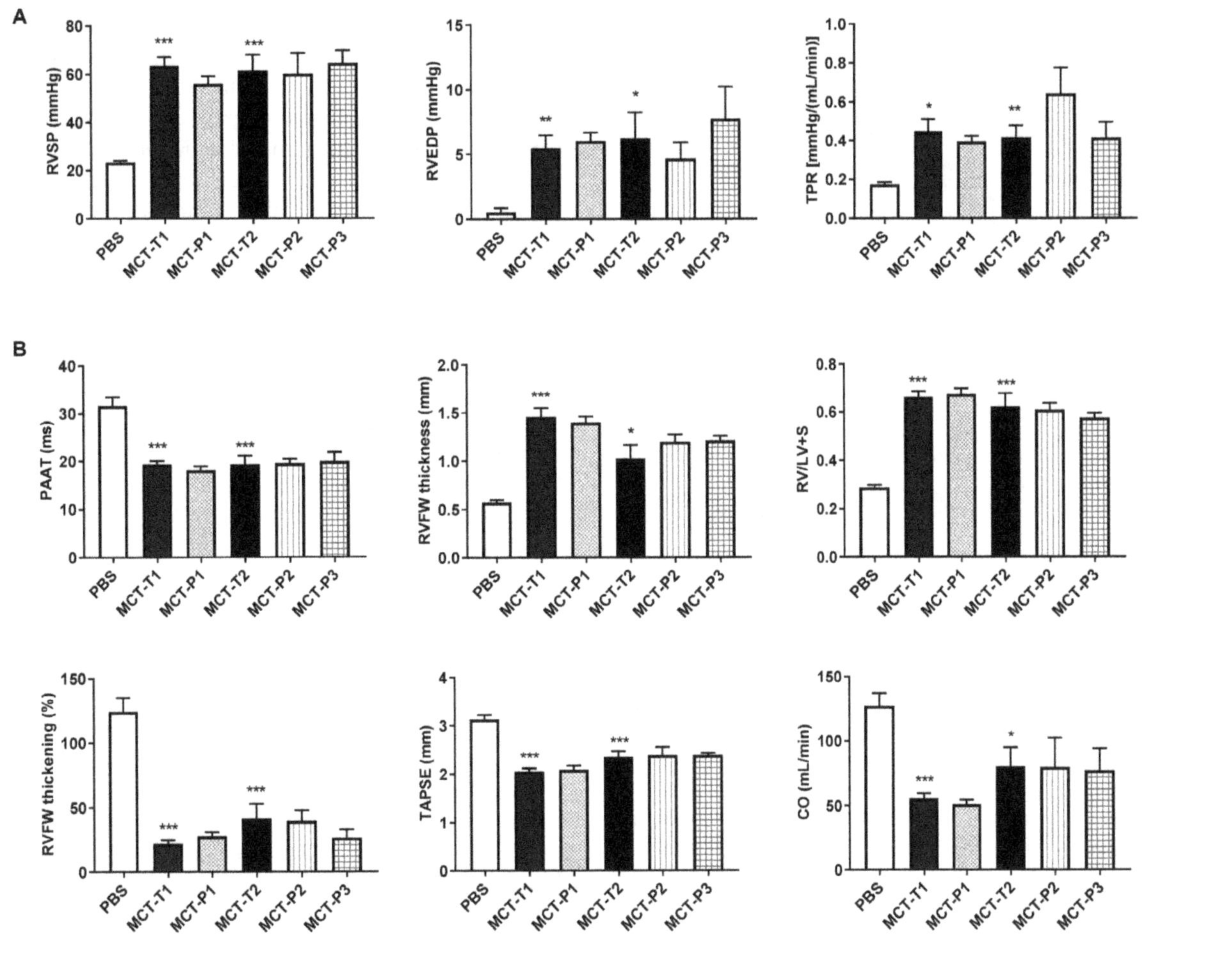

FIGURE 5 | Monocrotaline (MCT) rats developed RV hypertrophy and pulmonary hypertension and P110 did not improve RV function. **(A)** RV systolic and diastolic pressures (RVSP and RVEDP) and total pulmonary resistance (TPR) increased in MCT rats and were not changed by P110 treatment; **(B)** MCT decreased pulmonary artery acceleration time (PAAT) and caused increases in RV free wall (RVFW) thickness and the ratio of RV over LV plus septum weight (RV/LV+S). MCT rats had reduced RVFW thickening, tricuspid annular plane systolic excursion (TAPSE), and cardiac output (CO). Treatment of P110 did not change any of these parameters in MCT rats. MCT-T1 and MCT-P1, MCT rats treated with TAT and P110, respectively, on day 14 and 19; MCT-T2 and MCT-P2, MCT rats treated with TAT and P110, respectively, every other day starting from day 10; MCT-P3, MCT rats treated with P110 only once immediately before the injection of MCT. $^{*}P < 0.05$, $^{**}P < 0.01$, and $^{***}P < 0.001$ versus PBS group. $n = 4\sim10$ per group.

to PAH PASMC, we also found that RVfib in MCT-PAH display more mitochondrial fragmentation (**Figure 1**) and increased proliferation (**Figure 2**), confirming the persistence of a phenotype characterized by excess fission and rates of fibroblast proliferation in culture. To the best of our knowledge, this is the first study to demonstrate mitochondrial fission and show that it regulates the proliferation and collagen production of in RVfib in PAH, or indeed in any cardiac disease. We speculate that epigenetic mechanisms, triggered by MCT, are in play, since the phenotype persists through multiple passages of fibroblasts in culture of these cells, which are derived from genetically normal rodents.

Mechanistically, the mitochondrial network is regulated by fission mediator (Drp1) and fusion mediators (MFN1, MFN2, OPA1). Increases in Drp1 or decreases in fusion mediators result in mitochondrial fragmentation in both PASMC and pulmonary artery adventitial fibroblasts in PAH (Marsboom et al., 2012; Ryan et al., 2013; Plecita-Hlavata et al., 2016; Chen et al., 2018). Our group has previously found an increase in the phosphorylated Drp1 at Serine 616 and a decrease in MFN2 in PASMC in PAH (Marsboom et al., 2012; Ryan et al., 2013). Studies on pulmonary artery adventitial fibroblasts from the lungs in PAH found a decrease in both MFN2 and OPA1 (Plecita-Hlavata et al., 2016). Consistent with this we found an increase in the phosphorylated Drp1 at Serine 616 (**Figures 4A–D**) and a strong trend to decreased MFN2 expression (Supplementary Figures S3, S4) in RVfib in MCT-PAH, without significant changes in the other two fusion mediators (MFN1 and OPA1) (Supplementary Figure S3). Therefore, our data suggest that acquired activation of Drp1 promotes mitochondrial fragmentation in MCT-RVfib, perhaps reinforced by reduced expression of the fusion mediator MFN2.

Since Drp1 mediates mitochondrial mitotic fission, which is associated with accelerated cell cycle progression and increased

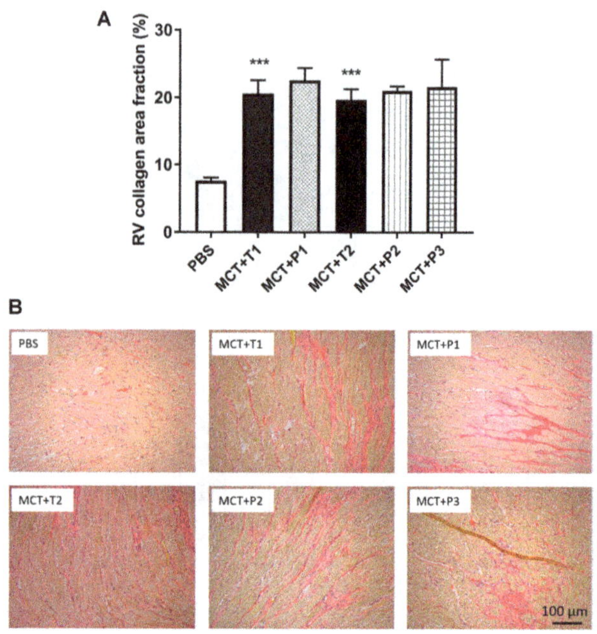

FIGURE 6 | Collagen deposition in RV is increased monocrotaline (MCT) rats and not changed by P110 treatment. **(A)** Representative images of RV stained with picrosirius red for collagen and **(B)** summary of collagen area fraction. MCT-T1 and MCT-P1, MCT rats treated with TAT and P110, respectively, on day 14 and 19; MCT-T2 and MCT-P2, MCT rats treated with TAT and P110, respectively, every other day starting from day 10; MCT-P3, MCT rats treated with P110 only once immediately before the injection of MCT. $^{***}P < 0.001$ versus PBS group. $n = 4{\sim}10$ per group.

cell proliferation, Drp1 has been proposed as a therapeutic target for PAH (Marsboom et al., 2012). Mdivi-1, which inhibits a conformational change of Drp1 required for self-assembly and GTP hydrolysis, is a selective Drp1 GTPase activity inhibitor (Cassidy-Stone et al., 2008). Inhibiting Drp1 via Mdivi-1 inhibits mitochondrial fission and reduces proliferation in PASMC in PAH (Marsboom et al., 2012). In agreement with the study on PASMC, the current study demonstrates the same effects of Mdivi-1 on RVfib in MCT-PAH *in vitro*, i.e., the inhibition of mitochondrial fission and reduction in proliferation (**Figures 1**, **2**). The inhibition of mitochondrial fission is also achieved by knocking down Drp1 (i.e., siDrp1; **Figure 1**), providing additional molecular certainty that it is Drp1 which is crucial to the fragmented mitochondrial morphology in MCT-RVfib.

Along with excessive mitochondrial fission and hyperproliferation, MCT-RVfib also have greater collagen production than Control-RVfib (**Figure 3**), consistent with the increased RV fibrosis observed in MCT versus control rats (**Figure 6**). Mdivi-1 also reduced collagen type III production in MCT-RVfib (**Figure 3**), indicating that mitochondrial fission is linked to collagen production and that Drp1 is a potential antifibrotic target.

Activated Drp1 translocates to the mitochondrion where it associates with its binding partners creating a ring-like, multimeric structure which constricts and divides the mitochondrion. The relevant binding partner varies by cell type. For example, in cardiomyocytes, Drp1 binds to Fis1 but not MiD51 or MFF under conditions of acute ischemia-reperfusion injury (Disatnik et al., 2013). In the MCT RV, P110 (1 μM) both inhibits mitochondrial fission and improves RV myocyte and cardiac diastolic function in ischemia-reperfusion injury (Tian et al., 2017). In contrast, in the current study, only 1000-fold higher doses of P110 were able to inhibit mitochondrial fission or reduce proliferation in MCT-RVfib *in vitro* (**Figures 1**, **2**). At these doses, the specificity of P110, a competitive peptide which theoretically only inhibits the interaction between Fis1 and Drp1, is unknown. This basis for the difference between the cardiomyocytes and RVfib studies is unknown. *In vivo* P110 failed to prevent or regress RV fibrosis. Our protocol involved repeated administration of P110 over 2 weeks. In contrast, Disatnik et al. (2013) gave P110 treatment immediately prior to a single point injury (acute ischemia-reperfusion injury) and observed a beneficial effect. We speculate that MCT, which causes a complex and sustained injury, may be less amenable to intervention (**Figures 5**, **6**). Previous studies have used a high dose of P110 at 3 mg/kg/day using Alzet osmotic mini-pumps on mouse models of Huntington's disease and amyotrophic lateral sclerosis and shown benefits of P110 (Guo et al., 2013; Joshi et al., 2018). In addition, the half-life of P110 is probably as short as 1 h (Qi et al., 2013), perhaps higher doses of P110 and use of continuous infusion protocols might have proven more effective. Alternatively, Fis1 may simply be less relevant as a Drp1 binding partner in MCT-RVfib than other binding partners, which we did not assess (MFF, MiD49, and MiD51).

Nonetheless, the fact that P110 at high dose also inhibited mitochondrial fission and cell proliferation (**Figures 1**, **2**) may indicate a role for Drp1–Fis1 interaction, as observed in the RV myocytes in this MCT model of PAH (Tian et al., 2017). However, we were only able to observe an effect of P110 at 1 mM dose and the effect required several days of incubation. This may indicate that the observed effects are nonspecific or that the interaction between Drp1 and Fis1 in RV fibroblasts is robust and hard to reverse. Certainly, at the doses of P110 that we could afford to test we could neither prevent nor regress RV fibrosis *in vivo* (**Figure 6**). This would favor the interpretation that the Drp1–Fis1 interaction may be less critical in RVfib than in RV myocytes.

The finding that P110 treatment did not change PAAT or pulmonary vascular resistance (or TPR) in MCT rats (**Figure 5**) indicates Drp1–Fis1 interaction is not important either for pulmonary vasculature at least in MCT-PAH. This confirms a recent study from our group. Although Fis1 is found to be upregulated in PASMC in human PAH patients (Marsboom et al., 2012; Ryan et al., 2013), knockdown of Fis1 using a small interfering RNA (siRNA) does not inhibit mitochondrial fission nor reduce proliferation in PASMC in human PAH patients (Chen et al., 2018).

Drp1 may use different binding partners to facilitate mitochondrial fission in RVfib in PAH. We recently showed that two Drp1 binding partners (MiD49 and MiD51) are upregulated in PASMC in PAH. The epigenetic upregulation of

MiDs (mediated by a reduced expression of microRNA 34a-3p) promotes a Drp1-dependent increase in mitochondrial fission and proliferation in PASMC in both human PAH patients and MCT rats (Chen et al., 2018). In this study, mRNA expression of MiD49 and MiD51 was not changed in MCT-RVfib (**Figure 4E**), although mRNA and protein expression levels are not always concordant. The role of MiDs on mitochondrial fission in RVfib remains unknown.

Limitations

Several limitations are acknowledged. First, we did not examine if Mdivi-1 can reduce RV fibrosis in MCT rats. Our group has previously shown that Mdivi-1 can improve RV function in MCT rats (Marsboom et al., 2012). In addition, another study demonstrates that Mdivi-1 can reduce LV fibrosis in aortic banding model in rats (Givvimani et al., 2012). We propose (but did not prove) that Mdivi-1 would reduce RV fibrosis in PAH. This requires direct confirmation in a future *in vivo* study.

Second, we did not measure the expression of Drp1 phosphorylated at Serine 637. Decreased phosphorylation of Drp1 at Serine 637 contributes to ischemia-reperfusion injury in cardiac arrest (Cereghetti et al., 2008; Chang and Blackstone, 2010; Sharp et al., 2014, 2015). In future studies, measurement of this phosphorylation of Drp1 in RVfib will be important to better determine the mechanism of Drp1 activation.

Third, we did not perform immunoprecipitation studies on RVfib to directly examine the role of Drp1–Fis1 interaction in MCT-RVfib. Indeed, previous *in vitro* studies (Disatnik et al., 2013) showed that P110 at 1 μM (which is a low dose) inhibited ischemia-induced mitochondrial fission in cardiac myocytes. In ischemia-reperfusion injury, the Drp1–Fis1 interaction is well established as an early step in the generation of the mitochondrial-derived reactive oxygen species that drives cardiac dysfunction. In contrast, in RV fibroblasts, P110 at this dose (1 μM) had no effect. This may be due to the difference in sensitivity of the Drp1–Fis1 interaction in different cell types (cardiomyocytes versus cardiac fibroblasts) and/or a different role for Fis1 in different pathologic situations (more important in acute ischemia than in the MCT model of chronic, pressure-volume overload). The reason why such high doses of P110 were required to have significant effects on RVfib *in vitro* is unclear. In the future, immunoprecipitation studies will be used to clarify the role of high dose P110 on Drp1–Fis1 interaction.

Fourth, because P110 only blocks the interaction between Drp1 and Fis1, the failure of P110 treatment *in vivo* may indicate either that adequate levels of P110 were not achieved *in vivo* and/or that the Drp1–Fis1 interaction is less important in the pathogenesis of the fragmented mitochondria-proliferative fibroblast phenotype than other Drp1-binding partner interactions (such as Drp1-MiD49 and Drp1-MiD51). The role of MiD49 and MiD51 in MCT-RVfib remains unknown and requires further study.

CONCLUSION

We conclude that in MCT-induced PAH, RV fibroblasts display mitochondrial fragmentation that reflects Drp1-mediated fission. Increased mitochondrial fission promotes a hyperproliferative state and results in excessive production of collagen type III. Inhibiting Drp1 can inhibit mitochondrial fission, and reduce fibroblast proliferation and collagen production, suggesting Drp1 is a potential antifibrotic target. Further *in vivo* preclinical studies are required to establish the translational relevance of these observations.

AUTHOR CONTRIBUTIONS

LT and SA designed the work. LT, FP, DW, AD, K-HC, JM, and PL performed the experiments. LT, FP, DW, AD, K-HC, JM, PL, and SA analyzed and interpreted the data. LT drafted the work. LT, FP, DW, AD, K-HC, JM, PL, and SA revised the work critically and performed the final approval of the version to be published.

REFERENCES

Agocha, A. E., and Eghbali-Webb, M. (1997). A simple method for preparation of cultured cardiac fibroblasts from adult human ventricular tissue. *Mol. Cell. Biochem.* 172, 195–198. doi: 10.1023/A:1006848512174

Archer, S. L. (2013). Mitochondrial dynamics–mitochondrial fission and fusion in human diseases. *N. Engl. J. Med.* 369, 2236–2251. doi: 10.1056/NEJMra1215233

Archer, S. L., Fang, Y. H., Ryan, J. J., and Piao, L. (2013). Metabolism and bioenergetics in the right ventricle and pulmonary vasculature in pulmonary hypertension. *Pulm. Circ.* 3, 144–152. doi: 10.4103/2045-8932.109960

Archer, S. L., Gomberg-Maitland, M., Maitland, M. L., Rich, S., Garcia, J. G., and Weir, E. K. (2008). Mitochondrial metabolism, redox signaling, and fusion: a mitochondria-ROS-HIF-1alpha-Kv1.5 O2-sensing pathway at the intersection of pulmonary hypertension and cancer. *Am. J. Physiol. Heart Circ. Physiol.* 294, H570–H578.

Bonnet, S., Michelakis, E. D., Porter, C. J., Andrade-Navarro, M. A., Thebaud, B., Bonnet, S., et al. (2006). An abnormal mitochondrial-hypoxia inducible factor-1alpha-Kv channel pathway disrupts oxygen sensing and triggers pulmonary arterial hypertension in fawn hooded rats: similarities to human pulmonary arterial hypertension. *Circulation* 113, 2630–2641. doi: 10.1161/CIRCULATIONAHA.105.609008

Bonnet, S., Rochefort, G., Sutendra, G., Archer, S. L., Haromy, A., Webster, L., et al. (2007). The nuclear factor of activated T cells in pulmonary arterial hypertension can be therapeutically targeted. *Proc. Natl. Acad. Sci. U.S.A.* 104, 11418–11423. doi: 10.1073/pnas.0610467104

Campo, A., Mathai, S. C., Le Pavec, J., Zaiman, A. L., Hummers, L. K., Boyce, D., et al. (2010). Hemodynamic predictors of survival in scleroderma-related pulmonary arterial hypertension. *Am. J. Respir. Crit. Care Med.* 182, 252–260. doi: 10.1164/rccm.200912-1820OC

Cassidy-Stone, A., Chipuk, J. E., Ingerman, E., Song, C., Yoo, C., Kuwana, T., et al. (2008). Chemical inhibition of the mitochondrial division dynamin reveals its role in Bax/Bak-dependent mitochondrial outer membrane permeabilization. *Dev. Cell* 14, 193–204. doi: 10.1016/j.devcel.2007.11.019

Cereghetti, G. M., Stangherlin, A., Martins de Brito, O., Chang, C. R., Blackstone, C., Bernardi, P., et al. (2008). Dephosphorylation by calcineurin regulates translocation of Drp1 to mitochondria. *Proc. Natl. Acad. Sci. U.S.A.* 105, 15803–15808. doi: 10.1073/pnas.0808249105

Chan, D. C. (2007). Mitochondrial dynamics in disease. *N. Engl. J. Med.* 356, 1707–1709. doi: 10.1056/NEJMp078040

Chang, C. R., and Blackstone, C. (2010). Dynamic regulation of mitochondrial fission through modification of the dynamin-related protein Drp1. *Ann. N. Y. Acad. Sci.* 1201, 34–39. doi: 10.1111/j.1749-6632.2010.05629.x

Chemla, D., Castelain, V., Humbert, M., Hebert, J. L., Simonneau, G., Lecarpentier, Y., et al. (2004). New formula for predicting mean pulmonary artery pressure using systolic pulmonary artery pressure. *Chest* 126, 1313–1317. doi: 10.1378/chest.126.4.1313

Chen, H., Detmer, S. A., Ewald, A. J., Griffin, E. E., Fraser, S. E., and Chan, D. C. (2003). Mitofusins Mfn1 and Mfn2 coordinately regulate mitochondrial fusion and are essential for embryonic development. *J. Cell Biol.* 160, 189–200. doi: 10.1083/jcb.200211046

Chen, K. H., Dasgupta, A., Lin, J., Potus, F., Bonnet, S., Iremonger, J., et al. (2018). Epigenetic dysregulation of the Drp1 binding partners MiD49 and MiD51 increases mitotic mitochondrial fission and promotes pulmonary arterial hypertension: mechanistic and therapeutic implications. *Circulation.* doi: 10.1161/CIRCULATIONAHA.117.031258 [Epub ahead of print].

D'Alonzo, G. E., Barst, R. J., Ayres, S. M., Bergofsky, E. H., Brundage, B. H., Detre, K. M., et al. (1991). Survival in patients with primary pulmonary hypertension. Results from a national prospective registry. *Ann. Intern. Med.* 115, 343–349. doi: 10.7326/0003-4819-115-5-343

Disatnik, M. H., Ferreira, J. C., Campos, J. C., Gomes, K. S., Dourado, P. M., Qi, X., et al. (2013). Acute inhibition of excessive mitochondrial fission after myocardial infarction prevents long-term cardiac dysfunction. *J. Am. Heart Assoc.* 2:e000461. doi: 10.1161/JAHA.113.000461

Fang, Y. H., Piao, L., Hong, Z., Toth, P. T., Marsboom, G., Bache-Wiig, P., et al. (2012). Therapeutic inhibition of fatty acid oxidation in right ventricular hypertrophy: exploiting Randle's cycle. *J. Mol. Med.* 90, 31–43. doi: 10.1007/s00109-011-0804-9

Ghio, S., Klersy, C., Magrini, G., D'Armini, A. M., Scelsi, L., Raineri, C., et al. (2010). Prognostic relevance of the echocardiographic assessment of right ventricular function in patients with idiopathic pulmonary arterial hypertension. *Int. J. Cardiol.* 140, 272–278. doi: 10.1016/j.ijcard.2008.11.051

Givvimani, S., Munjal, C., Tyagi, N., Sen, U., Metreveli, N., and Tyagi, S. C. (2012). Mitochondrial division/mitophagy inhibitor (Mdivi) ameliorates pressure overload induced heart failure. *PLOS One* 7:e32388. doi: 10.1371/journal.pone.0032388

Guo, X., Disatnik, M. H., Monbureau, M., Shamloo, M., Mochly-Rosen, D., and Qi, X. (2013). Inhibition of mitochondrial fragmentation diminishes Huntington's disease-associated neurodegeneration. *J. Clin. Invest.* 123, 5371–5388. doi: 10.1172/JCI70911

Hong, Z., Chen, K. H., DasGupta, A., Potus, F., Dunham-Snary, K., Bonnet, S., et al. (2017). MicroRNA-138 and MicroRNA-25 down-regulate mitochondrial calcium uniporter, causing the pulmonary arterial hypertension cancer phenotype. *Am. J. Respir. Crit. Care Med.* 195, 515–529. doi: 10.1164/rccm.201604-0814OC

Humbert, M., Sitbon, O., Chaouat, A., Bertocchi, M., Habib, G., Gressin, V., et al. (2010). Survival in patients with idiopathic, familial, and anorexigen-associated pulmonary arterial hypertension in the modern management era. *Circulation* 122, 156–163. doi: 10.1161/CIRCULATIONAHA.109.911818

Joshi, A. U., Saw, N. L., Vogel, H., Cunnigham, A. D., Shamloo, M., and Mochly-Rosen, D. (2018). Inhibition of Drp1/Fis1 interaction slows progression of amyotrophic lateral sclerosis. *EMBO Mol. Med.* doi: 10.15252/emmm.201708166 [Epub ahead of print].

Lee, Y. J., Jeong, S. Y., Karbowski, M., Smith, C. L., and Youle, R. J. (2004). Roles of the mammalian mitochondrial fission and fusion mediators Fis1, Drp1, and Opa1 in apoptosis. *Mol. Biol. Cell* 15, 5001–5011. doi: 10.1091/mbc.e04-04-0294

Loson, O. C., Song, Z., Chen, H., and Chan, D. C. (2013). Fis1, Mff, MiD49, and MiD51 mediate Drp1 recruitment in mitochondrial fission. *Mol. Biol. Cell* 24, 659–667. doi: 10.1091/mbc.E12-10-0721

Marsboom, G., Toth, P. T., Ryan, J. J., Hong, Z., Wu, X., Fang, Y. H., et al. (2012). Dynamin-related protein 1-mediated mitochondrial mitotic fission permits hyperproliferation of vascular smooth muscle cells and offers a novel therapeutic target in pulmonary hypertension. *Circ. Res.* 110, 1484–1497. doi: 10.1161/CIRCRESAHA.111.263848

McMurtry, M. S., Bonnet, S., Wu, X., Dyck, J. R., Haromy, A., Hashimoto, K., et al. (2004). Dichloroacetate prevents and reverses pulmonary hypertension by inducing pulmonary artery smooth muscle cell apoptosis. *Circ. Res.* 95, 830–840. doi: 10.1161/01.RES.0000145360.16770.9f

Michelakis, E. D., McMurtry, M. S., Wu, X. C., Dyck, J. R., Moudgil, R., Hopkins, T. A., et al. (2002). Dichloroacetate, a metabolic modulator, prevents and reverses chronic hypoxic pulmonary hypertension in rats: role of increased expression and activity of voltage-gated potassium channels. *Circulation* 105, 244–250. doi: 10.1161/hc0202.101974

Neuss, M., Regitz-Zagrosek, V., Hildebrandt, A., and Fleck, E. (1996). Isolation and characterisation of human cardiac fibroblasts from explanted adult hearts. *Cell Tissue Res.* 286, 145–153. doi: 10.1007/s004410050683

Otera, H., Wang, C., Cleland, M. M., Setoguchi, K., Yokota, S., Youle, R. J., et al. (2010). Mff is an essential factor for mitochondrial recruitment of Drp1 during mitochondrial fission in mammalian cells. *J. Cell Biol.* 191, 1141–1158. doi: 10.1083/jcb.201007152

Piao, L., Fang, Y. H., Cadete, V. J., Wietholt, C., Urboniene, D., Toth, P. T., et al. (2010). The inhibition of pyruvate dehydrogenase kinase improves impaired cardiac function and electrical remodeling in two models of right ventricular hypertrophy: resuscitating the hibernating right ventricle. *J. Mol. Med.* 88, 47–60. doi: 10.1007/s00109-009-0524-6

Piao, L., Sidhu, V. K., Fang, Y. H., Ryan, J. J., Parikh, K. S., Hong, Z., et al. (2013). FOXO1-mediated upregulation of pyruvate dehydrogenase kinase-4 (PDK4) decreases glucose oxidation and impairs right ventricular function in pulmonary hypertension: therapeutic benefits of dichloroacetate. *J. Mol. Med.* 91, 333–346. doi: 10.1007/s00109-012-0982-0

Plecita-Hlavata, L., Tauber, J., Li, M., Zhang, H., Flockton, A. R., Pullamsetti, S. S., et al. (2016). Constitutive reprogramming of fibroblast mitochondrial metabolism in pulmonary hypertension. *Am. J. Respir. Cell Mol. Biol.* 55, 47–57. doi: 10.1165/rcmb.2015-0142OC

Prins, K. W., Tian, L., Wu, D., Thenappan, T., Metzger, J. M., and Archer, S. L. (2017). Colchicine depolymerizes microtubules, increases junctophilin-2, and improves right ventricular function in experimental pulmonary arterial hypertension. *J. Am. Heart Assoc.* 6:e006195. doi: 10.1161/JAHA.117.006195

Qi, X., Qvit, N., Su, Y. C., and Mochly-Rosen, D. (2013). A novel Drp1 inhibitor diminishes aberrant mitochondrial fission and neurotoxicity. *J. Cell Sci.* 126, 789–802. doi: 10.1242/jcs.114439

Rehman, J., Zhang, H. J., Toth, P. T., Zhang, Y., Marsboom, G., Hong, Z., et al. (2012). Inhibition of mitochondrial fission prevents cell cycle progression in lung cancer. *FASEB J.* 26, 2175–2186. doi: 10.1096/fj.11-196543

Ryan, J. J., and Archer, S. L. (2014). The right ventricle in pulmonary arterial hypertension: disorders of metabolism, angiogenesis and adrenergic signaling in right ventricular failure. *Circ. Res.* 115, 176–188. doi: 10.1161/CIRCRESAHA.113.301129

Ryan, J. J., Marsboom, G., Fang, Y. H., Toth, P. T., Morrow, E., Luo, N., et al. (2013). PGC1alpha-mediated mitofusin-2 deficiency in female rats and humans with pulmonary arterial hypertension. *Am. J. Respir. Crit. Care Med.* 187, 865–878. doi: 10.1164/rccm.201209-1687OC

Sachdev, A., Villarraga, H. R., Frantz, R. P., McGoon, M. D., Hsiao, J. F., Maalouf, J. F., et al. (2011). Right ventricular strain for prediction of survival in patients with pulmonary arterial hypertension. *Chest* 139, 1299–1309. doi: 10.1378/chest.10-2015

Sandoval, J., Bauerle, O., Palomar, A., Gomez, A., Martinez-Guerra, M. L., Beltran, M., et al. (1994). Survival in primary pulmonary hypertension. Validation of a prognostic equation. *Circulation* 89, 1733–1744. doi: 10.1161/01.CIR.89.4.1733

Sharp, W. W., Beiser, D. G., Fang, Y. H., Han, M., Piao, L., Varughese, J., et al. (2015). Inhibition of the mitochondrial fission protein dynamin-related protein 1 improves survival in a murine cardiac arrest model. *Crit. Care Med.* 43, e38–e47. doi: 10.1097/CCM.0000000000000817

Sharp, W. W., Fang, Y. H., Han, M., Zhang, H. J., Hong, Z., Banathy, A., et al. (2014). Dynamin-related protein 1 (Drp1)-mediated diastolic dysfunction in myocardial ischemia-reperfusion injury: therapeutic benefits of Drp1 inhibition to reduce mitochondrial fission. *FASEB J.* 28, 316–326. doi: 10.1096/fj.12-226225

Suen, D. F., Norris, K. L., and Youle, R. J. (2008). Mitochondrial dynamics and apoptosis. *Genes Dev.* 22, 1577–1590. doi: 10.1101/gad.1658508

Sutendra, G., and Michelakis, E. D. (2014). The metabolic basis of pulmonary arterial hypertension. *Cell Metab.* 19, 558–573. doi: 10.1016/j.cmet.2014.01.004

Taguchi, N., Ishihara, N., Jofuku, A., Oka, T., and Mihara, K. (2007). Mitotic phosphorylation of dynamin-related GTPase Drp1 participates in mitochondrial fission. *J. Biol. Chem.* 282, 11521–11529. doi: 10.1074/jbc.M607279200

Tian, L., Neuber-Hess, M., Mewburn, J., Dasgupta, A., Dunham-Snary, K., Wu, D., et al. (2017). Ischemia-induced Drp1 and Fis1-mediated mitochondrial fission and right ventricular dysfunction in pulmonary hypertension. *J. Mol. Med.* 95, 381–393. doi: 10.1007/s00109-017-1522-8

Urboniene, D., Haber, I., Fang, Y. H., Thenappan, T., and Archer, S. L. (2010). Validation of high-resolution echocardiography and magnetic resonance imaging vs. high-fidelity catheterization in experimental pulmonary hypertension. *Am. J. Physiol. Lung Cell. Mol. Physiol.* 299, L401–L412. doi: 10.1152/ajplung.00114.2010

Voelkel, N. F., Bogaard, H. J., and Gomez-Arroyo, J. (2015). The need to recognize the pulmonary circulation and the right ventricle as an integrated functional unit: facts and hypotheses (2013 Grover Conference series). *Pulm. Circ.* 5, 81–89. doi: 10.1086/679702

Westermann, B. (2010). Mitochondrial fusion and fission in cell life and death. *Nat. Rev. Mol. Cell Biol.* 11, 872–884. doi: 10.1038/nrm3013

Youle, R. J., and van der Bliek, A. M. (2012). Mitochondrial fission, fusion, and stress. *Science* 337, 1062–1065. doi: 10.1126/science.1219855

Zhang, H., Wang, D., Li, M., Plecita-Hlavata, L., D'Alessandro, A., Tauber, J., et al. (2017). Metabolic and proliferative state of vascular adventitial fibroblasts in pulmonary hypertension is regulated through a microRNA-124/PTBP1 (polypyrimidine tract binding protein 1)/pyruvate kinase muscle axis. *Circulation* 136, 2468–2485. doi: 10.1161/CIRCULATIONAHA.117.028069

Zhao, J., Liu, T., Jin, S., Wang, X., Qu, M., Uhlen, P., et al. (2011). Human MIEF1 recruits Drp1 to mitochondrial outer membranes and promotes mitochondrial fusion rather than fission. *EMBO J.* 30, 2762–2778. doi: 10.1038/emboj.2011.198

Zhu, P. P., Patterson, A., Stadler, J., Seeburg, D. P., Sheng, M., and Blackstone, C. (2004). Intra- and intermolecular domain interactions of the C-terminal GTPase effector domain of the multimeric dynamin-like GTPase Drp1. *J. Biol. Chem.* 279, 35967–35974. doi: 10.1074/jbc.M404105200

12

Arrhythmic Burden and Outcomes in Pulmonary Arterial Hypertension

Jennifer T. Middleton[1,2,3], Angshuman Maulik[2,3], Robert Lewis[1,2], David G. Kiely[1], Mark Toshner[4,5], Athanasios Charalampopoulos[1], Andreas Kyriacou[3] and Alexander Rothman[1,2,3]*

[1] Sheffield Pulmonary Vascular Disease Unit, Royal Hallamshire Hospital, Sheffield Teaching Hospitals NHS Foundation Trust, Sheffield, United Kingdom, [2] Department of Infection, Immunity and Cardiovascular Disease, Medical School, University of Sheffield, Sheffield, United Kingdom, [3] Department of Cardiology, Northern General Hospital, Sheffield Teaching Hospitals NHS Foundation Trust, Sheffield, United Kingdom, [4] Department of Medicine, Addenbrooke's Hospital, University of Cambridge, Cambridge, United Kingdom, [5] Royal Papworth Hospital NHS Foundation Trust, Cambridgeshire, United Kingdom

***Correspondence:**
Alexander Rothman
a.rothman@sheffield.ac.uk

Pulmonary arterial hypertension (PAH) is a devastating, life-limiting disease driven by small vessel vascular remodeling leading to a rise in pulmonary vascular resistance (PVR). Patients present with a range of symptoms including shortness of breath, exercise intolerance, palpitations or syncope. Symptoms may be related to vascular disease progression or arrhythmia secondary to the adaptation of the right heart to pressure overload. Arrhythmic burden is high in patients with left heart disease and guideline-based treatment of arrhythmias improves quality of life and prognosis. In PAH the incidence and prevalence of arrhythmias is less well-defined and there are no PAH-specific guidelines for arrhythmia management. We undertook a literature search identifying 13 relevant papers; detection of arrhythmias was acquired from 12-lead electrocardiogram (ECG) or Holter monitors. In all forms of pulmonary hypertension (PH) the prevalence of supraventricular arrhythmias (SVA) was 26–31%, ventricular arrhythmias (VA) 24% and a 5-year incidence of SVA ~13.2–25.1%. Prevalence and incidence of arrhythmias in PAH is less clear due to limited study numbers and the heterogenous nature of the patient population studied. For arrhythmia treatment, only single-arm studies of therapeutic strategies were reported using antiarrhythmic drugs (AAD), direct current cardioversion (DCCV) and ablation. Periods between ECG or Holter have not been investigated, highlighting the possibility that significant arrhythmias may be undetected. Advances in monitoring allow long-term surveillance via implanted/non-invasive monitors. Use of such technologies may provide an accurate estimate of incidence and prevalence of arrhythmias in patients with PAH, further defining relationships to adverse outcomes, and therapeutic options.

Keywords: arrhythmia, pulmonary arterial hypertension, right heart failure, atrial fibrillation, atrial flutter, ventricular tachycardia

INTRODUCTION

The recent World Symposium classifies pulmonary hypertension into five groups based on underlying cause (1). Group one incorporates pulmonary arterial hypertension including familial and idiopathic causes; group two is secondary to left sided heart disease; group three to lung disease and hypoxia; group four is secondary to chronic thromboembolic disease (CTEPH) and group five includes miscellaneous causes including sarcoidosis and hematological disease (1). Increased right ventricular pressure and volume overload of the right heart leads to structural changes that impair left ventricular filling (2) and function which may predispose to the development of arrhythmias. In this review we will discuss the prevalence and incidence of arrhythmia in PAH and the potential treatment options.

CARDIAC ARRHYTHMIAS: CLASSIFICATION AND MECHANISM

Cardiac arrhythmias are caused by either disruption of the cardiac action potential or structural/functional changes to the heart that result in abnormalities of electrical conduction. Classification is made based on heart rate (bradycardic or tachycardic) and sub-divided based on site of origin (supraventricular or ventricular arrhythmia). In the left and right atrium, dilatation and stretch results in structural, and ion channel adaptations resulting in an increased development of SVA's including atrial fibrillation (AF) and atrial flutter (see **Figures 1A,B**). Subsequent loss of atrial contraction leads to underfilling of the ventricle and reduction in cardiac output (CO). VA's can be precipitated by a dilated, dysfunctional ventricle, or altered ventricular substrate in the form of scar (3), giving rise to pro-arrhythmic myocardium (see **Figures 2A,B**). In left sided heart failure there is an increased risk of arrhythmia, which when present often exacerbates left ventricular failure (3, 4). Impaired left ventricular function results in reduced CO due to inadequate filling and contraction leading to compensatory hypertrophy and dilatation of the left ventricle. These changes increase sarcomere length and alter sensitivity to calcium leading to more forceful ventricular contraction (5), the resultant ion channel remodeling (6) can make myocardium pro-arrhythmic (3). Bradyarrhythmia presents often secondary to changes in heart structure, nodal fibrosis, or rate-limiting medication used to treat heart failure.

Current guidelines for the treatment of arrhythmia specifically relate to patients with left sided heart disease (4–9). Management strategies include AAD's that alter the action of specific ion channels to stabilize myocardium; anticoagulation to reduce stroke risk in AF (6); synchronized DCCV to revert to normal sinus rhythm (NSR); electrophysiology studies (EPS); and/or ablation to identify abnormal heart rhythms using intracardiac catheters and ablation to disrupt abnormal conduction pathways and finally permanent pacemakers or internal defibrillator devices (7, 10). Guidance for the treatment of arrhythmias in patients with PAH is lacking despite the potential harmful/unknown effects of AAD's and or therapies in this cohort (7).

Arrhythmias in PAH

Patients with PAH often describe palpitations and/or syncope. The incidence and prevalence of cardiac arrhythmias in PAH is not well-described, however a number of recent studies describe a significant arrhythmic burden in all forms of PH, and a relationship to clinical outcome. These studies are based on "snapshots" in time using 12 lead ECGs or short-term Holter monitors. We undertook a literature-based review searching PubMed with the search terms "pulmonary arterial hypertension, supraventricular, and ventricular arrhythmias, atrial fibrillation/flutter, ventricular tachycardia, and mode of death," 13 relevant papers were reviewed as well as PAH registry data. A review of the REVEAL PAH registry data demonstrated a relationship between increased heart rate and adverse outcomes (11, 12) and during follow up, Burger et al. found 5.1% of patients were admitted secondary to an arrhythmia, however further details were not provided (13).

Supraventricular Arrhythmias

Prevalence

In a multi-center, observational study (14), patients with PAH/inoperable CTEPH attending routine outpatients had their notes reviewed retrospectively for evidence of AF or atrial flutter. 297 patients were identified as fulfilling criteria (PAH 266/CTEPH 31) with 90% on PAH specific medication. An ECG diagnosis of AF or atrial flutter was noted in 79 (26.5%), approximately 50% of those were deemed to be paroxysmal in nature. Patients with AF were as a group, of increased age, male gender with a higher systolic blood pressure (BP), a reduced left ventricular ejection fraction (LVEF), and had a higher rate of chronic obstructive lung disease (COPD). At right heart catheterization (RHC), the AF group had a higher pulmonary capillary wedge pressure (PCWP), and lower pulmonary vascular resistance, potentially suggesting a more elderly population with a greater burden of co-morbid condition. There was no difference found in mean pulmonary artery pressure (PAP) or CO. Results suggest that a diagnosis of permanent or paroxysmal AF/atrial flutter in PAH confers an increased mortality. The use of 12-lead ECGs alone and the unbalanced co-morbidities of patients with and without AF/atrial flutter masked the true burden of arrhythmias in patients with PAH (14).

Rottlaender et al. (15), investigated patients with all forms of PH who developed SVA in a retrospective study of 225 patients. Thirty one percentage of patients recruited were found to have AF (41% paroxysmal) and it was apparent that AF was more likely if secondary to PH-left heart disease and less common in CTEPH. All patients identified as having AF deteriorated clinically at the time of arrhythmia. The true prevalence of SVA was again difficult to determine due to the inclusion of all types of PH. In contrast Ruiz-Cano et al. retrospectively reviewed 282 patients with PAH. In total 28 SVA episodes were detected: AF 12 patients (42.8%); atrial flutter 12 (42.8%); other SVA 4 (14.2%), 82% of SVA episodes resulted in symptoms and clinical deterioration / worsening right heart failure (RHF).

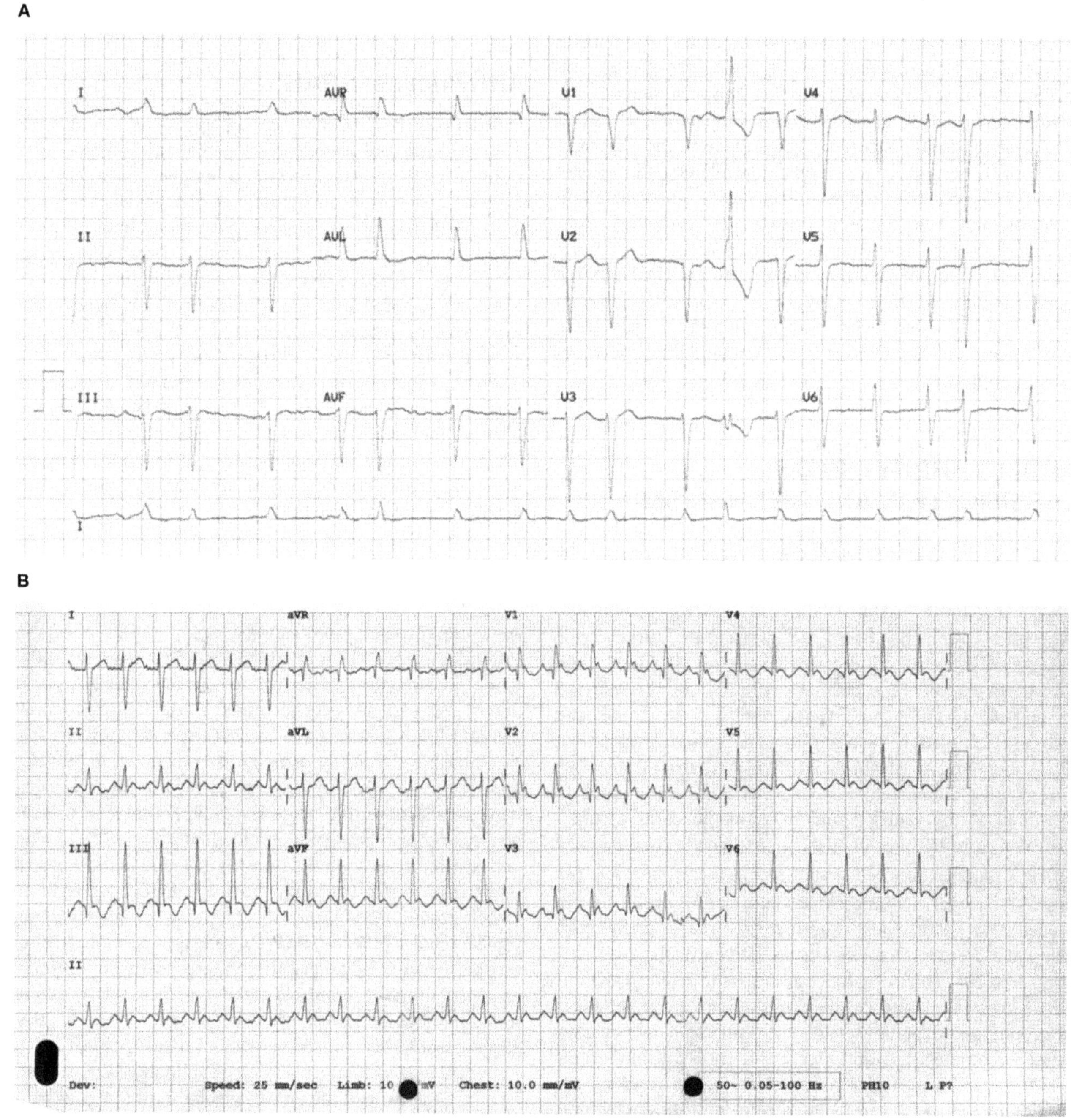

FIGURE 1 | (A) An ECG of atrial fibrillation. An example of an ECG taken from a patient with atrial fibrillation showing uncoordinated atrial activity resulting in an irregular ventricular rate. **(B)** An ECG of atrial flutter. An example of an ECG taken from a patient with atrial flutter. It is characterized by rapid, regular atrial depolarizations (typically, but not always at a rate of 300 bpm) resulting in a ventricular rate of 150 bpm.

Time from PAH diagnosis to SVA was approximately 60 months and time from SVA diagnosis to death/transplant was 17.8 months suggesting increased morbidity and mortality with the development of SVA.

Incidence

A number of studies investigated incidence through prospective/retrospective cohort studies (summarized in **Table 1**), with 6-year incidence of SVA in PAH approximately 15.8% and in all forms of PH a 5-year incidence of between 13.2 and 25.1% (17–21). In a retrospective, cohort study, Cannillo et al. examined patients with PAH, lung disease-associated PH, and CTEPH who had NSR at baseline on a 12-lead ECG, patients with previous SVA diagnosis were excluded (18). Retrospective analysis of ECG's was undertaken during follow-up, if admitted or if they developed palpitations. Holter monitors were only

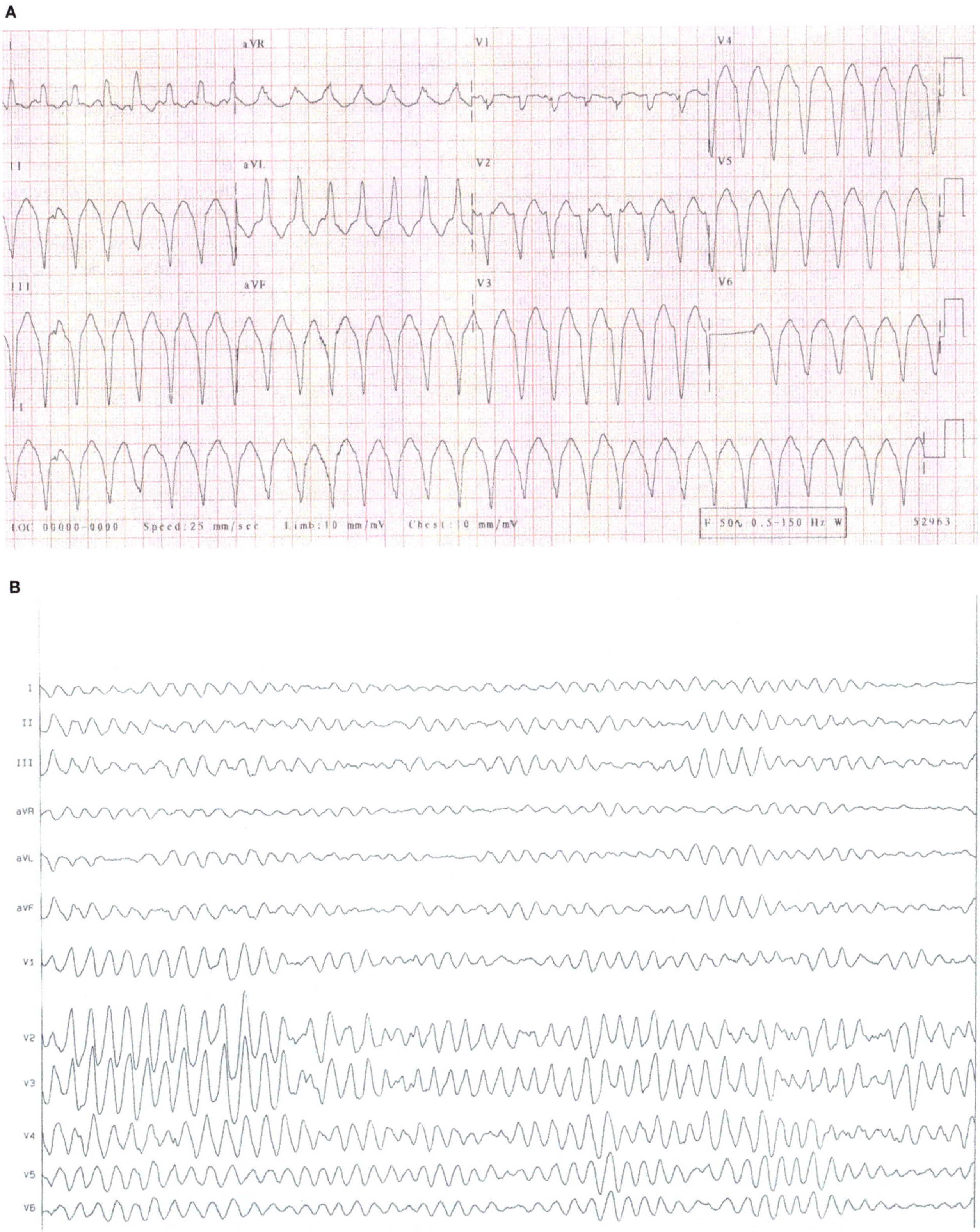

FIGURE 2 | (A) An ECG of ventricular tachycardia. An example of an ECG from a patient with sustained monomorphic ventricular tachycardia. It is characterized by regular, broad QRS complexes of similar morphology often over 100 bpm. **(B)** An ECG of Ventricular fibrillation. An example of an ECG from a patient with ventricular fibrillation. It is characterized by rapid, erratic ventricular activity as the heart fibrillates rather than pumps effectively. This rhythm quickly degenerates into cardiac arrest.

fitted in patients reporting palpitations, not as a screen for asymptomatic SVA's. 77 patients met criteria, 17 patients (22%) were newly diagnosed with SVA during the follow-up period (35 months). Patients were found to have persistent AF in 8 patients (47%), permanent AF 3 patients (17%), paroxysmal SVA 3 patients (17%), atrial ectopic tachycardia 2 patients (12%), right atrial flutter 2 patients (12%) and paroxysmal AF (PAF) in 1 patient (6%), other SVA 1 patient (6%). Diagnosis of SVA's occurred on average 15.1 months after PH diagnosis and was associated with worsening parameters (World health organization (WHO)-functional class/6-min walk test (6MWT)/brain natriuretic protein (BNP), and increased mortality. This suggests SVA to be a manifestation of more severe PAH [as per Tongers (21) and Ruiz-Cano (16)]. Severe PAH resulted in more hospital admissions and closer monitoring by default, potentially introducing detection bias of SVA in these patients. Consistent with these findings, Mercurio et al. (17) again looked at PAH only and specifically idiopathic PAH and systemic sclerosis-associated pulmonary hypertension (SSc-PH). A prospective, single center study recruited 317 patients in total (116 idiopathic PAH) and of these 42 developed SVA. In keeping with Smith et al. (14) these patients had higher baseline PCWP and in this case right atrial pressure (RAP). In 90.1% cases the onset of SVA resulted in clinical worsening and RHF. A 5-year incidence of SVA in idiopathic PAH and SSc-PAH was found to be 13.2%, lower than previously documented by Olsson et al. in a similar PH group (20). Olsson et al. described a 5-year incidence of 25.1% of SVA in PAH and inoperable CTEPH. Patients again had NSR at baseline and diagnosis of arrhythmia was based on 12-lead ECG's only. Forty-Eight patients (20%) had at least one episode of SVA. They also showed patients with persistent AF to have a worse prognosis than those with PAF or NSR (20). This followed on from a previous study by Tongers et al. (21), that retrospectively recruited 231 patients under follow-up for PAH and inoperable CTEPH. Thirty-one episodes of SVA were noted on 12-lead ECG in 27 patients (Atrial flutter 15, AF 13, and other SVA 3). Episodes were again associated with marked clinical deterioration and RHF (84% SVA episodes), improving if NSR was restored. Interestingly this study appears to show an increased mortality in AF patients where NSR could not be restored. All 15 patients with atrial flutter had NSR, restored with medication (1), DCCV (6), overdrive pacing (15) or ablation (5), with one death during follow-up. In the AF group only 2 patients had NSR restored by DCCV. NSR in the remaining 9 was not achieved despite multiple medications and DCCV, with 8 deaths during follow-up. This suggests an increased mortality in AF and PAH if NSR is not achieved. It would also appear that treatment measures in the AF group were less aggressive (ablation was not attempted) but the study was from 2007 so potentially now outdated as ablation is more common place today.

In patients with idiopathic PAH on disease specific therapies Wen et al. (19) undertook a prospective, cohort study with 280 patients recruited specifically with NSR at baseline. Forty patients developed SVA at least once during follow-up, 5-year incidence was calculated as 15.8%, potentially a more realistic reflection in PAH alone. Patients as with previous studies did not tolerate SVA and restoration of NSR correlated with clinical recovery. Studies again only diagnosed SVA on 12-lead ECG, potentially failing to diagnose asymptomatic SVA.

Treatment

AAD's, overdrive pacing, DCCV, and radiofrequency ablation are all guideline based therapies for SVA (6, 7), (although not PAH-specific). Existing data showed that rhythm control has been the most popular first line strategy and restoration of NSR demonstrated clinical improvement. Cannillo et al. (18) attempted rhythm control in 76% of patients diagnosed with SVA, NSR was restored in 11 (65%) cases but there was a high recurrence rate (~80%). Olsson et al. (20) diagnosed patients with SVA on 12-lead ECG and largely from patients presenting with deterioration of PAH/RHF symptoms rather than symptoms of arrhythmia [as per Cannillo et al. (18)]. Those with atrial flutter received ablation earlier with the concurrent use of AAD's with or without synchronized DCCV. For stable AF 10–14 days of oral amiodarone was prescribed pre DCCV and continued thereafter. If there were signs of RHF, amiodarone was given intravenously, and DCCV was performed. NSR was restored in 21/24 patients with atrial flutter and 16/24 patients with AF, resulting in clinical improvement. As such this observational study demonstrates that amiodarone was well-tolerated in PAH. Five-year survival in PAH/inoperable CTEPH was 68% with a fall to 58% if the patient developed a transient SVA and reduced further to 47% in permanent SVA. They also found that AF was more resistant to treatment than atrial flutter (similar to non-PAH disease). Consistent with these findings, Ruiz-Cano et al. (16) found that after the first episode of SVA (despite restoration of NSR/adequate rate control) 46.4% patients required an increase in PAH-specific medications secondary to progressive RHF, an interesting observation but not guideline directed. This data may suggest that the onset of SVA can be a prelude to RHF and/or clinical deterioration and that restoration of NSR or escalating PAH-specific therapy should be considered. Zhang et al. (22) specifically reviewed the efficacy and safety of electrophysiology studies and ablation in SVA and PAH. A retrospective study it reviewed 300 patients over 3 years [PAH 100 (observation) and non-PAH 200 (control)] with PAF undergoing ablation for the first time. All patients had a 24 h Holter monitor fitted immediately post ablation and AAD's were stopped 2 months later. EPS and ablation were found to be safe and reasonably effective in this cohort of patients. Bandorski et al. (23) agreed and found that 12/14 patients (all PH types) with a diagnosis of atrial flutter during EPS subsequently had successful ablation. Zhang et al. (22) noted that 11.3% of patients had an early recurrence PAF and 7.3% a late recurrence, with some correlation between a higher RAP and the incidence of late PAF recurrence.

In conclusion, incidence of SVA in PH (including PAH) ranges from 13.2 to 25.1% with a relationship to clinical worsening. As such this may be an indicator for restoration of NSR or alteration of PAH specific therapy. A range of therapeutic strategies have been investigated, however conclusions on efficacy are challenging to substantiate as the majority of studies were single arm. Little evidence of harm was identified. As in left heart disease NSR was easier to restore in atrial flutter vs. AF and all

TABLE 1 | Summary of literature reviewing SVA in PH.

Reference	Type of study	Pathology	Number of patients	Demographics in arrhythmia group	Prevalence/ incidence	Investigation	Rhythm identified	NSR restored?	Treatment given	Outcome
Smith et al. (14)	Retrospective 4-year study	PAH CTEPH	PAH 266 CTEPH 31	F:M 53:14% Age 61.8±14 MeanPAP 44±11	Prevalence	12-Lead ECG	AF/atrial flutter 50% paroxysmal	31 patients	86% AAD's 14% Not specified	
Rottlaender et al. (15)	Retrospective 4-year study	All types of PH	Total 225	F:M 36:64% Age 71.2±1.1 MeanPAP 40.8±1.6	Prevalence	12 Lead ECG	AF 41% paroxysmal	Not discussed	Not discussed	Permanent AF = Clinical deterioration.
Ruiz- Cano et al. (16)	Retrospective, 4-year, single center study	PAH	Total 282	F:M 61:39% Age 47.3±4.3	Prevalence	Medical notes/12-lead ECG	AF/atrial flutter /atrioventricular node re-entry tachycardia (AVNRT)	Attempted in all	All underwent EPS +/− ablation	Restoration of NSR = clinical improvement 4 SVA recurrence
Mercurio et al. (17)	Prospective, single center study	Idiopathic PAH PAH-SSc	116 IPAH 201 SSc-PH	F:M 71-29% Age 59+-12.1 MeanPAP 47.3+-14.3	Incidence at 5 years 13.2%		AF/atrial flutter/atrial tachycardia	Attempted in all	90.1% SVA = clinical worsening/RHF.	Restoration of NSR = clinical improvement
Cannillo et al. (18)	Retrospective, single center study? type of PH experienced SVA	PAH PH secondary to lung disease CTEPH (inoperable)	Total 77	F:M 55:45% Mean age 63 MeanPAP 43	Incidence	12 Lead ECG Holter if symptomatic	AF/atrial flutter 4 paroxysmal (23%).	13 patients	AAD's/DCCV/ablation SVA = worsening prognostic parameters and RHF. NSR restored in 11 cases	Recurrent SVA in 9 patients
Li-Wen et al. (19)	Prospective, cohort 6-year study	Idiopathic PAH (all taking PH meds)	Total 280	F:M 72.5:27.5% Age 39+-15 MeanPAP 64+-18	Incidence at 6 years (15.8%)		AF/atrial flutter /atrial tachycardia	21 patients	AAD's/DCCV/ablation SVA = clinical deterioration	NSR restored = clinical improvement 6 x recurrence
Olsson et al. (20)	Prospective 5-year, single center study	PAH or CTEPH (inoperable) NSR at baseline, all receiving PH meds	157 PAH 82 Inoperable CTEPH	F:M 65:35% Age 58+-9 MeanPAP 52+-8	Incidence at 5 years (25.1%)	12-Lead ECG	AF/atrial flutter	21/24 atrial flutter 16/24 AF	AAD's/overdrive pacing /DCCV/ablation	NSR = clinical improvement
Tongers et al. (21)	Retrospective 6-year study	PAH CTEPH (inoperable)	Total 231	F:M 65:35% Age 49+-13 MeanPAP 50+-10	Cumulative incidence of 11.7% and annual risk of 2.8%/ patient.	12 Lead ECG AVNRT diagnosed on EPS	AF/atrial flutter /AVNRT 4 SVA recurrence	15/15 atrial flutter 2/13 AF	AAD's/overdrive pacing /DCCV/ablation	Restoration of NSR = clinical improvement. Increased mortality in AF group
Zhang et al. (22)	Retrospective, 3-year, single center study	PAH Non- PAH PAF	PAH 100 Non-PAH 200	F:M 54.4:45.6% Age 62.9 + 6.8 MeanPAP 31.9+-6.2	X	Holter post ablation + 24-h Holter 3 monthly	11.3% early recurrence of PAF 7.3% Late recurrence of PAF	Attempted in all	All patients underwent radiofrequency ablation AAD's stopped 2 months post ablation	Suggests raised PAP increases chance of late recurrence PAF.

studies suggested that restoration of NSR resulted in improved clinical outcomes.

Ventricular Arrhythmias

The impact of ventricular arrhythmias in patients with PH is examined in a series of papers by Bandorski et al. An initial retrospective, two-center study (23) analyzed data from 55 PH patients presenting with indications for EPS (14 with group I PH). Fifteen had non-sustained ventricular tachycardia (NSVT) on a Holter monitor, however the prognostic relevance is unclear although likely to infer increased risk and extrapolation of prevalence from such a study is challenging due to small numbers and the large contribution of patients (23 in this study) with left heart disease-associated PH. There were no evidence suggesting EPS or ablation to be unsafe or ineffective in PH patients.

In a larger study, Bandorski et al. (24) sought to determine the incidence of VA in PH. Ninety two patients were enrolled in total (54 Group I, 10 Group 3, 26 Group 4, 2 Group 5), all of whom were on PAH-specific medication and in NSR at the time of enrolment. During 72-h Holter monitoring, 17 patients (18.5%) had a detectable arrhythmia [NSVT (12 patients), second degree atrioventricular block (1), intermittent complete heart block (1), and atrial flutter (1)]. Although small and including patients with all PH types, they undertook Holter monitoring and found arrhythmia in asymptomatic patients highlighting the potential inaccuracy of determining the incidence or prevalence of asymptomatic arrhythmia from 12-lead ECG. It highlighted that the use of Holter monitoring in this cohort was beneficial for arrhythmia diagnosis and this may be a useful tool in PAH patients also. To determine the prognostic significance of NSVT Bandorski et al. (25) examined 78 patients with PAH or inoperable CTEPH. Fifty-Five patients with PAH and 23 CTEPH underwent a clinical review, bloods, Holter monitoring, 6 MWT, echocardiography and RHC (25), of whom 12 had newly detected NSVT.

Relatively little evidence exists defining the prevalence and incidence of VA in PAH. Prevalence is estimated to be ~27% in all PH types with a considerable proportion of whom have co-existing left heart disease. Longer studies utilizing Holter monitoring rather than 12-lead ECG show higher rates of VA suggesting a bias in methods. The most reliable incidence of VA in all PH was ~15–18.5% based on Holter monitoring (25) suggesting a significant burden. Therapeutic options are unclear with only single arm studies available.

Bradyarrhythmia's

Limited data is available. Whilst determining the incidence of VA in PH Bandorski et al. (24), identified that 4/17 patients with newly diagnosed arrhythmias had intermittent heart block. Two patients, despite not taking rate limiting medication, progressed to complete heart block, and required pacemaker implantation. Studies are small and the relationship to poor outcome is uncertain.

Mode of Death

The predominant cause of death in patients with PAH is thought to be RHF or sudden cardiac death (SCD) (26). Hoeper et al. (27) undertook a retrospective, multi-center (17 referral centers in Europe and the United States) looking at patients with PAH who had developed cardiac arrest. 3130 patients with PAH were treated over 3 years and 513 had circulatory arrest. Cardiopulmonary resuscitation (CPR) was attempted in 132 (26%) but despite the majority occurring in a hospital setting only 8 patients (6%) survived to > 90 days. No apparent differences were found preceding cardiac arrest accounting for why a patient did or did not survive. It is difficult to fully assess cause of death, this data showed that 54% of patients were admitted with intercurrent illness; 49% died from progressive RHF; 18% respiratory failure, and 8% from other causes. Seventeen percent died from SCD and it is unclear as to whether this was secondary to PAH progression or potentially treatable arrhythmia.

CONCLUSION

Present data suggest that patients with PH have increased risk of arrhythmia, however accurate estimates of incidence and prevalence in patients with PAH remain elusive. PAH is a rare disease and as such patient numbers are often limited and the studies undertaken have grouped patients with PAH with other forms of related disease. As such, longitudinal studies with defined enrolment criteria are required to determine the arrhythmic burden of patients with PAH. The enrolment of patients with pre-existing symptoms is a potential source of bias exemplified by the increased rates of asymptomatic SVA and VA (24) identified with prolonged monitoring. Arrhythmias have been demonstrated to precede adverse clinical events and it is therefore of clinical importance to accurately define prevalence and incidence and examine potential therapeutic options. Current evidence highlights gaps in our knowledge as we only have "snapshots" of data from a 12-Lead ECG or Holter monitoring. Advances in technology now allow for long term monitoring of cardiac rhythm and as such a prospective study with continuous monitoring may further inform incidence, prevalence and relationships to adverse outcomes, prior to studies of therapeutic strategies.

AUTHOR CONTRIBUTIONS

JM and AR wrote the manuscript draft. All authors critically reviewed the paper and approved the final manuscript for submission.

REFERENCES

1. Galiè N, McLaughlin VV, Rubin LJ, Simonneau G. An overview of the 6th world symposium on pulmonary hypertension. *Europ Respirat J.* (2019) 53:3. doi: 10.1183/13993003.02148-2018
2. Peacock AJ, Naeije R, Rubin LJ. *Pulmonary Circulation: Diseases and Their Treatment. 3rd Ed.* Boca Raton, FL: CRC Press (2011). doi: 10.1201/b13219
3. Masarone D, Limongelli G, Rubino M, Valente F, Vastarella R, Ammendola

E, et al. Management of arrhythmias in heart failure. *Cardiovas Develop Dis.* (2017) 4:E3. doi: 10.3390/jcdd4010003

4. Ponikowski P, Voors AA, Anker SD, Bueno H, Cleland JG, Coats AJ, et al. 2016 ESC guidelines for the diagnosis and treatment of acute and chronic heart failure. *Europ Heart J.* (2016) 18:891–975. doi: 10.1002/ejhf.592
5. Braveny P. Editorial: heart, calcium and time. *J Exp Clin Cardiol.* (2002) 7:3–6.
6. Kirchhof P, Benussi S, Kotecha D, Ahlsson A, Atar D, Casadei B, et al. 2016 ESC guidelines for the management of atrial fibrillation developed in collaboration with EACTS. *Eur J Cardiothorac Surg.* (2017) 50:e1–e88. doi: 10.1016/j.rec.2016.11.033
7. Priori SG, Blomstrom-Lundqvist C, Mazzanti A, Bloma N, Borggrefe M, Camm J, et al. 2015 ESC guidelines for the management of patients with ventricular arrhythmias and the prevention of sudden cardiac death the task force for the management of patients with ventricular arrhythmias and the prevention of sudden cardiac death of the european society of cardiology (ESC). Endorsed by: association for european paediatric and congenital cardiology (AEPC). *Europ Heart J.* (2015) 36:2793–867l. doi: 10.1093/eurheartj/ehv316
8. Adler A. *Implantable Cardioverter Defibrillators and Cardiac Resynchronisation Therapy for Arrhythmias and Heart Failure.* London: NICE Guidance (2014).
9. Cowan C. *Atrial Fibrillation: Management Atrial Fibrillation: Management Clinical Guideline.* NICE Guidance (2014).
10. Brignole, M, Aurricchio A, Baron-Esquivias G, Bordachar P, Boriani G, Breithardt O-A, et al. ESC Guidelines on cardiac pacing and cardiac resynchronisation therapy. *Eur Heart J.* (2013) 34:2281–329. doi: 10.1093/eurheart/eht150
11. Malcolm MB. Systemic BP and heart rate as prognostic indicators in pulmonary arterial hypertension. *Chest.* (2013) 144:959–65. doi: 10.1378/chest.12-2572
12. Benza RL, Miller DP, Gomberg-Maitland M, Frantz RP, Foreman AJ, Coffey CS. Predicting survival in pulmonary arterial hypertension insights from the registry to evaluate early and long-term pulmonary arterial hypertension disease management (REVEAL). *Circulation.* (2010) 122:164–72. doi: 10.1161/CIRCULATIONAHA.109.898122
13. Burger CD, Long PK, Shah MR, McGoon MD, Miller DP, Romero AJ, et al. Characterization of first-time hospitalizations in patients with newly diagnosed pulmonary arterial hypertension in the reveal registry. *J Public Chestnet Org.* (2014) 146:1263–73. doi: 10.1378/chest.14-0193
14. Smith B, Genuardi MV, Koczo A, Zou RH, Thoma FW, Handen A, et al. EXPRESS: atrial arrhythmias are associated with increased mortality in pulmonary arterial hypertension. *Pulm Circ.* (2018) 8:204589401879031. doi: 10.1177/2045894018790316
15. Rottlaender D, Motloch LJ, Schmidt D, Reda S, Larbig R, Wolny M, et al. Clinical impact of atrial fibrillation in patients with pulmonary hypertension. *PLoS ONE.* (2012) 7:e33902. doi: 10.1371/journal.pone.0033902
16. Ruiz-Cano MJ, Gonzalez-Mansilla A, Escribano P, Delgado J, Arribas F, Torres J, et al. Clinical implications of supraventricular arrhythmias in patients with severe pulmonary arterial hypertension. *Int J Cardiol.* (2011) 146:105–6. doi: 10.1016/j.ijcard.2010.09.065
17. Mercurio V, Peloquin G, Bourji KI, Diab N, Sato T, Enobun B, et al. Pulmonary arterial hypertension and atrial arrhythmias: incidence, risk factors, and clinical impact. *Pulmonary Circulat.* (2018) 8:4–11. doi: 10.1177/2045894018769874
18. Cannillo M, Grosso Marra W, Gili S, D'Ascenzo F, Morello M, Mercante L, et al. Supraventricular arrhythmias in patients with pulmonary arterial hypertension. *Am J Cardiol.* (2015) 116:1883–9. doi: 10.1016/j.amjcard.2015.09.039
19. Wen L, Sun ML, An P, Jiang X, Sun K, Zheng L, et al. Frequency of supraventricular arrhythmias in patients with idiopathic pulmonary arterial hypertension. *Am J Cardiol.* (2014) 114:1420–5. doi: 10.1016/j.amjcard.2014.07.079
20. Olsson KM, Nickel NP, Tongers J, Hoeper MM. Atrial flutter and fibrillation in patients with pulmonary hypertension. *Int J Cardiol.* (2013) 167:2300–5. doi: 10.1016/j.ijcard.2012.06.024
21. Tongers J, Schwerdtfeger B, Klein G, Kempf T, Schaefer A, Knapp JM, et al. Incidence and clinical relevance of supraventricular tachyarrhythmias in pulmonary hypertension. *Am Heart J.* (2007) 153:127–32. doi: 10.1016/j.ahj.2006.09.008
22. Zhang Y-Q, Zhang F-L, Wang W-W, Chen X-H, Chen J-H, Chen LL. The correlation of pulmonary arterial hypertension with late recurrence of paroxysmal atrial fibrillation after catheter ablation. *J Thoracic Dis.* (2018) 10:2789–94. doi: 10.21037/jtd.2018.04.92
23. Bandorski D, Schmitt J, Kurzlechner C, Erkapic D, Hamm CW, Seeger W, et al. Electrophysiological studies in patients with pulmonary hypertension: a retrospective investigation. *Biomed Res Int.* (2014) 2014:617565. doi: 10.1155/2014/617565
24. Bandorski D, Erkapic D, Stempfl J, Höltgen R, Grünig E, Schmitt J, et al. Ventricular tachycardias in patients with pulmonary hypertension: an underestimated prevalence? *A Prospective Clinical Study. Herzschrittmachertherapie Elektrophysiologie.* (2015) 26:155–62. doi: 10.1007/s00399-015-0364-8
25. Bandorski D, Bogossian H, Stempfl J, Seeger W, Hecker M, Ghofrani A, et al. Prognostic relevance of nonsustained ventricular tachycardia in patients with pulmonary hypertension. *BioMed Res Int.* (2016) 2016:1327265. doi: 10.1155/2016/1327265
26. Galiè N, Hoeper MM, Humbert M, Torbicki A, Vachiery JL, Barbera J, et al. Guidelines for the diagnosis and treatment of pulmonary hypertension: the task force for the diagnosis and treatment of pulmonary hypertension of the european society of cardiology (ESC) and the european respiratory society (ERS), endorsed by the international Society of Heart and Lung Transplantation (ISHLT). *Euro Heart J.* (2009) 30:2493–537. doi: 10.1093/eurheartj/ehp297
27. Hoeper MM, Galié N, Murali S, Olschewski H, Rubenfire M, Robbins IM, et al. Outcome after cardiopulmonary resuscitation in patients with pulmonary arterial hypertension. *Am J Respir Crit Care Med.* (2002) 165:341–4. doi: 10.1164/ajrccm.165.3.200109-0130c

13

Switching-Off Adora2b in Vascular Smooth Muscle Cells Halts the Development of Pulmonary Hypertension

Tinne C. J. Mertens[1], *Ankit Hanmandlu*[1], *Ly Tu*[2,3], *Carole Phan*[2,3], *Scott D. Collum*[1], *Ning-Yuan Chen*[1], *Tingting Weng*[1], *Jonathan Davies*[4], *Chen Liu*[1], *Holger K. Eltzschig*[5], *Soma S. K. Jyothula*[6], *Keshava Rajagopal*[6], *Yang Xia*[1], *Ashrith Guha*[7], *Brian A. Bruckner*[7], *Michael R. Blackburn*[1], *Christophe Guignabert*[2,3] and *Harry Karmouty-Quintana*[1*]

[1] Department of Biochemistry and Molecular Biology, McGovern Medical School, The University of Texas Health Science Center at Houston, Houston, TX, United States, [2] Institut National de la Santé et de la Recherche Médicale UMR_S 999, Le Plessis-Robinson, France, [3] Université Paris-Sud and Université Paris-Saclay, Le Kremlin-Bicêtre, France, [4] Department of Pediatrics, Baylor College of Medicine, Houston, TX, United States, [5] Department of Anesthesiology, McGovern Medical School, The University of Texas Health Science Center at Houston, Houston, TX, United States, [6] Department of Internal Medicine, McGovern Medical School, The University of Texas Health Science Center at Houston, Houston, TX, United States, [7] Methodist Debakey Heart and Vascular Center, Houston Methodist Hospital, Houston, TX, United States

***Correspondence:**
Harry Karmouty-Quintana
harry.karmouty@uth.tmc.edu

Background: Pulmonary hypertension (PH) is a devastating and progressive disease characterized by excessive proliferation of pulmonary artery smooth muscle cells (PASMCs) and remodeling of the lung vasculature. Adenosine signaling through the ADORA2B receptor has previously been implicated in disease progression and tissue remodeling in chronic lung disease. In experimental models of PH associated with chronic lung injury, pharmacological or genetic inhibition of ADORA2B improved markers of chronic lung injury and hallmarks of PH. However, the contribution of ADORA2B expression in the PASMC was not fully evaluated.

Hypothesis: We hypothesized that adenosine signaling through the ADORA2B receptor in PASMC mediates the development of PH.

Methods: PASMCs from controls and patients with idiopathic pulmonary arterial hypertension (iPAH) were characterized for expression levels of all adenosine receptors. Next, we evaluated the development of PH in ADORA2B$^{f/f}$-Transgelin (Tagln)^{cre} mice. These mice or adequate controls were exposed to a combination of SUGEN (SU5416, 20 mg/kg/b.w. IP) and hypoxia (10% O_2) for 28 days (HX-SU) or to chronic low doses of bleomycin (BLM, 0.035U/kg/b.w. IP). Cardiovascular readouts including right ventricle systolic pressures (RVSPs), Fulton indices and vascular remodeling were determined. Using PASMCs we identified ADORA2B-dependent mediators involved in vascular remodeling. These mediators: IL-6, hyaluronan synthase 2 (HAS2) and tissue transglutaminase (Tgm2) were determined by RT-PCR and validated in our HX-SU and BLM models.

Results: Increased levels of ADORA2B were observed in PASMC from iPAH patients. ADORA2B$^{f/f}$-Tagln^{cre} mice were protected from the development of PH following HX-SU or BLM exposure. In the BLM model of PH, ADORA2B$^{f/f}$- Tagln^{cre} mice were not protected from the development of fibrosis. Increased expression of IL-6, HAS2 and

Tgm2 was observed in PASMC in an ADORA2B-dependent manner. These mediators were also reduced in ADORA2B$^{f/f}$- Tagln^{cre} mice exposed to HX-SU or BLM.

Conclusions: Our studies revealed ADORA2B-dependent increased levels of IL-6, hyaluronan and Tgm2 in PASMC, consistent with reduced levels in ADORA2B$^{f/f}$- Tagln^{cre} mice exposed to HX-SU or BLM. Taken together, our data indicates that ADORA2B on PASMC mediates the development of PH through the induction of IL-6, hyaluronan and Tgm2. These studies point at ADORA2B as a therapeutic target to treat PH.

Keywords: Group I PH, Group III PH, hyaluronan, tissue transglutaminase, lung fibrosis, vascular remodeling

INTRODUCTION

Pulmonary Hypertension (PH) is a condition of the pulmonary vasculature characterized by an mPAP of ≥25 mmHg at rest (Archer et al., 2010). The pathological diagnosis is portrayed as muscularization of previously non-muscular arteries, smooth muscle and endothelial cell proliferation, and the development of vascular lesions (Morrell et al., 2001). PH can be grouped into 5 subsets of hypertension based upon the etiology of the disease. Group I PH, or Pulmonary Arterial Hypertension (PAH), is PH that primarily affects the pre-capillary vasculature of the lungs (Ventetuolo and Klinger, 2012; Hansdottir et al., 2013). Group III PH is associated with chronic lung diseases such as chronic obstructive pulmonary disease (COPD) and idiopathic pulmonary fibrosis (IPF) (Farkas et al., 2011; Fell, 2012; Judge et al., 2012). Group III PH affects between 30 and 80% of patients (Poor et al., 2012; Hansdottir et al., 2013) where it is strongly associated with increased morbidity and mortality (Poor et al., 2012; Ventetuolo and Klinger, 2012; Hansdottir et al., 2013). In the vast majority of cases, PH is not curable. The pathogenesis of PH is poorly understood due to a lack of knowledge of the mechanisms governing its onset and progression. Consequently, research efforts aimed at uncovering the mechanisms involved in disease progression in PH are necessary to stimulate the development of novel therapies for this deadly disorder.

Adenosine is a nucleoside that is elevated following cell injury and stress (Fredholm, 2007). Under conditions of stress or cell injury, ATP is released from the cells and is converted by CD39 and CD73 (CD73 being the rate limiting enzyme) into adenosine (Lennon et al., 1998). Adenosine is then able to bind to one of its four G-protein coupled receptors: the adenosine A1 (ADORA1), A2A (ADORA2A), A2B (ADORA2B), and A3 (ADORA3) receptors (Fredholm et al., 2001). Adenosine is then metabolized extracellularly to inosine by adenosine deaminase (ADA) (Fredholm et al., 2001). In the context of chronic lung disease, increased expression of ADORA2B has been observed in patients with COPD and IPF (Zhou et al., 2010), although it is important to mention that protective effects of ADORA2B have been reported in acute lung injury settings (Karmouty-Quintana et al., 2013b).

In the context of PH, studies performed using explanted lungs from patients with a diagnosis of IPF with and without PH revealed increased expression levels of ADORA2B and enhanced capacity for the generation and accumulation of adenosine levels in patients with Group III PH (Garcia-Morales et al., 2016). Experiments using the ADORA2B antagonist (GS-6201) or *full* Adora2b knock-out mice revealed that genetic deletion or pharmacological inhibition of Adora2b subdued both the fibrotic deposition and the development of PH in a mouse model of chronic bleomycin (BLM)-induced lung fibrosis and PH (Karmouty-Quintana et al., 2012). Further studies revealed that conditional deletion of Adora2b from the myeloid lineage resulted in a reduction in fibrotic deposition and the absence of hallmarks of PH, including thickening of the vascular wall and elevated right ventricle systolic pressure (RVSP), in mice with conditional deletion of Adora2b in myeloid cells (Karmouty-Quintana et al., 2015). In experiments using pulmonary artery smooth muscle cells (PASMC), studies have shown that activation of ADORA2B can lead to increased expression of hyaluronan synthase (HAS) isozymes 1 and 2, enhancing levels of hyaluronan (Karmouty-Quintana et al., 2013a), the major glycosaminoglycan in the lungs that when fragmented has been implicated in modulating PH and lung fibrosis (Karmouty-Quintana et al., 2013a; Collum et al., 2017b). However, expression levels of CD39, CD73, ADA, and adenosine receptors in PAH has not yet been evaluated. In addition, the effects of conditional deletion of ADORA2B from vascular smooth muscle cells on the development of PH have not yet been determined. Here, we have assessed expression levels of mediators involved in the generation and metabolism of adenosine in PAH and evaluated the effects of conditional deletion of ADORA2B in vascular smooth muscle cells using the transgelin (Tagln) promoter, also known as smooth muscle protein 22-alpha promoter. In these *in vivo* experiments, mice were exposed to two distinct models of PH: the chronic hypoxia-SUGEN (HX-SU) model of PH and the BLM model of lung fibrosis and PH. In addition, we performed cell culture studies using human isolated PASMCs to identify ADORA2B-mediated mechanisms leading to PH.

MATERIALS AND METHODS

Isolation of Human Pulmonary Artery Smooth Muscle Cells (PASMCs)

Human PASMCs were isolated and cultured as previously described (Guignabert et al., 2005; Huertas et al., 2015). To identify PASMCs, we examined cultured cells for expression of muscle specific contractile and cytoskeletal proteins including smooth-muscle α actin, desmin, and Tagln. Cells were used between passages 3 and 6. A minimum N of 5 was used for all experiments using PASMCs. The clinical data from the donors were the PASMCs were isolated for western blots is available in Supplementary Table 1. The clinical data for PASMCs used for RT-PCR experiments can be found in the following publication: (Huertas et al., 2015, Table 2). Our studies using human material was reviewed by an institutional review board (IRB): HSC-MS-08-0354.

Cell Culture Experiments

Primary human pulmonary artery smooth muscle cells (PASMCs) were plated at 3,000 cells/cm^2 and grown in DMEM containing 10% FBS and antibiotics until 70–80% confluence. Next, PASMCs were serum starved overnight followed by 72 h exposure to normoxia or 2% O_2 (hypoxia) using a modular incubator chamber (Billups-Rothenberg, San Diego, CA, USA). PASMC were exposed for 72 h in combination with normoxia or hypoxia to the ADORA2B agonist BAY 60-6583 (10 μM) with or without the ADORA2B antagonist GS-6201 (100 nM) (both Tocris Bioscience, Bristol, UK). DMSO was used as a solvent control.

Animals

Adora2b$^{f/f}$-Tagln^{Cre} and Tagln^{Cre} mice on the C57/Bl6 background were used for all experiments. Animals were mated and genotyped as described previously (Zimmerman et al., 2013). All mice were housed in ventilated cages equipped with microisolator lids and maintained under strict containment protocols. N of 5 was used for all experimental groups (except for western blots). Mice were randomized to group treatment using a random number generator using www.graphpad.com/quickcalcs. For sample analysis, all mice were ear-tagged and researchers were blinded to the treatment group. In cases where data was normalized, this was performed to control for unwanted sources of variation. Mice were housed 5 per cage and were provided with variable free paper bedding (Pure-o'Cel The Andersons, Inc. Maumee, Ohio, USA) and Nestlets™ provided by Ancare (Bellmore, NY). The red mouse loft (Tecniplast, Buguggiate, Italy) was provided as amusement to all mouse cages. Mice were kept at an ambient temperature of 22°C and in a 12 h dark/light cycle. Animal care was in accordance with institutional and NIH guidelines. All studies were reviewed and approved by the University of Texas Health Science Center at Houston Animal Welfare Committee. Following consultation with a statistician, our experimental N number was set to 5 based on a power analysis (*F*-tests ANOVA:One Way) with the following criteria: alpha error: 0.05, Power: 0.95, number of groups 4, f:1.189. The Power and *f*-values were calculated *post-hoc* using previous data generated by our lab, including pulseox values, right ventricle systolic pressures, Fulton Indices and gene expression data for fibrotic markers. G*Power 3.1.9.2 Universität Düsseldorf, Germany was used for all the analysis.

In order to verify that Adora2b was depleted in PASMCs; primary cultures of pulmonary artery smooth muscle cells (PASMC) from mice were isolated as previously described (Lee et al., 2013) with some minor alterations. A mixture of 0.5% (w/v) agarose + 0.5% iron particles in DMEM containing antibiotics was infused through the right ventricle, resulting in lodging of 0.2 μM iron particles in PAs. The lungs were then inflated with 1% (w/v) agarose in DMEM containing antibiotics, removed, and dissociated. The iron-containing vessels were pulled down with a magnet, treated with 0.2% (w/v) collagenase, Type 2 (Worthington, Lakewood, NY, USA), and for 45 min. The resulting PASMC were maintained in DMEM media with 25 mM HEPES, 10% fetal bovine serum (FBS) and antibiotics at 37°C in a humidified atmosphere with 5% CO^2. After isolation and reaching 80–90% confluence, cells were lysed for RNA and protein extraction. Depletion of Adora2b was assessed on isolated primary pulmonary artery smooth muscle cells (PASMCs) from Tagln^{Cre} and Adora2b$^{f/f}$-Tagln^{Cre} mice where Cre expression was also determined (Supplementary Figure 1).

Experimental Design

In experiments involving chronic exposure to hypoxia-SUGEN (HX-SU), mice were placed in open cages inside a specifically designed chamber (A-Chamber, Biospherix, Lacona, NY) and exposed to 10% oxygen for 4 weeks. The oxygen levels were maintained using the Oxygen regulator from OKO Labs (Pozzuoli, NA, Italy). In our model, SUGEN (SU5416; Tocris, Bristol, BS11 9QD United Kingdom) was dissolved in a solution of 10% Kolliphor® HS 15 (Macrogol (15)-hydroxystearate, Sigma Aldrich, St Louis. MO) and administered once weekly via the intra-peritoneal route (20 mg/kg/b.w. IP). Control mice were housed in the same room and were exposed to ambient air (normoxia) for 4 weeks and received the vehicle for SUGEN (10% Kolliphor® once weekly IP). In our bleomycin (BLM) model of chronic lung injury, mice were exposed to BLM (0.035 U/kg/b.w. IP) or vehicle (PBS) twice weekly for 4 weeks as previously described (Karmouty-Quintana et al., 2012). Mice were euthanized on day 28 in the HX-SU model and on day 33 for the BLM model for histological analysis after physiological measurements were performed. A minimum N of 5 was used for experimental groups.

Hemodynamic Measurements: Right Ventricle Systolic Pressure (RVSP), Heart Rate, and RV Hypertrophy

This procedure was performed as previously described (Karmouty-Quintana et al., 2012). Briefly, mice were given 0.75 mg/g of 2.5% Avertin (a mixture of tert-amyl alcohol and 2-2-2 Tribromoethanol, Sigma Aldrich, ST. Louis, MO) to induce a surgical plane of anesthesia. Mice were placed on a heated pad (Deltaphase Isothermal pad model 39; Braintree Scientific, Braintree, MA) and secured with surgical tape. Mice were then tracheotomised with a 19G blunt needle (BRICO, Dayton, NJ) and attached to a small animal ventilator (MiniVent, Hugo-Sachs Elektronik, March-Hugstetten, Germany) and ventilated at a stroke volume of 250 μl at 60 strokes per minute. The surgical site was viewed using a surgical microscope (SMZ-2B, Nikon, Tokyo, Japan). An incision of ∼1 cm in length was made just below the xiphoid process. An alm retractor (ALM-112, Braintree Scientific, Braintree, MA) was used to expose the abdominal cavity to visualize the diaphragm and the liver. An incision was then made on the diaphragm to expose the heart and the pericardium was removed. The right ventricle was then identified and a puncture was made with a 27G needle. A 1 French pressure catheter (SPR-1000, Millar Instruments, Houston, TX) was then inserted through the puncture. The heart rate results were continuously recorded using a Powerlab 8-SP A/D (AD Instruments) converter, acquired at 1000 Hz. All RVSP results were recorded to a PC utilizing Chart5.3 software. After completion of the measurements, blood was collected and the lungs were excised and flash frozen in liquid nitrogen for RNA extraction. The heart was excised and the atria were removed. The right ventricle was then surgically removed and the dry weights of the RV were used to determine the Fulton Index: extent of RV-hypertrophy using the weight of the left ventricle and septum to normalize the data (RV/LV+S).

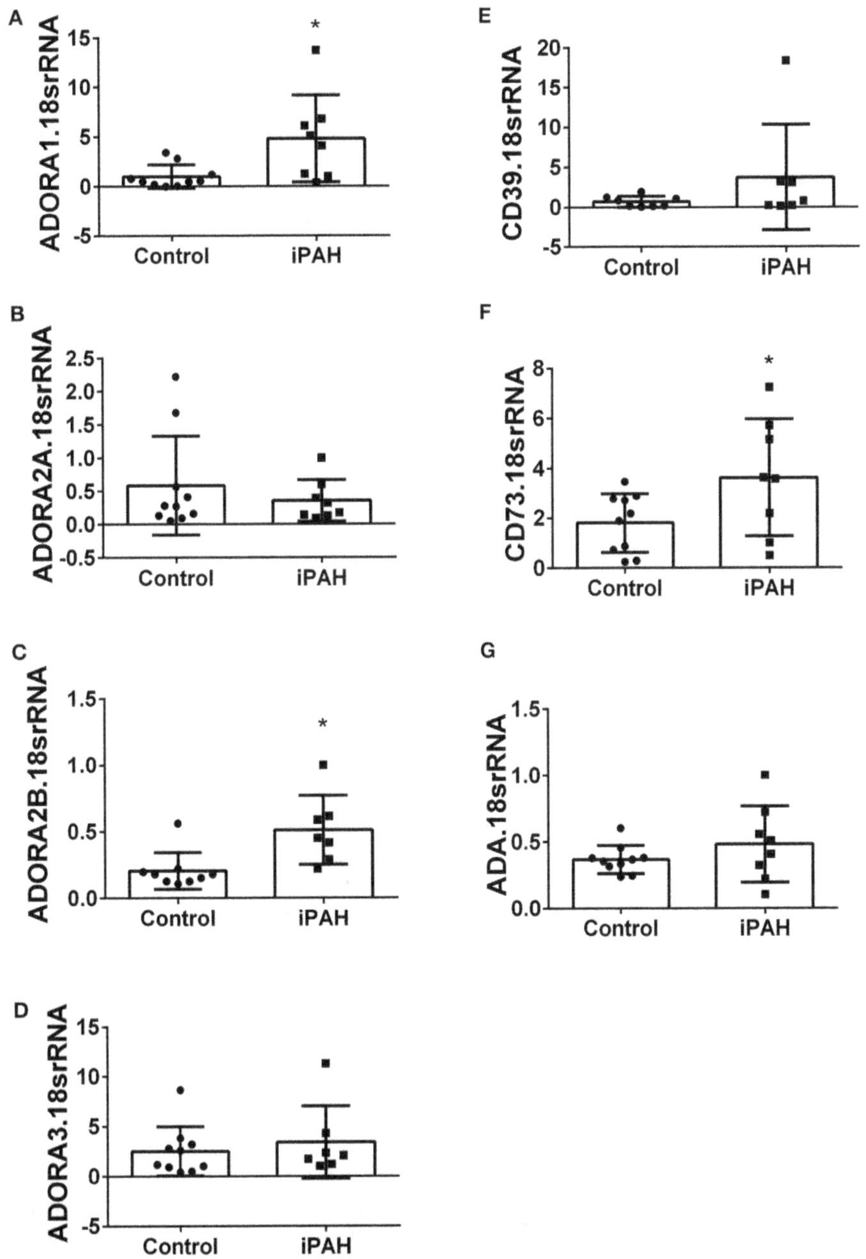

FIGURE 1 | Expression levels of adenosine receptors and genes associated with adenosine synthesis in pulmonary artery smooth muscle cells (PASMCs) derived from controls and idiopathic pulmonary hypertension (iPAH) lung tissue. ADORA1 **(A)**; ADORA2A **(B)**; ADORA2B **(C)**; ADORA3 **(D)**; CD39 **(E)**; CD73 **(F)**; and adenosine deaminase (ADA, **G**). Results are presented as means ± SE, $N = 10$ (control) or 8 (iPAH) and normalized to the expression of 18srRNA. $^{*}P < 0.05$ refers to comparisons between control vs. iPAH groups.

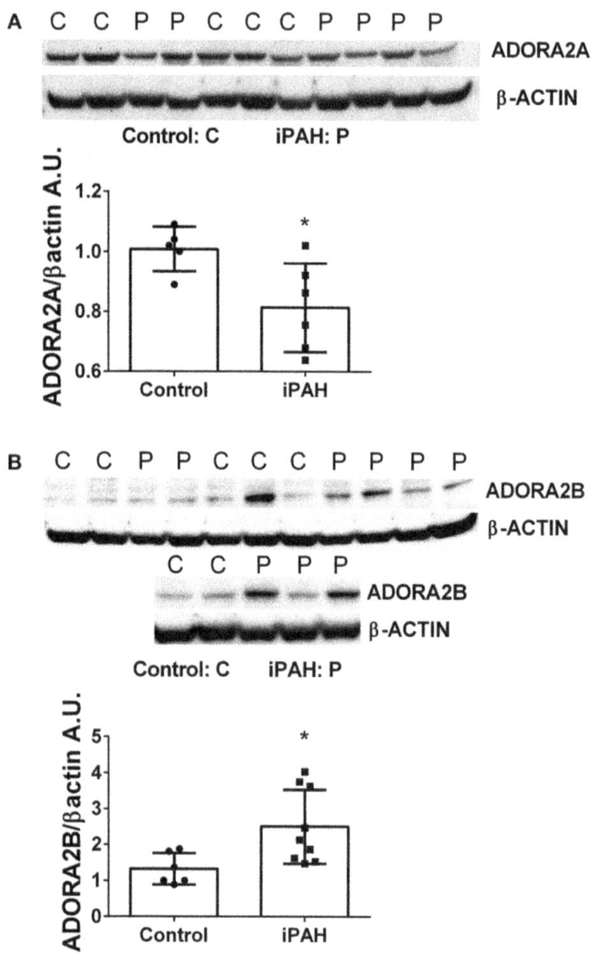

FIGURE 2 | Protein levels of adenosine receptors in pulmonary artery smooth muscle cells (PASMCs) derived from controls and idiopathic pulmonary hypertension (iPAH). Protein expression levels and quantification of ADORA2A **(A)** and ADORA2B **(B)** levels in isolated PASMCs from control or iPAH patients. β-ACTIN was used to normalize expression levels of ADORA2A and ADORA2B, blots are shown. $^{*}P < 0.05$ refers to comparisons between control vs. iPAH groups. $N = 7$ Control, $N = 6$ iPAH for **(A)** and $N = 6$ Control, $N = 9$ iPAH for **(B)**. Lane 6 from **(B)** was excluded from the analysis as it was determined as an outlier by the Grubb's Test.

Histology, Immunohistochemistry, and Western Blots

Mouse lungs were inflated with 10% buffered formalin at 25 cm of water and fixed at 4°C overnight. Lungs were dehydrated in ethanol gradients and embedded in paraffin, and 5-μm tissue sections were collected on microscope slides and stained with Masson's trichrome (EM Science, Gibbstown, NJ) according to manufacturer's instructions.

Immunohistochemistry was performed on 5 μm sections cut from formalin-fixed, paraffin-embedded lungs. Sections were rehydrated through graded ethanol to water, antigen retrieval was performed using a solution of 10 mM citric acid and heated for 2 min for 3 intervals at high power using a microwave, endogenous peroxidase and alkaline phosphatase were inactivated using BLOXALL (Vector Labs, Burlingame, CA) and 2.5% normal horse serum (Vector Labs) was used as a blocking solution prior to incubation with the primary antibody. Following overnight incubation with the primary antibody, sections were treated with the ImmPRESS polymer detection kits for alkaline phosphatase or horse-radish peroxidase (Vector Labs) based on the host of the primary antibody and development method. Slides were incubated with primary antibodies (see Supplementary Table 1). Sections were developed with VIP-HRP Substrate Kit or Vector Blue/Red or BCIP/NBT Alkaline Phosphatase Substrate Kits (Vector Laboratories). Slides were mounted using cytoseal or mountiung medium containing DAPI (Sigma Aldrich).

For Western blots, protein from lung tissue lysates or PASMCs was extracted with RIPA buffer (Thermo Scientific, Rockford, IL) containing 1 mM of protease and phosphatase inhibitor (Sigma Aldrich, St Louis, MO). Thirty microgram of protein per sample was loaded onto 4–12% Mini-Protean TGX gels (Bio-Rad, Hercules, CA) for electrophoresis and then transferred on polyvinylidene difluoride (PVDF) membranes (0.45 μm, GE Healthcare Piscataway, NJ). Membranes were then blocked in 5% Milk (Bio-Rad) for 1 h at room temperature and then incubated with the appropriate primary antibody overnight (see Supplementary Table 2). Secondary antibodies and an ECL kit (GE Healthcare) were applied for generating chemiluminescent signals. Isotype control images for all IHC staining is available in Supplementary Figure 2.

Morphometry

Muscularized arterioles of the lung parenchyma were observed under 20x magnification and noted as being different from both airways and non-muscularized arterioles. Muscularized arterioles were then photographed under 40x magnifications. Micropictographs were then analyzed using Image Pro-Plus software (MediaCybernetics Inc, Bethesda, MD). In short, the overall area of the muscularized portion was measured for each arteriole. To account for size, the largest diameter for each arteriole was also measured. The area of the arteriole was then divided by the largest diameter to give a relative measurement of muscularization. To determine fibrotic deposition, lung sections were stained for Masson's Tri-chrome and analyzed using a modified Ashcroft scale optimized for mouse lung sections (Hubner et al., 2008). Ten images per animal were analyzed by 3 individuals blinded to group status.

RT-PCR

Total RNA was isolated from frozen lung tissue using Trizol reagent (Life Technologies). RNA samples were then DNase treated (ArticZymes, Tromso, Norway) and subjected to quantitative real-time RT-PCR. The specific primers used is available in Supplementary Table 3. Data is presented as mean normalized transcript levels using the comparative Ct method ($2\Delta\Delta$Ct).

HPLC

Adenosine levels in bronchoalveolar lavage fluid (BALf) were measured as previously described (Wakamiya et al., 1995).

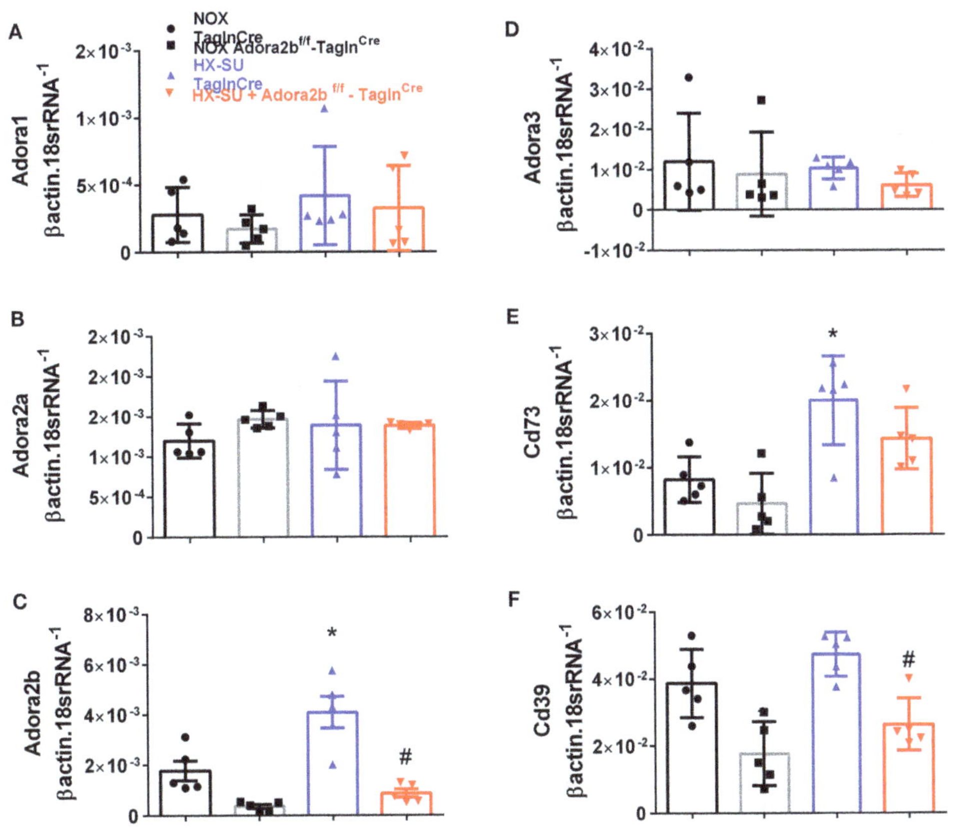

FIGURE 3 | Expression levels of adenosine receptors and genes associated with adenosine synthesis in TaglnCre and Adora2b$^{f/f}$-Tagln^{Cre} mice exposed to hypoxia-SUGEN (HX-SU) or normoxia (NOX). All analyses were performed on day 28 of HX-SU and NOX exposure. Adora1 **(A)**; Adora2a **(B)**; Adora2b **(C)**; Adora3 **(D)**; Cd73 **(E)**; Cd39 **(F)**; expression levels measured by RT-PCR and normalized to the Geo mean of expression levels of βactin and 18srRNA from NOX-Tagln^{Cre} mice (black circles and bar outline); NOX- Adora2b$^{f/f}$-Tagln^{Cre} mice (black squares and gray bar outline); HX-SU-Tagln^{Cre} mice (blue triangles and bar outline); HX-SU-Adora2b$^{f/f}$-Tagln^{Cre} mice (red triangles and bar outline). Significant values: $^{*}P < 0.05$ refer to comparisons between Tagln^{Cre} HX-SU and Tagln^{Cre} NOX treatment groups. $\#P < 0.05$, are for comparisons between Tagln^{Cre} HX-SU and Adora2b$^{f/f}$-Tagln^{Cre} + HX-SU treatment groups. $N = 5$ for all groups.

Briefly, to measure the nucleoside levels in BALF, mice were anesthetized with 2.5% avertin and the lungs were lavaged 4 times with 0.3 ml PBS containing 2 μM dipyridamole (Sigma-Aldrich, St. Louis, MO, USA) and 5 μM ADA-inhibitor deoxycoformycin (dCF, R&D Systems Inc, Minneapolis, MN, USA), which pooled 1.0 ml BALF. The BALF was then centrifuged to remove cells and debris. To measure nucleoside levels, 200 μl BALF supernatant were loaded to the HPLC meter per reading and the flow rate was set at 1 ml/min. The representative peaks were identified and quantitated by running known external standard curves.

Statistical Analysis

All analyses were blinded to the experimenter. A two-way analysis of variance (ANOVA) with a Tukey *post hoc* test was performed for all experiments with more than 2 groups. For experiments that consisted of two groups, an un-paired two-tailed Students *t*-test with a Welch correction was performed. Categorical data was analyzed using a Chi-Squared calculation. Statistical significance was defined as $P \leq 0.05$ by use of GraphPad Prism version 5 (GraphPad Software, La Jolla, CA). Densitometry analysis from Western blots were performed using ImageJ (National Institutes of Health, Bethesda, Maryland, USA). The Grubbs' test was used to detect outliers.

RESULTS

Enhanced Adenosinergic System in Idiopathic Pulmonary Arterial Hypertension (iPAH)

Using isolated PASMCs from normal controls or patients with a diagnosis of idiopathic pulmonary arterial hypertension (iPAH), we first profiled the expression levels of adenosine receptors (**Figures 1A–D**). In these experiments, we identified increased transcript levels of ADORA1 (**Figure 1A**) and ADORA2B (**Figure 1C**) but not ADORA2A or ADORA3 (**Figures 1B,D**). Subsequently, we determined expression levels of CD39 and CD73, key enzymes for the catabolism of ATP to adenosine. These experiments did not show significant changes for CD39 in iPAH PASMCs compared to controls (**Figure 1E**). CD73, the rate-limiting enzyme, was significantly elevated in iPAH vs. control PASMCs (**Figure 1F**); yet no

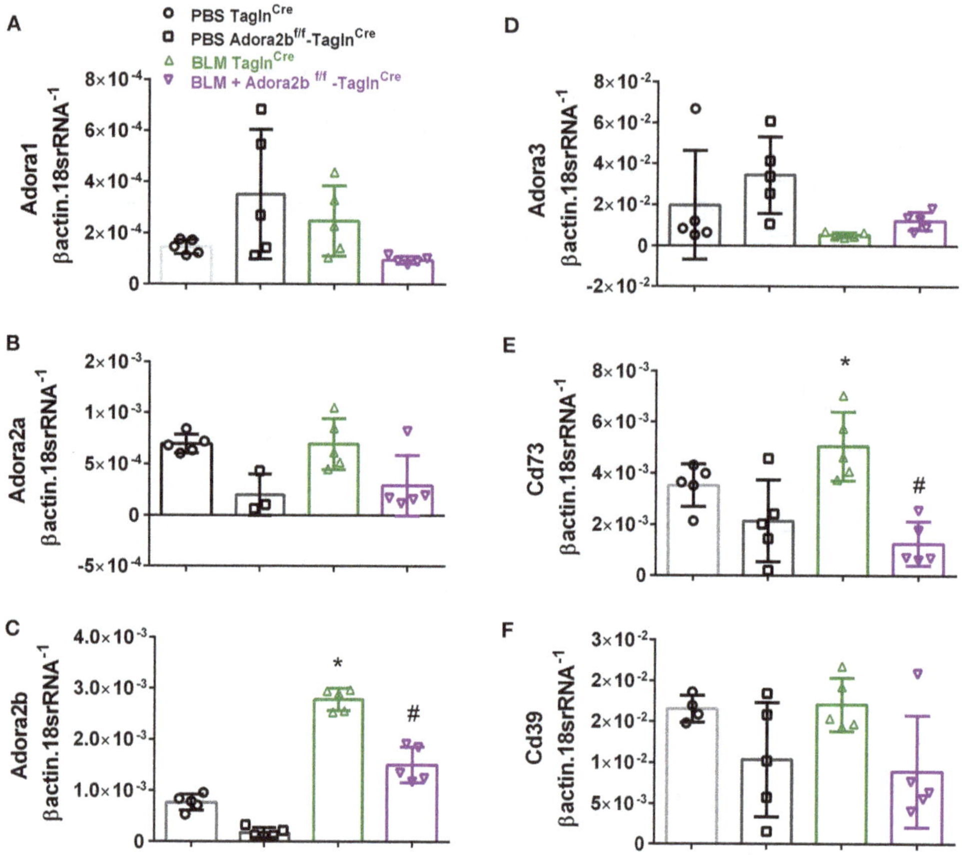

FIGURE 4 | Expression levels of adenosine receptors and genes associated with adenosine synthesis in TaglnCre and Adora2b$^{f/f}$–Tagln^{Cre} mice exposed to bleomycin (BLM) or vehicle phosphate-buffered saline (PBS). All analyses were performed on day 33 of PBS or BLM exposure. Adora1 **(A)**; Adora2a **(B)**; Adora2b **(C)**; Adora3 **(D)**; Cd73 **(E)**; Cd39 **(F)**; expression levels measured by RT-PCR and normalized to the Geo mean of expression levels of βactin and 18srRNA from PBS-Tagln^{Cre} mice (black circles and bar outline); PBS- Adora2b$^{f/f}$–Tagln^{Cre} mice (black squares and bar outline); BLM-Tagln^{Cre} mice (green triangles and bar outline); BLM-Adora2b$^{f/f}$–Tagln^{Cre} mice (magenta triangles and bar outline). Significant values: $^{*}P < 0.05$ refer to comparisons between Tagln^{Cre} BLM and Tagln^{Cre} PBS treatment groups. $\#P < 0.05$, are for comparisons between Tagln^{Cre} BLM and Adora2b$^{f/f}$-Tagln^{Cre} + BLM treatment groups. $N = 5$ for all groups.

changes in ADA expression were seen (**Figure 1G**). Expression levels of ADA did not appear altered in iPAH vs. control PASMCs.

We next used Western blots to validate expression levels of ADORA2A and ADORA2B. Remarkably, iPAH PASMCs showed attenuated levels of ADORA2A but elevated ADORA2B (**Figures 2A,B**); the latter consistent with transcript levels for ADORA2B. Collectively, these data point at enhanced capacity for the generation of adenosine in PASMCs from iPAH patients in addition to increased altered expression of adenosine receptors leading to increased ADORA2B, but reduced ADORA2A. These results point at altered adenosine receptor expression in human PASMCs from patients with iPAH.

Enhanced Adenosinergic System in Mice Exposed to Hypoxia-SUGEN (HX-SU) or Bleomycin (BLM)

In order to model pulmonary hypertension, we exposed mice for 4 weeks to hypoxia and treated them once weekly with SUGEN (SU5416, 20 mg/kg bw). This protocol was adapted from earlier studies (Ciuclan et al., 2011). RT-PCR from flash frozen lungs revealed no significant changes in Adora1 or Adora2a expression levels between mice exposed to HX-SU or normoxia (NOX) in Tagln^{Cre} or Adora2b$^{f/f}$-Tagln^{Cre} mice (**Figures 3A,B**). However, consistent with our observations in iPAH PASMCs, we report increased Adora2b transcripts in HX-SU–exposed Tagln^{Cre} mice compared to NOX exposed Tagln^{Cre} mice which were attenuated in HX-SU exposed Adora2b$^{f/f}$-Tagln^{Cre} mice (**Figure 3C**). No significant differences were observed in Adora3 expression levels between treatment groups (**Figure 3D**). Interestingly, increased expression levels of CD73 were observed between HX-SU–exposed Tagln^{Cre} compared to NOX exposed Tagln^{Cre} mice, albeit no differences between HX-SU exposed Adora2b$^{f/f}$-Tagln^{Cre} and HX-SU Tagln^{Cre} mice (**Figure 3E**). CD39 expression analysis revealed reduced levels in Adora2b$^{f/f}$-Tagln^{Cre} mice exposed to normoxia or HX-SU compared to Adora2b competent mice (**Figure 3F**). In summary HX-SU exposed Adora2b$^{f/f}$-Tagln^{Cre} mice showed reduced expression levels of Adora2b and CD39 compared to HX-SU exposed Tagln^{Cre} mice (**Figures 3C,F**).

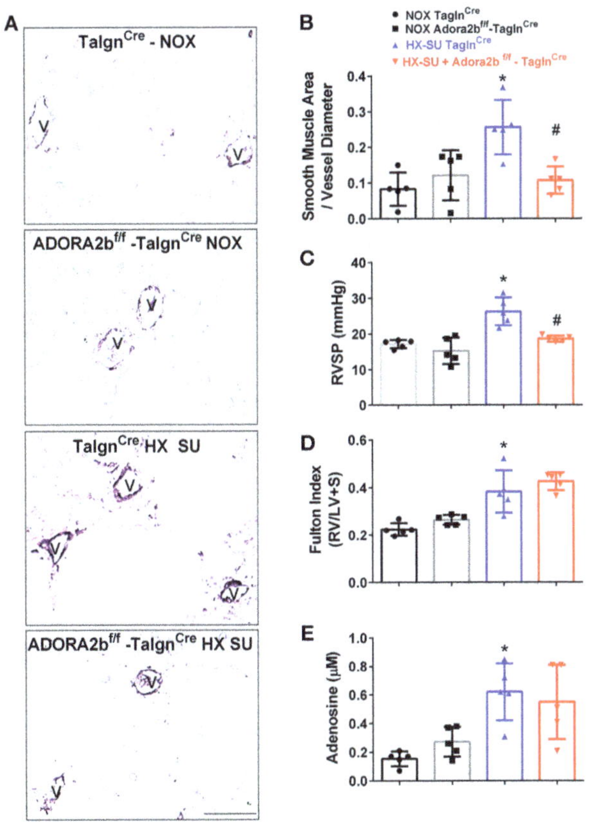

FIGURE 5 | Cardiovascular physiology in TaglnCre and Adora2b$^{f/f}$-Tagln^{Cre} mice exposed to hypoxia-SUGEN (HX-SU) or normoxia (NOX). All analyses were performed on day 28 of HX-SU and NOX exposure. **(A)** Representative immunohistochemistry for alpha smooth muscle actin (αSMA, violet-purple signals) vessels are demarked by a **V** from Tagln^{Cre} and Adora2b$^{f/f}$-Tagln^{Cre} mice exposed to NOX or HX-SU. Morphometric evaluation of αSMA deposition from 5-7 vessels for each mouse **(B)**; Right ventricle systolic pressure (RVSP) **(C)**; Fulton Index ratio determined by the measure of right ventricle and left ventricle with septum **(D)**; and broncho-alveolar lavage fluid (BALF) adenosine levels measured by HPLC **(E)**; from NOX-Tagln^{Cre} mice (black circles and bar outline); NOX- Adora2b$^{f/f}$-Tagln^{Cre} mice (black squares and gray bar outline); HX-SU-Tagln^{Cre} mice (blue triangles and bar outline); HX-SU-Adora2b$^{f/f}$-Tagln^{Cre} mice (red triangles and bar outline). Significant values: $^*P < 0.05$ refer to comparisons between Tagln^{Cre} HX-SU and Tagln^{Cre} NOX treatment groups. $^{\#}P < 0.05$, are for comparisons between Tagln^{Cre} HX-SU and Adora2b$^{f/f}$-Tagln^{Cre} + HX-SU treatment groups. $N = 5$ for all groups.

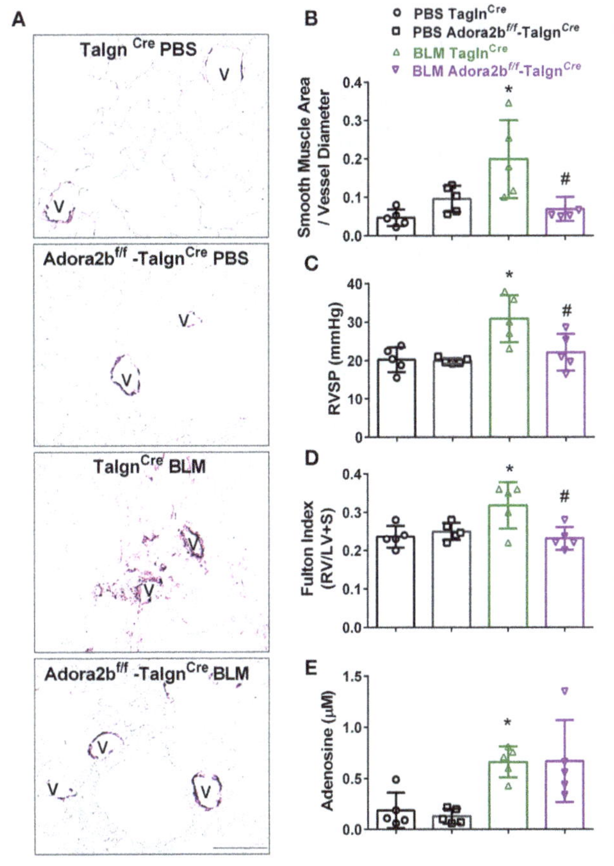

FIGURE 6 | Cardiovascular physiology in Tagln^{Cre} and Adora2b$^{f/f}$−Tagln^{Cre} mice exposed to bleomycin (BLM) or phosphate-buffered saline vehicle (PBS). All analyses were performed on day 33 of BLM and PBS exposure. **(A)** Representative immunohistochemistry for alpha smooth muscle actin (αSMA, violet-purple signals) vessels are demarked by a **V** from Tagln^{Cre} and Adora2b$^{f/f}$−Tagln^{Cre} mice exposed to PBS or BLM. Morphometric evaluation of αSMA deposition from 5 to 7 vessels for each mouse **(B)**; Right ventricle systolic pressure (RVSP) **(C)**; Fulton Index ratio determined by the measure of right ventricle and left ventricle with septum **(D)**; and broncho-alveolar lavage fluid (BALF) adenosine levels measured by HPLC **(E)**; from PBS-Tagln^{Cre} mice (black circles and bar outline); PBS- Adora2b$^{f/f}$−Tagln^{Cre} mice (black squares and bar outline); BLM-Tagln^{Cre} mice (green triangles and bar outline); BLM-Adora2b$^{f/f}$−Tagln^{Cre} mice (magenta triangles and bar outline). Significant values: $^*P < 0.05$ refer to comparisons between Tagln^{Cre} BLM and Tagln^{Cre} PBS treatment groups. $^{\#}P < 0.05$, are for comparisons between Tagln^{Cre} BLM and Adora2b$^{f/f}$-Tagln^{Cre} + BLM treatment groups. $N = 5$ for all groups.

These changes were consistent with mice chronically exposed to low doses of BLM IP where no significant changes in Adora1, Adora2a, or Adora3 expression levels were observed between Adora2b$^{f/f}$-Tagln^{Cre} or Tagln^{Cre} mice expose to either BLM or PBS (**Figures 4A,B,D**). In line with our HX-SU exposed mice and with our previous studies using BLM-treated mice (Karmouty-Quintana et al., 2012), increased levels of Adora2b were observed in BLM-exposed Tagln^{Cre} mice compared to PBS-treated mice (**Figure 4C**). Consistent with the depletion of Adora2b using the Tagln^{Cre} promoter, we report reduced expression levels of Adora2b in Adora2b$^{f/f}$-Tagln^{Cre} mice exposed to either BLM or PBS (**Figure 4C**). Expression levels of CD73 demonstrated increased levels in the BLM-Tagln^{Cre} group (**Figure 4E**). No significant changes in CD39 were reported between treatment groups (**Figure 4F**). BLM- exposed Adora2b$^{f/f}$-Tagln^{Cre} mice showed reduced expression levels of Adora2b and CD73 compared to HX-SU exposed Tagln^{Cre} mice **Figures 4C,E**). These results demonstrate Adora2b expression is augmented in Tagln^{Cre} mice following BLM-exposure, consistent with increased CD73 expression. Interestingly, expression levels of Adora2b were only partially attenuated in BLM-exposed Adora2b$^{f/f}$-Tagln^{Cre} mice. These results likely reflect Adora2b expression in non-Tagln^{Cre}-expressing cells.

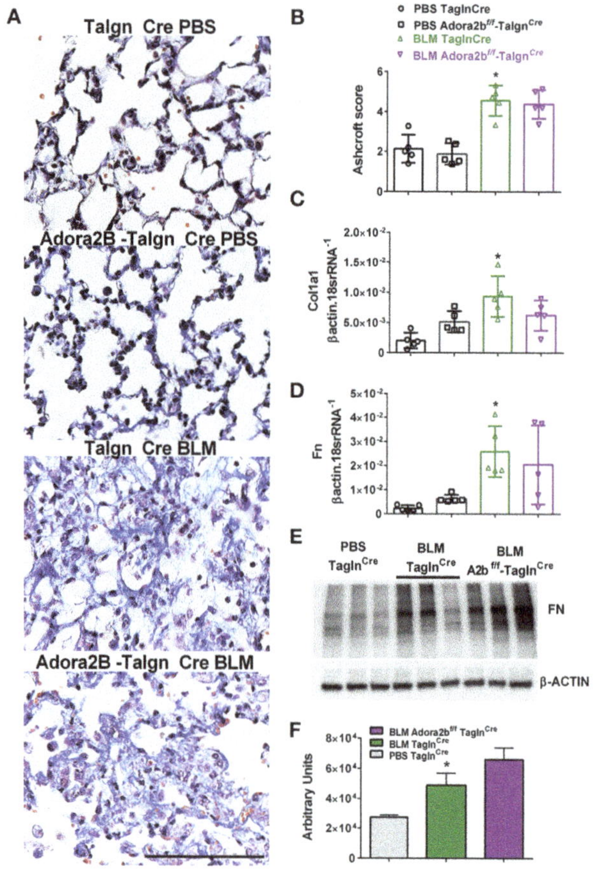

FIGURE 7 | Fibrotic injury in Tagln^{Cre} and Adora2b$^{f/f}$−Tagln^{Cre} mice exposed to bleomycin (BLM) or phosphate-buffered saline vehicle (PBS). All analyses were performed on day 33 of BLM and PBS exposure. **(A)** Representative Masson's Trichrome stained images showing fibrotic deposition in the parenchyma of PBS or BLM exposed Tagln^{Cre} or Adora2b$^{f/f}$−Tagln^{Cre} mice and corresponding Ashcroft scores **(B)**. **(C)** Expression levels of Collagen 1a1 (Col1a1 **C**) Fibronectin (FN, **D**) by RT-PCR from PBS-Tagln^{Cre} mice (black circles and bar outline); PBS- Adora2b$^{f/f}$−Tagln^{Cre} mice (black squares and bar outline); BLM-Tagln^{Cre} mice (green triangles and bar outline); BLM-Adora2b$^{f/f}$−Tagln^{Cre} mice (magenta triangles and bar outline). Significant values: $^{*}P < 0.05$ refer to comparisons between Tagln^{Cre} BLM and Tagln^{Cre} PBS treatment groups. **(E)** Western blot for FN and β-actin for Tagln^{Cre} mice exposed to PBS or BLM and BLM-treated Adora2b$^{f/f}$−Tagln^{Cre} mice. Densitometry analyses from Western Blot **(F)**. $N = 5$ for all groups for RT-PCR data an $N = 3$ for Western Blots.

Vascular Deletion of Adora2b Prevents the Development of Hypoxia-SUGEN (HX-SU)-Induced Pulmonary Hypertension (PH)

We next examined the role of vascular deletion of Adora2b in the development of HX-SU-induced PH. In these experiments, Tagln^{Cre} mice exposed to HX-SU presented with increased α-smooth muscle actin (αSMA) deposition, consistent with vascular remodeling, compared to Tagln^{Cre} and Adora2b$^{f/f}$-Tagln^{Cre} exposed to normoxia (**Figure 5A**). HX-SU-exposed Adora2b$^{f/f}$-Tagln^{Cre} mice showed reduced vascular αSMA deposition compared to HX-SU exposed Tagln^{Cre} mice (**Figure 5A**). These histological observations were consistent with morphometric analyses showing evidence of vascular remodeling in HX-SU-Tagln^{Cre} mice compared to mice exposed to normoxia. Adora2b$^{f/f}$-Tagln^{Cre} mice exposed to HX-SU showed a significant reduction in vascular remodeling compared to HX-SU exposed Tagln^{Cre} mice (**Figure 5B**). RVSP measurements revealed increased pressures in HX-SU exposed Tagln^{Cre} mice compared to mice exposed to normoxia. HX-SU exposed Adora2b$^{f/f}$-Tagln^{Cre} mice showed reduced RVSP levels in comparison with HX-SU exposed Tagln^{Cre} mice (**Figure 5C**). We next examined the extent of right ventricle hypertrophy (RVH) using the Fulton index. Here we report an increased Fulton index in Tagln^{Cre} mice exposed to HX-SU compared to normoxia-exposed mice. Remarkably, HX-SU-Adora2b$^{f/f}$-Tagln^{Cre} mice did not show a reduced extent of RVH compared to HX-SU Tagln^{Cre} mice (**Figure 5D**). Adenosine levels in BALF revealed increased levels in Tagln^{Cre} mice exposed to HX-SU compared to mice exposed to normoxia that remained elevated in HX-SU Adora2b$^{f/f}$-Tagln^{Cre} mice (**Figure 5E**). These observations are in line with RT-PCR data showing increased CD73 levels in HX-SU Tagln^{Cre} mice that are maintained in conditional KO mice lacking Adora2b. Taken together, these results demonstrate that conditional deletion of Adora2b from vascular smooth muscle cells attenuated the development of PH in mice despite increased levels of adenosine remaining unchanged. Interestingly, in this model, the Fulton index remained elevated in HX-SU exposed Adora2b$^{f/f}$-Tagln^{Cre} mice.

Vascular Deletion of Adora2b Prevents the Development of Bleomycin (BLM)-Induced Pulmonary Hypertension (PH)

We next used our BLM-induced model of lung fibrosis and PH to evaluate the effect of conditional deletion of Adora2b in vascular smooth muscle cells in a model mimicking features of Group III PH. Immunohistochemistry for αSMA revealed increased vascular αSMA deposition in BLM exposed Tagln^{Cre} mice compared to PBS-exposed Tagln^{Cre} mice, which appeared to be attenuated in the BLM-treated Adora2b$^{f/f}$-Tagln^{Cre} group (**Figure 6A**). No significant changes in αSMA deposition were observed in PBS-exposed Adora2b$^{f/f}$-Tagln^{Cre} mice compared to Tagln^{Cre} mice receiving PBS (**Figure 6A**). Morphometric determination of vascular remodeling showed thickening of the vascular wall in BLM-treated Tagln^{Cre} mice compared to mice receiving PBS. BLM-treated Adora2b$^{f/f}$-Tagln^{Cre} mice showed significantly reduced vascular remodeling, observed histologically and morphometrically, compared to BLM-exposed Tagln^{Cre} mice (**Figures 6A,B**). Determination of RVSP in these mice revealed increased pressures in Tagln^{Cre} mice exposed to BLM compared to PBS groups, which is consistent with our previous studies (Karmouty-Quintana et al., 2012, 2015). In line with our morphometric data, BLM-treated Adora2b$^{f/f}$-Tagln^{Cre} mice showed reduced RVSP levels compared to BLM-treated Tagln^{Cre} mice (**Figure 6C**). Determination of RVH using the Fulton index revealed evidence of RVH in BLM-treated Tagln^{Cre} mice that was attenuated in BLM-exposed Adora2b$^{f/f}$-Tagln^{Cre}

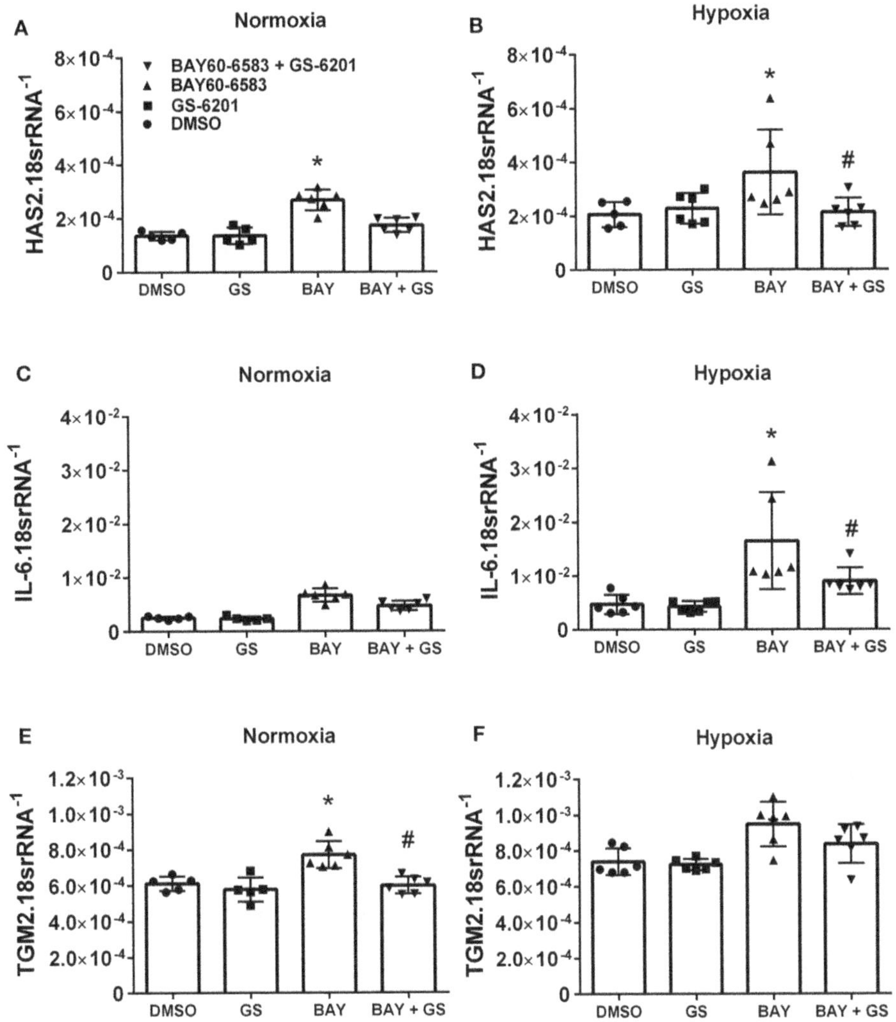

FIGURE 8 | Response of primary human pulmonary artery smooth muscle cells (PASMCs) to activation of ADORA2B). Expression levels of HAS2 **(A,B)**; IL-6 **(C,D)**; and TGM2 **(E,F)** under normoxia **(A–C)** or under hypoxia (2%O_2, **D–F**) of human PASMC exposed to DMSO (white bars); the ADORA2B antagonist: GS-6201 (light gray bars); the ADORA2B agonist: BAY60-6583 (black bars) or under the presence of both GS-6201 and BAY60-6583 (dark gray bars). $^*P < 0.05$ refers to comparisons between DMSO and BAY60-6583 treatment groups and $\#P < 0.05$, are for comparisons between BAY60-6583 and BAY60-6583 + GS-6201 treatment groups. $N = 5$ for all groups.

mice (**Figure 6D**). Consistent with previous publications (Sun et al., 2006; Zhou et al., 2010; Karmouty-Quintana et al., 2015), exposure to BLM led to increased levels of adenosine in BLM-treated $Tagln^{Cre}$ mice that remained elevated in BLM-exposed $Adora2b^{f/f}$-$Tagln^{Cre}$ mice (**Figure 6E**). Collectively, these results demonstrate that conditional deletion of Adora2b using the $Tagln^{Cre}$ promoter is able to attenuate markers of PH following BLM exposure.

Vascular Deletion of Adora2b Does Not Alter Fibrotic Deposition Following Bleomycin (BLM)-Induced Lung Injury

Most remarkably, $Adora2b^{f/f}$-$Tagln^{Cre}$ mice exposed to BLM did not appear to show a reduction in fibrotic deposition as observed histologically in Masson's Trichome (MT) stained sections (**Figure 7A**) and in Ashcroft scores (**Figure 7B**). Expression analysis for collagen 1a2 (Col1a2) also reveal increased levels in the BLM- $Tagln^{Cre}$ group that were not significantly reduced in the BLM-exposed $Adora2b^{f/f}$-$Tagln^{Cre}$ mice (**Figure 7C**). These observations are further supported by transcript levels for fibronectin (Fn), showing increased levels in BLM-exposed $Tagln^{Cre}$ mice that are maintained in $Adora2b^{f/f}$-$Tagln^{Cre}$ mice exposed to BLM (**Figure 7D**). In line with these results, Western blots for Fn revealed increased signals for BLM-$Tagln^{Cre}$ compared to PBS-$Tagln^{Cre}$ mice that were maintained in the BLM-$Adora2b^{f/f}$-$Tagln^{Cre}$ group (**Figures 7E,F**). These results indicate that Adora2b-expressing $Tagln^{Cre}$ cells plays a pivotal role in vascular remodeling in PH, but do not appear to modulate fibrotic responses in the lung, following BLM-exposure.

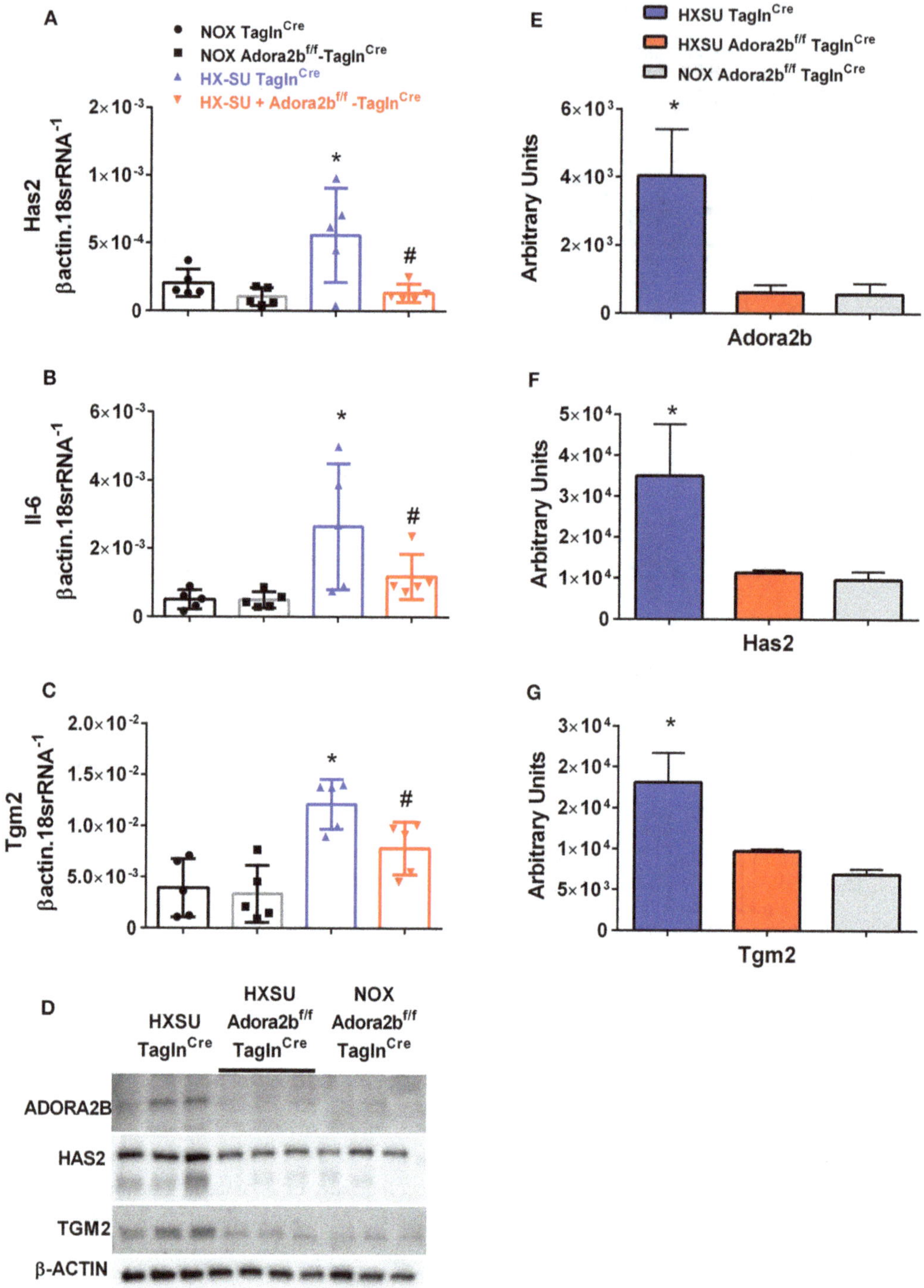

FIGURE 9 | Expression levels of hyaluronan synthase 2 (Has2), interleukin-6 (Il-6) and transglutaminase 2 (Tgm2) in $Tagln^{Cre}$ and $Adora2b^{f/f}$–$Tagln^{Cre}$ mice exposed to hypoxia-SUGEN (HX-SU) or normoxia (NOX). All analyses were performed on day 28 of HX-SU and NOX exposure. Has2 **(A)**; Il-6 **(B)**; Tgm2 **(C)**; expression levels measured by RT-PCR and normalized to the Geo mean of expression levels of βactin and 18srRNA from NOX-$Tagln^{Cre}$ mice (black circles and bar outline); NOX-$Adora2B^{f/f}$–$Tagln^{Cre}$ mice (black squares and gray bar outline); HX-SU-$Tagln^{Cre}$ mice (blue triangles and bar outline); HX-SU-$Adora2B^{f/f}$–$Tagln^{Cre}$ mice (red triangles and bar outline). Significant values: $^*P < 0.05$ refer to comparisons between $Tagln^{Cre}$ HX-SU and $Tagln^{Cre}$ NOX treatment groups. $^\#P < 0.05$, are for comparisons between $Tagln^{Cre}$ HX-SU and $Adora2b^{f/f}$–$Tagln^{Cre}$ + HX-SU treatment groups. **(D)** Western blot for Adora2b, Has2, Tgm2, and β-actin for $Tagln^{Cre}$ mice exposed to HX-SU, HX-SU exposed $Adora2b^{f/f}$–$Tagln^{Cre}$ mice and NOX-treated $Adora2b^{f/f}$–$Tagln^{Cre}$ mice. Densitometry data for Adora2b **(E)**, Has2 **(F)** and Tgm2 **(G)**: $^*P < 0.05$ refer to comparisons between Adora2b-$Tagln^{Cre}$ HX-SU and $Tagln^{Cre}$ HX-SU treatment groups. $N = 5$ for all RT-PCR experiments and $N = 3$ for western blots.

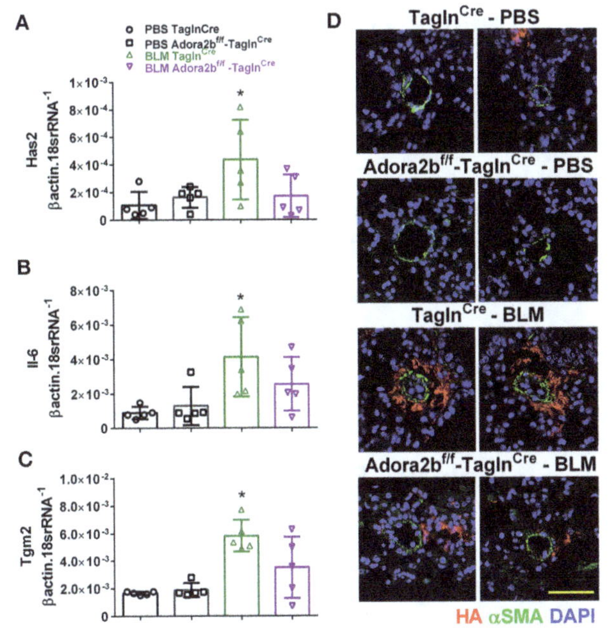

FIGURE 10 | Expression levels of hyaluronan synthase 2 (HAS2), interleukin-6 (IL-6) and transglutaminase 2 (Tgm2) in TaglnCre and Adora2b$^{f/f}$–Tagln^{Cre} mice exposed to bleomycin (BLM) or vehicle phosphate-buffered saline (PBS). Has2 **(A)**; IL-6 **(B)**; Tgm2 **(C)**; from PBS-Tagln^{Cre} mice (black circles and bar outline); PBS- Adora2b$^{f/f}$–Tagln^{Cre} mice (black squares and bar outline); BLM-Tagln^{Cre} mice (green triangles and bar outline); BLM-Adora2b$^{f/f}$–Tagln^{Cre} mice (magenta triangles and bar outline). Significant values: $^{*}P < 0.05$ refer to comparisons between TaglnCre BLM and TaglnCre PBS treatment groups. **(D)** Immunohistochemistry from representative vessels from PBS or BLM exposed Tagln^{Cre} and Adora2b$^{f/f}$–Tagln^{Cre} mice stained for alpha smooth muscle actin (αSMA, green signals), hyaluronan (red signals) and counter stained with DAPI (blue signals). Scale bar represents 50 μm. $N = 5$ for all groups.

Activation of ADORA2b in Human Pulmonary Artery Smooth Muscle Cells (PASMCs) Leads to Increased Pro-Remodeling Mediators

Interestingly, our results demonstrate that deletion of Adora2b from smooth muscle cells is able to prevent the development of pulmonary hypertension in two distinct experimental models of PH. Thus, in order to evaluate the ADORA2B-mediated mechanisms that lead to PH, we performed experiments with isolated primary pulmonary artery smooth muscle cells (PASMCs) from normal healthy donors. In these experiments we report that activation of ADORA2B by the selective agonist BAY 60-6583 leads to increased expression levels of hyaluronan synthase 2 (HAS2) under both normoxia and hypoxia (**Figures 8A,B**); interleukin (IL)-6 only under hypoxia but not in normoxia (**Figures 8C,D**) and transglutaminase 2 (TGM2) under normoxia but not hypoxia (**Figures 8E,F**). It is interesting to note that the responses for HAS2 and IL-6 but not TGM2 were augmented under hypoxic conditions (**Figures 7A–F**). Remarkably, BAY60-6583-induced increased HAS2 and IL-6 signals were attenuated following treatment with GS-6201, a selective ADORA2B antagonist, in conditions of hypoxia, but not normoxia (**Figures 8A–D**). GS-6201 was only able to inhibit BAY 60-6583-induced up-regulation of TGM2 under normoxia but not in hypoxia (**Figures 8E,F**). Taken together, these results demonstrate an ADORA2B-dependent up-regulation of the pro-remodeling mediators HAS2, IL6, and TGM2, and that this response is further augmented under hypoxic conditions.

Hyaluronan Synthase 2 (Has2), Il-6 and Transglutaminase 2 (Tgm2) Levels in PH

We next examined whether expression levels of hyaluronan synthase 2 (Has2), Il-6 and transglutaminase 2 (Tgm2) were altered in mice exposed to HX-SU. Consistent with our data, HX-SU-Tagln^{Cre} mice presented with higher levels of Has2, IL6, and Tgm2 that were attenuated in HX-SU-Adora2b$^{f/f}$-Tagln^{Cre} mice (**Figures 9A–C**). These observations are consistent with Western blots from mice showing reduced expression levels of ADORA2B, HAS2, and TGM2 in HX-SU-Adora2b$^{f/f}$-Tagln^{Cre} and NOX-Adora2b$^{f/f}$-Tagln^{Cre} mice compared to Adora2b-competent-HX-SU-exposed Tagln^{Cre} mice (**Figure 9D**) and subsequent densitometry analyses (**Figures 9E–G**).

In our experimental model of BLM-induced lung fibrosis and PH, we report increased levels of Has2, Il-6 and Tgm2 following BLM exposure compared to PBS exposure in Tagln^{Cre} mice (**Figures 10A–C**). No significant difference in Has2, Il-6 or Tgm2 transcript levels were observed between BLM exposed Adora2b$^{f/f}$-Talgn^{Cre} mice compared to the BLM Talgn^{Cre} group (**Figures 10A–C**). However, vascular hyaluronan deposition was reduced in BLM-exposed Adora2b$^{f/f}$-Talgn^{Cre} mice compared to BLM-exposed Talgn^{Cre} mice (**Figure 10D**). Our RT-PCR findings were consistent with increased signals from Western blots for P-STAT3 (but not STAT3) and HAS2 for BLM-exposed Talgn ^{Cre} mice compared to PBS exposed Talgn ^{Cre} mice that remained elevated in BLM exposed Adora2b$^{f/f}$-Talgn^{Cre} mice, albeit no differences in TGM2 were identified (Supplementary Figures 3A–E). IHC staining for P-STAT3 and TGM2 revealed increased signals in the vasculature of BLM-exposed Talgn^{Cre} mice compared to PBS-treated mice that were attenuated in BLM-exposed Adora2b$^{f/f}$-Talgn^{Cre} mice (**Figures 11A,C**). Consistent with the presence of fibrosis in these mice, we report increased signals for P-STAT3 and TGM2 in fibrotic areas rich in myofibroblasts (**Figures 11B,D**). In addition to augmented TGM2 levels in HX-SU and BLM-exposed mice, we report increased TGM2 signals within remodeled vessels in patients with a diagnosis of PAH or IPF + PH (**Figure 12A**). These observations were in line increased TGM2 transcripts from PAH patients compared to controls (**Figure 12B**) and with increased HAS2 mRNA in PAH vs. control PASMCs (**Figure 12C**). Taken together, our results show a likely mechanism where Adora2b activation promotes the development of PH through increased expression of Has2, Il6 and Tgm2 in experimental models of disease and in human patients with Group I or Group III PH.

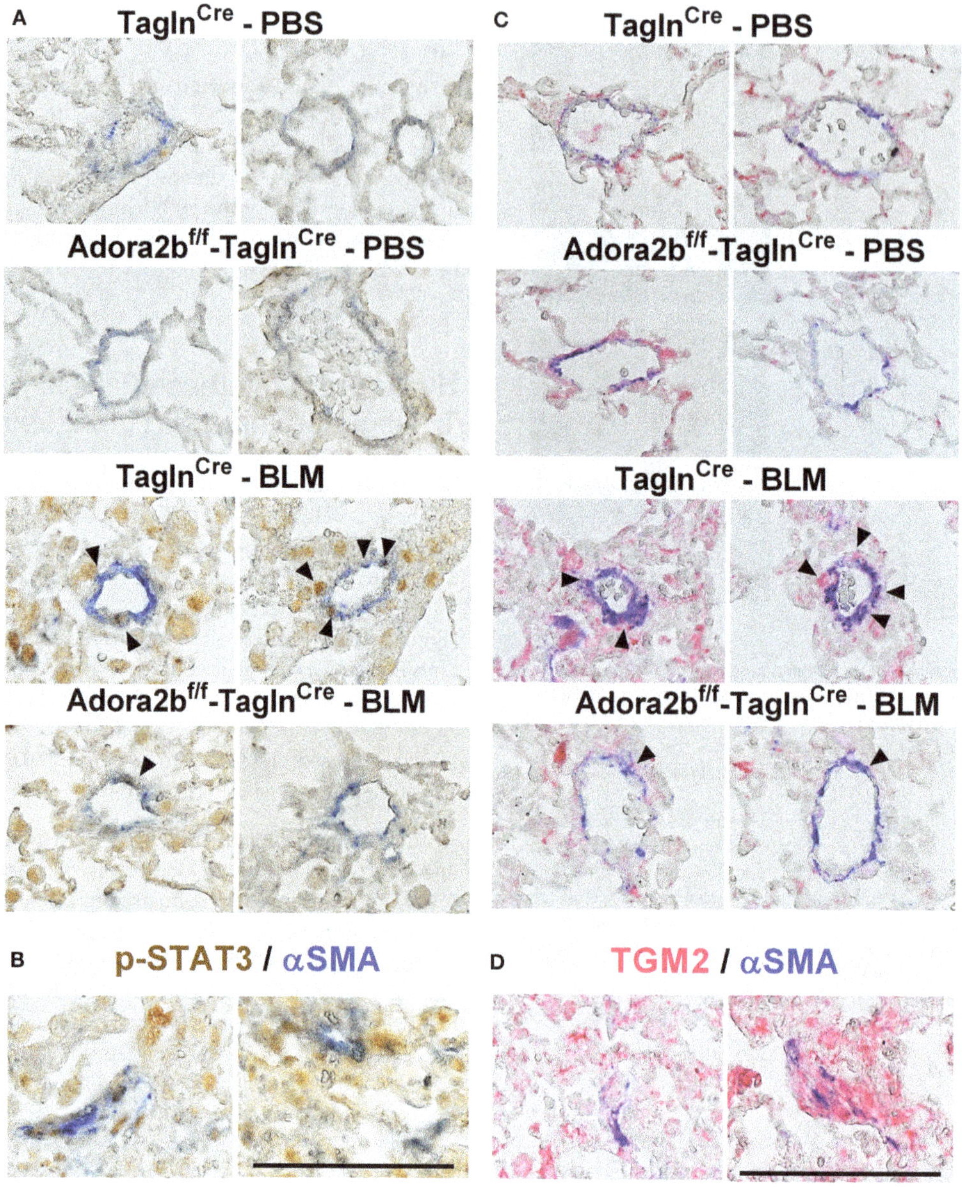

FIGURE 11 | Dual immunohistochemistry (IHC) from representative vessels from PBS or BLM exposed $Tagln^{Cre}$ and $Adora2b^{f/f}-Tagln^{Cre}$ mice stained for **(A)** alpha smooth muscle actin (αSMA, blue) and nuclear P-STAT3 (brown signals); **(B)** represent fibrotic areas rich in myofibroblasts (αSMA positive) where PSTAT is present; **(C)** αSMA, blue and transglutaminase (TGM2, red signals) **(D)** represents fibrotic areas rich in myofibroblasts (αSMA positive) where TGM2 is also present. Scale bar represents 200 μm. Arrow heads point and p-STAT3 or TGM2 positive cells in the vessel wall (αSMA positive).

DISCUSSION

The presence of pulmonary hypertension (PH) in the context of idiopathic pulmonary fibrosis (IPF) is associated with significantly increased morbidity and mortality rates (Behr and Ryu, 2008; Pitsiou et al., 2011; Collum et al., 2017a). Despite the detrimental consequences of PH, there are very limited therapies available that can treat PH in IPF patients (Collum et al., 2017a). Although anti-fibrotic agents have been shown to attenuate experimental fibrosis and PH (Hemnes et al., 2008; Schroll et al., 2010, 2013; Van Rheen et al., 2011; Karmouty-Quintana et al., 2012, 2015; Bei et al., 2013; Grasemann et al., 2015; Chen et al., 2016; Avouac et al., 2017), these therapies have not translated to the clinic. Moreover, standard therapies for PAH have failed to show a benefit in Group III PH and have been associated with worsening mortality (Ruggiero et al., 2012; Klinger, 2016).

A major finding of our study is that switching-off Adora2b in vascular smooth muscle cells using the Tagln promoter is able to prevent the development of PH in two distinct mouse

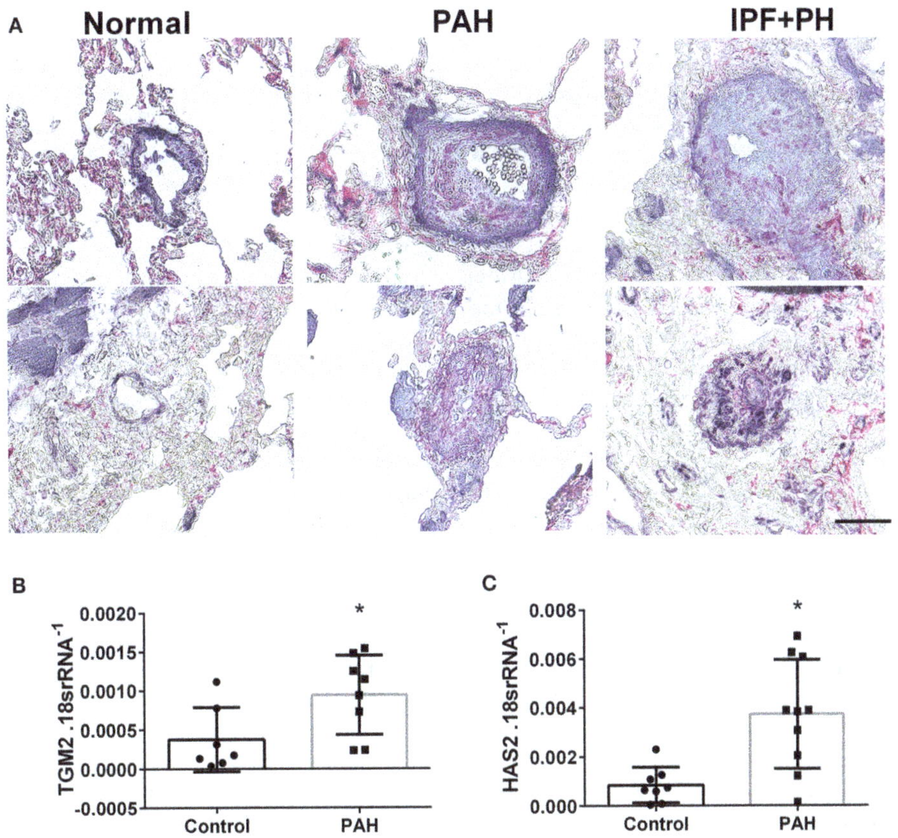

FIGURE 12 | (A) Dual immunohistochemistry (IHC) for alpha smooth muscle actin (αSMA, indigo-blue signals) and transglutaminase (TGM2, pink-magenta signals) from representative pulmonary arteries from normal (top), pulmonary arterial hypertension (PAH, middle), or IPF+PH (lower) lungs. Scale bar represents 200 μm. Expression levels of TGM2 **(B)** and HAS2 **(C)** from PASMCs isolated from controls and patients with iPAH. $^*P < 0.05$ refer to comparisons between Control and PAH groups. $N = 8$ for all groups.

models: the HX-SU and the BLM model. Most remarkably, we report that Adora2b$^{f/f}$-Tagln^{Cre} mice exposed to BLM still present with fibrotic lung injury that is not significantly different to that of control Tagln^{Cre} mice exposed to BLM. These results demonstrate that Adora2b expression in the vascular smooth muscle is a viable target to treat PH, either on its own or associated with chronic lung injury. Consistent with previous publications from our group, we demonstrate that the likely mechanism for Adora2b-mediated PH is through enhanced IL-6 and hyaluronic acid deposition (Karmouty-Quintana et al., 2012, 2013a, 2015; Collum et al., 2017b). In addition to these meditators, we also report the novel finding that Tgm2 can be modulated by Adora2b and that this is consistent with increased expression of vascular Tgm2 in experimental models of PH and in remodeled vessels of patients with a diagnosis of PAH or IPF+PH.

In response to injury or stress, the lung releases ATP that is then converted to adenosine by ecto-nucleotidases (Colgan et al., 2006). This response is part of a normal physiological reaction to high altitude (Song et al., 2017; Sun et al., 2017) and to acute lung injury (Van Linden and Eltzschig, 2007; Eckle et al., 2009). These ecto-nucleotidases include CD39 and CD73 that are regulated by hypoxia-inducible factor (HIF-1A) (Synnestvedt et al., 2002; Hart et al., 2010). Adenosine is then able to activate one of its four G-protein coupled receptors: the adenosine A1 (ADORA1), A2A (ADORA2A), A2B (ADORA2B), and A3 (ADORA3) receptors (Fredholm et al., 2001). All four of these receptors have been shown to be involved in cellular processes implicated in tissue injury (Karmouty-Quintana et al., 2013b). Under normal physiological conditions, adenosine is rapidly metabolized to inosine by adenosine deaminase (ADA) (Fredholm et al., 2001) or up-taken intracellularly through equilibrative nucleotide transporters (ENTs) (Eltzschig et al., 2005). Studies in CD73 and CD39 deficient mice have demonstrated that increased adenosine levels are critical for the resolution of acute lung injury (Volmer et al., 2006; Eckle et al., 2007; Davies et al., 2014). Yet, despite the protective effects of adenosine, sustained levels have been shown to mediate chronic lung injury (Blackburn, 2003; Blackburn and Kellems, 2005; Chunn et al., 2006). These studies are consistent with increased expression of CD73 and ADORA2B in experimental models and patients with lung injury (Chunn et al., 2006; Zhou et al., 2010; Wirsdörfer et al., 2016). Lowering extracellular adenosine through treatment with ADA or genetic deletion of CD73 have shown that these mice are protected from the development of chronic lung injury (Chunn et al., 2006; Zhou et al., 2010; Wirsdörfer et al., 2016). This dualistic action of adenosine can be explained by the concept of purinergic remodeling, where alterations in the expression levels of enzymes of adenosine metabolism (CD73, ADA), transport proteins such as ENTs, or adenosine receptors may influence the progression from acute to chronic responses (Zhou et al., 2009). A highly relevant example of purinergic remodeling is the altered levels of CD39, CD73, ENTs and adenosine receptors in IPF+PH (Garcia-Morales et al., 2016). Here, purinergic remodeling shifted the balance toward accumulation of adenosine and increased expression of ADORA2B (Garcia-Morales et al., 2016). Interestingly, in our study, although adenosine levels were maintained, vascular remodeling and RVSP were attenuated in both the HX-SU and the BLM model. Yet these increased levels of adenosine were likely responsible for the presence of RVH following HX-SU exposure (Toldo et al., 2012; Ferrari et al., 2016) and for the development of fibrosis (Blackburn and Kellems, 2005; Chunn et al., 2006; Sun et al., 2006).

Intriguingly, in the context of PH, reduced adenosine levels in the pulmonary circulation were reported in patients with COPD + PH and in Primary Pulmonary Hypertension (PPH) compared to normal individuals (Saadjian et al., 1999). Although the sample size is limited ($n = 7$ controls, $n = 8$ COPD+PH, and $n = 8$ PPH) these results suggest that reduced adenosine levels in the circulation are pathogenic (Saadjian et al., 1999). At face-value these observations are counterintuitive to our hypothesis that enhanced ADORA2B levels are pathogenic in PH since ADORA2B has the lowest affinity for adenosine (Fredholm et al., 2001). Despite this, it is important to consider that adenosine has a very low half-life and is rapidly metabolized *in vivo* and *in vitro* (Klabunde, 1983). Thus it is conceivable that local elevations of tissue adenosine near the vasculature lead to enhanced activation of vascular smooth cell ADORA2B and promote the development of PH. In line with these studies, we have reported increased activity of CD73 and reduced activity of ADA in tissue samples of patients with IPF+PH (Garcia-Morales et al., 2016) that point to a pathogenic accumulation of adenosine in PH. Similarly, we show that PASMCs from patients with PAH present with increased CD73 that point at an enhanced capacity to accumulate adenosine in remodeled vessels in PAH.

Augmented ADORA2B levels have been reported in patients with IPF and COPD (Zhou et al., 2010; Karmouty-Quintana et al., 2013b) that are consistent with increased Adora2b levels in experimental models of chronic lung injury that also present with PH (Sun et al., 2006; Pedroza et al., 2011; Karmouty-Quintana et al., 2012, 2013a). Using an Adora2b antagonist and *global* Adora2b-deficient mice, we have shown that abrogation of this receptor reduces PH associated with chronic lung disease (Karmouty-Quintana et al., 2012, 2013a). In these experiments, the attenuation of PH was linked with reduced severity of lung injury (Karmouty-Quintana et al., 2012, 2013a). Similarly, conditional deletion of myeloid ADORA2B resulted in reduced fibro-proliferative lesions and attenuated markers of PH following exposure to BLM (Karmouty-Quintana et al., 2015). Taken together, these results demonstrated the therapeutic potential of abrogation of ADORA2B signaling in lung injury and PH; however, it was not known whether vascular ADORA2B could contribute directly to the development of PH in an *in vivo* setting. Similarly, the role of ADORA2B in clinical or experimental models of PAH had not been addressed until now (Alencar et al., 2017). Strikingly, our results show that switching-off vascular smooth muscle ADORA2B is able to prevent HX-SU and BLM induced PH without altering fibrotic deposition levels in BLM-exposed mice. These results provide further rationale for the use of ADORA2B antagonists for the treatment of PAH and PH associated with chronic lung injury. We believe that this discrepancy is the result of the pleiotropic functions of ADORA2B; where ADORA2B activation in other cells such as fibroblasts and myeloid cells may continue to drive the fibrotic process (Sun et al., 2006; Karmouty-Quintana et al., 2013b, 2015). Further studies testing the effect of ADORA2B antagonists in established models replicating features of PAH would provide important pre-clinical data supporting the use of ADORA2B antagonists for the treatment of this fatal condition.

Regarding the ADORA2B mediated mechanisms, our data showed that activation of ADORA2B in PASMCs leads to increased levels of IL-6 and hyaluronan, two mediators that have been associated in the pathophysiology of lung fibrosis and PH (Karmouty-Quintana et al., 2012, 2015; Chen et al., 2016; Collum et al., 2017b). Indeed increased IL-6 has also been shown to play an important role in the development of PAH (Ricard et al., 2014). In fact, treatment with a hyaluronan synthase inhibitor attenuates BLM-induced PH independent from fibrotic deposition in the BLM model of lung injury (Collum et al., 2017b). Interestingly, we also show that activation of Adora2b modulates expression of Tgm2, a multifunctional enzyme (Gundemir et al., 2012; Eckert et al., 2014; Liu et al., 2017) that has been associated with PH (Diraimondo et al., 2014; Penumatsa et al., 2017) and pulmonary fibrosis (Oh et al., 2011; Olsen et al., 2011, 2014). Tgm2 likely contributes to the development of PH through serotonylation leading to enhanced cellular proliferation (Diraimondo et al., 2014; Penumatsa et al., 2014, 2017). However, Tgm2 can also crosslink with other ECM proteins that contribute to vascular stiffening (Gundemir et al., 2012; Eckert et al., 2014) similar to vascular expression of hyaluronan (Karmouty-Quintana et al., 2013a). Tgm2 could also promote pulmonary hypertension by other means (Liu et al., 2017) that may affect receptor levels by altering ubiquitination or influence the presence of auto-antibodies (Liu et al., 2014, 2015).

It is also important to consider that other adenosine receptors may a play a role in PH. An elegant review (Alencar et al., 2017) has recently summed up the most recent developments of adenosine receptors for the treatment of PAH. Most notably activation of Adora2a has been shown to be effective for the treatment of PAH (Alencar et al., 2017); this is consistent with our data showing reduced protein levels of Adora2a in PASMCs isolated from patients with iPAH.

In conclusion, our data show that conditional deletion of Adora2b from vascular smooth muscle cells prevents the development of PH through a mechanism that involves upregulation of IL-6, hyaluronan and Tgm2. Taken together, these results point at a role for inhibition of Adora2b for the treatment of Group I and Group III PH.

AUTHOR CONTRIBUTIONS

TM, AH, and HK-Q planned and performed experiments, acquired and analyzed data and wrote the manuscript. LT, CP, SC, N-YC, TW, and CL performed experiments, acquired and analyzed data. HE provided the floxed Adora2b mice and together with JD and YX contributed to the design of the study and interpretation of the results. SJ, KR, AG, and BB supervised the use of human samples for the study. MB, CG, and HK-Q conceived the idea, designed and supervised the study.

All authors discussed the results and contributed to the final manuscript.

ACKNOWLEDGMENTS

We would like to acknowledge the funding of the following organizations:

American Heart Association 14SDG18550039 to HK-Q, American Lung Association RG-414673 to HK-Q, National Institutes of Health (NIH) 1R01 HL138510-01 to HK-Q. NIH 1P01 HL114457-02 to MB, HE, and YX. We also acknowledge Kelly Volcik Ph.D., McGovern Medical School at UTHealth for proof-reading the manuscript.

REFERENCES

Alencar, A. K. N., Montes, G. C., Barreiro, E. J., Sudo, R. T., and Zapata-Sudo, G. (2017). Adenosine receptors as drug targets for treatment of pulmonary arterial hypertension. *Front. Pharmacol.* 8:858. doi: 10.3389/fphar.2017.00858

Archer, S. L., Weir, E. K., and Wilkins, M. R. (2010). Basic science of pulmonary arterial hypertension for clinicians: new concepts and experimental therapies. *Circulation* 121, 2045–2066. doi: 10.1161/CIRCULATIONAHA.108.847707

Avouac, J., Konstantinova, I., Guignabert, C., Pezet, S., Sadoine, J., Guilbert, T., et al. (2017). Pan-PPAR agonist IVA337 is effective in experimental lung fibrosis and pulmonary hypertension. *Ann. Rheum. Dis.* 76, 1931–1940. doi: 10.1136/annrheumdis-2016-210821

Behr, J., and Ryu, J. H. (2008). Pulmonary hypertension in interstitial lung disease. *Eur. Respir. J.* 31, 1357–1367. doi: 10.1183/09031936.00171307

Bei, Y., Hua-Huy, T., Duong-Quy, S., Nguyen, V. H., Chen, W., Nicco, C., et al. (2013). Long-term treatment with fasudil improves bleomycin-induced pulmonary fibrosis and pulmonary hypertension via inhibition of Smad2/3 phosphorylation. *Pulm. Pharmacol. Ther.* 26, 635–643. doi: 10.1016/j.pupt.2013.07.008

Blackburn, M. R. (2003). Too much of a good thing: adenosine overload in adenosine-deaminase-deficient mice. *Trends Pharmacol. Sci.* 24, 66–70. doi: 10.1016/S0165-6147(02)00045-7

Blackburn, M. R., and Kellems, R. E. (2005). Adenosine deaminase deficiency: metabolic basis of immune deficiency and pulmonary inflammation. *Adv. Immunol.* 86, 1–41. doi: 10.1016/S0065-2776(04)86001-2

Chen, N. Y., D Collum, S., Luo, F., Weng, T., Le, T. T., M Hernandez, A., et al. (2016). Macrophage bone morphogenic protein receptor 2 depletion in idiopathic pulmonary fibrosis and Group III pulmonary hypertension. *Am. J. Physiol. Lung Cell. Mol. Physiol.* 311, L238–254. doi: 10.1152/ajplung.00142.2016

Chunn, J. L., Mohsenin, A., Young, H. W., Lee, C. G., Elias, J. A., Kellems, R. E., et al. (2006). Partially adenosine deaminase-deficient mice develop pulmonary fibrosis in association with adenosine elevations. *Am. J. Physiol. Lung Cell. Mol. Physiol.* 290, L579–L587. doi: 10.1152/ajplung.00258.2005

Ciuclan, L., Bonneau, O., Hussey, M., Duggan, N., Holmes, A. M., Good, R., et al. (2011). A novel murine model of severe pulmonary arterial hypertension. *Am. J. Respir. Crit. Care Med.* 184, 1171–1182. doi: 10.1164/rccm.201103-0412OC

Colgan, S. P., Eltzschig, H. K., Eckle, T., and Thompson, L. F. (2006). Physiological roles for ecto-5′-nucleotidase (CD73). *Purinergic Signal.* 351–360. doi: 10.1007/s11302-005-5302-5

Collum, S. D., Amione-Guerra, J., Cruz-Solbes, A. S., DiFrancesco, A., Hernandez, A. M., Hanmandlu, A., et al. (2017a). Pulmonary hypertension associated with idiopathic pulmonary fibrosis: current and future perspectives. *Can. Respir. J.* 2017:1430350. doi: 10.1155/2017/1430350

Collum, S. D., Chen, N. Y., Hernandez, A. M., Hanmandlu, A., Sweeney, H., Mertens, T. C. J., et al. (2017b). Inhibition of hyaluronan synthesis attenuates pulmonary hypertension associated with lung fibrosis. *Br. J. Pharmacol.* 174, 3284–3301. doi: 10.1111/bph.13947

Davies, J., Karmouty-Quintana, H., Le, T. T., Chen, N. Y., Weng, T., Luo, F., et al. (2014). Adenosine promotes vascular barrier function in hyperoxic lung injury. *Physiol Rep* 2: e12155. doi: 10.14814/phy2.12155

Diraimondo, T. R., Klöck, C., Warburton, R., Herrera, Z., Penumatsa, K., Toksoz, D., et al. (2014). Elevated transglutaminase 2 activity is associated with hypoxia-induced experimental pulmonary hypertension in mice. *ACS Chem. Biol.* 9, 266–275. doi: 10.1021/cb4006408

Eckert, R. L., Kaartinen, M. T., Nurminskaya, M., Belkin, A. M., Colak, G., Johnson, G. V., et al. (2014). Transglutaminase regulation of cell function. *Physiol. Rev.* 94, 383–417. doi: 10.1152/physrev.00019.2013

Eckle, T., Füllbier, L., Wehrmann, M., Khoury, J., Mittelbronn, M., Ibla, J., et al. (2007). Identification of ectonucleotidases CD39 and CD73 in innate protection during acute lung injury. *J. Immunol.* 178, 8127–8137. doi: 10.4049/jimmunol.178.12.8127

Eckle, T., Koeppen, M., and Eltzschig, H. K. (2009). Role of extracellular adenosine in acute lung injury. *Physiology* 24, 298–306. doi: 10.1152/physiol.00022.2009

Eltzschig, H. K., Abdulla, P., Hoffman, E., Hamilton, K. E., Daniels, D., Schönfeld, C., et al. (2005). HIF-1-dependent repression of equilibrative nucleoside transporter (ENT) in hypoxia. *J. Exp. Med.* 202, 1493–1505. doi: 10.1084/jem.20050177

Farkas, L., Gauldie, J., Voelkel, N. F., and Kolb, M. (2011). Pulmonary hypertension and idiopathic pulmonary fibrosis: a tale of angiogenesis, apoptosis, and growth factors. *Am. J. Respir. Cell Mol. Biol.* 45, 1–15. doi: 10.1165/rcmb.2010-0365TR

Fell, C. D. (2012). Idiopathic pulmonary fibrosis: phenotypes and comorbidities. *Clin. Chest Med.* 33, 51–57. doi: 10.1016/j.ccm.2011.12.005

Ferrari, D., Gambari, R., Idzko, M., Müller, T., Albanesi, C., Pastore, S., et al. (2016). Purinergic signaling in scarring. *FASEB J.* 30, 3–12. doi: 10.1096/fj.15-274563

Fredholm, B. B. (2007). Adenosine, an endogenous distress signal, modulates tissue damage and repair. *Cell Death Differ.* 14, 1315–1323. doi: 10.1038/sj.cdd.4402132

Fredholm, B. B., IJzerman, A.P., Jacobson, K. A., Klotz, K. N., and Linden, J. (2001). International Union of Pharmacology. XXV. Nomenclature and classification of adenosine receptors. *Pharmacol. Rev.* 53, 527–552. doi: 10.1016/j.neuropharm.2015.12.001

Garcia-Morales, L. J., Chen, N. Y., Weng, T., Luo, F., Davies, J., Philip, K., et al. (2016). Altered hypoxic-adenosine axis and metabolism in group III pulmonary hypertension. *Am. J. Respir. Cell Mol. Biol.* 54, 574–583. doi: 10.1165/rcmb.2015-0145OC

Grasemann, H., Dhaliwal, R., Ivanovska, J., Kantores, C., Mcnamara, P. J., Scott, J. A., et al. (2015). Arginase inhibition prevents bleomycin-induced pulmonary hypertension, vascular remodeling, and collagen deposition in neonatal rat lungs. *Am. J. Physiol. Lung Cell. Mol. Physiol.* 308, L503–L510. doi: 10.1152/ajplung.00328.2014

Guignabert, C., Raffestin, B., Benferhat, R., Raoul, W., Zadigue, P., Rideau, D., et al. (2005). Serotonin transporter inhibition prevents and reverses monocrotaline-induced pulmonary hypertension in rats. *Circulation* 111, 2812–2819. doi: 10.1161/CIRCULATIONAHA.104.524926

Gundemir, S., Colak, G., Tucholski, J., and Johnson, G. V. (2012). Transglutaminase 2: a molecular Swiss army knife. *Biochim. Biophys. Acta* 1823, 406–419. doi: 10.1016/j.bbamcr.2011.09.012

Hansdottir, S., Groskreutz, D. J., and Gehlbach, B. K. (2013). WHO's in second?: A practical review of World Health Organization group 2 pulmonary hypertension. *Chest* 144, 638–650. doi: 10.1378/chest.12-2114

Hart, M. L., Gorzolla, I. C., Schittenhelm, J., Robson, S. C., and Eltzschig, H. K. (2010). SP1-dependent induction of CD39 facilitates hepatic ischemic preconditioning. *J. Immunol.* 184, 4017–4024. doi: 10.4049/jimmunol.0901851

Hemnes, A. R., Zaiman, A., and Champion, H. C. (2008). PDE5A inhibition attenuates bleomycin-induced pulmonary fibrosis and pulmonary hypertension through inhibition of ROS generation and RhoA/Rho kinase activation. *Am. J. Physiol. Lung Cell. Mol. Physiol.* 294, L24–L33. doi: 10.1152/ajplung.00245.2007

Hübner, R. H., Gitter, W., El Mokhtari, N. E., Mathiak, M., Both, M., Bolte, H., et al. (2008). Standardized quantification of pulmonary fibrosis in histological samples. *Biotechniques* 44, 507–511, 514–507. doi: 10.2144/000112729

Huertas, A., Tu, L., Thuillet, R., Le Hiress, M., Phan, C., Ricard, N., et al. (2015). Leptin signalling system as a target for pulmonary arterial hypertension therapy. *Eur. Respir. J.* 45, 1066–1080. doi: 10.1183/09031936.00193014

Judge, E. P., Fabre, A., Adamali, H. I., and Egan, J. J. (2012). Acute exacerbations and pulmonary hypertension in advanced idiopathic pulmonary fibrosis. *Eur. Respir. J.* 40, 93–100. doi: 10.1183/09031936.00115511

Karmouty-Quintana, H., Philip, K., Acero, L. F., Chen, N. Y., Weng, T., Molina, J. G., et al. (2015). Deletion of ADORA2B from myeloid cells dampens lung fibrosis and pulmonary hypertension. *FASEB J.* 29, 50–60. doi: 10.1096/fj.14-260182

Karmouty-Quintana, H., Weng, T., Garcia-Morales, L. J., Chen, N. Y., Pedroza, M., Zhong, H., et al. (2013a). ADORA2B and hyaluronan modulate pulmonary hypertension associated with chronic obstructive pulmonary disease. *Am. J. Respir. Cell Mol. Biol.* 49, 1038–1047. doi: 10.1165/rcmb.2013-0089OC

Karmouty-Quintana, H., Xia, Y., and Blackburn, M. R. (2013b). Adenosine signaling during acute and chronic disease states. *J. Mol. Med.* 91, 173–181. doi: 10.1007/s00109-013-0997-1

Karmouty-Quintana, H., Zhong, H., Acero, L., Weng, T., Melicoff, E., West, J. D., et al. (2012). The A2B adenosine receptor modulates pulmonary hypertension associated with interstitial lung disease. *FASEB J.* 26, 2546–2557. doi: 10.1096/fj.11-200907

Klabunde, R. E. (1983). Dipyridamole inhibition of adenosine metabolism in human blood. *Eur. J. Pharmacol.* 93, 21–26. doi: 10.1016/0014-2999(83)90026-2

Klinger, J. R. (2016). Group III pulmonary hypertension: pulmonary hypertension associated with lung disease: epidemiology, pathophysiology, and treatments. *Cardiol. Clin.* 34, 413–433. doi: 10.1016/j.ccl.2016.04.003

Lee, K. J., Czech, L., Waypa, G. B., and Farrow, K. N. (2013). Isolation of pulmonary artery smooth muscle cells from neonatal mice. *J. Vis. Exp.* e50889. doi: 10.3791/50889

Lennon, P. F., Taylor, C. T., Stahl, G. L., and Colgan, S. P. (1998). Neutrophil-derived 5'-adenosine monophosphate promotes endothelial barrier function via CD73-mediated conversion to adenosine and endothelial A2B receptor activation. *J. Exp. Med.* 188, 1433–1443. doi: 10.1084/jem.188.8.1433

Liu, C., Kellems, R. E., and Xia, Y. (2017). Inflammation, autoimmunity, and hypertension: the essential role of tissue transglutaminase. *Am. J. Hypertens.* 30, 756–764. doi: 10.1093/ajh/hpx027

Liu, C., Luo, R., Elliott, S. E., Wang, W., Parchim, N. F., Iriyama, T., et al. (2015). Elevated transglutaminase activity triggers angiotensin receptor activating autoantibody production and pathophysiology of Preeclampsia. *J Am Heart Assoc* 4:e002323. doi: 10.1161/JAHA.115.002323

Liu, C., Wang, W., Parchim, N., Irani, R. A., Blackwell, S. C., Sibai, B., et al. (2014). Tissue transglutaminase contributes to the pathogenesis of preeclampsia and stabilizes placental angiotensin receptor type 1 by ubiquitination-preventing isopeptide modification. *Hypertension* 63, 353–361. doi: 10.1161/HYPERTENSIONAHA.113.02361

Morrell, N. W., Yang, X., Upton, P. D., Jourdan, K. B., Morgan, N., Sheares, K. K., et al. (2001). Altered growth responses of pulmonary artery smooth muscle cells from patients with primary pulmonary hypertension to transforming growth factor-beta(1) and bone morphogenetic proteins. *Circulation* 104, 790–795. doi: 10.1161/hc3201.094152

Oh, K., Park, H. B., Byoun, O. J., Shin, D. M., Jeong, E. M., Kim, Y. W., et al. (2011). Epithelial transglutaminase 2 is needed for T cell interleukin-17 production and subsequent pulmonary inflammation and fibrosis in bleomycin-treated mice. *J. Exp. Med.* 208, 1707–1719. doi: 10.1084/jem.201 01457

Olsen, K. C., Epa, A. P., Kulkarni, A. A., Kottmann, R. M., Mccarthy, C. E., Johnson, G. V., et al. (2014). Inhibition of transglutaminase 2, a novel target for pulmonary fibrosis, by two small electrophilic molecules. *Am. J. Respir. Cell Mol. Biol.* 50, 737–747. doi: 10.1165/rcmb.2013-0092OC

Olsen, K. C., Sapinoro, R. E., Kottmann, R. M., Kulkarni, A. A., Iismaa, S. E., Johnson, G. V., et al. (2011). Transglutaminase 2 and its role in pulmonary fibrosis. *Am. J. Respir. Crit. Care Med.* 184, 699–707. doi: 10.1164/rccm.201101-0013OC

Pedroza, M., Schneider, D. J., Karmouty-Quintana, H., Coote, J., Shaw, S., Corrigan, R., et al. (2011). Interleukin-6 contributes to inflammation and remodeling in a model of adenosine mediated lung injury. *PLoS ONE* 6:e22667. doi: 10.1371/journal.pone.0022667

Penumatsa, K. C., Toksoz, D., Warburton, R. R., Hilmer, A. J., Liu, T., Khosla, C., et al. (2014). Role of hypoxia-induced transglutaminase 2 in pulmonary artery smooth muscle cell proliferation. *Am. J. Physiol. Lung Cell. Mol. Physiol.* 307, L576–L585. doi: 10.1152/ajplung.00162.2014

Penumatsa, K. C., Toksoz, D., Warburton, R. R., Kharnaf, M., Preston, I. R., Kapur, N. K., et al. (2017). Transglutaminase 2 in pulmonary and cardiac tissue remodeling in experimental pulmonary hypertension. *Am. J. Physiol. Lung Cell. Mol. Physiol.* 313, L752–Ll762. doi: 10.1152/ajplung.00170.2017

Pitsiou, G., Papakosta, D., and Bouros, D. (2011). Pulmonary hypertension in idiopathic pulmonary fibrosis: a review. *Respiration* 82, 294–304. doi: 10.1159/000327918

Poor, H. D., Girgis, R., and Studer, S. M. (2012). World Health Organization Group III pulmonary hypertension. *Prog. Cardiovasc. Dis.* 55, 119–127. doi: 10.1016/j.pcad.2012.08.003

Ricard, N., Tu, L., Le Hiress, M., Huertas, A., Phan, C., Thuillet, R., et al. (2014). Increased pericyte coverage mediated by endothelial-derived fibroblast growth factor-2 and interleukin-6 is a source of smooth muscle-like cells in pulmonary hypertension. *Circulation* 129, 1586–1597. doi: 10.1161/CIRCULATIONAHA.113.007469

Ruggiero, R. M., Bartolome, S., and Torres, F. (2012). Pulmonary hypertension in parenchymal lung disease. *Heart Fail. Clin.* 8, 461–474. doi: 10.1016/j.hfc.2012.04.010

Saadjian, A. Y., Paganelli, F., Gaubert, M. L., Levy, S., and Guieu, R. P. (1999). Adenosine plasma concentration in pulmonary hypertension. *Cardiovasc. Res.* 43, 228–236. doi: 10.1016/S0008-6363(99)00059-0

Schroll, S., Arzt, M., Sebah, D., Nüchterlein, M., Blumberg, F., and Pfeifer, M. (2010). Improvement of bleomycin-induced pulmonary hypertension and pulmonary fibrosis by the endothelin receptor antagonist Bosentan. *Respir. Physiol. Neurobiol.* 170, 32–36. doi: 10.1016/j.resp.2009. 11.005

Schroll, S., Lange, T. J., Arzt, M., Sebah, D., Nowrotek, A., Lehmann, H., et al. (2013). Effects of simvastatin on pulmonary fibrosis, pulmonary hypertension and exercise capacity in bleomycin-treated rats. *Acta Physiol.* 208, 191–201. doi: 10.1111/apha.12085

Song, A., Zhang, Y., Han, L., Yegutkin, G. G., Liu, H., Sun, K., et al. (2017). Erythrocytes retain hypoxic adenosine response for faster acclimatization upon re-ascent. *Nat. Commun.* 8:14108. doi: 10.1038/ncomms14108

Sun, C. X., Zhong, H., Mohsenin, A., Morschl, E., Chunn, J. L., Molina, J. G., et al. (2006). Role of A2B adenosine receptor signaling in adenosine-dependent pulmonary inflammation and injury. *J. Clin. Invest.* 116, 2173–2182. doi: 10.1172/JCI27303

Sun, K., Liu, H., Song, A., Manalo, J. M., D'alessandro, A., Hansen, K. C., et al. (2017). Erythrocyte purinergic signaling components underlie hypoxia adaptation. *J. Appl. Physiol.* 123, 951–956. doi: 10.1152/japplphysiol.00155.2017

Synnestvedt, K., Furuta, G. T., Comerford, K. M., Louis, N., Karhausen, J., Eltzschig, H. K., et al. (2002). Ecto-5'-nucleotidase (CD73) regulation by hypoxia-inducible factor-1 mediates permeability changes in intestinal epithelia. *J. Clin. Invest.* 110, 993–1002. doi: 10.1172/JCI0215337

Toldo, S., Zhong, H., Mezzaroma, E., Van Tassell, B. W., Kannan, H., Zeng, D., et al. (2012). GS-6201, a selective blocker of the A2B adenosine receptor, attenuates cardiac remodeling after acute myocardial infarction in the mouse. *J. Pharmacol. Exp. Ther.* 343, 587–595. doi: 10.1124/jpet.111.191288

Van Linden, A., and Eltzschig, H. K. (2007). Role of pulmonary adenosine during hypoxia: extracellular generation, signaling and metabolism by surface adenosine deaminase/CD26. *Expert Opin. Biol. Ther.* 7, 1437–1447. doi: 10.1517/14712598.7.9.1437

Van Rheen, Z., Fattman, C., Domarski, S., Majka, S., Klemm, D., Stenmark, K. R., et al. (2011). Lung extracellular superoxide dismutase overexpression lessens bleomycin-induced pulmonary hypertension and vascular remodeling. *Am. J. Respir. Cell Mol. Biol.* 44, 500–508. doi: 10.1165/rcmb.2010-0065OC

Ventetuolo, C. E., and Klinger, J. R. (2012). WHO Group 1 pulmonary arterial hypertension: current and investigative therapies. *Prog. Cardiovasc. Dis.* 55, 89–103. doi: 10.1016/j.pcad.2012.07.002

Volmer, J. B., Thompson, L. F., and Blackburn, M. R. (2006). Ecto-5′-nucleotidase (CD73)-mediated adenosine production is tissue protective in a model of bleomycin-induced lung injury. *J. Immunol.* 176, 4449–4458. doi: 10.4049/jimmunol.176.7.4449

Wakamiya, M., Blackburn, M. R., Jurecic, R., Mcarthur, M. J., Geske, R. S., Cartwright, J., et al. (1995). Disruption of the adenosine-deaminase gene causes hepatocellular impairment and perinatal lethality in mice. *Proc. Natl. Acad. Sci. U.S.A.* 92, 3673–3677. doi: 10.1073/pnas.92.9.3673

Wirsdörfer, F., De Leve, S., Cappuccini, F., Eldh, T., Meyer, A. V., Gau, E., et al. (2016). Extracellular adenosine production by ecto-5′-nucleotidase (CD73) enhances radiation-induced lung fibrosis. *Cancer Res.* 76, 3045–3056. doi: 10.1158/0008-5472.CAN-15-2310

Zhou, Y., Murthy, J. N., Zeng, D., Belardinelli, L., and Blackburn, M. R. (2010). Alterations in adenosine metabolism and signaling in patients with chronic obstructive pulmonary disease and idiopathic pulmonary fibrosis. *PLoS ONE* 5:e9224. doi: 10.1371/journal.pone.0009224

Zhou, Y., Schneider, D. J., and Blackburn, M. R. (2009). Adenosine signaling and the regulation of chronic lung disease. *Pharmacol. Ther.* 123, 105–116. doi: 10.1016/j.pharmthera.2009.04.003

Zimmerman, M. A., Grenz, A., Tak, E., Kaplan, M., Ridyard, D., Brodsky, K. S., et al. (2013). Signaling through hepatocellular A2B adenosine receptors dampens ischemia and reperfusion injury of the liver. *Proc. Natl. Acad. Sci. U.S.A.* 110, 12012–12017. doi: 10.1073/pnas.1221733110

14

Pathophysiology and Diagnosis of Pulmonary Hypertension Due to Left Heart Disease

*Athanasios Charalampopoulos**, Robert Lewis, Peter Hickey, Charlotte Durrington, Charlie Elliot, Robin Condliffe, Ian Sabroe and David G. Kiely*

Sheffield Pulmonary Vascular Disease Unit, Royal Hallamshire Hospital, Sheffield Teaching Hospitals NHS Foundation Trust, Sheffield, United Kingdom

***Correspondence:**
Athanasios Charalampopoulos
athanasios.charalampopoulos@sth.nhs.uk

Pulmonary hypertension due to left heart disease (PH-LHD) is the most common type of pulmonary hypertension, although an accurate prevalence is challenging. PH-LHD includes PH due to systolic or diastolic left ventricular dysfunction, mitral or aortic valve disease and congenital left heart disease. In recent years a new and distinct phenotype of "combined post-capillary and pre-capillary PH," based on diastolic pulmonary gradient and pulmonary vascular resistance, has been recognized. The roles of right ventricular dysfunction and pulmonary vascular compliance in PH-LHD have also been elucidated recently and they appear to have significant clinical implications. Echocardiography continues to play a seminal role in diagnosis of PH-LHD and heart failure with preserved LV ejection fraction, as it can identify valve disease and help to distinguish PH-LHD from pre-capillary PH. Right, and occasionally left heart catheterization, remains the gold-standard for diagnosis and phenotyping of PH-LHD, although Cardiac Magnetic Resonance Imaging is emerging as a useful alternative tool in non-invasive diagnostic and prognostic assessment of PH-LHD. In this review, the latest evidence for more recent advances will be discussed, including the role of fluid challenge and exercise during cardiac catheterization to unravel occult post-capillary and the role of vasoreactivity testing. The use of many or all of these diagnostic techniques will undoubtedly provide key information about sub-groups of patients with PH-LHD that might benefit from medical therapy previously considered to be only suitable for pulmonary arterial hypertension.

Keywords: pulmonary hypertension, left heart disease, heart failure with preserved ejection fraction, left ventricular diastolic dysfunction, right heart catheterization

INTRODUCTION

Pulmonary hypertension due to left heart disease (PH-LHD) is the most common type of pulmonary hypertension (PH). The prevalence of PH in patients with heart failure varies significantly with diagnostic criteria from 25 to 83% (1–4). PH-LHD is defined by post-capillary hemodynamics at right heart catheterization (RHC); that is a mean pulmonary arterial pressure ≥25 mmHg and a mean pulmonary arterial wedge pressure (PAWP) > 15 mmHg. PAWP is a surrogate marker of left atrial pressure (LAP). An elevated LAP causing PH can occur in systolic and/or diastolic left ventricular (LV) dysfunction and in left-sided valvular disease. In the most recent clinical classification of PH (5) two additional etiologies of PH-LHD have been recognized: PH due to congenital or acquired left ventricular outflow tract

TABLE 1 | Definitions.

Pre-capillary PH	Mean PAP ≥ 25 mmHg, mean PAWP ≤15 mmHg
Isolated post-capillary PH	Mean PAP ≥ 25 mmHg, mean PAWP >15 mmHg, DPG < 7 mmHg and/or PVR ≤ 3 Wood units
Combined pre-capillary and post-capillary PH	Mean PAP ≥ 25 mmHg, mean PAWP >15 mmHg, DPG ≥ 7 mmHg and/or PVR > 3 Wood units

PAP, pulmonary artery pressure; PAWP, pulmonary artery wedge pressure; DPG, diastolic pressure gradient; PVR, pulmonary vascular resistance. Modified from 2015 ESC/ERS Pulmonary Hypertension Guidelines (5).

obstruction and pulmonary vein stenosis. In the same guidelines, a new PH phenotype of "combined pre-capillary and post-capillary PH" (Cpc-PH) has been introduced on the grounds of a diastolic pressure gradient (DPG)-the difference between diastolic pulmonary arterial pressure and mean PAWP-equal or higher than 7 mmHg (**Table 1**). This new term came to replace the older "PH out of proportion to LHD." Although, pathophysiology of Cpc-PH is not entirely clear, a chronic elevation of LAP due to longstanding LHD is believed to cause a profound pulmonary artery remodeling and pulmonary vascular resistance (PVR) rise, which is not usually found in isolated post-capillary PH. Patients with Cpc-PH seem to be in the middle of a spectrum of which pre-capillary PH and isolated post-capillary PH are the two extremes, regarding their clinical and echocardiographic characteristics (6).The prevalence of Cpc-PH amongst patients with systolic and diastolic heart failure is believed to be within 12 and 14% (7). An adequate understanding of pathophysiology along with an accurate diagnosis and differentiation of PH-LHD from pre-capillary PH, such as pulmonary arterial hypertension (PAH) and chronic thromboembolic PH (CTEPH), are of paramount importance to select the appropriate treatment for the patient.

PATHOPHYSIOLOGY

The pathophysiological hallmark of PH-LHD is elevated LAP. LV systolic and diastolic dysfunction as well as aortic and/or mitral valve stenosis and/or regurgitation can raise left ventricular filling pressure and subsequently LAP over a period of time. LAP can then be transmitted backwards via pulmonary veins to the pulmonary vasculature leading to pulmonary arterial intimal thickening and medial hypertrophy and PH (**Figure 1**). Compliance in the pulmonary vasculature, unlike in the systemic circulation, is more evenly distributed across the pulmonary bed and the distal vessels are responsible for most of it (8). Hence, compliance is mostly determined by PVR. The relationship between PVR and compliance is an inverse hyperbolic one. "Passive" left-sided elevated pressures shift the hyperbole leftwards leading to an additional decline of compliance for a given PVR and thus enhanced pulmonary wave reflections which return during ventricular systole and increase the systolic (but not the diastolic) pulmonary artery pressure (9). In a recent study, pulmonary arterial compliance (or capacitance) defined as the ratio of stroke volume to pulmonary pulse pressure was the best predictor of mortality in PH-LHD associated with heart failure with preserved left ventricular ejection fraction (HFpEF) (10).

The Right Ventricle (RV)

The first compensatory mechanism of the RV to the elevated pulmonary pressure is hypertrophy. Thus, the RV can adapt with a 4- to 5-fold increase in myocardial contractility, a process which is described pathophysiologically as right ventricular-pulmonary artery (RV-PA) "coupling." In the next progressive stage the RV starts dilating, wall stress according to LaPlace's law increases, imbalance between oxygen demand and supply and RV ischemia occurs, contractility declines, the RV fails to maintain cardiac output and inevitably "uncoupling" and decompensation begins. The development of tricuspid (TR) and pulmonary regurgitation due to annular dilatation leads to RV volume overloading and decreases stroke volume even further. RV-PA coupling has been estimated by echocardiography as the ratio of tricuspid annular plane systolic excursion (TAPSE) to pulmonary artery systolic pressure (PASP) and a cut-off limit <0.36 has been shown to have prognostic value (11). Coupling has also been estimated by a hybrid method combining RHC and cardiac magnetic resonance (CMR) as the ratio of pulmonary artery effective elastance, which is a measure of arterial load, to the maximum end-systolic RV elastance, which is an index of contractility (12).

Up until recently the impact of PH-LHD on RV function had been underestimated. In recent years, however, its significance and prognostic value has been highlighted. RV systolic dysfunction assessed by echocardiography has been found in at least 1/5 of patients with HFpEF and potentially up to 30–50% (13). In addition, a decrease of TAPSE by 5 mm was associated with a 26% mortality rise (13), while in another study a decrease of RV fractional area change by 7% with a 2.2-fold increase of all-cause mortality after adjustment for pulmonary pressures in patients with HFpEF (14).

Ventricular Interdependence and Comorbidities

Other parameters such as ventricular interdependence may contribute to decreased cardiac output and heart failure. As RV pressure increases and interventricular dyssynchrony is established, the interventricular septum bows toward the LV moving "paradoxically" and leading to a decrease of LV diastolic filling and a further drop of stroke volume. In addition, atrial fibrillation, coronary artery disease via right coronary or circumflex artery stenosis leading to reduced RV oxygen supply, chronic obstructive pulmonary disease, obstructive sleep apnea, diabetes, and obesity, all comorbidities frequently seen in patients with LHD may increase pulmonary pressures and further compromise RV function.

The Role of DPG

DPG has been considered to be a more accurate indicator of pulmonary vascular remodeling in LHD than transpulmonary gradient (the difference between mean pulmonary artery pressure and mean PAWP [TPG]), as it is theoretically not influenced

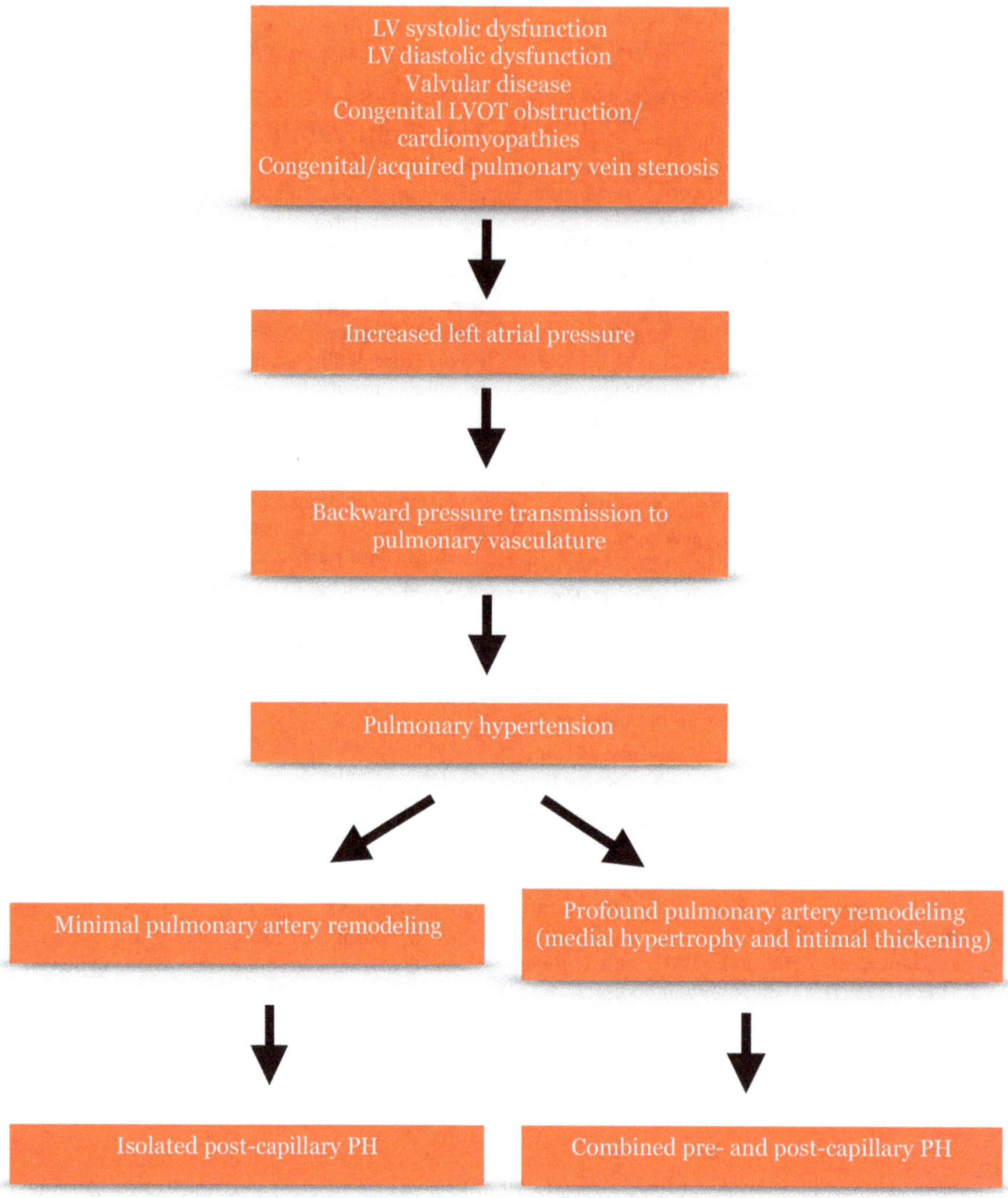

FIGURE 1 | Pathophysiological mechanisms of pulmonary hypertension due to left heart disease.

by the variability of cardiac output or the impact of LAP on pulmonary vascular compliance. In a retrospective large study in patients with PH-LHD an elevated DPG $\geq$ 7 mmHg was correlated with worse median survival compared with a DPG $<$ 7 mmHg and a high TPG $>$ 12 mmHg (15). In the same study, in a small number of patients high DPG was also correlated with greater pathological pulmonary vascular remodeling compared to patients with high TPG but normal DPG. Two further studies, retrospective as well, in patients who had undergone orthotopic heart transplantation and in patients with unexplained cardiomyopathy did not confirm the prognostic value of DPG (16, 17). In a more recent study the risk of death in Cpc-PH and isolated post-capillary PH after adjustment of relevant covariates was similar, however the researchers identified 75 common exonic single-nucleotide polymorphisms between Cpc-PH and pre-capillary PH in pathways pertinent with cell structure, extracellular matrix and immune function (6).

DIAGNOSIS

Risk Factors, Clinical Symptoms, and Signs

Features of metabolic syndrome such as obesity, systemic hypertension, diabetes and dyslipidemia, are more prevalent in patients with PH-LHD than PAH. Researchers have shown that two or more of these features were present in 94.1% of PH-LHD patients vs. only 34.3% of PAH (18). The findings were confirmed in another study, which showed that older age, the presence of systemic hypertension and coronary artery disease are more frequent in PH-LHD and can best differentiate from PAH along with other echocardiographic and hemodynamic parameters (19). In the same study there was a similarly high female predominance in the PH-LHD and PAH groups but more pronounced than in the HFpEF without PH group. In addition to these risk factors, the prevalence of permanent atrial fibrillation in PH-LHD seems to be significantly higher than in patients with PAH and risk factors for LHD (20).

The symptoms and clinical signs of patients with PH-LHD are these of heart failure. Exertional dyspnea, orthopnea, and/or paroxysmal nocturnal dyspnea, anginal chest pain typically on exertion, palpitations, dry cough, pre-syncope and/or syncope, hepatomegaly, ascites, elevated jugular venous pressure, and peripheral edema are the most common ones. Right ventricular heave, a loud pulmonary component of the second heart sound and a pansystolic murmur of tricuspid regurgitation may also be present. In a retrospective study which compared patients with PAH with or without cardiovascular comorbidities to PH-LHD, patients with PH-LHD were more likely to have peripheral edema, whilst there was a trend toward a worse functional class after adjustment for age but no difference in 6-min walking test distance (20). Patients with PH-LHD usually have normal resting oxygen saturations with a possible drop on exercise, unless if they also have respiratory comorbidity or a right-to-left shunt.

Chest X-Ray, ECG, and Pulmonary Function Test

The chest X-ray may show signs of cardiomegaly and enlarged pulmonary artery branches. Pleural effusions may be seen more frequently in PH-LHD than PAH, although they are not uncommon in severe PAH as well (21).

Left QRS axis deviation, atrial fibrillation and signs of left ventricular hypertrophy are more likely on ECG in PH-LHD than in pre-capillary PH, whereas right axis, sinus rhythm, R wave dominant in lead V1, ST-T segment depression, and T-wave inversion in the right precordial and inferior leads are more frequently seen in pre-capillary PH. Right bundle branch block does not appear to differentiate the two conditions (20, 22). These ECG findings have been recently incorporated in predictive score models to discriminate non-invasively between PH-LHD and PAH (23, 24).

It is well-known that pulmonary alveolar diffusion is impaired in patients with congestive heart failure. Gas transfer factor for carbon monoxide (TLco) is reduced in this population compared to controls (25). In addition, TLco and end-tidal CO_2 have been found to be lower in PAH patients compared to PH-LHD (26, 27). In the ASPIRE registry, mean TLco in the PAH group was 55 vs. 62% predicted in the PH-LHD one (26).

Natriuretic Peptides

Brain natriuretic peptide (BNP) and its N-terminal fragment NT-proBNP can both be elevated in heart failure with reduced LV ejection fraction and HFpEF. They can be secreted from the cardiomyocytes of both ventricles due to stretching from volume overload. The upper limit of normal for BNP is 35 pg/mL and for NT-proBNP 125 pg/mL (28). Natriuretic peptides may be elevated in elderly people, atrial fibrillation and renal impairment without heart failure. They can also be disproportionally low in obese patients. In addition, they cannot differentiate between pre-capillary PH and PH-LHD as they may be raised in both conditions. Their role in patients' follow-up, assessment of response to treatment and detection of progression of the underlying disease as well as their prognostic role can be very important.

Echocardiography

Echocardiography plays a seminal role in the detection of signs of PH-LHD. It can diagnose LV systolic and diastolic dysfunction, aortic and mitral valve disease, LV outflow tract obstruction, restrictive and hypertrophic cardiomyopathy and constrictive pericarditis. In all these conditions, LV diastolic dysfunction usually occurs and may lead to PH-LHD. The estimation of PASP, which raises the suspicion of PH when elevated, derives from applying continuous Doppler and the modified Bernoulli equation: *4 x peak TR velocity (TRV)*^{2} + *estimated right atrial pressure*. Right atrial pressure can be estimated from the size and collapsibility during respiration/sniff of the inferior vena cava on the subcostal view (29). According to the current ESC/ERS guidelines a threshold of peak TRV higher than 2.8 m/s is considered suspicious of PH with or without the presence of other echocardiographic signs of PH and risk factors for PH (5). However, peak TRV is angle and flow-dependent and it can frequently be under- or overestimated (30). Peak TRV should be measured from several different acoustic windows and views, while in atrial fibrillation an average of measurements from the view with the highest velocities should be taken and only a well-defined, spade-shaped, dense spectral profile should be measured. In cases with no or trivial TR when TRV cannot accurately be estimated, mean pulmonary artery pressure can be calculated instead from the peak velocity of a pulmonary regurgitant jet at the beginning of diastole or from the acceleration time (time from onset to peak) of the forward flow at the right ventricular outflow tract (29).

Diagnosing LV diastolic dysfunction with echocardiography sometimes can be challenging. Four parameters have been recently included in an algorithm to determine diastolic dysfunction: an average (of septal and lateral) E/e' $>$ 14, a septal e' $<$ 7 cm/s or lateral $<$10 cm/s, a TRV $>$ 2.8 m/s and a left atrial volume index $>$34 ml/m^2. If $<$50% of these parameters are present, diastolic function is normal, if $>$50%, there is diastolic dysfunction and when exactly 50%, diastolic function is indeterminate (31). Other echocardiographic signs such as mitral "L" velocity $>$20 cm/s (ongoing LV filling in mid-diastole due to markedly delayed LV relaxation), mitral inflow E/A wave velocity ratio and E wave deceleration time, as well as a higher diastolic wave velocity than the systolic one in the pulmonary vein Pulsed Doppler profile may also be useful (31). Unlike PH-LHD, significant LV diastolic dysfunction in PAH is very unlikely. In a small study, 88% of PAH patients demonstrated grade I (mild) diastolic dysfunction and 10% normal diastolic function (32).

Left atrial dilatation is considered to be one of the most useful indicators of LHD. However, in the presence of atrial fibrillation may not always represent elevated LAP. In atrial fibrillation, an average E/e' $\geq$11 instead of 14 should be used as a marker of diastolic dysfunction (31). Researchers in the past have described conditions such as severe mitral regurgitation with a dilated left atrium but normal LAP. Left atrial compliance seems to play a pivotal role in these cases (33). The absence of mid-systolic "notching" in the right ventricular outflow tract Pulsed Doppler envelope has also been shown to be highly predictive of a PVR < 3 Wood units and a PAWP >15 mmHg (34). On the other hand, a PASP > 70 mmHg is more likely to represent PAH than PH-LHD (35). The severity of TR cannot differentiate between PH-LHD and PAH. In a prospective cohort of patients with PAH and PH-LHD, 45% had mild, 34% moderate, and 21% severe TR. The mechanisms causing TR were annular dilatation, RV remodeling-tethering and inadequate tricuspid valve leaflet area (36). Finally, a RV end-diastolic diameter to LV end-diastolic diameter ratio (measured in the 4-chamber apical view at the tips of the atrioventricular valves) <1 and the absence of pericardial effusion seem to be more likely in PH-LHD than PAH (20). **Table 2** summarizes the distinct echocardiographic characteristics in pre-capillary PH and PH-LHD. An echocardiographic score based on LA dimension, mid-systolic notching and E/e' to differentiate between PH-LHD and PAH has been proposed (37). More recently another echocardiographic score, which seems to be useful in discriminating between isolated and Cpc-PH as well, has been published (38).

CMR

CMR may play an important role in making diagnosis and identifying prognosis of PH in general and PH-LHD in particular. Especially in cases where visualization or accuracy of measurements is limited, CMR should be strongly considered. CMR remains the gold standard imaging modality for RV assessment (39). Beyond RV size and function, CMR can quantify the curvature of interventricular septum and more recently pulmonary arterial stiffness, which may detect early stages of pulmonary vascular remodeling (40, 41). In the ASPIRE registry, patients with PH-LHD had lower RV mass, a better-preserved cardiac function and less gadolinium hinge-point enhancement compared to pre-capillary PH (42). In addition, CMR is an excellent tool for myocardial tissue characterization and with the use of late gadolinium enhancement it can diagnose infiltrative cardiomyopathies e.g., amyloidosis, hypertrophic cardiomyopathy, as well as systolic and diastolic LV dysfunction. CMR can also play a significant role in diagnosis of congenital heart diseases, which may be related to both PAH and PH-LHD.

TABLE 2 | Echocardiographic features likely to be present in pre- and post-capillary pulmonary hypertension.

Pre-capillary PH	PH-LHD
Normal sized or small LV cavity	Normal sized or dilated LV cavity
No LV hypertrophy	LV hypertrophy
Preserved LVEF	Variable LVEF
Normal sized or small left atrium	Dilated left atrium
Grade I LV diastolic dysfunction or normal LV diastolic function	≥ Grade II LV diastolic dysfunction
Presence of mid-systolic notching	Absence of mid-systolic notching
RV/LV ratio > 1	RV/LV ratio < 1
PASP > 70 mmHg	Typically PASP < 70 mmHg
Pericardial effusion	No pericardial effusion
No mitral and/or aortic valve disease	Mitral and/or aortic valve disease

PH-LHD, pulmonary hypertension due to left heart disease; LV, left ventricle; LVEF, left ventricular ejection fraction; RV/LV ratio, right ventricular to left ventricular end-diastolic diameter ratio; PASP, pulmonary artery systolic pressure. Modified from Roberts JD and Forfia PR. Pulm Circ. 2011;1:160-181.

Predictive Non-invasive Score Models

Over the last few years, score models to assess the pre-RHC probability of PH-LHD have been created aspiring to avoid potentially unnecessary catheterizations. Bonderman et al. proposed a model based on RV strain on ECG and BNP (23). Jacobs et al. suggested a risk model including history of LHD, the sum of S deflection in V1 and R deflection in V6 on the ECG, left atrial dilatation and left valve disease worse than mild on echocardiogram (24). Finally, Richter et al. suggested a prediction score for elevated PAWP based on age >68 years, BMI > 30 kg/m^2, absence of RV enlargement and presence of left atrial dilatation on echocardiography (43).

RHC-Fluid Challenge-Exercise-Vasoreactivity Testing

The gold standard method for the diagnosis of PH-LHD remains RHC. All pulmonary pressures should be measured at end-expiration with the patient breathing spontaneously. The mean PAWP has been better correlated with mean LAP than the LV end-diastolic pressure (LVEDP) in patients with LV disease, except for very high PAWP over 25 mmHg (44, 45). However, a LVEDP > 15 mmHg on left heart catheterization can be used to define PH-LHD, when an accurate PAWP is not feasible (e.g., in chronic thromboembolic disease). An accurate PAWP may be challenging to obtain. A waveform consistent with atrial waveform, a PAWP $\leq$ diastolic pulmonary arterial pressure, blood easily aspirated and highly oxygenated in the wedge position and the placement of the tip of the catheter in West zone 3 (at the lung base, where pulmonary artery and venous pressure exceeds pulmonary alveolar pressure, which represents lung areas with the greatest blood flow rates), below left atrial level, can eliminate technical difficulties. Mitral regurgitation may cause large "v" waves that can be mistakenly interpreted as an elevated PAWP. This can be accounted for by reading the PAWP at the time of the "a" wave. Patients with PH-LHD tend to have a higher mean right atrial pressure, cardiac output and right ventricular end-diastolic pressure, as well as lower PVR compared with PAH (19, 20).

Patients with clinical and echocardiographic features suggestive of PH-LHD may sometimes have pre-capillary PH, especially if they have been previously heavily diuresed. Fluid challenge, which is the rapid intravenous administration of a high volume of normal saline, is believed to be helpful to unpick cases of occult PH-LHD with resting pre-capillary hemodynamics and unmask LV diastolic dysfunction. The current ESC/ERS PH guidelines do not recommend fluid loading at RHC due to lack of standardization as well as the theoretical risk of a rapid significant PAWP elevation to result in pulmonary edema. Three studies with fluid challenge in PH patients have been conducted since the publication of these guidelines though. In the first one, the infusion of 500 mL of saline within 5–10 min led to the reclassification of 22.2% of patients as occult PH-LHD (defined as a mean PAWP > 15 mmHg), while in another small study in patients with systemic sclerosis a similar percentage of patients with pre-capillary baseline hemodynamics were found to have a LVEDP > 15 mmHg post-infusion of 500 mL within 5–10 min (46, 47). In the most recent one, rapid infusion of saline at a rate of 7 mL/kg reclassified 8% of patients with no PH and 6% of patients with pre-capillary PH at baseline. A cut-off limit of PAWP ≥ 18 mmHg was used in the latter study (48). In all three studies, fluid loading was safe. Of note, even in healthy subjects a rapid fluid infusion will lead to a PAWP > 15 mmHg in a percentage >60%, however with a larger than 500 mL volume of saline (49). Likewise, exercise during RHC may unmask diastolic dysfunction in patients with suspected HFpEF and a baseline PAWP < 15 mmHg. Exercise can be performed on a supine or upright bike (the latter would be feasible when the RHC is done from the neck or the arm) or with leg lifting. In normal subjects and athletes, an increase of PAWP up to 25 mmHg in a broadly linear fashion with cardiac output has been shown (50). However, significant increases of PAWP at a cardiac output <10 L/min is uncommon in normal individuals. Exercise during RHC seems to be particularly helpful in obese patients with a borderline, between 12 and 15 mmHg, PAWP (51).

According to the ESC/ERS guidelines vasoreactivity testing is only recommended in patients with suspected idiopathic, familial, or drug-induced PAH (5). In the context of PH-LHD vasodilator challenge can be used in the evaluation of patients for listing for cardiac transplantation, especially those with a TPG > 12–15 mmHg and/or PVR > 3 Wood units. The preferable vasodilator agent is inhaled nitric oxide. An increase of PAWP post-nitric oxide may be seen but pulmonary edema is very rare.

Treatment

PAH targeted therapies act on three distinct pathophysiological pathways. The first one is the nitric oxide-soluble guanylate cyclase (sGC)-cGMP pathway which includes drugs like phosphodiesterase type 5 inhibitors (Sildenafil, Tadalafil) and stimulators of cGC like Riociguat. The second one is the endothelin-1 pathway with drugs like endothelin receptor antagonists (Bosentan, Ambrisentan, and Macitentan) and the third is the prostacyclin pathway with prostacyclin analogs (Epoprostenol, Treprostinil, Iloprost) and an oral selective IP prostacyclin-receptor agonist (Selexipag). These drugs have proven to be efficacious in PAH and CTEPH patients in several randomized, controlled, double-blind trials. On the other hand, trials of the same drugs in patients with PH-LHD have not shown any benefit and some of them have also been related with increased mortality (52–54). In the recent SIOVAC trial (55), where Sildenafil was tested vs. placebo in patients with post-capillary PH and history of correction of valvular heart disease, median PVR in the Sildenafil group was 3.4 Wood units, TPG 16 mmHg, but DPG only 2 mmHg. Of note, the study did not meet its primary end-point. Further trials need to be conducted in patients with Cpc-PH hemodynamics to answer the question about a possible efficacy of pulmonary vasodilator drugs in this specific PH phenotype.

CONCLUSIONS

Up to now, no pulmonary vasodilator treatment has proven to be efficacious in PH-LHD. Some of the PAH drugs have even been detrimental when given in patients with LHD. Hence, it is apparent that the accurate identification of the major driver of PH in each patient is essential. In clinical practice the diagnosis and phenotyping of PH cannot be based on a single test, even if that test is the RHC, but rather on a combination of clinical data, imaging and hemodynamics. A better understanding of pathophysiology and further clinical trials are required to clarify whether Cpc-PH is a distinct clinical entity or part of a spectrum of PH phenotypes and identify potential treatments for the future.

AUTHOR CONTRIBUTIONS

All authors listed have made a substantial, direct and intellectual contribution to the work, and approved it for publication.

REFERENCES

1. Lam CS, Roger VL, Borlaug BA, Enders FT, Redfield MM. Pulmonary hypertension in heart failure with preserved ejection fraction: a community-based study. *J Am Coll Cardiol.* (2009) **53**:1119–26. doi: 10.1016/j.jacc.2008.11.051
2. Leung CC, Moondra V, Catherwood E, Andrus BW. Prevalence and risk factors of pulmonary hypertension in patients with elevated pulmonary venous pressure and preserved ejection fraction. *Am J Cardiol.* (2010) **106**:284–6. doi: 10.1016/j.amjcard.2010.02.039
3. Damy T, Goode KM, Kallvikbacka-Bennett A, Lewinter C, Hobkirk J, Nikitin NP, et al. Determinants and prognostic value of pulmonary arterial hypertension in patients with chronic heart failure. *Eur Heart J.* (2010) **31**:2280–90. doi: 10.1093/eurheartj/ehq245
4. Bursi F, McNallan SM, Redfield MM, Nkomo VT, Lam CS, Weston SA, et al. Pulmonary pressures and death in heart failure: a community study. *J Am Coll Cardiol.* (2012) **59**:222–31. doi: 10.1016/j.jacc.2011.06.076
5. Galiè N, Humbert M, Vachiery J-L, Gibbs S, Lang I, Torbicki A, et al. 2015 ESC/ERS Guidelines for the diagnosis and treatment of pulmonary

hypertension: The Joint Task Force for the Diagnosis and Treatment of Pulmonary Hypertension of the European Society of Cardiology (ESC) and the European Respiratory Society (ERS): Endorsed by: Association for European Paediatric and Congenital Cardiology (AEPC), International Society for Heart and Lung Transplantation (ISHLT). *Eur Heart J.* (2016) **37**:67–119. doi: 10.1093/eurheartj/ehv317

6. Assad TR, Hemnes AR, Larkin EK, Glazer AM, Xu M, Wells QS, et al. Clinical and biological insights into combined post- and pre-capillary pulmonary hypertension. *J Am Coll Cardiol.* (2016) **68**:2525–36. doi: 10.1016/j.jacc.2016.09.942
7. Gerges M, Gerges C, Pistritto AM, Lang MB, Trip P, Jakowitsch J, et al. Pulmonary hypertension in heart failure: epidemiology, right ventricular function, and survival. *Am J Respir Crit Care Med.* (2015) **192**:1234–46. doi: 10.1164/rccm.201503-0529OC
8. Saouti N, Westerhof N, Helderman F, Marcus JT, Stergiopulos N, Westerhof BE, et al. RC time constant of single lung equals that of both lungs together: a study in chronic thromboembolic pulmonary hypertension. *Am J Physiol Heart Circ Physiol.* (2009) **297**:H2154–60. doi: 10.1152/ajpheart.00694.2009
9. Tedford RJ, Hassoun PM, Mathai SC, Girgis RE, Russell SD, Thiemann DR, et al. Pulmonary capillary wedge pressure augments right ventricular pulsatile loading. *Circulation* (2012) **125**:289–97. doi: 10.1161/CIRCULATIONAHA.111.051540
10. Al-Naamani N, Preston IR, Paulus JK, Hill NS, Roberts KE. Pulmonary arterial capacitance is an important predictor of mortality in heart failure with a preserved ejection fraction. *JACC Heart Fail* (2015) **3**:467–74. doi: 10.1016/j.jchf.2015.01.013
11. Guazzi M, Bandera F, Pelissero G, Castelvecchio S, Menicanti L, Ghio S, et al. Tricuspid annular plane systolic excursion and pulmonary arterial systolic pressure relationship in heart failure: an index of right ventricular contractile function and prognosis. *Am J Physiol Heart Circ Physiol.* (2013) **305**:H1373–81. doi: 10.1152/ajpheart.00157.2013
12. Sanz J, García-Alvarez A, Fernández-Friera L, Nair A, Mirelis JG, Sawit ST, et al. Right ventriculo-arterial coupling in pulmonary hypertension: a magnetic resonance study. *Heart* (2012) **98**:238–43. doi: 10.1136/heartjnl-2011-300462
13. Gorter TM, Hoendermis ES, van Veldhuisen DJ, Voors AA, Lam CS, Geelhoed B, et al. Right ventricular dysfunction in heart failure with preserved ejection fraction: a systematic review and meta-analysis. *Eur J Heart Fail* (2016) **18**:1472–87. doi: 10.1002/ejhf.630
14. Melenovsky V, Hwang SJ, Lin G, Redfield MM, Borlaug BA. Right heart dysfunction in heart failure with preserved ejection fraction. *Eur Heart J.* (2014) **35**:3452–62. doi: 10.1093/eurheartj/ehu193
15. Gerges C, Gerges M, Lang MB, Zhang Y, Jakowitsch J, Probst P, et al. Diastolic pulmonary vascular pressure gradient: a predictor of prognosis in "out-of-proportion" pulmonary hypertension. *Chest* (2013) **1433**:758–66. doi: 10.1378/chest.12-1653
16. Tampakakis E, Leary PJ, Selby VN, De Marco T, Cappola TP, Felker GM, et al. The diastolic pulmonary gradient does not predict survival in patients with pulmonary hypertension due to left heart disease. *JACC Heart Fail* (2015) **3**:9–16. doi: 10.1016/j.jchf.2014.07.010
17. Tedford RJ, Beaty CA, Mathai SC, Kolb TM, Damico R, Hassoun PM, et al. Prognostic value of the pre-transplant diastolic pulmonary artery pressure-to-pulmonary capillary wedge pressure gradient in cardiac transplant recipients with pulmonary hypertension. *J Heart Lung Transplant* (2014) **33**:289–197. doi: 10.1016/j.healun.2013.11.008
18. Robbins IM, Newman JH, Johnson RF, Hemnes AR, Fremont RD, Piana RN, et al. Association of the metabolic syndrome with pulmonary venous hypertension. *Chest* (2009) **136**:31–36. doi: 10.1378/chest.08-2008
19. Thenappan T, Shah SJ, Gomberg-Maitland M, Collander B, Vallakati A, Shroff P, et al. Clinical characteristics of pulmonary hypertension in patients with heart failure and preserved ejection fraction. *Circ Heart Fail* (2011) **4**:257–65. doi: 10.1161/CIRCHEARTFAILURE.110.958801
20. Charalampopoulos A, Howard LS, Tzoulaki I, Gin-Sing W, Grapsa J, Wilkins MR, et al. Response to pulmonary arterial hypertension drug therapies in patients with pulmonary arterial hypertension and cardiovascular risk factors. *Pulm Circ.* (2014) **4**:669–78. doi: 10.1086/678512
21. Milne EN. Forgotten gold in diagnosing pulmonary hypertension: the plain chest radiograph. *Radiographics* (2012) **32**:1085–7. doi: 10.1148/rg.324125021
22. McMurray JJ, Carson PE, Komajda M, McKelvie R, Zile MR, Ptaszynska A, et al. Heart failure with preserved ejection fraction: clinical characteristics of 4133 patients enrolled in the I-PRESERVE trial. *Eur J Heart Fail.* (2008) **10**:149–56. doi: 10.1016/j.ejheart.2007.12.010
23. Bonderman D, Wexberg P, Martischnig AM, Heinzl H, Lang MB, Sadushi R, et al. A noninvasive algorithm to exclude pre-capillary pulmonary hypertension. *Eur Respir J.* (2011) **37**:1096–103. doi: 10.1183/09031936.00089610
24. Jacobs W, Konings TC, Heymans MW, Boonstra A, Bogaard HJ, van Rossum AC, et al. Noninvasive identification of left-sided heart failure in a population suspected of pulmonary arterial hypertension. *Eur Respir J.* (2015) **46**:422–30. doi: 10.1183/09031936.00202814
25. Smith AA, Cowburn PJ, Parker ME, Denvir M, Puri S, Patel KR, et al. Impaired pulmonary diffusion during exercise in patients with chronic heart failure. *Circulation* (1999) **100**:1406–10.
26. Hurdman J, Condliffe R, Elliot CA, Davies C, Hill C, Wild JM, et al. ASPIRE registry: assessing the Spectrum of Pulmonary hypertension Identified at a referral centre. *Eur Respir J.* (2012) **39**:945–55. doi: 10.1183/09031936.00078411
27. Hemnes AR, Pugh ME, Newman AL, Robbins IM, Tolle J, Austin ED, et al. End tidal CO_2 tension: pulmonary arterial hypertension vs pulmonary venous hypertension and response to treatment. *Chest* (2011) **140**:1267–73. doi: 10.1378/chest.11-0155
28. Ponikowski P, Voors AA, Anker SD, Bueno H, Cleland JGF, Coates AJS, et al. 2016 ESC Guidelines for the diagnosis and treatment of acute and chronic heart failure. *Eur Heart J.* (2016) **37**:2129–200. doi: 10.1093/eurheartj/ehw128
29. Rudski LG, Wyman WL, Afilalo J, Hua L, Handschumacher MD, Chandrasekaran K, et al. Guidelines for the echocardiographic assessment of the right heart in adults: a report from the american society of echocardiography. endorsed by the european association of echocardiography, a registered branch of the European Society of Cardiology, and the Canadian Society of Echocardiography. *J Am Soc Echocardiogr.* (2010) **23**:685–713. doi: 10.1016/j.echo.2010.05.010
30. Fisher MR, Forfia PR, Chamera E, Housten-Harris T, Champion HC, Girgis RE, et al. Accuracy of Doppler echocardiography in the hemodynamic assessment of pulmonary hypertension. *Am J Respir Crit Care Med.* (2009) **179**:615–21. doi: 10.1164/rccm.200811-1691OC
31. Nagueh SF, Smiseth OA, Appleton CP, Byrd BF III, Dokainish H, Edvardsen T, et al. Recommendations for the evaluation of left ventricular diastolic function by echocardiography: an update from the American Society of Echocardiography and the European Association of Cardiovascular Imaging. *Eur Heart J Cardiovasc Imaging* (2016) **17**:1321–60. doi: 10.1016/j.echo.2016.01.011
32. Tonelli AR, Plana JC, Heresi GA, Dweik RA. Prevalence and prognostic value of left ventricular diastolic dysfunction in idiopathic and heritable pulmonary arterial hypertension. *Chest* (2012) **141**:1457–65. doi: 10.1378/chest.11-1903
33. Braunwald E, Awe W. The syndrome of severe mitral regurgitation with normal left atrial pressure. *Circulation* (1963) **27**:29–35.
34. Arkles JS, Opotowsky AR, Ojeda J, Rogers F, Liu T, Prassana V, et al. Shape of the right ventricular Doppler envelope predicts hemodynamics and right heart function in pulmonary hypertension. *Am J Respir Crit Care Med.* (2011) **183**:268–76. doi: 10.1164/rccm.201004-0601OC
35. Hussain N, Ramjug S, Hurdman J, Elliot C, Kiely D. Non-invasive testing can help differentiate idiopathic pulmonary arterial hypertension and pulmonary hypertension associated with heart failure with preserved ejection fraction. *Am J Respir Crit Care Med.* (2014) **189**:A1891. doi: 10.1164/ajrccm-conference. 2014.189.1_MeetingAbstracts.A1891
36. Afilalo J, Grapsa J, Nihoyannopoulos P, Beaudoin J, Gibbs JS, Channick RN, et al. Leaflet area as a determinant of tricuspid regurgitation severity in patients with pulmonary hypertension. *Circ Cardiovasc Imaging* (2015) **8**: e002714. doi: 10.1161/CIRCIMAGING.114.002714
37. Opotowsky AR, Ojeda J, Rogers F, Prasanna V, Clair M, Moko L, et al. A simple echocardiographic prediction rule for hemodynamics in pulmonary hypertension. *Circ Cardiovasc Imaging* (2012) **5**:765–75. doi: 10.1161/CIRCIMAGING.112.976654
38. D'Alto M, Romeo E, Argiento P, Pavelescu A, D'Andrea A, Di Marco GM, et al. A simple echocardiographic score for the diagnosis of pulmonary vascular disease in heart failure. *J Cardiovasc Med.* (2017) **18**:237–43. doi: 10.2459/JCM.0000000000000485
39. Mooij CF, de Wit CJ, Graham DA, Powell AJ, Geva T. Reproducibility of MRI measurements of right ventricular size and function in patients with normal and dilated ventricles. *J Magn Reson Imaging* (2008) **28**:67–73. doi: 10.1002/jmri.21407
40. Marcus JT, Vonk Noordegraaf A, Roeleveld RJ, Postmus PE, Heethaar RM, Van Rossum AC, et al. Impaired left ventricular filling due to right ventricular pressure overload in primary pulmonary hypertension:

noninvasive monitoring using MRI. *Chest* (2001) **119**:1761–5

41. Sanz J, Kariisa M, Dellegrottaglie S, Prat-González S, Garcia MJ, Fuster V, et al. Evaluation of pulmonary artery stiffness in pulmonary hypertension with cardiac magnetic resonance. *JACC Cardiovasc Imaging* (2009) **2**:286–95. doi: 10.1016/j.jcmg.2008.08.007
42. Swift AJ, Rajaram S, Condliffe R, Capener D, Hurdman J, Elliot CA, et al. Diagnostic accuracy of cardiovascular magnetic resonance imaging of right ventricular morphology and function in the assessment of suspected pulmonary hypertension results from the ASPIRE registry. *J Cardiovasc Magn Reson.* (2012) **14**:40. doi: 10.1186/1532-429X-14-40
43. Richter SE, Roberts KE, Preston IR, Hill NS. A simple derived prediction score for the identification of an elevated pulmonary artery wedge pressure using precatheterization clinical data in patients referred to a Pulmonary Hypertension center. *Chest* (2016) **149**:1261–8. doi: 10.1378/chest.1 5-0819
44. Braunwald E, Frahm C. Studies on Starling's law of the heart. IV. Observations on the hemodynamic functions of the left atrium in man. *Circulation* (1961) **24**:633–42.
45. Walston A 2nd, Kendall ME. Comparison of pulmonary wedge and left atrial pressure in man. *Am Heart J.* (1973) **86**:159–64.
46. Robbins IM, Hemnes AR, Pugh ME, Brittain EL, Zhao DX, Piana RN, et al. High prevalence of occult pulmonary venous hypertension revealed by fluid challenge in pulmonary hypertension. *Circ Heart Fail* (2014) **7**:116–22. doi: 10.1161/CIRCHEARTFAILURE.113.000468
47. Fox BD, Shimony A, Langleben D, Hirsch A, Rudski L, Schlesinger R, et al. High prevalence of occult left heart disease in scleroderma-pulmonary hypertension. *Eur Respir J.* (2013) **42**:1083–91. doi: 10.1183/09031936.00091212
48. D'Alto M, Romeo E, Argiento P, Motoji Y, Correra A, Di Marco GM, et al. Clinical relevance of fluid challenge in patients evaluated for pulmonary hypertension. *Chest* (2017) **151**:119–26. doi: 10.1016/j.chest.2016.08.1439
49. Fujimoto N, Borlaug BA, Lewis GD, Hastings JL, Shafer KM, Bhella PS, et al. Hemodynamic responses to rapid saline loading: the impact of age, sex, and heart failure. *Circulation* (2013) **127**:55–62. doi: 10.1161/CIRCULATIONAHA.112.111302
50. Naeije R, Vanderpool R, Dhakal BP, Saggar R, Saggar R, Vachiery J-L, et al. Exercise-induced pulmonary hypertension. physiological basis and methodology concerns. *Am J Respir Crit Care Med.* (2013) **187**:576–83. doi: 10.1164/rccm.201211-2090CI
51. Maor E, Grossman Y, Balmor RG, Segel M, Fefer P, Ben-Zekry S, et al. Exercise haemodynamics may unmask the diagnosis of diastolic dysfunction among patients with pulmonary hypertension. *Eur J Heart Fail* (2015) **17**:151–8. doi: 10.1002/ejhf.198
52. Califf RM, Adams KF, McKenna WJ, Gheorghiade M, Uretsky BF, McNulty SE, et al.A randomized controlled trial of epoprostenol therapy for severe congestive heart failure: The Flolan International Randomized Survival Trial (FIRST). *Am Heart J.* (1997) **134**:44–54.
53. Kalra PR, Moon JC, Coats AJ. Do results of the ENABLE (Endothelin Antagonist Bosentan for Lowering Cardiac Events in Heart Failure) spell the end for non-selective endothelin antagonism in heart failure? *Int J Cardiol.* (2002) **85**:195–97. doi: 10.1016/S0167-5273(02)00182-1
54. Bonderman D, Ghio S, Felix SB, Ghofrani HA, Michelakis E, Mitrovic V, et al. Riociguat for patients with pulmonary hypertension caused by systolic left ventricular dysfunction: a phase IIb double-blind, randomized, placebo-controlled, dose-ranging hemodynamic study. *Circulation* (2013) **128**:502–11. doi: 10.1161/CIRCULATIONAHA.113.001458
55. Bermejo J, Yotti R, García-Orta R, Sánchez-Fernández PL, Castaño M, Segovia-Cubero J, et al. Sildenafil for improving outcomes in patients with corrected valvalar heart disease and persistent pulmonary hypertension: a multicenter, double-blind, randomized, controlled trial. *Eur Heart J.* (2018) 39:1255–64. doi: 10.1093/eurheartj/ehx700

15

Inflammatory Mediators Drive Adverse Right Ventricular Remodeling and Dysfunction and Serve as Potential Biomarkers

Akylbek Sydykov[1,2†], Argen Mamazhakypov[1†], Aleksandar Petrovic[1], Djuro Kosanovic[1], Akpay S. Sarybaev[2], Norbert Weissmann[1], Hossein A. Ghofrani[1] and Ralph T. Schermuly[1]*

[1] *Excellence Cluster Cardio-Pulmonary System, Universities of Giessen and Marburg Lung Center, German Center for Lung Research, Justus Liebig University of Giessen, Giessen, Germany,* [2] *Department of Mountain and Sleep Medicine and Pulmonary Hypertension, National Center of Cardiology and Internal Medicine, Bishkek, Kyrgyzstan*

Correspondence:
Ralph T. Schermuly
Ralph.Schermuly@innere.med.uni-giessen.de

† These authors have contributed equally to this work.

Adverse right ventricular (RV) remodeling leads to ventricular dysfunction and failure that represents an important determinant of outcome in patients with pulmonary hypertension (PH). Recent evidence indicates that inflammatory activation contributes to the pathogenesis of adverse RV remodeling and dysfunction. It has been shown that accumulation of inflammatory cells such as macrophages and mast cells in the right ventricle is associated with maladaptive RV remodeling. In addition, inhibition of inflammation in animal models of RV failure ameliorated RV structural and functional impairment. Furthermore, a number of circulating inflammatory mediators have been demonstrated to be associated with RV performance. This work reviews the role of inflammation in RV remodeling and dysfunction and discusses anti-inflammatory strategies that may attenuate adverse structural alterations while promoting improvement of RV function.

Keywords: right ventricle, adverse remodeling, dysfunction, failure, inflammation

INTRODUCTION

Pulmonary arterial hypertension (PAH) is a severe and debilitating disease characterized by progressive remodeling of small pulmonary arteries leading to sustained pressure elevation in the pulmonary circulation. The resulting chronic pressure overload induces remodeling of the right ventricle. Although increased pulmonary pressure is caused by changes in the pulmonary vasculature, severity of symptoms and survival of patients with PAH are strongly dependent on the ability of the right ventricle to cope with chronically increased afterload (Chin et al., 2005).

Cardiac remodeling in general is defined as "genome expression, molecular, cellular, and interstitial changes that are manifested clinically as changes in size, shape and function of the heart after cardiac injury" (Cohn et al., 2000). Cardiac remodeling is a complex process that affects every cell type comprising the heart tissue and involves cardiomyocyte hypertrophy, fibrosis, metabolic changes, and angiogenesis. Right ventricular (RV) remodeling in response to pressure overload represents a number of adaptations in the size, shape, structure, and function of the right ventricle. Hypertrophy of the RV wall allows compensating for increased afterload and helps maintain cardiac output in PAH patients. However, geometric adaptation of the right ventricle in PAH is heterogeneous. Although PAH is associated with a spectrum of RV geometric adaptation, two patterns of RV hypertrophy can be distinguished based on the RV mass to volume (M/V) ratio: eccentric hypertrophy with low M/V ratio and concentric hypertrophy with high M/V ratio (Badagliacca et al., 2015). Concentric hypertrophy represents a more favorable RV adaptive remodeling pattern in patients with PAH and is associated with minimal fibrosis and preserved RV function and cardiac output (Vonk-Noordegraaf et al., 2013). In contrast, eccentric hypertrophy represents maladaptive RV remodeling and is associated with excessive RV fibrosis, RV dysfunction, and decreased cardiac output (Vonk-Noordegraaf et al., 2013). However, the mechanisms underlying adverse RV remodeling and dysfunction are poorly understood. A better understanding of the mechanisms of the RV remodeling may help identify candidate targets for novel therapeutic strategies directed specifically at the right ventricle and thus improve survival in these patients.

There is substantial evidence for the important role of inflammation in the pathogenesis of PAH (Hassoun et al., 2009; El Chami and Hassoun, 2011; Price et al., 2012). Furthermore, elevated levels of circulating mediators of inflammation correlate with disease severity, symptom burden and survival in PAH patients (Humbert et al., 1995; Quarck et al., 2009; Soon et al., 2010; Cracowski et al., 2014; Heresi et al., 2014; Matura et al., 2015; Al-Naamani et al., 2016). Moreover, circulating inflammatory mediators released from the pulmonary vasculature might trigger or contribute to inflammatory processes in the right ventricle and thus adversely affect RV remodeling and function. Consistent with this view, chronic RV pressure overload without concomitant pulmonary vascular disease in patients with pulmonary stenosis is often associated with adaptive RV remodeling and preserved RV function, which remains compensated for decades (Haddad et al., 2008; Jurcut et al., 2011; Driessen et al., 2016, 2017).

Another line of evidence suggesting the role of inflammation as a driver of adverse RV remodeling and dysfunction comes from studies of patients with systemic sclerosis or scleroderma-associated (SSc) PAH. Scleroderma is a systemic connective tissue disease characterized by chronic inflammation, fibrosis, and immune abnormalities (Furue et al., 2017). Although various mechanisms may underlie pulmonary hypertension (PH) in scleroderma patients, PAH due to vasculopathy of the small pulmonary arteries secondary to inflammation and fibrosis is one of the most frequent forms of PH in these patients (Launay et al., 2017). Patients with SSc-PAH have worse survival than patients with idiopathic PAH (Kato and Atsumi, 2017). Further, RV function strongly predicts survival in SSc-PAH patients (Mathai et al., 2011). Moreover, SSc-PAH patients have more impaired RV function compared with idiopathic PAH patients despite comparable afterload (Tedford et al., 2013; Mukherjee et al., 2017). Remarkably, significantly more inflammatory cells were found in RV tissue samples from SSc-PAH patients as compared to those from patients with idiopathic PAH thus confirming increased local inflammation in these patients (Overbeek et al., 2010). Contribution of inflammatory pathways to the pathogenesis of RV adverse remodeling and dysfunction is further supported by the association of circulatory mediators of inflammation with RV function in patients with PAH (Sztrymf et al., 2010; Yang et al., 2014; Prins et al., 2017). Interestingly, a recent magnetic resonance imaging investigation in individuals free of clinical cardiovascular disease has demonstrated that plasma levels of pro-inflammatory C-reactive protein (CRP) and interleukin-6 (IL-6) are independently associated with RV morphology, suggesting that systemic inflammation may contribute to RV structural changes (Harhay et al., 2013).

ACUTE RIGHT VENTRICULAR PRESSURE OVERLOAD

Acute pulmonary embolism (PE) can produce a rapid and excessive elevation in afterload leading to acute RV dilatation, dysfunction and failure (Vitarelli et al., 2014; Grignola and Domingo, 2017). Importantly, RV dilatation and dysfunction in patients with acute PE are strong predictors of adverse clinical outcome (Coutance et al., 2011; Trujillo-Santos et al., 2013; Cho et al., 2014; Meinel et al., 2015). Interestingly, examination of autopsy RV tissue samples from patients who died from acute PE showed increased accumulation of neutrophilic granulocytes, lymphocytes, and macrophages in the RV wall suggesting that acute pressure overload-induced inflammatory response might contribute to RV failure after PE (Iwadate et al., 2001, 2003; Begieneman et al., 2008).

Experimental models of acute RV pressure overload induced by PE or pulmonary artery banding (PAB) confirmed that inflammation is one of the earliest events following pressure overload. In a rat model of acute PE induced by infusion of microspheres, RV failure after PE was associated with tissue infiltration of neutrophils and monocyte/macrophages (Watts et al., 2006, 2009). Neutrophil and macrophage infiltration in the right ventricle has also been demonstrated in a different model of acute RV failure induced by transient PAB in dogs (Dewachter et al., 2015). Increased mRNA expression of various chemokines (CCL-2, -3, -4, -6, -7, -9, -17, -20, -27; CXCL-1, -2, -3, -9, -10, -16; receptors CCR1 and CXCR4 in the right ventricle following acute elevation of afterload has been demonstrated (Watts et al., 2006, 2009; Zagorski et al., 2007, 2008; Dewachter et al., 2015). Notably, alterations in gene expression were more profound with increasing PH (Zagorski et al., 2008). Chemokines play important chemotactic roles for the recruitment of leukocytes to the site of inflammation and thus might promote leukocyte recruitment into the right ventricle during acute pressure overload. In addition, experimental acute RV failure was also associated with increased local expression of pro-inflammatory cytokines [IL-1β, IL-6, tumor necrosis factor α (TNF-α)] (Dewachter et al., 2010, 2015). Moreover, there was an inverse correlation between the right ventricle–pulmonary artery coupling and RV gene and protein expressions of IL-6 as well as to the RV neutrophil and macrophage infiltration (Dewachter et al., 2010).

CHRONIC RIGHT VENTRICULAR REMODELING AND FAILURE

Accumulating evidence from various experimental models of chronic RV pressure overload shows association of RV remodeling and dysfunction with increased inflammatory mediators in the right ventricle (Campian et al., 2010; Waehre et al., 2012; Belhaj et al., 2013; Guihaire et al., 2017; Luitel et al., 2017). The inflammatory mediators include pro-inflammatory cytokines, chemokines, as well as molecules secreted/released by inflammatory cells. The findings of studies investigating inflammatory markers in the RV tissue are summarized in **Table 1**.

INFLAMMATORY CELLS

Numerous studies have demonstrated that recruitment of immune cells from the circulatory system is important for the induction and maintenance of inflammatory processes in the

TABLE 1 | Summary of studies investigating inflammatory mediators in the right ventricular tissue.

Disease model	Species/subjects	Findings	References
Acute RVF following transient PAB	Dogs	Increased expression of CCL2, CCR2, IL-1β, IL-6, TNF-α mRNA.	Dewachter et al., 2010, 2015
Acute RVF following PE	Rats	Increased expression of the CC-chemokines (CCL-2, -3, -4, -6, -7, -9, -17, -20, -27), the CXC-chemokines (CXCL-1, -2, -3, -9, -10, -16), the receptors CCR1 and CXCR4, ICAM-1, selectin E, the cytokines IL-1β and IL-6 mRNA. Elevation of CCL2 protein expression. Increased MPO activity. Accumulation of neutrophils and monocyte/macrophages (CD68).	Watts et al., 2006, 2009; Zagorski et al., 2007, 2008
Acute RVF following PE	Autopsy tissues from patients	Increased recruitment of macrophages (CD68).	Iwadate et al., 2003
Acute RVF following transplantation	Human donors	Eight of 26 recipients (30.8%) developed RVF. Seven of these eight (87.5%) expressed TNF-α, but only 4 of the 18 (22.2%) who did not develop RVF expressed TNF-α. Higher TNF-α protein expression in the myocardium of donor hearts that developed RVF.	Birks et al., 2000
Chronic hypoxic PH	Mice	Increased accumulation of CD68 positive cells.	Nergui et al., 2014
MCT-induced PH	Rats	Increased TNF-α, IL-1, IL-6 mRNA expression. Elevated protein expression of TNF-α, NF-κB subunits p100/p52, and Rel-B. Increased accumulation of $CD45^{+}$ cells enhanced MPO activity.	Handoko et al., 2009; Campian et al., 2010; de Man et al., 2012; Ahmed et al., 2014; Moreira-Goncalves et al., 2015; Paulin et al., 2015; Nogueira-Ferreira et al., 2016; Rice et al., 2016; Wang et al., 2016; Alencar et al., 2017; Brown et al., 2017
Sugen-injection induced PH	Athymic rats	Macrophage infiltration.	Guihaire et al., 2017
PH due to blockade of VEGF receptor and exposure to chronic hypoxia	Female ovariectomized rats	Increased IL-6 mRNA expression.	Frump et al., 2015
PH due to prolonged systemic-to-pulmonary shunting	Growing piglets	Increased TNF-α, IL-1α, IL-1b, and ICAM2 mRNA expression.	Rondelet et al., 2012; Belhaj et al., 2013
Chronic RVF remodeling following PAB	Mice	Increased mRNA expression of CCL-2, CCL-5, CX3CL-1, CXCL-6, CXCL-10, CXCL-16, CD45R, CD3, CD4, CD8, IL-6, TNF-α, Fn14, mMCP-2, 4, -5, -6, and CPA3. Increased density and activity of mast cells.	Vistnes et al., 2010; Waehre et al., 2012; Luitel et al., 2017
Chronic RVF following PAB	Rats	Increased expression of activated p65 (NF-κB). Increased density and activity of mast cells, enhanced accumulation of CD68-positive macrophages.	Olivetti et al., 1989; Yoshida et al., 2016
PAH	Autopsy tissues from patients	Increased tissue content of CD68 positive macrophages.	Nergui et al., 2014
SSc-PAH, IPAH and controls	Autopsy tissues from patients	RV's from SSc-PAH patients showed significantly more inflammatory cells than those from IPAH and then of controls.	Overbeek et al., 2010

PE, pulmonary embolism; PAB, pulmonary artery banding; MCT, monocrotaline; PH, pulmonary hypertension; PAH, pulmonary arterial hypertension; SSc-PAH, pulmonary arterial hypertension due to systemic sclerosis; IPAH, idiopathic pulmonary arterial hypertension; RV, right ventricle; RVF, right ventricular failure; ICAM2, intercellular adhesion molecule 2; CXCL, chemokine (C-X-C motif) ligand; CCL, CC-chemokine; CX3CL, chemokine (C-X3-C motif) ligand; CCR2, chemokine C-C receptor 2; IL, interleukin; TNF-α, tumor necrosis factor α; NF-κB, nuclear factor "kappa-light-chain-enhancer" of activated B-cells; mMCP, mouse mast cell protease; CPA3, mast cell carboxypeptidase A3; MPO, myeloperoxidase; Fn14, fibroblast growth factor-inducible molecule 14; VEGF, vascular endothelial growth factor.

heart (Sanchez-Trujillo et al., 2017). Although the precise role of inflammatory cells in the pathophysiology of maladaptive RV remodeling and dysfunction is not well established, accumulating evidence suggests that these cells might represent a potentially important target for management of RV adverse remodeling and failure.

Macrophages

Resident macrophages are present in all tissues including the heart (Mylonas et al., 2015; Pinto et al., 2016). Expansion of cardiac macrophages has been documented in various experimental models of pressure overload-induced left ventricular remodeling and failure (Xia et al., 2009; Velten et al., 2012; Weisheit et al., 2014).

In contrast, data regarding the role of macrophages in RV remodeling and failure are still very limited. Similar to the left ventricular pressure overload, recruitment of macrophages into the right ventricle has been shown to be triggered by increased RV afterload induced by PAB in rats (Yoshida et al., 2016). Moreover, in a model of severe PH caused by a single injection of vascular endothelial growth factor (VEGF) receptors blocker in athymic rats, macrophage infiltration was associated with adverse RV remodeling and dysfunction (Guihaire et al., 2017). Increased macrophage recruitment has also been demonstrated in RV autopsy samples from PAH patients with RV failure (Nergui et al., 2014). Notably, autopsy samples from patients with SSc-associated PAH exhibited significantly more macrophage infiltration in the right ventricle as compared with those from patients with idiopathic PAH (Overbeek et al., 2010). The role of macrophage recruitment in the pathogenesis of pressure overload-induced RV remodeling has not yet been well studied. However, based on studies in left ventricular remodeling and failure, the potential mechanisms through which macrophages might contribute to RV remodeling and dysfunction include production of reactive oxygen species, regulation of cardiac inflammation and mediation of extracellular matrix alterations (Glezeva et al., 2015).

Mast Cells

Mast cells are immune cells of the myeloid lineage and are residing in various tissues throughout the body including the heart (Dvorak, 1986; Rakusan et al., 1990). Mast cells play an important role in many inflammatory settings. Moreover, a growing body of evidence implicates mast cells in various cardiovascular diseases including left ventricular remodeling and failure (Levick et al., 2011). Enhanced accumulation of mast cells in hypertrophied and failing hearts suggests that mast cells play a role in the pathogenesis of these diseases (Panizo et al., 1995; Shiota et al., 2003; Batlle et al., 2006). Studies utilizing mast cell stabilizers, inhibitors of mast cell proteases, and mast cell deficient mice provided further evidence of the importance of mast cells for left ventricular remodeling and failure (Hara et al., 2002; Matsumoto et al., 2003; Levick et al., 2009; Li et al., 2016).

An early accumulation of mast cells in both left and right ventricles has been documented in a rat model of biventricular volume overload (Forman et al., 2006). Interestingly, the time course of the responses in the density of myocardial mast cells in this model was similar for the left and right ventricles (Brower et al., 2002). However, the number of mast cells after an initial increase returned to normal values by day 14 post-fistula. In rats, long-term pressure overload induced by PAB was associated with an increased mast cell density in the right ventricle (Olivetti et al., 1989). Similarly, in mice subjected to PAB, there was a time-dependent accumulation and activation of mast cells in the right ventricle (Luitel et al., 2017). In contrast, significant RV hypertrophy in rats born at simulated high altitude was not associated with an increase in cardiac mast cells density (Rakusan et al., 1990). Adaptive nature of RV remodeling in hypoxic PH may account for the unaltered mast cells density in the right ventricle in rat exposed to chronic hypoxia.

Mast cells granules contain proteases tryptase and chymase (Gilfillan and Beaven, 2011). In addition, mast cells generate a wide variety of cytokines, including IL-3, IL-4, IL-5, IL-6, IL-10, IL-13, IL-33, and TNFα; and chemokines, including CCL2, CCL3, CCL5, and CXCL8 (Gilfillan and Beaven, 2011). Mast cell mediators have been implicated in the stimulation of collagen synthesis leading to myocardial fibrosis or activation of matrix metalloproteinases causing collagen degradation and resulting in left ventricular dilatation (Levick et al., 2011). However, the role of mast cells in the pathogenesis of pressure overload-induced RV remodeling and dysfunction has not yet been studied in detail. Interestingly, elevated mRNA levels of mast cell proteases (Mcp)-2, 4, 5, 6, and carboxypeptidase A3 in the right ventricle have been observed in mice subjected to PAB suggesting their potential contribution to RV remodeling process (Luitel et al., 2017).

Leukocytes

Numerous studies have shown that leukocytes play critical roles in the pathogenesis of left ventricular remodeling and failure in experimental models of left ventricular pressure overload (Damilano et al., 2011; Laroumanie et al., 2014; Nevers et al., 2015; Salvador et al., 2016). However, data on the leukocyte involvement in the RV remodeling and failure are limited. Several reports have demonstrated increased accumulation of $CD45^{+}$ cells in the right ventricle of rats with monocrotaline-induced PH (Handoko et al., 2009; de Man et al., 2012; Brown et al., 2017). Notably, no leukocyte infiltration in the right ventricle was detected in compensated RV remodeling in rats with mild PH induced by injection of low doses of monocrotaline (Handoko et al., 2009; Brown et al., 2017). In mice subjected to PAB, pressure overload was associated with increased mRNA expression of leukocyte cell-surface gene markers, including CD45R, CD3, CD4, and CD8, in the right ventricle (Waehre et al., 2012).

INFLAMMATORY MEDIATORS: CHEMOKINES AND CYTOKINES

The inflammatory mediators involved in ventricular remodeling and dysfunction can be produced by cells in the heart tissue, by infiltrating immune cells, or can be of extra-cardiac origin (Van Linthout and Tschope, 2017). Multiple factors may be responsible for the induction of inflammatory genes in the pressure-overloaded heart, including neurohumoral mediators, reactive oxygen species, as well as direct activation of mechanosensitive pro-inflammatory signals in the myocardium (Van Linthout and Tschope, 2017). Chemokines can recruit inflammatory cells into the pressure-overloaded myocardium. In addition to their chemotactic role, chemokines can stimulate release of pro-inflammatory cytokines, thus contributing to the amplified activation of inflammatory processes. Pro-inflammatory cytokines and chemokines can contribute to ventricular remodeling and dysfunction through various mechanisms, including negative inotropic effects on the myocardium, cardiomyocyte hypertrophy, cardiomyocyte apoptosis, and extracellular matrix alterations (Mann, 2015).

Chemokines

Elevated plasma levels of the chemokines CXCL10, CXCL12, CXCL13, and CXCL16 have been observed in PAH patients (Heresi et al., 2010). Importantly, CXCL10, CXCL12, and CXCL16 levels significantly correlated with RV function (Yang et al., 2014). Elevated plasma levels of a chemokine CXCL9 have been observed in a murine model of PAB-induced RV pressure overload (Vistnes et al., 2010). Further, marked upregulation of several chemokines, including CCL2, CCL5, CXCL6, CXCL10, CXCL16, and CX3CL1, was detected in the right ventricle of mice subjected to PAB (Waehre et al., 2012). Similarly, in female ovariectomized rats with severe angioproliferative PH due to blockade of VEGF receptor and exposure to chronic hypoxia, upregulation of CCL2 mRNA in the right ventricle has been reported (Frump et al., 2015).

TNF-α

TNF-α is a key multifunctional cytokine with pleiotropic actions in various inflammatory processes (Feldman et al., 2000). Although the normal heart does not express TNF-α, its mRNA and protein expression is rapidly induced in response to pressure overload (Kapadia et al., 1997). High levels of TNF-α have been shown to lead to left ventricular remodeling and dysfunction in animal models with long-term infusion of TNF-α, as well as in transgenic animals with targeted cardiac overexpression (Kubota et al., 1997; Bozkurt et al., 1998; Bryant et al., 1998). In contrast, TNF-α deficiency was associated with attenuation of cardiac inflammation and amelioration of adverse left ventricular remodeling and dysfunction in mice subjected to transverse aortic constriction (Sun et al., 2007). Consistent with findings from animal studies implicating TNF-α in the pathogenesis of heart failure, circulating levels of TNF-α have consistently been shown to be elevated in patients with chronic heart failure (Liu et al., 2014).

Involvement of TNF-α in the pathogenesis of RV failure has been suggested by demonstrating a relationship between TNF-α mRNA and protein expression in right ventricles of donor hearts immediately before implantation and the development of right heart failure early after transplantation (Birks et al., 2000). Further, a relationship between circulating levels of TNF-α and several parameters of RV failure, including severity of peripheral edema, RV ejection fraction and NYHA functional class, has been shown in patients with right heart failure related to ischemic heart disease or idiopathic dilated cardiomyopathy (Odeh et al., 2006). In line with these observations, expression of TNF-α has been shown to be upregulated in the right ventricle in various animal models of pressure overload-induced RV remodeling and failure, including PAB in mice (Luitel et al., 2017), monocrotaline-induced PH in rats (Ahmed et al., 2014; Moreira-Goncalves et al., 2015; Nogueira-Ferreira et al., 2016; Rice et al., 2016; Wang et al., 2016; Alencar et al., 2017), and prolonged overcirculation-induced PH in piglets (Rondelet et al., 2012; Belhaj et al., 2013). Notably, decompensated RV failure in monocrotaline-injected rats was associated with higher serum and RV myocardial TNF-α expression levels compared with compensated RV hypertrophy (Campian et al., 2010; Paulin et al., 2015).

The TNF superfamily comprises several members, including TNF-like weak inducer of apoptosis and its receptor fibroblast growth factor-inducible molecule 14 (Fn14), which have been implicated in pathological ventricular remodeling and heart failure (Novoyatleva et al., 2014). Recently, increased mRNA and protein expression of Fn14 in the pressure-overloaded right ventricles has been demonstrated (Novoyatleva et al., 2013). Moreover, mice deficient for Fn14 developed substantially less RV fibrosis and dysfunction following PAB compared to wild-type mice (Novoyatleva et al., 2013).

IL-1

IL-1 cytokines consist of 11 members, including pro-inflammatory cytokines IL-1α and IL-1β that induce synthesis and expression of several hundreds of secondary inflammatory mediators (Dinarello, 2018). Upregulation of IL-1 has been consistently demonstrated in heart failure and is associated with worse prognosis (Van Tassell et al., 2015). Increased levels of IL-1β have also been shown in PAH patients (Humbert et al., 1995; Soon et al., 2010; Duncan et al., 2012; Cracowski et al., 2014; McMahan et al., 2015). Similarly, RV pressure overload in mice was associated with elevated plasma levels of IL-1α (Vistnes et al., 2010). Further, expression of IL-1α and IL-1b was upregulated in right ventricles of piglets subjected to prolonged systemic-to-pulmonary shunting (Rondelet et al., 2012; Belhaj et al., 2013) and rats with monocrotaline-induced PH (Rice et al., 2016) suggesting potential contribution of IL-1 cytokines to RV remodeling and dysfunction.

IL-6

IL-6 is a multi-functional cytokine with a variety of biological activities, which has been implicated in left ventricular remodeling and failure (Fontes et al., 2015). Chronic IL-6 infusion in rats has been shown to lead to left ventricular dilatation and dysfunction (Janssen et al., 2005). In contrast, genetic deletion of IL-6 ameliorated pressure overload-induced adverse left ventricular remodeling and dysfunction in mice (Zhao et al., 2016). In patients with chronic heart failure, elevated circulating levels of IL-6 have been reported (Liu et al., 2014).

Numerous studies have documented increased levels of IL-6 in PAH patients (Humbert et al., 1995; Selimovic et al., 2009; Soon et al., 2010; Duncan et al., 2012; Cracowski et al., 2014; Heresi et al., 2014; Matura et al., 2015; Al-Naamani et al., 2016; Prins et al., 2017). Notably, increased expression of IL-6 mRNA has been detected in right ventricles of failing hearts (Plenz et al., 2001). In addition, IL-6 mRNA expression in the right ventricles inversely correlated with cardiac index in patients with advanced heart failure (Plenz et al., 2001). Similar findings were made in experimental models of RV pressure overload. Thus, elevated plasma levels of IL-6 and increased IL-6 expression in right ventricles has been demonstrated in rats with monocrotaline-induced PH (Wang et al., 2016), in mice subjected to PAB (Vistnes et al., 2010; Luitel et al., 2017), and in female ovariectomized rats with severe angioproliferative PH due to blockade of VEGF receptor and exposure to chronic hypoxia (Frump et al., 2015). Interestingly, in a recent study, a strong, independent, inverse relationship between IL-6 and RV morphology was demonstrated in asymptomatic individuals without documented cardiovascular disease (Harhay et al., 2013).

Nuclear Factor-κB

The nuclear factor-κB (NF-κB) super family of transcription factors has been implicated in the regulation of a variety of physiological processes and plays a key role in regulation of inflammatory responses (Begalli et al., 2017). However, preclinical studies provided conflicting evidence for the role of NF-κB in left ventricular remodeling and failure. Several studies have demonstrated a critical role of NF-κB in promoting adverse cardiac remodeling and failure (Gupta et al., 2008; Maier et al., 2012), whereas other studies have suggested its importance in the development of compensatory hypertrophy following pressure overload (Andersen et al., 2012; Javan et al., 2015).

There have been only a few studies investigating the role of NF-κB in RV remodeling and dysfunction. In rats subjected to PAB, elevated expression of activated NF-κB has been found in right ventricles (Yoshida et al., 2016). Further, activation of the non-canonical NF-κB pathway with upregulation NF-κB subunits p100/p52 and Rel-B in right ventricles has been reported in rats with monocrotaline-induced PH (Nogueira-Ferreira et al., 2016). Interestingly, treatment of PAB rats with the NF-κB inhibitor pyrrolidine dithiocarbamate ameliorated RV inflammation and fibrosis and improved RV function (Yoshida et al., 2015).

INFLAMMATORY MEDIATORS AS BIOMARKERS

Circulating biomarkers serve as a non-invasive tool for diagnosis, assessment of the severity of the disease, prognosis, and response to treatment (Foris et al., 2013). A variety of inflammatory mediators, including IL-1α, IL-1b, IL-2, IL-4, IL-6, IL-8, IL-10, IL-13, IL-12p70, TNF-α, and CRP are upregulated in PAH (Quarck et al., 2009; Selimovic et al., 2009; Sztrymf et al., 2010; Duncan et al., 2012; Heresi et al., 2014; Matura et al., 2015; Al-Naamani et al., 2016; Prins et al., 2017). Importantly, markers of inflammation are associated with disease severity and mortality in these patients (Humbert et al., 1995;

TABLE 2 | Summary of studies evaluating the relationship of circulating inflammatory biomarkers with the parameters of right ventricular performance.

Disease	Sample	Population	Inflammatory mediators	Findings	References
CTEPH and CHF	Serum	Patients with CTEPH (*n* = 49), CHF (*n* = 17), Control (*n* = 34)	TNF-α, sTNFR-1 and -2, IL-10, hs-CRP, and NT-proBNP	High serum levels of TNF-α sTNFR1, sTNFR2, NT-proBNP, and IL-10 in CTEPH and CHF patients. Correlations between sTNFR1, sTNFR2, IL-6, hs-CRP, and NT-proBNP and magnetic resonance imaging-derived RVEF.	von Haehling et al., 2010
IPAH	Plasma	Patients with IPAH (*n* = 61), Control (*n* = 20)	CXCL-10, CXCL-12, and CXCL-16	Association of increased levels of CXCL-10, CXCL-12 and CXCL-16 with RVEF and TAPSE.	Yang et al., 2014
PAH	Serum	Patients with PAH (*n* = 40)	IL-6	Inverse correlation of serum IL-6 levels with echocardiography-derived RV FAC, TAPSE, and right ventricle–pulmonary artery coupling parameters. Negative relationship between circulating IL-6 and cardiac magnetic resonance imaging-derived RV ejection fraction.	Prins et al., 2017
HF patients presenting with RVF	Serum	HF patients with RVF (*n* = 83), Control (*n* = 15)	TNF-α	Correlation of TNF-α levels with severity of peripheral edema and multigated acquisition (MUGA) technique-derived RVEF.	Odeh et al., 2006

PAH, pulmonary arterial hypertension; IPAH, idiopathic pulmonary arterial hypertension; CTEPH, chronic thromboembolic pulmonary arterial hypertension; CHF, chronic heart failure; RV, right ventricular; RVF, right ventricular failure; RVEF, right ventricular ejection fraction; RV FAC, right ventricular fractional area change; TAPSE, tricuspid annular plane systolic excursion; TNF-α, tumor necrosis factor alpha; sTNFR, soluble tumor necrosis factor receptors; IL, interleukin; CXCL, chemokine (C-X-C motif) ligand; NT-proBNP, N-terminal pro b-type natriuretic peptide; hs-CRP, high-sensitivity C-reactive protein.

RV, right ventricular; TNF-α, tumor necrosis factor alpha; sTNFR, soluble tumor necrosis factor receptors; NT-proBNP, N-terminal pro b-type natriuretic peptide; hs-CRP, high-sensitivity C-reactive protein; IL, interleukin; PTX3, pentraxin 3; CXCL, chemokine (C-X-C motif) ligand.

Soon et al., 2010; Cracowski et al., 2014; Karakurt et al., 2014; McMahan et al., 2015). However, there have been only a few studies that specifically addressed the relationship between circulating markers of inflammation and parameters of RV performance in patients with PAH. In patients with idiopathic PAH, elevated plasma levels of chemokines CXCL10, CXCL12, and CXCL16 correlated negatively with echocardiographic parameters of RV function such as tricuspid annular plane systolic excursion (TAPSE) and RV ejection fraction (Yang et al., 2014). In addition, CXCL10 and CXCL12 correlated significantly with RV end-diastolic diameter, mean right atrial pressure, and cardiac index (Yang et al., 2014). Recently, relationships between increased circulating IL-6 levels and RV function in PAH patients have been analyzed (Prins et al., 2017). Serum IL-6 levels correlated inversely with echocardiography-derived measures of RV function, including RV fractional area change, TAPSE and right ventricle–pulmonary artery coupling parameters (Prins et al., 2017). Importantly, these relationships remained significant, even after excluding patients with SSc-PAH (Prins et al., 2017). Remarkably, a negative relationship between circulating IL-6 and cardiac magnetic resonance imaging-derived RV ejection fraction was described (Prins et al., 2017). A significant relationship has also been demonstrated between circulating levels of TNF-α and severity of peripheral edema in patients with right heart failure related to ischemic heart disease or idiopathic dilated cardiomyopathy (Odeh et al., 2006). Further, a significant inverse correlation was found between serum TNF-α and multigated acquisition (MUGA) technique-derived RV ejection fraction (Odeh et al., 2006). In **Table 2**, we reported a list of inflammatory markers, which reflect adverse RV remodeling and dysfunction.

TARGETING INFLAMMATION

Low-level graded aerobic exercise is recommended as a general measure in the treatment of PH by the current European Society of Cardiology – European Respiratory Society Guidelines on Pulmonary Hypertension (Galie et al., 2016). There is substantial evidence for anti-inflammatory effects of physical activity in patients with various cardiovascular, metabolic, or pulmonary diseases (Pedersen, 2017). Beneficial effects of exercise training on pulmonary hemodynamics and functional capacity has also been shown in patients with PH (Arena et al., 2015; Buys et al., 2015; Babu et al., 2016; Ehlken et al., 2016). Moreover, acute effects of exercise on the inflammatory state in patients with idiopathic PAH have recently been reported (Harbaum et al., 2016). In a recent study using monocrotaline-induced PH in rats, high intensity interval training lowered RV systolic pressure, RV hypertrophy and fibrosis, and increased

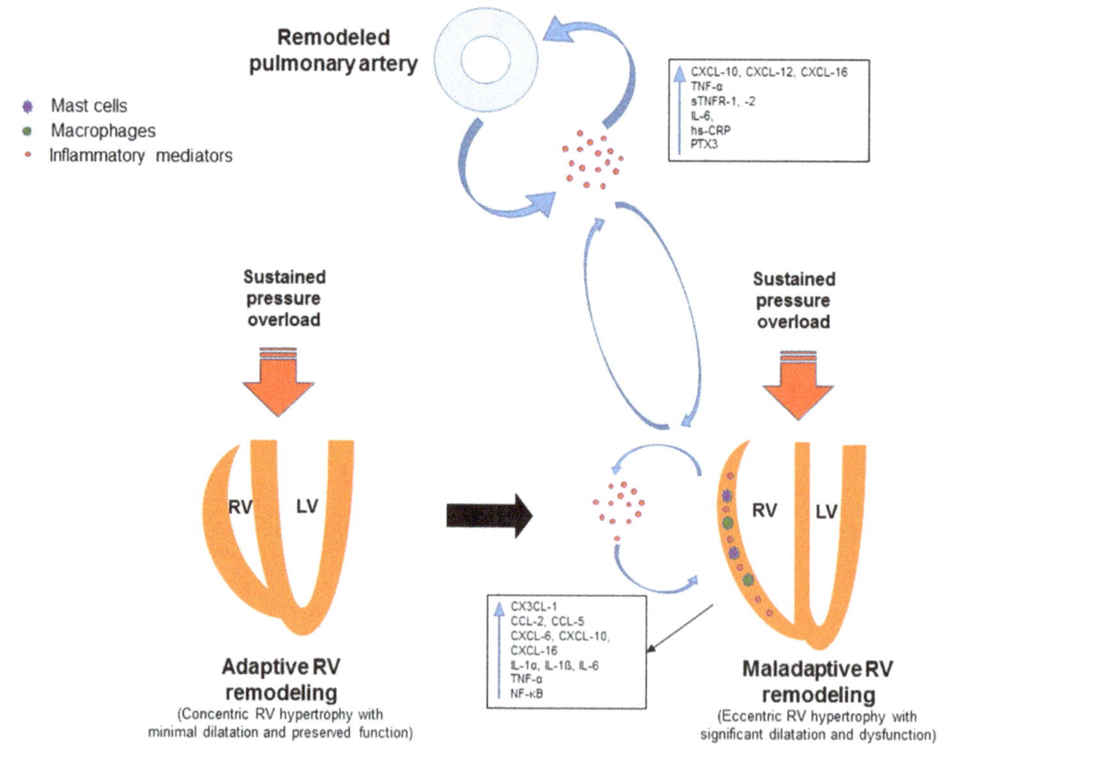

FIGURE 1 | Schematic view of the involvement of inflammatory mediators in adverse right ventricular remodeling and dysfunction. Remodeling of pulmonary vessels in PAH is induced by various pathological mechanisms including inflammatory and autoimmune processes. Circulating inflammatory mediators originating from the pulmonary vasculature may trigger or contribute to inflammatory processes in the pressure-overloaded right ventricle. Inflammation in the right ventricle is characterized by upregulation of pro-inflammatory cytokines and chemokines, expansion of leukocytes, macrophages and mast cells. Upregulated inflammatory mediators contribute to adverse right ventricular remodeling and dysfunction through various mechanisms.

cardiac output (Brown et al., 2017). In another study, effects of continuous exercise training were found to be beneficial only in adaptive RV remodeling (Handoko et al., 2009). In contrast, in progressive PH with maladaptive RV remodeling, continuous exercise training worsened survival and dramatically increased RV leukocyte infiltration (Handoko et al., 2009). It is obvious that effects of exercise training depend on frequency, duration, and intensity of exercise. More studies are therefore necessary to explore a potentially more optimal exercise regimen and to investigate effects of training on RV adaptation/maladaptation. A randomized controlled trial to evaluate the effect of exercise training program on hemodynamics and cardiac magnetic resonance-derived parameters of RV function in patients with PAH (the ExPAH study) is currently underway (Chia et al., 2017).

Currently approved drugs used in the medical management of PAH target endothelin 1, nitric oxide, and prostacyclin pathways, which are important in the control of pulmonary vasomotor tone and vascular cell proliferation (Galie et al., 2016). Although none of the currently approved PAH-specific therapies primarily targets inflammatory mechanisms, there is evidence for anti-inflammatory properties of these drugs (Stasch et al., 2011; Stitham et al., 2011; Watzinger et al., 2016). There are several preclinical studies suggesting that PAH-targeted drugs might influence inflammatory processes in the pressure overloaded right ventricle. In dogs subjected to transient PAB, epoprostenol infusion limited activation of inflammatory processes in the right ventricle (Dewachter et al., 2015). Further, chronic treatment of rats with monocrotaline-induced PH with the endothelin-1 antagonist bosentan was associated with improved RV function and preserved right ventricle-pulmonary artery coupling and reduced cytokine levels in the right ventricle (Fontoura et al., 2014).

Recent experimental studies have demonstrated efficacy of direct anti-inflammatory drugs, including TNF-α antagonists (Wang et al., 2013), anti-CD20 antibodies (Mizuno et al., 2012; Breitling et al., 2017), an inhibitor of T helper 17 cell development SR1001 (Maston et al., 2017), and mast cell stabilizers (Dahal et al., 2011; Bartelds et al., 2012), in attenuating PH. Phase II clinical trials investigating novel drugs targeting inflammation and immune dysfunction in PAH (ubenimex, rituximab, and tocilizumab) are currently underway (Lau et al., 2017). However, data on the effects of anti-inflammatory agents on adverse RV remodeling and dysfunction are scarce. In experimental acute RV failure following PE, several studies have shown that various anti-inflammatory strategies, including treatment with antibodies against polymorphonuclear leukocytes, antibodies to CXCL-1, or anti-inflammatory drug ketorolac can decrease expression of RV inflammatory genes, reduce neutrophil influx, and prevent RV dysfunction (Watts et al., 2006, 2009; Zagorski et al., 2007). Similarly, in rats with chronic RV pressure overload following PAB, treatment with the NF-κB inhibitor pyrrolidine dithiocarbamate decreased macrophage accumulation in the right ventricle, which was associated with improved RV remodeling and function (Yoshida et al., 2016).

CONCLUDING REMARKS

A plethora of inflammatory mediators are upregulated in the right ventricle in response to pressure overload along with accumulation of inflammatory cells (**Figure 1**). However, the exact role of the inflammatory mediators in this context is not established yet. Further studies are required to gain mechanistic insight into how these mediators contribute to maladaptive RV remodeling and dysfunction. A better understanding of the role of inflammation in the pathogenesis of adverse RV remodeling and failure may lead to novel anti-inflammatory therapies for selected patients. Biomarker strategies identifying patient subpopulations with overactive pro-inflammatory signaling may contribute to rational implementation of anti-inflammatory therapies to prevent or reverse RV maladaptive remodeling and dysfunction. Preliminary evidence from preclinical studies suggests that therapeutic approaches targeting specific components of the inflammatory response may be promising for patients with pressure overload-induced adverse RV remodeling and dysfunction.

AUTHOR CONTRIBUTIONS

AS, AM, AP, and DK drafted the manuscript. AS, AM, AP, DK, ASS, HG, NW, and RS revised the manuscript critically for important intellectual content. AS, AM, AP, DK, ASS, HG, NW, and RS approved the final version of the manuscript submitted.

REFERENCES

Ahmed, L. A., Obaid, A. A., Zaki, H. F., and Agha, A. M. (2014). Role of oxidative stress, inflammation, nitric oxide and transforming growth factor-beta in the protective effect of diosgenin in monocrotaline-induced pulmonary hypertension in rats. *Eur. J. Pharmacol.* 740, 379–387. doi: 10.1016/j.ejphar.2014.07.026

Alencar, A. K., Montes, G. C., Montagnoli, T., Silva, A. M., Martinez, S. T., Fraga, A. G., et al. (2017). Activation of GPER ameliorates experimental pulmonary hypertension in male rats. *Eur. J. Pharm. Sci.* 97, 208–217. doi: 10.1016/j.ejps.2016.11.009

Al-Naamani, N., Palevsky, H. I., Lederer, D. J., Horn, E. M., Mathai, S. C., Roberts, K. E., et al. (2016). Prognostic significance of biomarkers in pulmonary arterial hypertension. *Ann. Am. Thorac. Soc.* 13, 25–30. doi: 10.1513/AnnalsATS.201508-543OC

Andersen, N. M., Tang, R., Li, L., Javan, H., Zhang, X. Q., and Selzman, C. H. (2012). Inhibitory κ-B kinase-beta inhibition prevents adaptive left ventricular hypertrophy. *J. Surg. Res.* 178, 105–109. doi: 10.1016/j.jss.2012.03.003

Arena, R., Cahalin, L. P., Borghi-Silva, A., and Myers, J. (2015). The effect of exercise training on the pulmonary arterial system in patients with pulmonary hypertension. *Prog. Cardiovasc. Dis.* 57, 480–488. doi: 10.1016/j.pcad.2014.03.008

Babu, A. S., Padmakumar, R., Maiya, A. G., Mohapatra, A. K., and Kamath, R. L. (2016). Effects of exercise training on exercise capacity in pulmonary arterial hypertension: a systematic review of clinical trials. *Heart Lung Circ.* 25, 333–341. doi: 10.1016/j.hlc.2015.10.015

Badagliacca, R., Poscia, R., Pezzuto, B., Nocioni, M., Mezzapesa, M., Francone, M., et al. (2015). Right ventricular remodeling in idiopathic pulmonary arterial hypertension: adaptive versus maladaptive morphology. *J. Heart Lung Transplant.* 34, 395–403. doi: 10.1016/j.healun.2014.11.002

Bartelds, B., van Loon, R. L. E., Mohaupt, S., Wijnberg, H., Dickinson, M. G., Boersma, B., et al. (2012). Mast cell inhibition improves pulmonary vascular remodeling in pulmonary hypertension. *Chest* 141, 651–660. doi: 10.1378/chest.11-0663

Batlle, M., Roig, E., Perez-Villa, F., Lario, S., Cejudo-Martin, P., Garcia-Pras, E., et al. (2006). Increased expression of the renin-angiotensin system and mast cell density but not of angiotensin-converting enzyme II in late stages of human heart failure. *J. Heart Lung Transplant.* 25, 1117–1125. doi: 10.1016/j.healun.

2006.04.012

Begalli, F., Bennett, J., Capece, D., Verzella, D., D'Andrea, D., Tornatore, L., et al. (2017). Unlocking the NF-κB conundrum: embracing complexity to achieve specificity. *Biomedicines* 5:E50. doi: 10.3390/biomedicines5030050

Begieneman, M. P., van de Goot, F. R., van der Bilt, I. A., Vonk Noordegraaf, A., Spreeuwenberg, M. D., Paulus, W. J., et al. (2008). Pulmonary embolism causes endomyocarditis in the human heart. *Heart* 94, 450–456. doi: 10.1136/hrt.2007.118638

Belhaj, A., Dewachter, L., Kerbaul, F., Brimioulle, S., Dewachter, C., Naeije, R., et al. (2013). Heme oxygenase-1 and inflammation in experimental right ventricular failure on prolonged overcirculation-induced pulmonary hypertension. *PLoS One* 8:e69470. doi: 10.1371/journal.pone.0069470

Birks, E. J., Owen, V. J., Burton, P. B., Bishop, A. E., Banner, N. R., Khaghani, A., et al. (2000). Tumor necrosis factor-alpha is expressed in donor heart and predicts right ventricular failure after human heart transplantation. *Circulation* 102, 326–331. doi: 10.1161/01.CIR.102.3.326

Bozkurt, B., Kribbs, S. B., Clubb, FJ Jr, Michael, L. H., Didenko, V. V., Hornsby, P. J., et al. (1998). Pathophysiologically relevant concentrations of tumor necrosis factor-alpha promote progressive left ventricular dysfunction and remodeling in rats. *Circulation* 97, 1382–1391. doi: 10.1161/01.CIR.97.14.1382

Breitling, S., Hui, Z., Zabini, D., Hu, Y., Hoffmann, J., Goldenberg, N. M., et al. (2017). The mast cell-B cell axis in lung vascular remodeling and pulmonary hypertension. *Am. J. Physiol. Lung Cell. Mol. Physiol.* 312, L710–L721. doi: 10.1152/ajplung.00311.2016

Brower, G. L., Chancey, A. L., Thanigaraj, S., Matsubara, B. B., and Janicki, J. S. (2002). Cause and effect relationship between myocardial mast cell number and matrix metalloproteinase activity. *Am. J. Physiol. Heart Circ. Physiol.* 283, H518–H525. doi: 10.1152/ajpheart.00218.2000

Brown, M. B., Neves, E., Long, G., Graber, J., Gladish, B., Wiseman, A., et al. (2017). High-intensity interval training, but not continuous training, reverses right ventricular hypertrophy and dysfunction in a rat model of pulmonary hypertension. *Am. J. Physiol. Regul. Integr. Comp. Physiol.* 312, R197–R210. doi: 10.1152/ajpregu.00358.2016

Bryant, D., Becker, L., Richardson, J., Shelton, J., Franco, F., Peshock, R., et al. (1998). Cardiac failure in transgenic mice with myocardial expression of tumor necrosis factor-alpha. *Circulation* 97, 1375–1381. doi: 10.1161/01.CIR.97.14.1375

Buys, R., Avila, A., and Cornelissen, V. A. (2015). Exercise training improves physical fitness in patients with pulmonary arterial hypertension: a systematic review and meta-analysis of controlled trials. *BMC Pulm. Med.* 15:40. doi: 10.1186/s12890-015-0031-1

Campian, M. E., Hardziyenka, M., de Bruin, K., van Eck-Smit, B. L., de Bakker, J. M., Verberne, H. J., et al. (2010). Early inflammatory response during the development of right ventricular heart failure in a rat model. *Eur. J. Heart Fail.* 12, 653–658. doi: 10.1093/eurjhf/hfq066

Chia, K. S., Faux, S. G., Wong, P. K., Holloway, C., Assareh, H., McLachlan, C. S., et al. (2017). Randomised controlled trial examining the effect of an outpatient exercise training programme on haemodynamics and cardiac MR parameters of right ventricular function in patients with pulmonary arterial hypertension: the ExPAH study protocol. *BMJ Open* 7:e014037. doi: 10.1136/bmjopen-2016-014037

Chin, K. M., Kim, N. H., and Rubin, L. J. (2005). The right ventricle in pulmonary hypertension. *Coron. Artery Dis.* 16, 13–18. doi: 10.1097/00019501-200502000-00003

Cho, J. H., Kutti Sridharan, G., Kim, S. H., Kaw, R., Abburi, T., Irfan, A., et al. (2014). Right ventricular dysfunction as an echocardiographic prognostic factor in hemodynamically stable patients with acute pulmonary embolism: a meta-analysis. *BMC Cardiovasc. Disord.* 14:64. doi: 10.1186/1471-2261-14-64

Cohn, J. N., Ferrari, R., and Sharpe, N. (2000). Cardiac remodeling–concepts and clinical implications: a consensus paper from an international forum on cardiac remodeling. Behalf of an International Forum on Cardiac Remodeling. *J. Am. Coll. Cardiol.* 35, 569–582. doi: 10.1016/S0735-1097(99)00630-0

Coutance, G., Cauderlier, E., Ehtisham, J., Hamon, M., and Hamon, M. (2011). The prognostic value of markers of right ventricular dysfunction in pulmonary embolism: a meta-analysis. *Crit. Care* 15:R103. doi: 10.1186/cc10119

Cracowski, J. L., Chabot, F., Labarere, J., Faure, P., Degano, B., Schwebel, C., et al. (2014). Proinflammatory cytokine levels are linked to death in pulmonary arterial hypertension. *Eur. Respir. J.* 43, 915–917. doi: 10.1183/09031936.00151313

Dahal, B. K., Kosanovic, D., Kaulen, C., Cornitescu, T., Savai, R., Hoffmann, J., et al. (2011). Involvement of mast cells in monocrotaline-induced pulmonary hypertension in rats. *Respir. Res.* 12:60. doi: 10.1186/1465-9921-12-60

Damilano, F., Franco, I., Perrino, C., Schaefer, K., Azzolino, O., Carnevale, D., et al. (2011). Distinct effects of leukocyte and cardiac phosphoinositide 3-kinase gamma activity in pressure overload-induced cardiac failure. *Circulation* 123, 391–399. doi: 10.1161/circulationaha.110.950543

de Man, F. S., Handoko, M. L., van Ballegoij, J. J., Schalij, I., Bogaards, S. J., Postmus, P. E., et al. (2012). Bisoprolol delays progression towards right heart failure in experimental pulmonary hypertension. *Circ. Heart Fail.* 5, 97–105. doi: 10.1161/circheartfailure.111.964494

Dewachter, C., Belhaj, A., Rondelet, B., Vercruyssen, M., Schraufnagel, D. P., Remmelink, M., et al. (2015). Myocardial inflammation in experimental acute right ventricular failure: effects of prostacyclin therapy. *J. Heart Lung Transplant.* 34, 1334–1345. doi: 10.1016/j.healun.2015.05.004

Dewachter, C., Dewachter, L., Rondelet, B., Fesler, P., Brimioulle, S., Kerbaul, F., et al. (2010). Activation of apoptotic pathways in experimental acute afterload-induced right ventricular failure. *Crit. Care Med.* 38, 1405–1413. doi: 10.1097/CCM.0b013e3181de8bd3

Dinarello, C. A. (2018). Overview of the IL-1 family in innate inflammation and acquired immunity. *Immunol. Rev.* 281, 8–27. doi: 10.1111/imr.12621

Driessen, M. M., Hui, W., Bijnens, B. H., Dragulescu, A., Mertens, L., Meijboom, F. J., et al. (2016). Adverse ventricular-ventricular interactions in right ventricular pressure load: Insights from pediatric pulmonary hypertension versus pulmonary stenosis. *Physiol. Rep.* 4:e12833. doi: 10.14814/phy2.12833

Driessen, M. M. P., Meijboom, F. J., Hui, W., Dragulescu, A., Mertens, L., and Friedberg, M. K. (2017). Regional right ventricular remodeling and function in children with idiopathic pulmonary arterial hypertension vs those with pulmonary valve stenosis: Insights into mechanics of right ventricular dysfunction. *Echocardiography* 34, 888–897. doi: 10.1111/echo.13529

Duncan, M., Wagner, B. D., Murray, K., Allen, J., Colvin, K., Accurso, F. J., et al. (2012). Circulating cytokines and growth factors in pediatric pulmonary hypertension. *Mediators Inflamm.* 2012:143428. doi: 10.1155/2012/143428

Dvorak, A. M. (1986). Mast-cell degranulation in human hearts. *N. Engl. J. Med.* 315, 969–970. doi: 10.1056/NEJM198610093151515

Ehlken, N., Lichtblau, M., Klose, H., Weidenhammer, J., Fischer, C., Nechwatal, R., et al. (2016). Exercise training improves peak oxygen consumption and haemodynamics in patients with severe pulmonary arterial hypertension and inoperable chronic thrombo-embolic pulmonary hypertension: a prospective, randomized, controlled trial. *Eur. Heart J.* 37, 35–44. doi: 10.1093/eurheartj/ehv337

El Chami, H., and Hassoun, P. M. (2011). Inflammatory mechanisms in the pathogenesis of pulmonary arterial hypertension. *Compr. Physiol.* 1, 1929–1941. doi: 10.1002/cphy.c100028

Feldman, A. M., Combes, A., Wagner, D., Kadakomi, T., Kubota, T., Li, Y. Y., et al. (2000). The role of tumor necrosis factor in the pathophysiology of heart failure. *J. Am. Coll. Cardiol.* 35, 537–544. doi: 10.1016/S0735-1097(99)00600-2

Fontes, J. A., Rose, N. R., and Cihakova, D. (2015). The varying faces of IL-6: from cardiac protection to cardiac failure. *Cytokine* 74, 62–68. doi: 10.1016/j.cyto.2014.12.024

Fontoura, D., Oliveira-Pinto, J., Tavares-Silva, M., Leite, S., Vasques-Nóvoa, F., Mendes-Ferreira, P., et al. (2014). Myocardial and anti-inflammatory effects of chronic bosentan therapy in monocrotaline-induced pulmonary hypertension. *Rev. Port. Cardiol.* 33, 213–222. doi: 10.1016/j.repce.2013.09.019

Foris, V., Kovacs, G., Tscherner, M., Olschewski, A., and Olschewski, H. (2013). Biomarkers in pulmonary hypertension: what do we know? *Chest* 144, 274–283. doi: 10.1378/chest.12-1246

Forman, M. F., Brower, G. L., and Janicki, J. S. (2006). Rat cardiac mast cell maturation and differentiation following acute ventricular volume overload. *Inflamm. Res.* 55, 408–415. doi: 10.1007/s00011-006-6016-z

Frump, A. L., Goss, K. N., Vayl, A., Albrecht, M., Fisher, A., Tursunova, R., et al. (2015). Estradiol improves right ventricular function in rats with severe angioproliferative pulmonary hypertension: effects of endogenous and exogenous sex hormones. *Am. J. Physiol. Lung Cell. Mol. Physiol.* 308, L873–L890. doi: 10.1152/ajplung.00006.2015

Furue, M., Mitoma, C., Mitoma, H., Tsuji, G., Chiba, T., Nakahara, T., et al. (2017). Pathogenesis of systemic sclerosis-current concept and emerging treatments. *Immunol. Res.* 65, 790–797. doi: 10.1007/s12026-017-8926-y

Galie, N., Humbert, M., Vachiery, J. L., Gibbs, S., Lang, I., Torbicki, A., et al. (2016). 2015 ESC/ERS guidelines for the diagnosis and treatment of pulmonary hypertension: the joint task force for the diagnosis and treatment of pulmonary hypertension of the European society of cardiology (ESC) and the European respiratory society (ERS): endorsed by: association for European paediatric and congenital cardiology (AEPC), international society for heart and lung transplantation (ISHLT). *Eur. Heart J.* 37, 67–119. doi: 10.1093/eurheartj/ehv317

Gilfillan, A. M., and Beaven, M. A. (2011). Regulation of mast cell responses in health and disease. *Crit. Rev. Immunol.* 31, 475–529. doi: 10.1615/CritRevImmunol.v31.i6.30

Glezeva, N., Horgan, S., and Baugh, J. A. (2015). Monocyte and macrophage subsets along the continuum to heart failure: misguided heroes or targetable villains? *J. Mol. Cell. Cardiol.* 89(Pt B), 136–145. doi: 10.1016/j.yjmcc.2015.10.029

Grignola, J. C., and Domingo, E. (2017). Acute right ventricular dysfunction in intensive care unit. *BioMed Res. Int.* 2017:8217105. doi: 10.1155/2017/8217105

Guihaire, J., Deuse, T., Wang, D., Fadel, E., Reichenspurner, H., Robbins, R. C., et al. (2017). Pulmonary hypertension: macrophage infiltration corelates with right ventricular remodeling in an experimental model of pulmonary hypertension. *J. Heart Lung Transplant.* 36, S370–S370. doi: 10.1016/j.healun.2017.01.1050

Gupta, S., Young, D., Maitra, R. K., Gupta, A., Popovic, Z. B., Yong, S. L., et al. (2008). Prevention of cardiac hypertrophy and heart failure by silencing of NF-κB. *J. Mol. Biol.* 375, 637–649. doi: 10.1016/j.jmb.2007.10.006

Haddad, F., Doyle, R., Murphy, D. J., and Hunt, S. A. (2008). Right ventricular function in cardiovascular disease, part II: pathophysiology, clinical importance, and management of right ventricular failure. *Circulation* 117, 1717–1731. doi: 10.1161/circulationaha.107.653584

Handoko, M. L., de Man, F. S., Happe, C. M., Schalij, I., Musters, R. J., Westerhof, N., et al. (2009). Opposite effects of training in rats with stable and progressive pulmonary hypertension. *Circulation* 120, 42–49. doi: 10.1161/circulationaha.108.829713

Hara, M., Ono, K., Hwang, M. W., Iwasaki, A., Okada, M., Nakatani, K., et al. (2002). Evidence for a role of mast cells in the evolution to congestive heart failure. *J. Exp. Med.* 195, 375–381. doi: 10.1084/jem.20002036

Harbaum, L., Renk, E., Yousef, S., Glatzel, A., Luneburg, N., Hennigs, J. K., et al. (2016). Acute effects of exercise on the inflammatory state in patients with idiopathic pulmonary arterial hypertension. *BMC Pulm. Med.* 16:145. doi: 10.1186/s12890-016-0301-6

Harhay, M. O., Tracy, R. P., Bagiella, E., Barr, R. G., Pinder, D., Hundley, W. G., et al. (2013). Relationship of CRP, IL-6, and fibrinogen with right ventricular structure and function: the MESA-Right Ventricle Study. *Int. J. Cardiol.* 168, 3818–3824. doi: 10.1016/j.ijcard.2013.06.028

Hassoun, P. M., Mouthon, L., Barbera, J. A., Eddahibi, S., Flores, S. C., Grimminger, F., et al. (2009). Inflammation, growth factors, and pulmonary vascular remodeling. *J. Am. Coll. Cardiol.* 54(1 Suppl), S10–S19. doi: 10.1016/j.jacc.2009.04.006

Heresi, G. A., Aytekin, M., Hammel, J. P., Wang, S., Chatterjee, S., and Dweik, R. A. (2014). Plasma interleukin-6 adds prognostic information in pulmonary arterial hypertension. *Eur. Respir. J.* 43, 912–914. doi: 10.1183/09031936.00164713

Heresi, G. A., Aytekin, M., Newman, J., and Dweik, R. A. (2010). CXC-chemokine ligand 10 in idiopathic pulmonary arterial hypertension: marker of improved survival. *Lung* 188, 191–197. doi: 10.1007/s00408-010-9232-9

Humbert, M., Monti, G., Brenot, F., Sitbon, O., Portier, A., Grangeot-Keros, L., et al. (1995). Increased interleukin-1 and interleukin-6 serum concentrations in severe primary pulmonary hypertension. *Am. J. Respir. Crit. Care Med.* 151, 1628–1631. doi: 10.1164/ajrccm.151.5.7735624

Iwadate, K., Doi, M., Tanno, K., Katsumura, S., Ito, H., Sato, K., et al. (2003). Right ventricular damage due to pulmonary embolism: examination of the number of infiltrating macrophages. *Forensic Sci. Int.* 134, 147–153. doi: 10.1016/S0379-0738(03)00138-5

Iwadate, K., Tanno, K., Doi, M., Takatori, T., and Ito, Y. (2001). Two cases of right ventricular ischemic injury due to massive pulmonary embolism. *Forensic Sci. Int.* 116, 189–195. doi: 10.1016/S0379-0738(00)00367-4

Janssen, S. P., Gayan-Ramirez, G., Van den Bergh, A., Herijgers, P., Maes, K., Verbeken, E., et al. (2005). Interleukin-6 causes myocardial failure and skeletal muscle atrophy in rats. *Circulation* 111, 996–1005. doi: 10.1161/01.cir.0000156469.96135.0d

Javan, H., Szucsik, A. M., Li, L., Schaaf, C. L., Salama, M. E., and Selzman, C. H. (2015). Cardiomyocyte p65 nuclear factor-kappaB is necessary for compensatory adaptation to pressure overload. *Circ. Heart Fail.* 8, 109–118. doi: 10.1161/circheartfailure.114.001297

Jurcut, R., Giusca, S., Ticulescu, R., Popa, E., Amzulescu, M. S., Ghiorghiu, I., et al. (2011). Different patterns of adaptation of the right ventricle to pressure overload: a comparison between pulmonary hypertension and pulmonary stenosis. *J. Am. Soc. Echocardiogr.* 24, 1109–1117. doi: 10.1016/j.echo.2011.07.016

Kapadia, S. R., Oral, H., Lee, J., Nakano, M., Taffet, G. E., and Mann, D. L. (1997). Hemodynamic regulation of tumor necrosis factor-alpha gene and protein expression in adult feline myocardium. *Circ. Res.* 81, 187–195. doi: 10.1161/01.RES.81.2.187

Karakurt, C., Baspinar, O., Celik, F. S., Taskapan, C., Sahin, A. D., and Yologlu, S. (2014). Serum pentraxin 3 and hs-CRP levels in children with severe pulmonary hypertension. *Balkan Med. J.* 31, 219–223. doi: 10.5152/balkanmedj.2014.13307

Kato, M., and Atsumi, T. (2017). Pulmonary arterial hypertension associated with connective tissue diseases: a review focusing on distinctive clinical aspects. *Eur. J. Clin. Invest.* 48:e12876. doi: 10.1111/eci.12876

Kubota, T., McTiernan, C. F., Frye, C. S., Slawson, S. E., Lemster, B. H., Koretsky, A. P., et al. (1997). Dilated cardiomyopathy in transgenic mice with cardiac-specific overexpression of tumor necrosis factor-alpha. *Circ. Res.* 81, 627–635. doi: 10.1161/01.RES.81.4.627

Laroumanie, F., Douin-Echinard, V., Pozzo, J., Lairez, O., Tortosa, F., Vinel, C., et al. (2014). CD4+ T cells promote the transition from hypertrophy to heart failure during chronic pressure overload. *Circulation* 129, 2111–2124. doi: 10.1161/circulationaha.113.007101

Lau, E. M. T., Giannoulatou, E., Celermajer, D. S., and Humbert, M. (2017). Epidemiology and treatment of pulmonary arterial hypertension. *Nat. Rev. Cardiol.* 14, 603–614. doi: 10.1038/nrcardio.2017.84

Launay, D., Sobanski, V., Hachulla, E., and Humbert, M. (2017). Pulmonary hypertension in systemic sclerosis: different phenotypes. *Eur. Respir. Rev.* 26:170056. doi: 10.1183/16000617.0056-2017

Levick, S. P., McLarty, J. L., Murray, D. B., Freeman, R. M., Carver, W. E., and Brower, G. L. (2009). Cardiac mast cells mediate left ventricular fibrosis in the hypertensive rat heart. *Hypertension* 53, 1041–1047. doi: 10.1161/hypertensionaha.108.123158

Levick, S. P., Melendez, G. C., Plante, E., McLarty, J. L., Brower, G. L., and Janicki, J. S. (2011). Cardiac mast cells: the centrepiece in adverse myocardial remodelling. *Cardiovasc. Res.* 89, 12–19. doi: 10.1093/cvr/cvq272

Li, J., Jubair, S., Levick, S. P., and Janicki, J. S. (2016). The autocrine role of tryptase in pressure overload-induced mast cell activation, chymase release and cardiac fibrosis. *IJC Metab. Endocr.* 10, 16–23. doi: 10.1016/j.ijcme.2015.11.003

Liu, M., Chen, J., Huang, D., Ke, J., and Wu, W. (2014). A meta-analysis of proinflammatory cytokines in chronic heart failure. *Heart Asia* 6, 130–136. doi: 10.1136/heartasia-2013-010484

Luitel, H., Sydykov, A., Schymura, Y., Mamazhakypov, A., Janssen, W., Pradhan, K., et al. (2017). Pressure overload leads to an increased accumulation and activity of mast cells in the right ventricle. *Physiol. Rep.* 5:e13146. doi: 10.14814/phy2.13146

Maier, H. J., Schips, T. G., Wietelmann, A., Kruger, M., Brunner, C., Sauter, M., et al. (2012). Cardiomyocyte-specific IkappaB kinase (IKK)/NF-κB activation induces reversible inflammatory cardiomyopathy and heart failure. *Proc. Natl. Acad. Sci. U.S.A.* 109, 11794–11799. doi: 10.1073/pnas.1116584109

Mann, D. L. (2015). Innate immunity and the failing heart: the cytokine hypothesis revisited. *Circ. Res.* 116, 1254–1268. doi: 10.1161/circresaha.116.302317

Maston, L. D., Jones, D. T., Giermakowska, W., Howard, T. A., Cannon, J. L., Wang, W., et al. (2017). Central role of T helper 17 cells in chronic hypoxia-induced pulmonary hypertension. *Am. J. Physiol. Lung Cell. Mol. Physiol.* 312, L609–L624. doi: 10.1152/ajplung.00531.2016

Mathai, S. C., Sibley, C. T., Forfia, P. R., Mudd, J. O., Fisher, M. R., Tedford, R. J., et al. (2011). Tricuspid annular plane systolic excursion is a robust outcome measure in systemic sclerosis-associated pulmonary arterial hypertension. *J. Rheumatol.* 38, 2410–2418. doi: 10.3899/jrheum.110512

Matsumoto, T., Wada, A., Tsutamoto, T., Ohnishi, M., Isono, T., and Kinoshita, M. (2003). Chymase inhibition prevents cardiac fibrosis and improves diastolic dysfunction in the progression of heart failure. *Circulation* 107, 2555–2558. doi: 10.1161/01.cir.0000074041.81728.79

Matura, L. A., McDonough, A., Hanlon, A. L., and Carroll, D. L. (2015). Development and initial psychometric properties of the pulmonary arterial hypertension symptom scale (PAHSS). *Appl. Nurs. Res.* 28, 42–47. doi: 10.1016/j.apnr.2014.04.001

McMahan, Z., Schoenhoff, F., Van Eyk, J. E., Wigley, F. M., and Hummers, L. K. (2015). Biomarkers of pulmonary hypertension in patients with scleroderma: a case-control study. *Arthritis Res. Ther.* 17:201. doi: 10.1186/s13075-015-0712-4

Meinel, F. G., Nance, J. W. Jr., Schoepf, U. J., Hoffmann, V. S., Thierfelder, K. M., Costello, P., et al. (2015). Predictive value of computed tomography in acute pulmonary embolism: systematic review and meta-analysis. *Am. J. Med.* 128, 747.e–759.e. doi: 10.1016/j.amjmed.2015.01.023

Mizuno, S., Farkas, L., Al Husseini, A., Farkas, D., Gomez-Arroyo, J., Kraskauskas, D., et al. (2012). Severe pulmonary arterial hypertension induced by SU5416 and ovalbumin immunization. *Am. J. Respir. Cell Mol. Biol.* 47, 679–687. doi: 10.1165/rcmb.2012-0077OC

Moreira-Goncalves, D., Ferreira, R., Fonseca, H., Padrao, A. I., Moreno, N., Silva, A. F., et al. (2015). Cardioprotective effects of early and late aerobic exercise training in experimental pulmonary arterial hypertension. *Basic Res. Cardiol.* 110:57. doi: 10.1007/s00395-015-0514-5

Mukherjee, M., Mercurio, V., Tedford, R. J., Shah, A. A., Hsu, S., Mullin, C. J., et al. (2017). Right ventricular longitudinal strain is diminished in systemic sclerosis compared with idiopathic pulmonary arterial hypertension. *Eur. Respir. J.* 50:1701436. doi: 10.1183/13993003.01436-2017

Mylonas, K. J., Jenkins, S. J., Castellan, R. F., Ruckerl, D., McGregor, K., Phythian-Adams, A. T., et al. (2015). The adult murine heart has a sparse, phagocytically active macrophage population that expands through monocyte recruitment and adopts an 'M2' phenotype in response to Th2 immunologic challenge. *Immunobiology* 220, 924–933. doi: 10.1016/j.imbio.2015.01.013

Nergui, S., Fukumoto, Y., Do, E. Z., Nakajima, S., Shimizu, T., Ikeda, S., et al. (2014). Role of endothelial nitric oxide synthase and collagen metabolism in right ventricular remodeling due to pulmonary hypertension. *Circ. J.* 78, 1465–1474. doi: 10.1253/circj.CJ-13-1586

Nevers, T., Salvador, A. M., Grodecki-Pena, A., Knapp, A., Velazquez, F., Aronovitz, M., et al. (2015). Left ventricular T-cell recruitment contributes to the pathogenesis of heart failure. *Circ. Heart Fail.* 8, 776–787. doi: 10.1161/circheartfailure.115.002225

Nogueira-Ferreira, R., Moreira-Goncalves, D., Silva, A. F., Duarte, J. A., Leite-Moreira, A., Ferreira, R., et al. (2016). Exercise preconditioning prevents MCT-induced right ventricle remodeling through the regulation of TNF superfamily cytokines. *Int. J. Cardiol.* 203, 858–866. doi: 10.1016/j.ijcard.2015.11.066

Novoyatleva, T., Sajjad, A., and Engel, F. B. (2014). TWEAK-Fn14 cytokine-receptor axis: a new player of myocardial remodeling and cardiac failure. *Front. Immunol.* 5:50. doi: 10.3389/fimmu.2014.00050

Novoyatleva, T., Schymura, Y., Janssen, W., Strobl, F., Swiercz, J. M., Patra, C., et al. (2013). Deletion of Fn14 receptor protects from right heart fibrosis and dysfunction. *Basic Res. Cardiol.* 108:325. doi: 10.1007/s00395-012-0325-x

Odeh, M., Sabo, E., and Oliven, A. (2006). Circulating levels of tumor necrosis factor-alpha correlate positively with severity of peripheral oedema in patients with right heart failure. *Eur. J. Heart Fail.* 8, 141–146. doi: 10.1016/j.ejheart.2005.05.010

Olivetti, G., Lagrasta, C., Ricci, R., Sonnenblick, E. H., Capasso, J. M., and Anversa, P. (1989). Long-term pressure-induced cardiac hypertrophy: capillary and mast cell proliferation. *Am. J. Physiol.* 257(6 Pt 2), H1766–H1772. doi: 10.1152/ajpheart.1989.257.6.H1766

Overbeek, M. J., Mouchaers, K. T., Niessen, H. M., Hadi, A. M., Kupreishvili, K., Boonstra, A., et al. (2010). Characteristics of interstitial fibrosis and inflammatory cell infiltration in right ventricles of systemic sclerosis-associated pulmonary arterial hypertension. *Int. J. Rheumatol.* 2010:604615. doi: 10.1155/2010/604615

Panizo, A., Mindan, F. J., Galindo, M. F., Cenarruzabeitia, E., Hernandez, M., and Diez, J. (1995). Are mast cells involved in hypertensive heart disease? *J. Hypertens.* 13, 1201–1208. doi: 10.1097/00004872-199510000-00015

Paulin, R., Sutendra, G., Gurtu, V., Dromparis, P., Haromy, A., Provencher, S., et al. (2015). A miR-208-Mef2 axis drives the decompensation of right ventricular function in pulmonary hypertension. *Circ. Res.* 116, 56–69. doi: 10.1161/circresaha.115.303910

Pedersen, B. K. (2017). Anti-inflammatory effects of exercise: role in diabetes and cardiovascular disease. *Eur. J. Clin. Invest.* 47, 600–611. doi: 10.1111/eci.12781

Pinto, A. R., Ilinykh, A., Ivey, M. J., Kuwabara, J. T., D'Antoni, M. L., Debuque, R., et al. (2016). Revisiting cardiac cellular composition. *Circ. Res.* 118, 400–409. doi: 10.1161/circresaha.115.307778

Plenz, G., Song, Z. F., Tjan, T. D., Koenig, C., Baba, H. A., Erren, M., et al. (2001). Activation of the cardiac interleukin-6 system in advanced heart failure. *Eur. J. Heart Fail.* 3, 415–421. doi: 10.1016/S1388-9842(01)00137-4

Price, L. C., Wort, S. J., Perros, F., Dorfmuller, P., Huertas, A., Montani, D., et al. (2012). Inflammation in pulmonary arterial hypertension. *Chest* 141, 210–221. doi: 10.1378/chest.11-0793

Prins, K. W., Archer, S. L., Pritzker, M., Rose, L., Weir, E. K., Sharma, A., et al. (2017). Interleukin-6 is independently associated with right ventricular function in pulmonary arterial hypertension. *J. Heart Lung Transplant.* 37, 376–384. doi: 10.1016/j.healun.2017.08.011

Quarck, R., Nawrot, T., Meyns, B., and Delcroix, M. (2009). C-reactive protein: a new predictor of adverse outcome in pulmonary arterial hypertension. *J. Am. Coll. Cardiol.* 53, 1211–1218. doi: 10.1016/j.jacc.2008.12.038

Rakusan, K., Sarkar, K., Turek, Z., and Wicker, P. (1990). Mast cells in the rat heart during normal growth and in cardiac hypertrophy. *Circ. Res.* 66, 511–516. doi: 10.1161/01.RES.66.2.511

Rice, K. M., Manne, N. D., Kolli, M. B., Wehner, P. S., Dornon, L., Arvapalli, R., et al. (2016). Curcumin nanoparticles attenuate cardiac remodeling due to pulmonary arterial hypertension. *Artif. Cells Nanomed. Biotechnol.* 44, 1909–1916. doi: 10.3109/21691401.2015.1111235

Rondelet, B., Dewachter, C., Kerbaul, F., Kang, X., Fesler, P., Brimioulle, S., et al. (2012). Prolonged overcirculation-induced pulmonary arterial hypertension as a cause of right ventricular failure. *Eur. Heart J.* 33, 1017–1026. doi: 10.1093/eurheartj/ehr111

Salvador, A. M., Nevers, T., Velazquez, F., Aronovitz, M., Wang, B., Abadia Molina, A., et al. (2016). Intercellular adhesion molecule 1 regulates left ventricular leukocyte infiltration, cardiac remodeling, and function in pressure overload-induced heart failure. *J. Am. Heart Assoc.* 5:e003126. doi: 10.1161/jaha.115.003126

Sanchez-Trujillo, L., Vazquez-Garza, E., Castillo, E. C., Garcia-Rivas, G., and Torre-Amione, G. (2017). Role of adaptive immunity in the development and progression of heart failure: new evidence. *Arch. Med. Res.* 48, 1–11. doi: 10.1016/j.arcmed.2016.12.008

Selimovic, N., Bergh, C. H., Andersson, B., Sakiniene, E., Carlsten, H., and Rundqvist, B. (2009). Growth factors and interleukin-6 across the lung circulation in pulmonary hypertension. *Eur. Respir. J.* 34, 662–668. doi: 10.1183/09031936.00174908

Shiota, N., Rysa, J., Kovanen, P. T., Ruskoaho, H., Kokkonen, J. O., and Lindstedt, K. A. (2003). A role for cardiac mast cells in the pathogenesis of hypertensive heart disease. *J. Hypertens.* 21, 1935–1944. doi: 10.1097/01.hjh.0000084766.37215.f2

Soon, E., Holmes, A. M., Treacy, C. M., Doughty, N. J., Southgate, L., Machado, R. D., et al. (2010). Elevated levels of inflammatory cytokines predict survival in idiopathic and familial pulmonary arterial hypertension. *Circulation* 122, 920–927. doi: 10.1161/circulationaha.109.933762

Stasch, J. P., Pacher, P., and Evgenov, O. V. (2011). Soluble guanylate cyclase as an emerging therapeutic target in cardiopulmonary disease. *Circulation* 123, 2263–2273. doi: 10.1161/circulationaha.110.981738

Stitham, J., Midgett, C., Martin, K. A., and Hwa, J. (2011). Prostacyclin: an inflammatory paradox. *Front. Pharmacol.* 2:24. doi: 10.3389/fphar.2011.00024

Sun, M., Chen, M., Dawood, F., Zurawska, U., Li, J. Y., Parker, T., et al. (2007). Tumor necrosis factor-alpha mediates cardiac remodeling and ventricular dysfunction after pressure overload state. *Circulation* 115, 1398–1407. doi: 10.1161/circulationaha.106.643585

Sztrymf, B., Souza, R., Bertoletti, L., Jais, X., Sitbon, O., Price, L. C., et al. (2010). Prognostic factors of acute heart failure in patients with pulmonary arterial hypertension. *Eur. Respir. J.* 35, 1286–1293. doi: 10.1183/09031936.00070209

Tedford, R. J., Mudd, J. O., Girgis, R. E., Mathai, S. C., Zaiman, A. L., Housten-Harris, T., et al. (2013). Right ventricular dysfunction in systemic sclerosis-associated pulmonary arterial hypertension. *Circ. Heart Fail.* 6, 953–963. doi: 10.1161/circheartfailure.112.000008

Trujillo-Santos, J., den Exter, P. L., Gomez, V., Del Castillo, H., Moreno, C., van der Hulle, T., et al. (2013). Computed tomography-assessed right ventricular dysfunction and risk stratification of patients with acute non-massive pulmonary embolism: systematic review and meta-analysis. *J. Thromb. Haemost.* 11, 1823–1832. doi: 10.1111/jth.12393

Van Linthout, S., and Tschope, C. (2017). Inflammation - cause or consequence of heart failure or both? *Curr. Heart Fail. Rep.* 14, 251–265. doi: 10.1007/s11897-017-0337-9

Van Tassell, B. W., Raleigh, J. M., and Abbate, A. (2015). Targeting interleukin-1 in heart failure and inflammatory heart disease. *Curr. Heart Fail. Rep.* 12, 33–41. doi: 10.1007/s11897-014-0231-7

Velten, M., Duerr, G. D., Pessies, T., Schild, J., Lohner, R., Mersmann, J., et al. (2012). Priming with synthetic oligonucleotides attenuates pressure overload-induced inflammation and cardiac hypertrophy in mice. *Cardiovasc. Res.* 96, 422–432. doi: 10.1093/cvr/cvs280

Vistnes, M., Waehre, A., Nygard, S., Sjaastad, I., Andersson, K. B., Husberg, C., et al. (2010). Circulating cytokine levels in mice with heart failure are etiology dependent. *J. Appl. Physiol.* 108, 1357–1364. doi: 10.1152/japplphysiol.01084.2009

Vitarelli, A., Barilla, F., Capotosto, L., D'Angeli, I., Truscelli, G., De Maio, M., et al. (2014). Right ventricular function in acute pulmonary embolism: a combined assessment by three-dimensional and speckle-tracking echocardiography. *J. Am. Soc. Echocardiogr.* 27, 329–338. doi: 10.1016/j.echo.2013.11.013

von Haehling, S., von Bardeleben, R. S., Kramm, T., Thiermann, Y., Niethammer, M., Doehner, W., et al. (2010). Inflammation in right ventricular dysfunction due to thromboembolic pulmonary hypertension. *Int. J. Cardiol.* 144, 206–211. doi: 10.1016/j.ijcard.2009.04.019

Vonk-Noordegraaf, A., Haddad, F., Chin, K. M., Forfia, P. R., Kawut, S. M., Lumens, J., et al. (2013). Right heart adaptation to pulmonary arterial hypertension: physiology and pathobiology. *J. Am. Coll. Cardiol.* 62, D22–D33. doi: 10.1016/j.jacc.2013.10.027

Waehre, A., Vistnes, M., Sjaastad, I., Nygard, S., Husberg, C., Lunde, I. G., et al. (2012). Chemokines regulate small leucine-rich proteoglycans in the extracellular matrix of the pressure-overloaded right ventricle. *J. Appl. Physiol.* 112, 1372–1382. doi: 10.1152/japplphysiol.01350.2011

Wang, J. J., Zuo, X. R., Xu, J., Zhou, J. Y., Kong, H., Zeng, X. N., et al. (2016). Evaluation and treatment of endoplasmic reticulum (ER) stress in right ventricular dysfunction during monocrotaline-induced rat pulmonary arterial hypertension. *Cardiovasc. Drugs Ther.* 30, 587–598. doi: 10.1007/s10557-016-6702-1

Wang, Q., Zuo, X. R., Wang, Y. Y., Xie, W. P., Wang, H., and Zhang, M. (2013). Monocrotaline-induced pulmonary arterial hypertension is attenuated by TNF-α antagonists via the suppression of TNF-α expression and NF-κB pathway in rats. *Vascul. Pharmacol.* 58, 71–77. doi: 10.1016/j.vph.2012.07.006

Watts, J. A., Gellar, M. A., Stuart, L. K., Obraztsova, M., and Kline, J. A. (2009). Proinflammatory events in right ventricular damage during pulmonary embolism: effects of treatment with ketorolac in rats. *J. Cardiovasc. Pharmacol.* 54, 246–252. doi: 10.1097/FJC.0b013e3181b2b699

Watts, J. A., Zagorski, J., Gellar, M. A., Stevinson, B. G., and Kline, J. A. (2006). Cardiac inflammation contributes to right ventricular dysfunction following experimental pulmonary embolism in rats. *J. Mol. Cell. Cardiol.* 41, 296–307. doi: 10.1016/j.yjmcc.2006.05.011

Watzinger, K., Tancevski, I., Sonnweber, T., and Löffler-Ragg, J. (2016). Antiinflammatory properties of PAH drugs. *Eur. Respir. J.* 48(Suppl. 60), A1818. doi: 10.1183/13993003.congress-2016.PA1818

Weisheit, C., Zhang, Y., Faron, A., Kopke, O., Weisheit, G., Steinstrasser, A., et al. (2014). Ly6C(low) and not Ly6C(high) macrophages accumulate first in the heart in a model of murine pressure-overload. *PLoS One* 9:e112710. doi: 10.1371/journal.pone.0112710

Xia, Y., Lee, K., Li, N., Corbett, D., Mendoza, L., and Frangogiannis, N. G. (2009). Characterization of the inflammatory and fibrotic response in a mouse model of cardiac pressure overload. *Histochem. Cell Biol.* 131, 471–481. doi: 10.1007/s00418-008-0541-5

Yang, T., Li, Z. N., Chen, G., Gu, Q., Ni, X. H., Zhao, Z. H., et al. (2014). Increased levels of plasma CXC-Chemokine Ligand 10, 12 and 16 are associated with right ventricular function in patients with idiopathic pulmonary arterial hypertension. *Heart Lung* 43, 322–327. doi: 10.1016/j.hrtlng.2014.04.016

Yoshida, K., Abe, K., Saku, K., and Sunagawa, K. (2016). Inhibition of nuclear factor-kappaB-mediated inflammation reverses fibrosis and improves rv function in rats with pulmonary artery banding. *J. Card. Fail.* 22:S198. doi: 10.1016/j.cardfail.2016.07.244

Yoshida, K., Abe, K., Tanaka, M., Shinoda, M., Kuwabara, Y., Saku, K., et al. (2015). Abstract 15221: Pulmonary artery banding induces NF-κB activated inflammation and deteriorates rv function. *Circulation* 132(Suppl. 3), A15221–A15221.

Zagorski, J., Gellar, M. A., Obraztsova, M., Kline, J. A., and Watts, J. A. (2007). Inhibition of CINC-1 decreases right ventricular damage caused by experimental pulmonary embolism in rats. *J. Immunol.* 179, 7820–7826. doi: 10.4049/jimmunol.179.11.7820

Zagorski, J., Sanapareddy, N., Gellar, M. A., Kline, J. A., and Watts, J. A. (2008). Transcriptional profile of right ventricular tissue during acute pulmonary embolism in rats. *Physiol. Genomics* 34, 101–111. doi: 10.1152/physiolgenomics.00261.2007

Zhao, L., Cheng, G., Jin, R., Afzal, M. R., Samanta, A., Xuan, Y. T., et al. (2016). Deletion of interleukin-6 attenuates pressure overload-induced left ventricular hypertrophy and dysfunction. *Circ. Res.* 118, 1918–1929. doi: 10.1161/circresaha.116.308688

16

Pulmonary Arterial Stiffness: An Early and Pervasive Driver of Pulmonary Arterial Hypertension

*Wei Sun and Stephen Y. Chan**

Division of Cardiology, Department of Medicine, Center for Pulmonary Vascular Biology and Medicine, Pittsburgh Heart, Lung, Blood, and Vascular Medicine Institute, University of Pittsburgh School of Medicine and University of Pittsburgh Medical Center, Pittsburgh, PA, United States

***Correspondence:**
Stephen Y. Chan
chansy@pitt.edu

Pulmonary arterial hypertension (PAH) is a historically neglected and highly morbid vascular disease that leads to right heart failure and, in some cases, death. The molecular origins of this disease have been poorly defined, and as such, current pulmonary vasodilator therapies do not cure or reverse this disease. Although extracellular matrix (ECM) remodeling and pulmonary arterial stiffening have long been associated with end-stage PAH, recent studies have reported that such vascular stiffening can occur early in pathogenesis. Furthermore, there is emerging evidence that ECM stiffening may represent a key first step in pathogenic reprogramming and molecular crosstalk among endothelial, smooth muscle, and fibroblast cells in the remodeled pulmonary vessel. Such processes represent the convergence of activation of a number of specific mechanoactivated signaling pathways, microRNAs, and metabolic pathways in pulmonary vasculature. In this review, we summarize the contemporary understanding of vascular stiffening as a driver of PAH, its mechanisms, potential therapeutic targets and clinical perspectives. Of note, early intervention targeting arterial stiffness may break the vicious cycle of PAH progression, leading to outcome improvement which has not been demonstrated by current vasodilator therapy.

Keywords: pulmonary arterial hypertension, arterial stiffness, endothelium, extracellular matrix, vascular metabolism

INTRODUCTION

Pulmonary hypertension (PH) is defined as an elevation of the mean pulmonary artery pressure above 25 mmHg at rest. It can be divided into 5 clinical groups according to the World Health Organization (WHO) Classification of PH, last updated in 2013 (1) and scheduled to be revised later in 2018. Briefly, Group 1 PH is pulmonary arterial hypertension (PAH), often familial or heritable, related to connective tissue disease or toxins, with unknown underlying etiology (idiopathic PH). Group 2 refers to PH caused by left heart disease (pulmonary vein hypertension). Group 3 includes pulmonary hypertension resulting from lung diseases or hypoxia, such as chronic obstructive lung disease or sleep apnea. Group 4 disease is related to chronic thromboembolic obstruction in pulmonary arteries. Group 5 includes other less-common causes such as hematological or metabolic disorders that do not fit into any of the other four groups. The different groups of PH differ not only in fundamental pathogenesis but also patients' prognosis and corresponding treatment strategies. As a severe form of PH, PAH (WHO clinical Group 1) is a devastating condition characterized by progressive pulmonary vascular remodeling and gradual obstruction of pulmonary arterioles (at times, from pathognomonic plexiform lesions), resulting in increased pulmonary vascular resistance and pressure. The increase in pulmonary arterial pressure can lead to right ventricular heart hypertrophy, failure, and premature death.

PAH has idiopathic, heritable, and comorbid etiologies, associated with other chronic diseases. Although PAH is a highly morbid disease, it has been historically neglected since symptoms such as dyspnea and right heart failure often present late in disease. The onset of PH symptoms is unfortunately associated with a markedly impaired prognosis, and the historical survival rate of PAH without treatment is only 34% at 5 years (2). The current treatment options for PAH—including calcium-channel blockers, prostanoids, endothelin receptor antagonists, and phosphodiesterase inhibitors/soluble guanylyl cyclase agonists—primarily target pulmonary vascular dilation, thus lowering pulmonary arterial pressure, providing symptom relief and prolonging of the time to clinical deterioration. These treatments, however, are not curative and do not stop or reverse this disease. This may stem from the fact that these medications largely do not target to molecular origins of PAH (3), many of which still remain poorly defined. As such, there are obvious and critical needs, both scientifically and clinically, for advanced insights into the mechanisms of PAH pathogenesis in order to identify novel biomarkers for the early detection of PAH, to offer valid prognosis estimation, and to define novel targets for specific molecular therapeutics.

In this article, we will focus on the emerging appreciation of pulmonary vascular and extracellular matrix (ECM) stiffening as a distinct and early initiating cause of PAH. We will summarize the current understanding of pulmonary vascular stiffening, which serves not only as a consequence of PAH but also a critical driver of disease. We will review the progress in the studies on the mechanisms of pulmonary vascular stiffening, the potential therapeutic targets, and relevant clinical perspectives.

PULMONARY ARTERIAL STIFFENING AND ECM REMODELING IN PAH

Pulmonary Arterial Remodeling and Stiffening

Pulmonary arterial stiffening is a key component in the pathogenesis of PAH. Stiffness occurs in the proximal and distal pulmonary arteries in multiple subtypes of PAH (4, 5), and stiffness can serve as an index of disease progression (6). At the histologic level, pulmonary vessel stiffening in PAH is characterized by the activation and proliferation of all cellular subtypes in the three layers of the pulmonary arterial wall, including endothelial cells of the tunica intima, vascular smooth muscle cells of the tunica media, as well as adventitial fibroblasts. Spatially and functionally associated with the endothelial cell layer in the intima, the fibroblasts and myofibroblasts in the media and adventitia are activated, resulting in the synthesis and stromal deposition of ECM components. Within the tunica media, activated smooth muscle cells together with myofibroblasts derived from the adventitia can also migrate into the endothelial cell layer. As a result of this complex interplay between cells and ECM components, a concentric hyperplasia of the tunica intima develops (7). Of note, there is convincing evidence to suggest the active interaction between inflammatory cells especially macrophages with pulmonary arterial cells which plays important roles in the pathogenesis of PAH (8). Interestingly, the histopathological feature of this remodeling can resemble allograft vasculopathy as found after heart transplantation (9). The expression of some fetal variants of certain cell adhesion modulating proteins such as fibronectin or tenascin-C, as well as the impact of fibroblast to myofibroblast trans-differentiation and vascular smooth muscle cell activation have been extensively described in both settings of allograft vasculopathy and PAH. This remodeling process in the pulmonary vasculature results in a progressive decrease in arterial compliance and an increase in vascular stiffening.

Clinically, pulmonary arterial stiffening can be assessed by pulse wave velocity measurement via non-invasive ultrasound or magnetic resonance imaging, based on the pulsatile characteristics of the pulmonary arteries. Pulse wave velocity is the speed of flow waves propagate along the lumen, which depend on the stiffness and dimensions of the blood vessels. Concomitant measurement of pulmonary arterial stiffness indices could allow for more precise prediction for risk of developing severe PAH and mortality, especially in the early stage of the disease (10). For example, in children with congenital heart disease, increased pulmonary arterial stiffening predicts the progression into advanced PAH even in the patients with low pulmonary vascular resistance, suggesting intrinsic pulmonary arterial stiffness may serve as an independent index that may enhance predictions of disease progression and survival (11).

Pulmonary arterial compliance (PACa), as measured invasively or more recently via non-invasive means, is another pulmonary arterial stiffening index (6, 12). PACa refers the change in pulmonary arterial cross-sectional area or volume over change in pressure. Unlike pulmonary arterial resistance, which is calculated by the pressure difference across the pulmonary vasculature under a certain cardiac output, PACa reflects the pulmonary arterial stiffness more directly. PACa is increasingly appreciated as a parameter of prognostic relevance in patients with various subtypes and severities of PH (13, 14). In chronic thromboembolic PH (WHO Group 4), reduced PACa is a determinant of poor functional capacity and is a marker of poor prognosis in the patients. Reduced PACa may even serve as the most prominent hemodynamic feature found in early stages of PAH. Furthermore, in PH due to left heart disease (WHO Group 2), reduced PACa has been found to offer prognostic value, both in those with elevated and normal pulmonary vascular resistance (15).

ECM Stiffening

At the histologic level, ECM remodeling plays a central role in pulmonary arterial stiffening. The ECM network provides biophysical support for various cells in the vessel wall, thus maintaining the mechanical stability and elastic recoil of the arteries. Biochemical and biophysical signals induced by the ECM direct vascular cellular function, differentiation, migration and apoptosis, enable intracellular communication, playing a decisive role in vascular development, remodeling processes and maintenance of vascular homeostasis, as previously reviewed (16). The pulmonary arterial ECM is highly dynamic, consisting mostly of collagens, elastins, and laminins as well as other components such as fibronectin, tenascin C, and glucosaminoglycans. Dynamic balance of the ECM is dictated by bidirectional alterations of proteolytic enzymes such as a disintegrin and metalloproteases (ADAMs), matrix metalloproteinases (MMPs), and their endogenous inhibitors, tissue inhibitors of metalloproteinases (TIMPs). In PAH, buildup of collagen, neutrophil-elastase and MMPs, along with decrease of their modulating counterparts TIMPs causes an imbalance of ECM turnover and subsequently a pathogenic alteration of the structure and stiffness of the pulmonary vessel wall. A landmark of this remodeling process, endothelial-to-mesenchymal transition, is controlled by a complex upstream intracellular signaling network including TGF-β, Wnt, and Notch pathways (17). The restoration of ECM kinetics has been promoted as a strategy to prevent or ameliorate vascular remodeling processes but only recently have the molecular control points of this balance begun to be clarified.

ECM remodeling and stiffening can be triggered by various PAH pathogenic factors, such as vascular injury, pro-inflammation factors, abnormal growth factor expression, and/or hypoxia exposure. It has been shown that accumulation of ECM is a key pathologic change notable across the vascular wall in PH (18). Vascular-specific serine elastase activity in the ECM has been implicated in PAH (19). In parallel with elastase activity, MMPs exhibit an elevated activity, especially MMP-2/9, leading to accelerated turnover of ECM and play an important role in the initial remodeling of ECM in pulmonary vessels in both patients and animal models of PAH (20–22). Since the function of MMPs is tightly controlled by endogenous inhibitors TIMPs, the loss of balance between MMPs and TIMPs has been shown to induce ECM remodeling in patients with idiopathic PAH. As an example, Wang et al. found that vascular collagen buildup promotes hypoxia-induced pulmonary vascular remodeling in both small and large arteries (23). ECM remodeling could also delay the recovery of pulmonary hemodynamics and subsequently worsen right ventricular function (24). In regard of pulmonary vascular adventitial remodeling, the expression of type I collagen in cultured fibroblasts is upregulated by hypoxia (25). In rodent hypoxia-induced PH models, the expression of ECM proteins, especially the collagens that contribute to arterial stiffening, has been found to be elevated, even after hypoxic stress has been removed. This process is thought to be mediated by impaired degradation of type I collagen (26).

Approaches to target ECM remodeling in experimental animal models have shown efficacy in reducing PAH. Zhang et al. demonstrated that the extension of arterial stiffening is alleviated by inhibiting 15-lipoxygenase (15-LO) and consequent collagen accumulation in pulmonary arteries in hypoxia mouse models (25). Alternatively, in monocrotaline (MCT)-induced PAH in rats, the activation of AMP activated protein kinase (AMPK) by the AMPK agonist metformin inhibited ECM remodeling in pulmonary arteries, thus reducing the elevated right ventricle systolic pressure and right ventricle hypertrophy (27). The mechanisms underlying AMPK-induced suppression of ECM remodeling in pulmonary arteries were coupled to decreased MMP-2/9 activity and TIMP-1 expression. Importantly, however, the known pleiotropy of AMPK agonism in PAH likely extends far beyond the direct effects on pulmonary vascular stiffness (28, 29). Thus, while these results suggest the potential therapeutic value of AMPK activation in PAH, these studies did not fully prove the causative role of matrix stiffening *per se* in this disease. Phosphodiesterase type 5 enzyme (PDE-5) inhibitors are widely used in the clinical management of PH through the mechanism of NO mediated vasodilatation. As mentioned above, it is generally thought that the vasodilators present no significant effect in stopping or reversing the progression of PAH. However, data exist that show the PDE-5 inhibitor sildenafil restores BMP signaling in cultured BMPR2 deficient smooth muscle cells, and also reduces pulmonary vascular remodeling in the MCT-induced PAH rat model (30).

ARTERIAL AND ECM STIFFENING AS EARLY DRIVER OF PAH

Although the connection of pulmonary vascular stiffening/ECM remodeling to PAH has been well established, until recently, the question remained unanswered as to whether ECM remodeling represented simply an end-stage consequence of PAH. Contemporary studies, including work from our group, have advanced the concept that vascular stiffening and ECM remodeling are early and potent pathogenic triggers in PAH, occurring at time points prior to typical hemodynamic and histologic evidence of PAH or medial thickening (31–33). Several major mechanisms have been identified in this process, especially the activation of mechanosensitive metabolic pathways, the pro-inflammatory phenotype switch of activated fibroblasts and macrophages, and the involvement of certain groups of mechanosensitive microRNAs.

Metabolic Mechanisms Involved in Pulmonary Vascular Stiffening in PAH

Metabolic reprogramming in both the diseased pulmonary vasculature and right ventricle is increasingly appreciated as a crucial mediator of the pro-proliferative condition in PAH. Not only hypoxia but also other PAH-inducing factors, such as genetic mutations, congenital heart disease, scleroderma, and HIV infection, are all related to profound metabolic dysregulation in the pulmonary vasculature. For instance, broad metabolic reprogramming, beyond aerobic glycolysis and independent of hypoxia, has been identified through metabolomic screening in pulmonary endothelial cells carrying a bone morphogenetic protein receptor type 2 (BMPR2) mutation, a known genetic driver of PAH (34). The utilization and metabolism of glutamine have also been found to be increased in the course of rat right ventricle remodeling and human PAH (35).

The shift of energy production from mitochondrial oxidative phosphorylation to glycolysis chronically (Warburg-like effect), represents a central feature of the extensive reprogramming found in pulmonary arterial endothelial cells and smooth muscle cells in PAH, as reviewed previously (36). Furthermore, such metabolic reprogramming has also been linked to a pathophenotypic switch of both pulmonary vascular macrophages and fibroblasts which then can contribute extensively to pulmonary arterial stiffening and matrix remodeling in PAH. In both experimental hypoxic PH in rodents and human PAH, a model of cellular crosstalk has emerged whereby adventitial fibroblasts can recruit, retain, and activate naive macrophages into a hyper-proliferative, apoptosis-resistant, and proinflammatory phenotype (37–39). To drive this process in adventitial fibroblasts, pathogenic suppression of mitochondrial bioenergetics was found to be accompanied by increased mitochondrial fragmentation, resulting in less-efficient ATP synthesis, hyperpolarized mitochondria, and increased mitochondrial superoxide production. In contexts both dependent and independent of hypoxia, these changes resulted in a pro-oxidative and pro-inflammatory status in the pulmonary vascular micro-environment (38, 40), thus driving matrix alterations and resulting in pulmonary vascular stiffening. Metabolic reprogramming in activated macrophages has also been described in PAH, highly dependent on increased aerobic glycolysis, altered TCA cycle activity, and reduced mitochondrial respiration (Warburg-like effect). Such reprogramming has been linked to a number of distinct and complicated mechanisms involving a cohort of metabolic enzymes and accumulated metabolites, as well as transcriptional regulatory factors such as the hypoxia inducible factor (HIF)-1α and downstream signaling molecules such as STAT3 [see reviews by (41, 42)].

Of note, the energy production from the increased glycolysis alone is not sufficient to fulfill the metabolic demands for the cells that are actively proliferating during the process of vascular remodeling in PAH. The energy generated from the classic tricarboxylic acid (TCA) cycle is necessary to maintain the cellular reprogramming process. Additionally, large amounts of various precursor substrates are produced via TCA cycle activity. These substrates are critical for amino acid, carbohydrate and lipid biosynthesis which supports rapid cell growth and proliferation. In doing so, a large quantity of carbon intermediates are consumed continuously and requires replenishment. This replenishment of TCA carbon intermediates, also termed anaplerosis, depends on two major mechanisms. One is glutaminolysis, which deamidates glutamine via the enzyme glutaminase 1 (GLS1). The other pathway is the carboxylation of pyruvate to oxaloacetate, which is mediated by ATP-dependent pyruvate carboxylase. Particularly, GLS1-mediated glutaminolysis in the proliferating cells during pulmonary vascular remodeling serves as a critical mechanism to support not only the mobilization of cellular energy, carbon and nitrogen to maintain cellular biomass but also the metabolic switch from oxidative phosphorylation to glycolysis.

Recently, emerging evidence, including findings from our group, has demonstrated a link between matrix mechanotransduction (i.e., mechanisms by which cells sense and react to external mechanical forces and convert extracellular mechanical cues into intracellular signaling) and pulmonary vascular metabolic reprogramming, thus triggering the initiation and development of PAH (31, 33). We previously defined the pulmonary vascular function of YAP (Yes Associated Protein 1) and TAZ (Transcriptional Coactivator with PDZ-Binding Motif, or WWRT1), which serve as transcriptional coactivators in the Hippo signaling pathway. YAP/TAZ are mechanoactivated by stiff ECM in pulmonary vascular cell types and function as central regulators of cellular proliferation. They do so by activating the enzyme GLS1 which promotes glutaminolysis and anaplerosis and downstream effects on cellular proliferation, migration, and apoptosis among multiple vascular cell types in a timed and stage-specific manner. As such, YAP/TAZ-dependent control of glutaminolysis may act as a central mechanism of the pulmonary vascular dysfunction induced by the change of the extracellular environment in PAH (**Figure 1**) (33).

Besides YAP/TAZ–GLS1 activation, some additional mechanisms may also be involved in the metabolic switch in the setting of pulmonary arterial stiffening. The enzymes lactate dehydrogenase A (LDHA) and the ATP-dependent pyruvate carboxylase (PC) have both been identified as associated checkpoints in stiffness-induced alterations of glycolysis and anaplerosis, respectively (33). Furthermore, YAP/TAZ signaling has been linked to AMPK activation, resulting in the induction of aerobic glycolysis (43). These findings suggest broader control over metabolic reprogramming in PAH by YAP/TAZ and vascular stiffness. Future work will be important to delineate more completely the connections of pulmonary vascular stiffness and glutaminolysis with cellular reprogramming, crosstalk, and also the timed evolution of cellular function and identity in PAH. These findings may also endorse the application of novel pharmacologic agents targeting the metabolic effects of vascular stiffness to prevent or even reverse PAH, which will be further discussed below.

MicroRNA-Related Mechanisms in Pulmonary Arterial Stiffening

MicroRNAs (miRNAs) are non-coding RNAs that vary in length between 19 and 25 nucleotides. They regulate gene expression by affecting mRNA stability and translation into protein, and they serve as essential mediators of multiple cellular processes involving cell-cell and cell-matrix interactions (44). Although many crucial roles of miRNAs in the cardiovascular system have been well established, studies of miRNAs in PAH are still advancing (3, 45). Until recently, the interaction between miRNAs and pulmonary arterial stiffening/ECM remodeling had not been well established, and the targets and downstream mechanisms of miRNAs were largely unexplored.

Numerous miRNAs have been found to function in the pathogenesis and progression of PAH, as previously reviewed (46). Among them, the miR-130/301 family has been shown to regulate the systems-wide, proliferative and vasoconstrictive actions in pulmonary vasculature. The involvement of miRNAs in pulmonary ECM biology, their targets and mechanisms, have been recently studied as an early driver of PAH progression. Specifically, mechanosensitive YAP/TAZ signaling has been found to activate miR-130/301 to form a feedback loop, thus

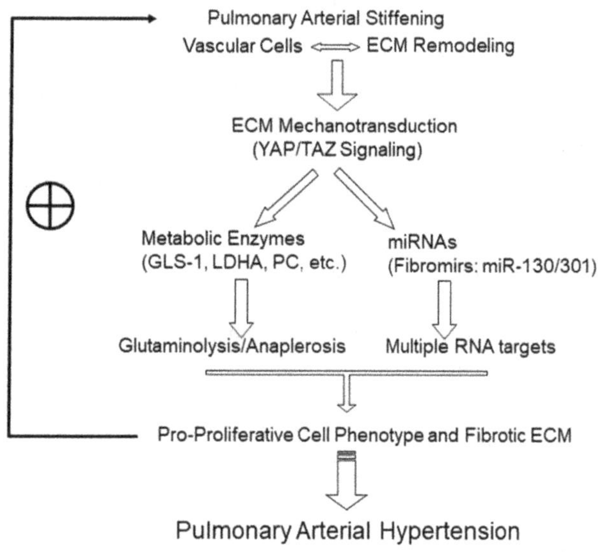

FIGURE 1 | Model of the positive feedback loop and vicious cycle triggered by pulmonary arterial and matrix stiffening in PAH inception and development. Pulmonary arterial stiffening and matrix remodeling activate mechanosensitive signaling. A prominent example includes YAP/TAZ-dependent reprogramming, which induces the key metabolic enzymes to promote glutaminolysis and glycolysis and sustains the metabolic needs of hyperproliferative vascular cells. In the other hand, mechanoactive YAP/TAZ signaling also induces miRNAs that are related to tissue fibrosis and remodeling ("fibromirs"), through interacting with multiple, and potentially synergistic, target mRNAs. These mechanisms drive pro-proliferative vascular cell phenotypes and ECM remodeling and in turn further enhance mechanotransduction, forming a vicious cycle underlying the progression of PAH. ECM, extracellular matrix. The symbol ⊕ indicates a positive feedback effect to maintain the vicious cycle.

promoting PAH via ECM remodeling and vascular stiffening (31). The downstream mediators of the YAP/TAZ-miR-130/301 circuit relevant to ECM remodeling were found to involve predominantly the pro-proliferative PPARγ-APOE-LRP8-LOX pathway. Overexpression or knockdown of PPARγ or its direct target ApoE, disrupted miR130/301 mediated vascular collagen disposition and remodeling (31). Other secreted factors, such as fibroblast growth factor 2 (FGF2), interleukin-6 (IL-6), and endothelin 1 (EDN1), as well as miRNAs such as miR-21 and miR-27a, have further defined an overlapping molecular hierarchy important to the remodeled ECM in PAH [as reviewed in Negi and Chan (3)]. The early development of ECM remodeling in PAH and the positive feedback loop connecting the ECM to the YAP/TAZ-miR-130/301 circuit suggest the pathogenic relevance of this axis both early and late in disease as well as present a model of self-sustained propagation of ECM remodeling throughout the pulmonary vascular tree as PAH progresses.

Much future work remains in studying the roles of miRNAs in pulmonary arterial stiffening. It is likely that an even more complex and broad interactome is active among YAP/TAZ, a cohort of fibrosis-related miRNAs including miR-130/301, and their targets. For example, independent of YAP/TAZ, pulmonary vessel stiffening has also been found to be regulated by a miRNA-dependent process involving the Runt-related transcription factor 2 (Runx2) to promote vascular calcification (47). Moreover, mechanoactivation of YAP/TAZ independent of miR-130/301 can promote increased matrix deposition and stiffening, thus propagating vessel stiffness throughout the pulmonary vascular tree in PAH (48). Recent studies have implicated the control of metabolic, inflammatory, and proliferative regulatory programs in diseased adventitial fibroblasts in PAH to miR-124 (49, 50) and transcriptional regulators, such as the C-terminal binding protein-1 (CtBP1) (51) and the polypyrimidine tract binding protein 1 (PTBP1)-pyruvate kinase muscle (PKM) axis (49).

Thus, a set of mechanosensitive and ECM-related miRNAs ("fibromirs") may comprise an important link in the complex regulation of ECM stiffening in PAH (**Figure 1**). Future work will be required to define additional mechanisms of RNA-dependent control of this process in PAH, specifically in regard to other aspects of ECM remodeling beyond biogenesis, such as matrix degradation and turnover.

NOVEL TRANSLATIONAL APPROACHES TARGETING PULMONARY ARTERIAL STIFFENING IN PAH

Diagnostic and Therapeutic Targets in the ECM for PAH

Given the pathogenic importance of vascular ECM reorganization in PAH, investment is ongoing to identify matrix components that may serve either as biomarkers for diagnosis and prognostic estimation in PAH or as true therapeutic targets. The translational value of measuring fetal ECM components, such as tenascin-C variants, as biomarkers, both in tissue and in circulating blood, has been proposed (52, 53). Due to the stable extracellular deposition, these matrix components could also be considered as target molecules for specific therapeutic modulation in PAH. For example, fibronectin and tenascin-C have been considered as feasible molecular targets for antibody-based delivery of diagnostic agents (e.g., radionuclides) or direct therapeutics (i.e., bioactive payloads such as cytokines or small molecule inhibitors). Such agents, in particular immunocytokines or antibody-drug conjugates, have been successfully administered in a variety of animal models of neoplastic and non-neoplastic chronic-inflammatory diseases (54–56). Applications of these approaches in PAH could advance considerably in the near future.

Therapeutic Strategy Targeting miRNA-Dependent or Metabolic Mechanisms of Pulmonary Arterial Stiffening

Multiple novel therapeutic gene targets in adventitial fibroblasts have shown promise recently in experimental rodent models of PH, including the CtBP1 inhibitor 4-methylthio-2-oxobutyric acid (MTOB) (51) and the PKM2 inhibitors TEPP-46 and shikonin (49) among others. Importantly, however, similar to targeting AMPK activity, the therapeutic effects of these pleiotropic agents may not solely be dependent on their effects on pulmonary vascular stiffness alone. On the other hand, the description of a true mechanosensitive YAP/TAZ-GLS1 circuit regulating glutaminolysis and cellular proliferation sets the stage for developing novel clinical management strategies in PAH that target pulmonary arterial stiffening more directly. As a historical example, the lysyl oxidase (Lox) inhibitor β-aminopropionitrile (BAPN) has been used to improve both hemodynamic and histologic indices of PAH in experimental rodent models, thus reinforcing the therapeutic feasibility of targeting collagen cross-linking and ECM reprogramming in PH (33, 57–59). Consistent with more recent evidence supporting the important roles of YAP and GLS1 in the pathogenesis of PAH, a YAP inhibitor such as verteporfin (33, 60), an oligonucleotide inhibitor of the miR-130/301 family (61), as well as GLS1 inhibitors such as CB-839 and C968 (33) have all been shown to mediate robust improvement of rodent PAH. Downstream of YAP, a liver X receptor (LXR) agonist GW3965, which upregulates ApoE level when administered orally to hypoxia treated mice, was shown to ameliorate ECM remodeling and PAH through interaction with YAP/TAZ-miR-130/301 circuit *in vivo* (31, 62). Importantly, verteporfin is already approved for use intravenously in treatment of age-related macular degeneration (63). Cyclic YAP-like peptides that interrupt YAP-TEAD interactions in oncogenesis (64) could also be applied to PAH. Moreover, CB-839, acting as oral GLS1 inhibitor, is developed for cancer therapy and currently under evaluation in an early human clinical trial (Clinical Trial NCT02071862) (65). Notably, since LXR along with the sterol regulatory element-binding protein (SREBP) also act together to mediate the actions of AMPK (66), there may exist an even greater interdependence and convergence of YAP with AMPK than already appreciated. Therefore, a strategy of repurposing these inhibitors for YAP, GLS1, or miR-130/301, potentially along with a LXR agonist and/or AMPK modulator, may provide a rare opportunity to offer novel "matrix" therapeutics for PAH without the delay of needing to develop new inhibitors *de novo*.

SUMMARY

ECM remodeling and pulmonary arterial stiffening have long been associated with PAH. However, only recently have we begun to appreciate that pulmonary vascular and ECM stiffening act as crucial early triggers in pathogenesis of this mysterious disease. Emerging evidence has demonstrated that pulmonary vascular stiffening activates mechanosensitive signaling such as YAP/TAZ signaling which in turn regulates downstream miRNAs and metabolic targets essential for PAH development (**Figure 1**). Further understanding of this and other novel mechanisms related to pulmonary arterial stiffening will strengthen the development of diagnostic, therapeutic, and potentially preventative, approaches targeting the early initiation of arterial stiffness. As such, it is hoped that the vicious cycle of PAH progression may be broken or entirely avoided, thus leading to disease prevention or reversal, which has not been possible thus far with current therapies.

AUTHOR CONTRIBUTIONS

All authors listed have made a substantial, direct and intellectual contribution to the work, and approved it for publication.

ACKNOWLEDGMENTS

This work was supported by NIH grants R01 HL124021, HL 122596, HL 138437, and UH2 TR002073 as well as AHA Established Investigator Award 18EIA339600027 (SYC).

REFERENCES

1. Simonneau G, Gatzoulis MA, Adatia I, Celermajer D, Denton C, Ghofrani A, et al. Updated clinical classification of pulmonary hypertension. *J Am Coll Cardiol.* (2013) 62:D34–41. doi: 10.1016/j.jacc.2013.10.029
2. D'Alonzo GE, Barst RJ, Ayres SM, Bergofsky EH, Brundage BH, Detre KM, et al. Survival in patients with primary pulmonary hypertension. Results from a national prospective registry. *Ann Intern Med.* (1991) 115:343–9. doi: 10.7326/0003-4819-115-5-343
3. Negi V, Chan SY. Discerning functional hierarchies of microRNAs in pulmonary hypertension. *JCI Insight* (2017) 2:e91327. doi: 10.1172/jci.insight.91327
4. Wang Z, Chesler NC. Pulmonary vascular wall stiffness: an important contributor to the increased right ventricular afterload with pulmonary hypertension. *Pulm Circ.* (2011) 1:212–23. doi: 10.4103/2045-8932.83453
5. Lammers S, Scott D, Hunter K, Tan W, Shandas R, Stenmark KR. Mechanics and function of the pulmonary vasculature: implications for pulmonary vascular disease and right ventricular function. *Compr Physiol.* (2012) 2:295–319. doi: 10.1002/cphy.c100070
6. Gan CT, Lankhaar JW, Westerhof N, Marcus JT, Becker A, Twisk JW, et al. Noninvasively assessed pulmonary artery stiffness predicts mortality in pulmonary arterial hypertension. *Chest* (2007) 132:1906–12. doi: 10.1378/chest.07-1246
7. Tuder RM, Archer SL, Dorfmuller P, Erzurum SC, Guignabert C, Michelakis E, et al. Relevant issues in the pathology and pathobiology of pulmonary hypertension. *J Am Coll Cardiol.* (2013) 62:D4–12. doi: 10.1016/j.jacc.2013.10.025
8. Savai R, Pullamsetti SS, Kolbe J, Bieniek E, Voswinckel R, Fink L, et al. Immune and inflammatory cell involvement in the pathology of idiopathic pulmonary arterial hypertension. *Am J Respir Crit Care Med.* (2012) 186:897–908. doi: 10.1164/rccm.201202-0335OC
9. Suzuki J, Isobe M, Morishita R, Nagai R. Characteristics of chronic rejection in heart transplantation: important elements of pathogenesis and future treatments. *Circ J.* (2010) 74:233–9. doi: 10.1253/circj.CJ-09-0809
10. Hunter KS, Lammers SR, Shandas R. Pulmonary vascular stiffness: measurement, modeling, and implications in normal and hypertensive pulmonary circulations. *Compr Physiol.* (2011) 1:1413–35. doi: 10.1002/cphy.c100005
11. Ploegstra MJ, Brokelman JG, Roos-Hesselink JW, Douwes JM, van Osch-Gevers LM, Hoendermis ES, et al. Pulmonary arterial stiffness indices assessed by intravascular ultrasound in children with early pulmonary vascular disease: prediction of advanced disease and mortality during 20-year follow-up. *Eur Heart J Cardiovasc Imaging* (2017) 19:216–24. doi: 10.1093/ehjci/jex015
12. Sanz J, Kariisa M, Dellegrottaglie S, Prat-Gonzalez S, Garcia MJ, Fuster V, et al. Evaluation of pulmonary artery stiffness in pulmonary hypertension with cardiac magnetic resonance. *JACC Cardiovasc Imaging* (2009) 2:286–95. doi: 10.1016/j.jcmg.2008.08.007
13. Mahapatra S, Nishimura RA, Sorajja P, Cha S, McGoon MD. Relationship of pulmonary arterial capacitance and mortality in idiopathic pulmonary arterial hypertension. *J Am Coll Cardiol.* (2006) 47:799–803. doi: 10.1016/j.jacc.2005.09.054
14. Ghio S, D'Alto M, Badagliacca R, Vitulo P, Argiento P, Mule M, et al. Prognostic relevance of pulmonary arterial compliance after therapy initiation

or escalation in patients with pulmonary arterial hypertension. *Int J Cardiol.* (2017) 230:53–8. doi: 10.1016/j.ijcard.2016.12.099

15. Pellegrini P, Rossi A, Pasotti M, Raineri C, Cicoira M, Bonapace S, et al. Prognostic relevance of pulmonary arterial compliance in patients with chronic heart failure. *Chest* (2014) 145:1064–70. doi: 10.1378/chest.13-1510
16. Wagenseil JE, Mecham RP. Vascular extracellular matrix and arterial mechanics. *Physiol Rev.* (2009) 89:957–89. doi: 10.1152/physrev.00041.2008
17. Arciniegas E, Frid MG, Douglas IS, Stenmark KR. Perspectives on endothelial-to-mesenchymal transition: potential contribution to vascular remodeling in chronic pulmonary hypertension. *Am J Physiol Lung Cell Mol Physiol.* (2007) 293:L1–8. doi: 10.1152/ajplung.00378.2006
18. Chelladurai P, Seeger W, Pullamsetti SS. Matrix metalloproteinases and their inhibitors in pulmonary hypertension. *Eur Respir J.* (2012) 40:766–82. doi: 10.1183/09031936.00209911
19. Rabinovitch M. Molecular pathogenesis of pulmonary arterial hypertension. *J Clin Invest.* (2012) 122:4306–13. doi: 10.1172/JCI60658
20. Dodson RB, Rozance PJ, Petrash CC, Hunter KS, Ferguson VL. Thoracic and abdominal aortas stiffen through unique extracellular matrix changes in intrauterine growth restricted fetal sheep. *Am J Physiol Heart Circ Physiol.* (2014) 306:H429–37. doi: 10.1152/ajpheart.00472.2013
21. Wetzl V, Tiede SL, Faerber L, Weissmann N, Schermuly RT, Ghofrani HA, et al. Plasma MMP2/TIMP4 ratio at follow-up assessment predicts disease progression of idiopathic pulmonary arterial hypertension. *Lung* (2017) 195:489–96. doi: 10.1007/s00408-017-0014-5
22. Lepetit H, Eddahibi S, Fadel E, Frisdal E, Munaut C, Noel A, et al. Smooth muscle cell matrix metalloproteinases in idiopathic pulmonary arterial hypertension. *Eur Respir J.* (2005) 25:834–42. doi: 10.1183/09031936.05.00072504
23. Wang Z, Lakes RS, Eickhoff JC, Chesler NC. Effects of collagen deposition on passive and active mechanical properties of large pulmonary arteries in hypoxic pulmonary hypertension. *Biomech Model Mechanobiol.* (2013) 12:1115–25. doi: 10.1007/s10237-012-0467-7
24. Schreier D, Hacker T, Song G, Chesler N. The role of collagen synthesis in ventricular and vascular adaptation to hypoxic pulmonary hypertension. *J Biomech Eng.* (2013) 135:021018. doi: 10.1115/1.4023480
25. Zhang L, Li Y, Chen M, Su X, Yi D, Lu P, et al. 15-LO/15-HETE mediated vascular adventitia fibrosis via p38 MAPK-dependent TGF-beta. *J Cell Physiol.* (2014) 229:245–57. doi: 10.1002/jcp.24443
26. Ooi CY, Wang Z, Tabima DM, Eickhoff JC, Chesler NC. The role of collagen in extralobar pulmonary artery stiffening in response to hypoxia-induced pulmonary hypertension. *Am J Physiol Heart Circ Physiol.* (2010) 299:H1823–31. doi: 10.1152/ajpheart.00493.2009
27. Li S, Han D, Zhang Y, Xie X, Ke R, Zhu Y, et al. Activation of AMPK prevents monocrotaline-induced extracellular matrix remodeling of pulmonary artery. *Med Sci Monit Basic Res.* (2016) 22:27–33. doi: 10.12659/MSMBR.897505
28. Wang W, Xiao ZD, Li X, Aziz KE, Gan B, Johnson RL, et al. AMPK modulates Hippo pathway activity to regulate energy homeostasis. *Nat Cell Biol.* (2015) 17:490–9. doi: 10.1038/ncb3113
29. Lai YC, Tabima DM, Dube JJ, Hughan KS, Vanderpool RR, Goncharov DA, et al. SIRT3-AMP-activated protein kinase activation by nitrite and metformin improves hyperglycemia and normalizes pulmonary hypertension associated with heart failure with preserved ejection fraction. *Circulation* (2016) 133:717–31. doi: 10.1161/CIRCULATIONAHA.115.018935
30. Yang J, Li X, Al-Lamki RS, Wu C, Weiss A, Berk J, et al. Sildenafil potentiates bone morphogenetic protein signaling in pulmonary arterial smooth muscle cells and in experimental pulmonary hypertension. *Arterioscler Thromb Vasc Biol.* (2013) 33:34–42. doi: 10.1161/ATVBAHA.112.300121
31. Bertero T, Cotrill KA, Lu Y, Haeger CM, Dieffenbach P, Annis S, et al. Matrix remodeling promotes pulmonary hypertension through feedback mechanoactivation of the YAP/TAZ-miR-130/301 circuit. *Cell Rep.* (2015) 13:1016–32. doi: 10.1016/j.celrep.2015.09.049
32. Bertero T, Cottrill KA, Annis S, Bhat B, Gochuico BR, Osorio JC, et al. A YAP/TAZ-miR-130/301 molecular circuit exerts systems-level control of fibrosis in a network of human diseases and physiologic conditions. *Sci Rep.* (2015) 5:18277. doi: 10.1038/srep18277
33. Bertero T, Oldham WM, Cottrill KA, Pisano S, Vanderpool RR, Yu Q, et al. Vascular stiffness mechanoactivates YAP/TAZ-dependent glutaminolysis to drive pulmonary hypertension. *J Clin Invest.* (2016) 126:3313–35. doi: 10.1172/JCI86387
34. Fessel JP, Hamid R, Wittmann BM, Robinson LJ, Blackwell T, Tada Y, et al. Metabolomic analysis of bone morphogenetic protein receptor type 2 mutations in human pulmonary endothelium reveals widespread metabolic reprogramming. *Pulm Circ.* (2012) 2:201–13. doi: 10.4103/2045-8932.97606
35. Piao L, Fang YH, Parikh K, Ryan JJ, Toth PT, Archer SL. Cardiac glutaminolysis: a maladaptive cancer metabolism pathway in the right ventricle in pulmonary hypertension. *J Mol Med.* (2013) 91:1185–97. doi: 10.1007/s00109-013-1064-7
36. Cottrill KA, Chan SY. Metabolic dysfunction in pulmonary hypertension: the expanding relevance of the warburg effect. *Eur J Clin Invest.* (2013) 43:855–65. doi: 10.1111/eci.12104
37. Anwar A, Li M, Frid MG, Kumar B, Gerasimovskaya EV, Riddle SR, et al. Osteopontin is an endogenous modulator of the constitutively activated phenotype of pulmonary adventitial fibroblasts in hypoxic pulmonary hypertension. *Am J Physiol Lung Cell Mol Physiol.* (2012) 303:L1–11. doi: 10.1152/ajplung.00050.2012
38. Li M, Riddle SR, Frid MG, El Kasmi KC, McKinsey TA, Sokol RJ, et al. Emergence of fibroblasts with a proinflammatory epigenetically altered phenotype in severe hypoxic pulmonary hypertension. *J Immunol.* (2011) 187:2711–22. doi: 10.4049/jimmunol.1100479
39. El Kasmi KC, Pugliese SC, Riddle SR, Poth JM, Anderson AL, Frid MG, et al. Adventitial fibroblasts induce a distinct proinflammatory/profibrotic macrophage phenotype in pulmonary hypertension. *J Immunol.* (2014) 193:597–609. doi: 10.4049/jimmunol.1303048
40. Plecita-Hlavata L, Tauber J, Li M, Zhang H, Flockton AR, Pullamsetti SS, et al. Constitutive reprogramming of fibroblast mitochondrial metabolism in pulmonary hypertension. *Am J Respir Cell Mol Biol.* (2016) 55:47–57. doi: 10.1165/rcmb.2015-0142OC
41. El Kasmi KC, Stenmark KR. Contribution of metabolic reprogramming to macrophage plasticity and function. *Semin Immunol.* (2015) 27:267–75. doi: 10.1016/j.smim.2015.09.001
42. Stenmark KR, Tuder RM, El Kasmi KC. Metabolic reprogramming and inflammation act in concert to control vascular remodeling in hypoxic pulmonary hypertension. *J Appl Physiol.* (2015) 119:1164–72. doi: 10.1152/japplphysiol.00283.2015
43. Santinon G, Pocaterra A, Dupont S. Control of YAP/TAZ activity by metabolic and nutrient-sensing pathways. *Trends Cell Biol.* (2016) 26:289–99. doi: 10.1016/j.tcb.2015.11.004
44. Valastyan S, Weinberg RA. Roles for microRNAs in the regulation of cell adhesion molecules. *J Cell Sci.* (2011) 124:999–1006. doi: 10.1242/jcs.081513
45. Chun HJ, Bonnet S, Chan SY. Translating MicroRNA biology in pulmonary hypertension: it will take more than "miR" words. *Am J Respir Crit Care Med.* (2016) 195:167–78. doi: 10.1164/rccm.201604-0886PP
46. Boucherat O, Potus F, Bonnet S. microRNA and pulmonary hypertension. *Adv Exp Med Biol.* (2015) 888:237–52. doi: 10.1007/978-3-319-22671-2_12
47. Ruffenach G, Chabot S, Tanguay VF, Courboulin A, Boucherat O, Potus F, et al. Role for runt-related transcription factor 2 in proliferative and calcified vascular lesions in pulmonary arterial hypertension. *Am J Respir Crit Care Med.* (2016) 194:1273–85. doi: 10.1164/rccm.201512-2380OC
48. Liu F, Haeger CM, Dieffenbach PB, Sicard D, Chrobak I, Coronata AM, et al. Distal vessel stiffening is an early and pivotal mechanobiological regulator of vascular remodeling and pulmonary hypertension. *JCI Insight* (2016) 1:e86987. doi: 10.1172/jci.insight.86987
49. Zhang H, Wang D, Li M, Plecita-Hlavata L, D'Alessandro A, Tauber J, et al. The metabolic and proliferative state of vascular adventitial fibroblasts in pulmonary hypertension is regulated through a MiR-124/PTBP1/PKM Axis. *Circulation* (2017) 136:2468–85. doi: 10.1161/CIRCULATIONAHA.117.028069
50. Caruso P, Dunmore BJ, Schlosser K, Schoors S, Dos Santos CC, Perez-Iratxeta C, et al. Identification of miR-124 as a major regulator of enhanced endothelial cell glycolysis in pulmonary arterial hypertension via PTBP1 and PKM2. *Circulation* (2017) 136:2451–67. doi: 10.1161/CIRCULATIONAHA.117.028034
51. Li M, Riddle S, Zhang H, D'Alessandro A, Flockton A, Serkova NJ, et al. Metabolic reprogramming regulates the proliferative and inflammatory phenotype of adventitial fibroblasts in pulmonary hypertension through the transcriptional corepressor C-terminal binding protein-1. *Circulation* (2016) 134:1105–21. doi: 10.1161/CIRCULATIONAHA.116.023171
52. Baldinger A, Brehm BR, Richter P, Bossert T, Gruen K, Hekmat K, et al. Comparative analysis of oncofetal fibronectin and tenascin-C expression in right atrial auricular and left ventricular human cardiac tissue from patients with coronary artery disease and aortic valve stenosis. *Histochem Cell Biol.*

(2011) 135:427–41. doi: 10.1007/s00418-011-0809-z

53. Nozato T, Sato A, Hikita H, Takahashi A, Imanaka-Yoshida K, Yoshida T, et al. Impact of serum tenascin-C on the aortic healing process during the chronic stage of type B acute aortic dissection. *Int J Cardiol.* (2015) 191:97–9. doi: 10.1016/j.ijcard.2015.05.009
54. Franz M, Doll F, Grun K, Richter P, Kose N, Ziffels B, et al. Targeted delivery of interleukin-10 to chronic cardiac allograft rejection using a human antibody specific to the extra domain A of fibronectin. *Int J Cardiol.* (2015) 195:311–22. doi: 10.1016/j.ijcard.2015.05.144
55. Casi G, Neri D. Antibody-drug conjugates: basic concepts, examples and future perspectives. *J Control Release* (2012) 161:422–8. doi: 10.1016/j.jconrel.2012.01.026
56. Bootz F, Neri D. Immunocytokines: a novel class of products for the treatment of chronic inflammation and autoimmune conditions. *Drug Discov Today* (2016) 21:180–9. doi: 10.1016/j.drudis.2015.10.012
57. Kerr JS, Riley DJ, Frank MM, Trelstad RL, Frankel HM. Reduction of chronic hypoxic pulmonary hypertension in the rat by beta-aminopropionitrile. *J Appl Physiol Respir Environ Exerc Physiol.* (1984) 57:1760–6. doi: 10.1152/jappl.1984.57.6.1760
58. Kerr JS, Ruppert CL, Tozzi CA, Neubauer JA, Frankel HM, Yu SY, et al. Reduction of chronic hypoxic pulmonary hypertension in the rat by an inhibitor of collagen production. *Am Rev Respir Dis.* (1987) 135:300–6.
59. Nave AH, Mizikova I, Niess G, Steenbock H, Reichenberger F, Talavera ML, et al. Lysyl oxidases play a causal role in vascular remodeling in clinical and experimental pulmonary arterial hypertension. *Arterioscler Thromb Vasc Biol.* (2014) 34:1446–58. doi: 10.1161/ATVBAHA.114.303534
60. Kudryashova TV, Goncharov DA, Pena A, Kelly N, Vanderpool R, Baust J, et al. HIPPO-integrin-linked kinase cross-talk controls self-sustaining proliferation and survival in pulmonary hypertension. *Am J Respir Crit Care Med.* (2016) 194:866–77. doi: 10.1164/rccm.201510-2003OC
61. Bertero T, Lu Y, Annis S, Hale A, Bhat B, Saggar R, et al. Systems-level regulation of microRNA networks by miR-130/301 promotes pulmonary hypertension. *J Clin Invest.* (2014) 124:3514–28. doi: 10.1172/JCI 74773
62. Im SS, Osborne TF. Liver x receptors in atherosclerosis and inflammation. *Circ Res.* (2011) 108:996–1001. doi: 10.1161/CIRCRESAHA.110.2 26878
63. Kent DL. Age-related macular degeneration: beyond anti-angiogenesis. *Mol Vis.* (2014) 20:46–55.
64. Zhou Z, Hu T, Xu Z, Lin Z, Zhang Z, Feng T, et al. Targeting Hippo pathway by specific interruption of YAP-TEAD interaction using cyclic YAP-like peptides. *FASEB J.* (2015) 29:724–32. doi: 10.1096/fj.14-262980
65. Katt WP, Lukey MJ, Cerione RA. A tale of two glutaminases: homologous enzymes with distinct roles in tumorigenesis. *Future Med Chem.* (2017) 9:223–43. doi: 10.4155/fmc-2016-0190
66. Zhou G, Myers R, Li Y, Chen Y, Shen X, Fenyk-Melody J, et al. Role of AMP-activated protein kinase in mechanism of metformin action. *J Clin Invest.* (2001) 108:1167–74. doi: 10.1172/JCI13505

17

Biomarkers for Pulmonary Vascular Remodeling in Systemic Sclerosis: A Pathophysiological Approach

Balazs Odler [1,2]***, Vasile Foris*** [1,2]***, Anna Gungl*** [1,3]***, Veronika Müller*** [4]***, Paul M. Hassoun*** [5]***,***
Grazyna Kwapiszewska [1,3]***, Horst Olschewski*** [1,2*] ***and Gabor Kovacs*** [1,2]

[1] Ludwig Boltzmann Institute for Lung Vascular Research, Graz, Austria, [2] Division of Pulmonology, Department of Internal Medicine, Medical University of Graz, Graz, Austria, [3] Physiology, Otto Loewi Research Center, Medical University of Graz, Graz, Austria, [4] Department of Pulmonology, Semmelweis University, Budapest, Hungary, [5] Division of Pulmonary & Critical Care Medicine, Johns Hopkins University, Baltimore, MD, United States

****Correspondence:***
Horst Olschewski
horst.olschewski@medunigraz.at

Pulmonary arterial hypertension (PAH) is a severe complication of systemic sclerosis (SSc) associated with high morbidity and mortality. There are several biomarkers of SSc-PAH, reflecting endothelial physiology, inflammation, immune activation, extracellular matrix, metabolic changes, or cardiac involvement. Biomarkers associated with diagnosis, disease severity and progression have been identified, however, very few have been tested in a prospective setting. Some antinuclear antibodies such as nucleosome antibodies (NUC), anti-centromere antibodies (CENP-A/B) and anti-U3-ribonucleoprotein (anti-U3-RNP) are associated with PAH while anti-U1-ribonucleoprotein (anti-U1-RNP) is associated with a reduced PAH risk. Anti-endothelin receptor and angiotensin-1 receptor antibodies might be good markers of SSc-PAH and progression of pulmonary vasculopathy. Regarding the markers reflecting immune activation and inflammation, there are many inconsistent results. CXCL-4 was associated with SSc progression including PAH and lung fibrosis. Growth differentiation factor (GDF)-15 was associated with PAH and mortality but is not specific for SSc. Among the metabolites, kynurenine was identified as diagnostic marker for PAH, however, its pathologic role in the disease is unclear. Endostatin, an angiostatic factor, was associated with heart failure and poor prognosis. Established heart related markers, such as N-terminal fragment of A-type natriuretic peptide/brain natriuretic peptide (NT-proANP, NT-proBNP) or troponin I/T are elevated in SSc-PAH but are not specific for the right ventricle and may be increased to the same extent in left heart disease. Taken together, there is no universal specific biomarker for SSc-PAH, however, there is a pattern of markers that is strongly associated with a risk of vascular complications in SSc patients. Further comprehensive, multicenter and prospective studies are warranted to develop reliable algorithms for detection and prognosis of SSc-PAH.

Keywords: systemic sclerosis, autoimmune, vascular, fibrosis, pulmonary hypertension, PAH, biomarker

INTRODUCTION

Systemic sclerosis (SSc) is an autoimmune, multiorgan disease characterized by autoimmunity, fibrosis and vascular damage of the skin and other organs, including the lungs. Clinically, SSc is a heterogeneous disease which is classified in two major subtypes based on the extent of skin involvement: limited cutaneous (lcSSc) and diffuse cutaneous SSc (dcSSc) (Leroy et al., 1988). DcSSc patients are characterized by a generalized skin involvement with sometimes rapidly progressive and often fatal organ involvement, while lcSSc patients generally show a slower progression with isolated cutaneous involvement. A third phenotype called systemic sclerosis sine scleroderma (ssSSc) can also be differentiated, if the patients have any of the characteristics features of internal organ involvement without skin involvement. In addition, SSc may overlap with other rheumatic or autoimmune disorders such as rheumatoid arthritis (RA), dermatomyositis or systemic lupus erythematosus (SLE). To make a definitive classification, the criteria of the American College of Rheumatology/European League against Rheumatism (ACR/EULAR) should be applied (van den Hoogen et al., 2013; Jordan et al., 2015).

Pulmonary arterial hypertension (PAH) is a devastating disease which develops on the basis of proliferative vasculopathy of small and medium-sized pulmonary arteries, leading to an increase in mean pulmonary artery pressure (mPAP $\geq$25 mmHg) at rest. The diagnosis must be confirmed by right heart catheterization (RHC), which besides measuring pulmonary arterial pressure (PAP) allows the determination of pulmonary arterial wedge pressure (PAWP), pulmonary vascular resistance (PVR), and cardiac output (Galiè et al., 2015). Based on the values of the PAWP a pre- (PAWP $\leq$15 mmHg) and post-capillary (PAWP $\geq$15 mmHg) pulmonary hypertension can be distinguished (Galiè et al., 2015). The life-time prevalence of PAH in SSc patients ranges from 5 to 12% (Avouac et al., 2010; Hao et al., 2015; Kovacs et al., 2017; Morrisroe et al., 2017), while the prognosis of these patients is very poor with about 50% 3-year mortality after PAH diagnosis (Chaisson and Hassoun, 2013; Chung et al., 2014b). SSc-PAH patients have a worse outcome compared to idiopathic (IPAH) or PAH associated with other collagen vascular diseases, such as mixed connective tissue disease (MCTD) or SLE and PAH represents one of the leading causes of death in SSc (Chung et al., 2010, 2014b; Tyndall et al., 2010; Sobanski et al., 2016). Despite the extended involvement of internal organs in dcSSc, PAH occurs more commonly in patients with lcSSc (Denton and Khanna, 2017). In the setting of SSc, primary pulmonary vasculopathy is not the unique cause of pulmonary hypertension (PH). Significant lung disease, which might lead to PH due to hypoxaemia was identified in up to 30–75% of SSc patients complicated by elevated pulmonary arterial pressure (group 3 of the World Classification of PH) (Kowal-Bielecka et al., 2010), although a clear delineation from PAH (group 1) is sometimes difficult to establish. In addition, left ventricular systolic or diastolic dysfunction, which is frequently found in SSc patients, may cause postcapillary PH (group 2).

Finally, pulmonary venoocclusive disease, a rare variant of PAH, may be also associated with SSc (Dorfmüller et al., 2007).

There are some differences in the pathogenesis of SSc-PAH as compared to IPAH. As an example, the expression of bone morphogenetic protein receptor 2 (BMPR2) is highly associated with heritable PAH and is often present in IPAH (Rubin, 2017), but this mutation has not been found in SSc-PAH patients, at least in two small genetic studies (Morse et al., 2002).

Recent studies provided novel insight into the key signaling pathways of PAH including the role of endothelial dysfunction, growth factors, inflammation, immune activation, metabolic changes, extracellular remodeling, and the development of heart failure (**Figure 1**). Considering the fact that PAH is a life-threatening complication of SSc, blood biomarkers of pulmonary vascular involvement, either alone, or in combination with other prognostic clinical parameters may be important tools contributing to earlier diagnosis and targeted treatment. In this review we summarize blood biomarkers associated with key changes reflecting the molecular pathology of pulmonary vascular abnormalities in SSc.

INFLAMMATION AND IMMUNE ACTIVATION

There is an increasing body of evidence for an inflammatory component in the patomechanism of pulmonary hypertension. The presence and exubarence of inflammatory cells and their interactive interplay may provide a missing link between PAH, autoimmunity, and inflammation (Marsh et al., 2018). However, the detailed and comprehensive description of the interaction between the inflammatory cells and proinflammatory processes is still difficult.

The imbalance and dysregulation of immune function and tolerance may lead to autoimmunity and chronic inflammation involving different types of immune cells and chemokines. Autoimmunity and immune activation of both the innate and adaptive immune system may play a role in the early development of SSc. The subsequent activation of immune cells and fibroblasts may contribute to the pathogenesis of SSc

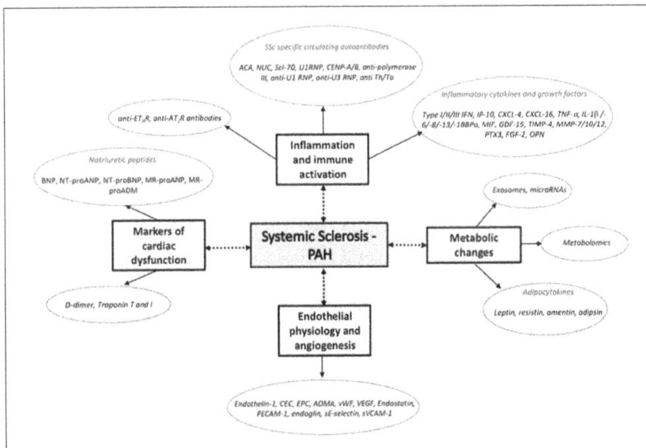

FIGURE 1 | Molecular changes and associated biomarker candidates in the development of pulmonary vascular remodeling.

and accelerated fibrogenesis and extracellular matrix deposition (Varga and Abraham, 2007). Immunological and inflammatory aspects of the disease may be therefore correlated with vascular and fibrotic manifestations and reflected by changes in the levels of corresponding circulating biomarkers (Gu et al., 2008; Denton, 2015), although most of these markers are not specific and often not based on robust studies.

SSc Specific Circulating Autoantibodies

As recently added to the ECR/EULAR criteria, the presence of highly SSc-specific circulating autoantibodies such as anti-topoisomerase 1 (ATA), anti-centromere (CENP, ACA), and anti-RNA polymerase III are used for the diagnosis of the disease (van den Hoogen et al., 2013). Specific autoantibodies indicating pulmonary vascular involvement, pulmonary disease progression or treatment response have not been included in this statement because they have not been confirmed in prospective studies. Over 85% of SSc patients present with circulating antibodies and there is emerging evidence that these antibodies are present in early stages of the disease highlighting their role as both pathogenetically important factors and early diagnostic biomarkers (Choi and Fritzler, 2016).

Over 90% of SSc patients present with antinuclear antibodies (ANAs), however, there is no association with the development of PAH (Sweiss et al., 2010). According to data from the Pulmonary Hypertension Assessment and Recognition of Outcomes in Scleroderma (PHAROS) Registry, the prevalence of anticentromere (ACA) and nucleolar antibodies (NUC), in SSc-PAH as compared to SSc without PAH, was elevated (35–37 and 24%, respectively) but not the prevalence of Scl-70 (7%) and U1RNP (5%) antibodies. No association was found between any of these biomarkers and survival (Chung et al., 2014a; Hinchliff et al., 2015). Accordingly, patients having ACA, CENP-A and/or CENP-B were more likely to have PAH but less likely to have ILD (Hudson et al., 2012).

There have been conflicting results regarding anti-polymerase III and PAH. A large longitudinal study showed that the presence of anti-polymerase III is a positive predictor for PAH (Nihtyanova et al., 2014). However, this could not be confirmed in another prospective patient cohort (Hoffmann-Vold et al., 2017). A study investigating 342 CTD-associated PAH patients found that Anti-U1 RNP positivity was associated with decreased mortality in CTD-associated PAH patients, even after correction for hemodynamic impairment (Sobanski et al., 2016). In contrast, SSc patients with anti-U3 RNP positivity were more frequently affected by PAH which was the most common cause of death in this patient group (Okano et al., 1992; Aggarwal et al., 2009). A study comparing lcSSc patients with anti-Th/To-positivity and CENP-positivity found that both groups presented with a high frequency of PAH, while the frequency of ILD was higher in the anti-Th/To group (Mitri et al., 2003). Among the larger PAH screening algorithms, only the DETECT (Evidence-Based Detection of Pulmonary Arterial Hypertension in Systemic Sclerosis) algorithm included an autoantibody (ACA) as criteria for identification of PAH in SSc (Hao et al., 2015). Autoantibody positivity and their association with survival in SSc-ILD and SSc-PAH patients are listed in **Table 1**.

Endothelin-1 Type a Receptor and Angiotensin Receptor Type-1 Antibodies

Autoantibodies against endothelin receptor type A (anti-ET_AR Ab) and angiotensin receptor type-1 (anti-AT_1R Ab) may affect inflammation and fibrotic processes by direct receptor activation thus causing vasoconstriction and proliferation (Kill et al., 2014; Cabral-Marques and Riemekasten, 2016). These autoantibodies are more frequent in patients with CTD-PAH compared to other forms of PH and might be diagnostic and prognostic biomarkers in SSc-PAH and/or CTD-PAH (Becker et al., 2014). In addition, it has been shown that anti-ET_AR Ab may identify patients at risk for the development of subsequent digital ulceration. Furthermore, SSc patients with loss of capillaries showed a strong

TABLE 1 | Autoantibody positivity and association with survival in SSc-ILD and SSc-PAH patients.

Reference	Antibody	Prevalence of PAH in patients with antibody positivity (No. of patients)	Prevalence of ILD in patients with antibody positivity (No. of patients)	Association with survival	Independent predictive ability for PAH (Odds ratio)
Hinchliff et al., 2015*	ACA	37% (162)	–	No	–
	ANA	24%	–	No	–
	Scl-70	7%	–	No	–
	U1RNP	5%	–	No	–
	RNA pol III	6%	–	No	–
Sobanski et al., 2016#	Anti-U1 RNP	11% (342)	–	No ($p = 0.055$)	
Okano et al., 1992	Anti-U3 RNP	17% (24)	25% (24)	–	–
Aggarwal et al., 2009	Anti-U3 RNP	31% (86)	36% (97)	–	–
Mitri et al., 2003	Anti Th/To	28% (87)	48% (87)	–	–
	ACA	19% (306)	13% (306)	–	–
Becker et al., 2014	Anti-ET_AR	–	–	Yes	2.7
	Anti-AT_1R	–	–	Yes	1.053

*ACA, anticentromere antibody; anti-ETAR, endothelin-1 type A receptor; AT1R, angiotensin II type 1 receptor; ANA, antinucleolar antibody; ILD, interstitial lung disease; PAH, pulmonary arterial hypertension; RNA pol III, RNA polymerase III; Scl-70, antitopoisomerase antibody. *SSc vs. SSc-PAH. #CTD-PAH patients.*

association between the presence of an antibody titer and digital ulcerations or PH (Avouac et al., 2015b).

Interferons

A member of the interferon family, the type I interferon (type I IFN) has a central role in the innate immune response to viral infections, while type I IFN therapy may represent a risk factor for PAH (Galiè et al., 2015). In a recent study, investigating the role of type I IFN in PAH, serum levels of type I, II, and III IFN were found to be increased in patients with SSc-PAH (George et al., 2014). In addition, the serum interferon γ inducible protein 10 (IP10/CXCL10) was positively correlated with hemodynamic parameters, 6 minute walking distance test (6MWT), brain natriuretic peptide (BNP) and cardiac index (CI) (George et al., 2014). In another study there was also an association between IP-10 and PAH in SSc patients (Eloranta et al., 2010).

Chemokines

Chemokines belong to a protein family with a major role in leukocyte activation and chemoattraction, but they may also play an important role in angiogenesis (Koch et al., 1992; Strieter et al., 1995). CXCL4 is a chemokine with potent antiangiogenic properties which is secreted by megakaryocytes and plasmocytoid dendritic cells. The serum level of CXCL4 was markedly elevated in SSc patients and associated with PAH and lung fibrosis development (van Bon et al., 2014). The proangiogenic receptor CXCR6 ligand CXCL16 was also elevated in patients with SSc-PAH, however, correlation analysis with hemodynamic parameters was not performed (Rabquer et al., 2011).

Inflammatory Cytokines and Growth Factors

In SSc-PAH patients, a large number of pro-inflammatory cytokines have been recorded to be increased. The tumor necrosis factor alpha (TNF-α), interleukin (IL)-1β, IL-6, IL-8, and IL-13 are elevated in the serum and plasma of lcSSc-PAH patients (Pendergrass et al., 2010; Christmann et al., 2011). IL-6 is increased in MCTD-PAH patients compared to those without PAH (Nishimaki et al., 1999). The IL-18-binding isoform a (IL-18BPa) is elevated in SSc patients compared to healthy controls and positively correlated with SPAP and mPAP (Nakamura et al., 2016a). The macrophage migration inhibitory factor (MIF)—a pleiotropic cytokine with proinflammatory properties—is also elevated in SSc-PAH patients (Stefanantoni et al., 2015). The level of IL-5, IL-8, and IL-12 show no difference between SSc patients with and without PH (McMahan et al., 2015). Bosentan, a drug used for PAH therapy, causes a significant decrease of the serum levels of IL-2, IL-6, IL-8, and IFN-γ (Bellisai et al., 2011).

The growth differentiation factor (GDF)-15—a member of the transforming growth factor (TGF)-β superfamily- is strongly elevated in remodeled pulmonary arteries of SSc-PAH patients (Nickel et al., 2011). Accordingly, serum levels are increased in SSc-PAH patients compared with SSc patients without PAH and positively correlate with SPAP (Meadows et al., 2011). Importantly, an increased level of GDF-15 is associated with increased mortality (Nickel et al., 2008).

The level of acute phase response protein pentraxin-3 (PTX3), which act as an antiangiogenic factor by binding to fibroblast growth factor-2 (FGF-2) and inhibiting FGF-2-dependent neovascularization and extracellular matrix (ECM) proliferation is increased, while the level of fibroblast growth factor-2 (FGF-2) is decreased in SSc-PAH (Rusnati et al., 2004). Moreover, both changes are independently associated with the presence of PAH (Shirai et al., 2015). Markers associated with inflammation and immune activation are indicated in **Table 2**.

EXTRACELLULAR MATRIX COMPONENTS

Matrix metalloproteinases (MMPs) together with their inhibitors (TIMPs) are responsible for the degradation of ECM proteins and lead to the release and activation of cytokines, growth factors but also ECM degradation products (Nagase et al., 2006).

Osteopontin (OPN) is an extracellular matrix protein involved in bone remodeling, but it is also involved in pro-inflammatory and pro-fibrotic properties via modulation of a variety of cell types, including endothelial and vascular smooth muscle cells (Anborgh et al., 2011). It is elevated in SSc patients with PH, however, the same is true in SSc patients with ILD (Lorenzen et al., 2010). Unfortunately, there are no data comparing OPN serum or plasma levels between SSc-PAH and SSc-ILD patients. OPN has also been associated with IPAH (Lorenzen et al., 2011) and is therefore not specific for SSc-PAH. Circulating pro-MMP-10 was increased, in SSc-PH patients in comparison with SSc patients without PH or controls, which is consistent with MMP-10 overexpression in the pulmonary arteries of SSc-PAH patients (Avouac et al., 2017). The matrix metalloproteinase tissue inhibitor-4 (TIMP-4) may contribute to extracellular matrix deposition in SSc and its level is correlated with elevated SPAP in SSc patients (Gialafos et al., 2008). However, such correlations have also been found in PAH patients without SSc (Tiede et al., 2016). MMP-12 was elevated in capillary vessels of SSc-ILD patients, while MMP-7 in blood of SSc-ILD patients. However, the blood level of them were not analyzed in SSc-PAH patients (Moinzadeh et al., 2011; Manetti et al., 2012).

MMPs seem to be increased in SSc-ILD patients, while TIMPs are more likely associated with vascular changes. However, there are no prospective studies comparing these molecules between SSc-ILD and SSc-PAH patients.

ENDOTHELIAL PHYSIOLOGY AND ANGIOGENESIS

Microvascular endothelial cell injury plays a pivotal role in the pathogenesis of SSc (Altorok et al., 2014). The disease is characterized by an elevated number of activated monocytes/macrophages or T-lymphocytes in the circulation and tissues (Hasegawa et al., 2014). The infiltration of internal organs by these cells may provoke endothelial damage, fibroblast abnormalities, and alternatively activated macrophages, through the release of a variety of chemokines, cytokines, or growth factors (Abraham et al., 2009; Ueda-Hayakawa et al., 2013). Clinical and pathological findings of vascular destruction and endothelial cell activation

TABLE 2 | Markers of inflammation and immune activation in SSc-PAH patients.

Reference	Marker	No. SSc patients with PAH	No. SSc patients without PAH	No. control subjects	*P*-value
George et al., 2014	IFN	28	35	9	n.s.*
	IP-10				<0.05*,**
	ET-1				<0.05*,**
	IL-6				<0.05**
	IL-12p70				<0.05*
	TNF-α				<0.05**
van Bon et al., 2014	CXCL-4	n.d.	n.d.	n.d.	<0.001**
Christmann et al., 2011	IL-13	13	22	10	<0.001*
McMahan et al., 2015	IL-5	37	40	–	n.s.
	IL-8				n.s.
	IL-12				n.s.
Meadows et al., 2011	GDF-15	30	24	13	=0.004**
Gialafos et al., 2008	TIMP-4	37#	69	–	=0.003
Shirai et al., 2015	PTX3	21	150	–	=0.006
Lorenzen et al., 2010	OPN	8	62	–	=0.001

ET-1, endothelin 1; GDF-15, growth differentiation factor-15; IFN, interferon; IL, interleukin; IP-10, interferon gamma (symbol) inducible protein 10; n.d., no data available; n.s., no significant; OPN, osteopontin; PTX3, pentraxin 3; TIMP, tissue inhibitor of matrix metalloproteinase-4; TNF-alpha(symbol), tumor necrosis factor alpha(symbol).
**SSc-PAH vs. Control.*
***SSc vs. SSc-PAH.*
#SSc patients with elevated pulmonary artery systolic pressure (> = 40 mmHg).

strongly support the hypothesis of a unique vascular disease accompanied by the presence of inflammatory and redox potential changes (Abraham and Distler, 2007). Several soluble markers associated with endothelial damage, including a wide spectrum of adhesion molecules, anti-endothelial antibodies, or endothelial progenitor cells are increased in the circulation of SSc-PAH patients and thus may serve as potential biomarkers of a pulmonary vascular involvement.

Endothelin 1

Cell adhesion molecules located on the surface of endothelial cells are involved in cell adhesion and endothelial cell-smooth muscle cell interactions. Endothelin 1 (ET-1) is a potent vasoconstrictor peptide that is mainly secreted from endothelial cells (Hickey et al., 1985). This mechanism is triggered by protein kinase C (PKC) activation via enhancing the production of 1,2-diacylglycerol in vascular muscle cells (Barman, 2007). However, in pathological conditions ET-1 is secreted by many other cells, including fibroblasts, epithelial cells, smooth muscle cells, or inflammatory cells, such as macrophages and leukocytes (Böhm and Pernow, 2007). In fibroblasts, the expression of the peptide is induced by TGF-β causing also fibroblast migration, myofibroblast differentiation and proliferation of smooth muscle cells. Endothelin exerts its biological activity by interacting with two cell membrane-bound receptors called ET receptor A (ET_AR) and B (ET_BR). ET receptor antagonists are approved as targeted medications for PAH and one of them, bosentan, is also approved for the prevention of new digital ulcers in SSc patients (Hamaguchi et al., 2017).

An early study showed that ET-1 is elevated in the plasma of SSc patients (Yamane et al., 1991). Additionally, its level is increased in SSc patients with PAH (Coral-Alvarado et al., 2009; Kim et al., 2010) and correlates with echocardiographic parameters of right ventricular (RV) overload (Ciurzynski et al., 2014). According to a prospective observational study, the peptide level could reflect the presence and severity of PH and may indicate the response to bosentan therapy in patients with SSc-PH (Kawashiri et al., 2014). However, circulating ET-1 levels depend very much on ET-1 clearance by ET_BR on endothelial cells and may not represent the ET-1 levels in the tissues of interest.

Circulating Endothelial Cells and Endothelial Progenitor Cells

Circulating endothelial cells (CECs) and endothelial progenitor cells (EPCs) may play a role in endothelial repair and neovascularization and serve as biomarkers of PAH (Foris et al., 2016). Moreover, there is an evidence of dysfunction of these cells in PAH (Toshner et al., 2009). Regarding CECs in SSc, they were significantly correlated with PAP and DLCO in lcSSc patients (Del Papa et al., 2004). Previous studies suggested that EPC-derived endothelial cells (ECs) may play a role in the progression of vascular complications in SSc (Avouac et al., 2008a,b). A reduced number of EPCs was associated with PAH in SSc (Nevskaya et al., 2008). EPC-derived ECs showed an upregulation of the matrix metalloproteinase-10 (MMP-10) gene in SSc-PAH.

Asymmetric Dimethylarginine

Asymmetric dimethylarginine (ADMA) is an endogenous inhibitor of eNOS, which may contribute to endothelial dysfunction. In a small cohort of SSc-PAH patients, ADMA levels were significantly associated with PAH after adjustment for specific disease characteristics, cardiovascular risk factors, and other related vascular complications (Thakkar et al., 2016). An ADMA level ≥0.7 ng/mL in combination with an NT-proBNP ≥210 ng/mL showed 100% sensitivity and 90% specificity for the identification of SSc-PAH (Thakkar et al., 2016). However, other studies did not find any significant correlations between ADMA and echocardiographic markers of PH, (Dag et al., 2014; Foris et al., 2016), although they found a negative correlation with the 6-minute walking test (6MWT) (Dimitroulas et al., 2008). Taken together, the role of ADMA as a biomarker is currently controversial.

Von Willebrand Factor, Vascular Endothelial Growth Factor, Endostatin

Von Willebrand Factor (vWF) is a circulating glycoprotein and a marker of endothelial cell activation or damage, secreted by endothelial cells and megakaryocytes. It plays an important role in the coagulation cascade as a carrier for coagulation factor VIII (Lip and Blann, 1997). Elevated levels of vWF were found in IPAH and in CTEPH patients (Bonderman et al., 2003) and also in lcSSc patients with PAH which was associated with an increased risk for a PAP elevation (Pendergrass et al., 2010; Barnes et al., 2012). In contrast, in another study, there was no difference between SSc and SSc-PAH patients in vWF levels (Iannone et al., 2008). In addition, the vWF antigen was elevated in MCTD-PAH patients, as compared to MCTD patients without PAH (Vegh et al., 2006). Thus, vWF may be a marker of increased PAH risk in lcSSc and MCTD patients. No data, however, are available for dcSSc patients.

The angiogenic factor vascular endothelial growth factor (VEGF) is increased in SSc patients with elevated SPAP as assessed by echocardiography. Additionally, there is a positive correlation between VEGF and SPAP (Papaioannou et al., 2009).

Endostatin is a potent angiostatic peptide, which is a cleavage product of the extracellular matrix protein, collagen 18. Indeed, it may be considered as an endogenous antagonist of VEGF. It is massively upregulated in the intima of remodeled pulmonary arteries from SSc-PAH patients, and circulating levels of endostatin are correlated with markers of right ventricular failure (Hoffmann et al., 2015). Endostatin levels were elevated in SSc patients as compared to control subjects and a multivariable analysis in SSc patients showed an association between elevated endostatin levels and PAH. Endostatin was also a strong predictor of mortality (Reiseter et al., 2015). There is a polymorphism of collagen 18a1 which alters circulating endostatin levels and is also strongly associated with mortality in SSc patients. Finally, endostatin serum levels are correlated with exercise capacity, World Health Organization (WHO) functional class, and pulmonary hemodynamics (Damico et al., 2015).

Other Endothelial Markers

Other factors associated with endothelial physiology, such as platelet endothelial cellular adhesion molecule-1 (PECAM-1) and endoglin were also investigated in SSc-PAH. Increased PECAM-1 was found in SSc patients with digital ulceration and PAH, however, correlations with clinical parameters were not significant (Riccieri et al., 2011). In SSc-PAH compared to healthy controls, the endoglin level was increased and correlated with circulating ET-1 levels (Coral-Alvarado et al., 2009). However, the diagnostic and predictive value of these markers has not been confirmed in prospective studies. The soluble forms of E-selectin (sE-selectin) and vascular cell adhesion molecule-1 (sVCAM-1) serum levels were not elevated in lcSSc patients (Stratton et al., 1998). In accordance, another study found also no difference between the sVCAM levels of SSc and SSc-PAH patients (Iannone et al., 2008). Endothelial cells not only secrete various mediators but they can also release exosomes, a cell-derived vesicles. Exosomes can contain various macromolecules including proteins, lipids, and nucleic acids such as microRNA. Therefore, either their content or exosomes *per se* can serve as biomarkers. They may play a role in extension of fibrotic SSc process in non-affected tissues (Wermuth et al., 2017). The blood level of exosomes in SSc patients with vascular involvements were decreased (Nakamura et al., 2016b). However, further studies are required to prove their role in the vascular pathological processes of SSc-PAH patients.

METABOLIC CHANGES

There is strong experimental and epidemiological evidence supporting a "metabolic theory" of PAH development. Accordingly, several organs of PAH patients share mitochondria-based metabolic changes (Paulin and Michelakis, 2014; Michelakis et al., 2017).

Adipocytokines

In SSc-PAH, dysregulated adipose tissue and adipokine dysbalance have been found. The adipocytokines such as resistin, leptin, adiponectine, adipsin, or omentin are soluble and circulating factors. They are mainly produced by adipocytes and have pro-inflammatory and pro-angiogenic properties (Tilg and Moschen, 2006). Leptin has been considered as a mediator of immunological disorders in IPAH. Its level was elevated in IPAH and SSc-PAH patients compared to healthy controls and the function of leptin expressing T-lymphocytes was impaired in a leptin-dependent manner. However, leptin levels were not different between IPAH and SSc-PAH patients (Huertas et al., 2012). Omentin was also elevated in SSc patients with increased SPAP, however, it was not correlated with any fibrotic or inflammatory parameters (Miura et al., 2015). In SSc patients, SPAP was also associated with elevated resistin levels (Masui et al., 2014). Elevated circulating levels of adipsin were associated with SSc-PAH and adipsin gene single-nucleotide polymorphisms (Korman et al., 2017).

25(OH)-D Vitamin

In patients with SSc, low serum 25(OH)-D Vitamin levels were associated with increased SPAP as assessed by echocardiography (Atteritano et al., 2016) and there was a significant correlation between serum levels and diastolic dysfunction (Groseanu et al., 2016), but not with pulmonary arterial pressure (Groseanu et al.,

2016). However, there are few diseases that have not been associated with decreased 25(OH)-D vitamin levels. Therefore, this is certainly not specific for SSc or for PAH.

Metabolomics

In recent years, metabolomics showed promising results in the field of pulmonary vascular research. In an exploratory approach, numerous metabolites were associated with pulmonary arterial pressure and the elevation of kynurenine appeared quite specific for PH (Lewis et al., 2016). Indeed, kynurenine is a strong endogenous pulmonary vasodilator increasing both cAMP and cGMP levels in the target cells (Nagy et al., 2017). This suggests that the kynurenine system represents a negative feedback mechanism for PH, similar to the natriuretic peptides. In addition, the kynurenine system has a strong impact on immunologic signaling (Jasiewicz et al., 2016). Moreover, a recent analysis based on orthogonal signal correction (OSC), combined with a method of two dimensional separation of NMR data, highlighting possible clusters, trends, or outliers, confirmed a change in the metabolic profile of SSc-PAH as compared to SSc without PAH (Deidda et al., 2017). Altogether this suggests that many metabolic factors are changed in PAH, however, it is not clear if they are cause or consequence of the disease and what is their role in the pathogenesis of SSc-PAH.

MICRORNAS

Epigenetic changes are heritable alterations of the human genome affecting the gene expression without involving changes of the underlying DNA sequences. As the pathogenesis of SSc is thought to be influenced by environmental factors affecting human genome, these stimuli have been considered to be responsible for epigenetic regulatory complex changes which can manifest in alterations in disease outcomes (Aslani et al., 2018). RNA interference via microRNAs is considered to be one of the potential mechanisms to initiate and maintain epigenetic changes. Alterations in the regulation of microRNAs may lead to pathway alterations playing a role in the development of PAH (Thenappan et al., 2018). Moreover, they might contribute in processes of right ventricular remodeling (Batkai et al., 2017).

According to these concepts, microRNAs can be identified in the circulation, and circulating miRNA levels vary according to the severity of PH (Wei et al., 2013; Zhao et al., 2017). In patients with PH, the level of circulating miR-424(322) was elevated and was associated with more severe symptoms and hemodynamic changes, while miR-4632 has been identified as a possible serum PAH biomarker (Qian et al., 2017; Baptista et al., 2018). Regarding SSc miR-193b, it has been described as a possible contributor to proliferative vasculopathy (Iwamoto et al., 2016). In addition, microRNA let-7d from skin biopsies showed a negative association with the severity of PAP measured by echocardiography in patients with SSc (Izumiya et al., 2015). In summary, based on results in PAH and SSc patients, micro RNAs might represent attractive biomarkers as well as future therapeutic targets in PH and SSc. However, their role in the pathogenesis of SSc-PAH needs further investigation.

MARKERS OF CARDIAC DYSFUNCTION

Microvascular alterations may play a pivotal role both in the impairment of myocardial function and the development of pulmonary vascular disease in SSc. These changes, directly or indirectly may cause right ventricular failure. Several studies investigated the potential role of different markers released by the heart, including the natriuretic peptide family, D-dimer as well as Troponin T and I as diagnostic and prognostic tools for PH in SSc patients. Studies investigating heart-related markers in SSc associated PH are listed in **Table 3**.

Natriuretic Peptides

Natriuretic peptides are well established, clinically useful markers of right ventricular dysfunction in PH. A-type natriuretic peptide (ANP) is secreted from granula in the atrial cardiomyocytes in response to an increased RV afterload. Any release of afterload causes an immediate decrease of the secretion (Wiedemann et al., 2001). The major disadvantage of ANP lies in its complicated handling methods. The N-terminal fragment of A-type natriuretic peptide (NT-proANP) is the inactive form of ANP, which is more stable and has a longer life-time in the circulation. In a prospective study, NT-proANP revealed a prognostic value for cardiac involvement, including PH in SSc (Költo et al., 2014).

Most of the studies focused on the investigation of BNP and its terminal fragment NT-proBNP. NT-proBNP is a 32-amino acid polypeptide attached to a 76-amino acid N-terminal fragment and it is secreted but not stored by ventricular cardiomyocytes (Janda and Swiston, 2010). BNP does not need cooled handling or transportation after blood drawn and the metabolic clearance of NT-proBNP is slow in comparison with ANP or BNP (Foris et al., 2013). As a consequence, the levels depend considerably on renal function.

Several studies found significant correlations between hemodynamic parameters, exercise capacity and natriuretic peptides in SSc-PAH (Mukerjee et al., 2003; Ciurzynski et al., 2008; Dimitroulas et al., 2010). In screening for PAH, both BNP and NT-proBNP were correlated with PAP, and BNP was an independent predictor of PAH in SSc patients (Cavagna et al., 2010). NT-proBNP combined with pulmonary function test and other markers had a high sensitivity and specificity in a screening model for PH (Thakkar et al., 2016). Importantly, NT-proBNP has been included in the 2015 risk stratification for IPAH as a prognostic marker (Galiè et al., 2015). A study in 101 SSc patients found that an increased NT-proBNP level together with a decreased DLCO/VA ratio was highly predictive for PAH development in the next 29-months (Allanore et al., 2008). Moreover, in a prospective study, the peptide level alone was strongly related to the severity of PAH and its increase during therapy was associated with high mortality (Williams et al., 2006). Another study found no relation between the changes of NT-proBNP and the clinical status (Rotondo et al., 2017). A retrospective study in 432 SSc patients with PH due to left heart disease from a French-Canadian cohort suggested mid-regional pro-atrial natriuritic peptide (MR-proANP) and mid-regional

TABLE 3 | Overview of heart related markers in patients with SSc-PAH or at risk of PH, correlation with hemodynamic parameters, predictive value, cut-off values, and association with survival.

Reference	Marker	No. SSc-PAH patients	RVSP	mPAP	PVR	Independent predictive ability for PAH (Odds ratio)	Cut-off value for identification of PAH	Association with survival
Költo et al., 2014	NT-proANP	144*	–	–	–	–	822.5 pmol/l (Sensitivity: 56.3% Specificity: 79.5%)	yes
	NT-proBNP						154.5 pmol/l (Sensitivity: 50% Specificity: 76.8%)	
Mukerjee et al., 2003	NT-proBNP	23	$r = 0.59$	$r = 0.53$	$r = 0.49$	–	395.34 pg/ml (Sensitivity:0.69 Specificity: 1.0)	–
Ciurzynski et al., 2008	NT-proBNP	51*	–	–	–	29.5	115 pg/ml (Sensitivity: 92% Specificity: 44%)	–
Cavagna et al., 2010	NT-proBNP	20	–	$r = 0.61$	$r = 0.61$	–	239.4 pg/ml (Sensitivity: 45% Specificity: 90%)	–
	BNP		–	$r = 0.72$	$r = 0.61$	2.1	64 pg/ml (Sensitivity: 60% Specificity: 87%)	–
Thakkar et al., 2016	NT-proBNP	15 (all 94)	$r = 0.65$**	$r = 0.63$**	$r = 0.76$**	–	209.8 pg/ml (Sensitivity: 92.9% Specificity: 100%)	–
Allanore et al., 2008	NT-proBNP	8	–	–	–	6.35 (p=0.053)	–	–
Williams et al., 2006	NT-proBNP	68	–	$r = 0.62$	$r = 0.81$	–	91 pg/ml (Sensitivity: 90% Specificity: 51%)	yes
Rotondo et al., 2017	NT-proBNP	21	$r = 0.30$	–	–	–	–	–
Kiatchoosakun et al., 2007	D-dimer	47	n.s.	–	–	–	–	–
Nordin et al., 2017	NT-proBNP	44#	–	–	–	1.9	–	–
	Hs-cTnI		–	–	–	3.2	–	–
Avouac et al., 2015a	NT-proBNP	89&	–	–	–	26.6	–	–
	Hs-cTnT		–	–	–	2.0	–	–
	NT-proBNP + Hs-cTnT		–	–	–	50.0	–	–

BNP, brain natriuretic peptide; Hs-cTnI, high-sensitivity cardiac troponin I; Hs-cTnI, high-sensitivity cardiac troponin T; NT-proANP, N-terminal atrial natriuretic peptide; NT-proBNP, N-terminal pro brain natriuretic peptide. All values reached the significance level of $p < 0.05$.
**SSc patients with heart involvement, including PH.*
***The analysis involved all the patients.*
#SSc patients with abnormal echocardiographic findings.
&SSc patients with cardiovascular risk factors.

pro-adrenomedullin (MR-proADM) may be more reliable than NT-proBNP as a biomarker for early PH (Miller et al., 2014).

D-Dimer, Troponin T and I

There is some indication from epidemiological and experimental studies that microvascular thrombosis may be involved in the pathogenesis of PAH. However, a cross-sectional study in SSc-PAH patients found no correlation between plasma D-dimer and RVSP assessed by echocardiography (Kiatchoosakun et al., 2007).

Troponin T (TnT) and high-sensitive Troponin I (hs-cTnI) are well-known markers of acute ischemic heart disease and have been identified as independent markers of mortality in PAH (Foris et al., 2013). A small study in SSc patients found a significant association between hs-cTnI and elevated echocardiographic SPAP (Nordin et al., 2017). The high-sensitive TnT (HS-cTnT) was even elevated in SSc patients without relevant cardiovascular risk factors and an HS-cTnT level of >14 ng/L was independently associated with PAH. The combination of this marker with NT-proBNP was strongly associated with PAH (Avouac et al., 2015a). Therefore, the combination of TnT subtypes and NT-proBNP might serve as predictor for PH in SSc. Unfortunately, these markers are not specific for the right ventricle and may be increased to the same extent by left heart disease. They are also not specific for SSc or any other cause of PH.

FUTURE CLINICAL AND RESEARCH NEEDS

The diagnosis of SSc-PAH needs an invasive method, therefore the inauguration of a well-established non-invasive diagnostic method would be crucial. The number of studies evaluating biomarkers in blood samples as diagnostic tools for PAH detection in SSc is progressively increasing, however very few of them have demonstrated solid diagnostic performance. Recent advances in the understanding of pathophysiological processes are promising for further therapies; nevertheless, the most important point for now is the early diagnosis as a mean to early treatment. The combination of biomarkers which help to differentiate between pulmonary parenchymal and vascular complications in SSc at an early stage would be very important. However, these biomarkers have to be validated in prospective multicenter studies involving a large series of patients. In addition, there are no unified definitions to segregate PAH (group 1 of the World Classification of PH) from PH-ILD (group 3 of the World Classification of PH). Different studies apply different definitions that make it difficult to compare the data about potential biomarkers. Thus, selection criteria for patients must be defined well and prospectively. Finally, an extended research interest is needed implicating underlying mechanisms described in systemic sclerosis. One example may be the association between adipocytokines and malabsorbtion, as latter molecules can be associated with the disease pathogenesis. It is likely that in the future some of the discussed biomarkers will be employed, alone or in combination with other already established biomarkers or clinical parameters, to improve the accuracy of early diagnosis and guide therapy.

CONCLUSIONS

PAH is a severe complication of SSc and associated with high morbidity and mortality. There are several biomarkers of SSc-PAH, reflecting endothelial physiology, inflammation, immune activation, extracellular matrix, metabolic changes, or cardiac involvement. Biomarkers in form of antibodies, cytokines, chemokines, metabolites, and natriuretic peptides were associated with diagnosis, disease severity, and progression. However, very few have been tested in a prospective setting. Prospective studies in well-defined patient cohorts are warranted to develop reliable algorithms for detection and prognosis of SSc-PAH.

AUTHOR CONTRIBUTIONS

All authors conceptualized and designed the review. BO, HO, and GK wrote the paper. VF, AG, VM, GKW and PH provided critical feedback and input. All authors agree to be accountable for the content of the work and approved the manuscript.

REFERENCES

Abraham, D., and Distler, O. (2007). How does endothelial cell injury start? The role of endothelin in systemic sclerosis. *Arthritis Res. Ther.* 9(Suppl. 2):S2. doi: 10.1186/ar2186

Abraham, D. J., Krieg, T., Distler, J., and Distler, O. (2009). Overview of pathogenesis of systemic sclerosis. *Rheumatology* 48(Suppl. 3), iii3–7. doi: 10.1093/rheumatology/ken481

Aggarwal, R., Lucas, M., Fertig, N., Oddis, C. V., and Medsger, T. A. Jr. (2009). Anti-U3 RNP autoantibodies in systemic sclerosis. *Arthritis Rheum.* 60, 1112–1128. doi: 10.1002/art.24409

Allanore, Y., Borderie, D., Avouac, J., Zerkak, D., Meune, C., Hachulla, E., et al. (2008). High N-terminal pro-brain natriuretic peptide levels and low diffusing capacity for carbon monoxide as independent predictors of the occurance of precapillary pulmonary arterial hypertension in patients with systemic sclerosis. *Arthritis Rheum.* 58, 284–291. doi: 10.1002/art.23187

Altorok, N., Wang, Y., and Kahaleh, B. (2014). Endothelial dysfunction in systemic sclerosis. *Curr. Opin. Rheumatol.* 26, 615–620. doi: 10.1097/BOR.0000000000000112

Anborgh, P. H., Mutrie, J. C., Tuck, A. B., and Chambers, A. F. (2011). Pre- and post-translational regulation of osteopontin in cancer. *J. Cell. Commun. Signal.* 5, 111–122. doi: 10.1007/s12079-011-0130-6

Aslani, S., Sobhani, S., Gharibdoost, F., Jamshidi, A., and Mahmoudi, M. (2018). Epigenetics and pathogenesis of systemic sclerosis; the ins and outs. *Hum. Immunol.* 79, 178–187. doi: 10.1016/j.humimm.2018.01.003

Atteritano, M., Santoro, D., Corallo, G., Visalli, E., Buemi, M., Catalano, A., et al. (2016). Skin invovement and pulmonary hypertension are associated with vitamin D insufficiency in scleroderma. *Int. J. Mol. Sci.* 17:2103. doi: 10.3390/ijms17122103

Avouac, J., Airo, P., Meune, C., Beretta, L., Dieude, P., Caramaschi, P., et al. (2010). Prevalence of pulmonary hypertension in systemic sclerosis in European Caucasians and meta-analysis of 5 studies. *J. Rheumatol.* 37, 2290–2298. doi: 10.3899/jrheum.100245

Avouac, J., Guignabert, C., Hoffmann-Vold, A. M., Ruiz, B., Dorfmuller, P., Pezet, S., et al. (2017). Stromelysin-2 (MMP-10), a novel mediator of vascular remodeling underlying pulmonary hypertension associated with systemic sclerosis. *Arthritis Rheumatol.* 69, 2209–2221. doi: 10.1002/art.40229

Avouac, J., Juin, F., Wipff, J., Couraud, P. O., Chiocchia, G., Kahan, A., et al. (2008a). Circulating endothelial progenitor cells in systemic sclerosis: association with disease severity. *Ann. Rheum. Dis.* 67, 1455–1460. doi: 10.1136/ard.2007.082131

Avouac, J., Meune, C., Chenevier-Gobeaux, C., Borderie, D., Lefevre, G., Kahan, A., et al. (2015a). Cardiac biomarkers in systemic sclerosis: contribution of high-sensitive cardiac troponin in addition to N-terminal pro-brain natriuretic peptide. *Arthritis Care Res.* 67, 1022–1030. doi: 10.1002/acr.22547

Avouac, J., Riemekasten, G., Meune, C., Ruiz, B., Kahan, A., and Allanore, Y. (2015b). Autoantibodies against Endothelin 1 Type A Receptor are strong predictors of digital ulcers in systemic sclerosis. *J. Rheumatol.* 42, 1801–1807. doi: 10.3899/jrheum.150061

Avouac, J., Wipff, J., Goldman, O., Ruiz, B., Couraud, P. O., Chiocchia, G., et al. (2008b). Angiogenesis in systemic sclerosis: impaired expression of vascular endothelial growth factor receptor 1 in endothelial progenitor-derived cells under hypoxic conditions. *Arthritis Rheum.* 58, 3550–3561. doi: 10.1002/art.23968

Baptista, R., Marques, C., Catarino, S., Enquita, F. J., Costa, M. C., Matafome, P., et al. (2018). MicroRNA-424(322) as a new marker of disease progression in pulmonary arterial hypertension and its role in right ventricular hypertrophy by targeting SMURF1. *Cardivasc. Res.* 114, 53–64. doi: 10.1093/cvr/cvx187

Barman, S. A. (2007). Vasoconstrictor effect of endothelin-1 on hypertensive pulmonary arterial smooth muscle involves Rho-kinase and protein kinase C. *Am. J. Physiol. Lung Cell. Mol. Physiol.* 293, L472–L479. doi: 10.1152/ajplung.00101.2006

Barnes, T., Giddon, A., Doré, C. J., Maddison, P., Moots, R. J., and the QUINs Trial Study Group (2012). Baseline vWF factor predicts the development of elevated pulmonary artery pressure in systemic sclerosis. *Rheumatology* 51, 1606–1609. doi: 10.1093/rheumatology/kes068

Batkai, S., Bär, C., and Thum, T. (2017). MicroRNAs in right ventricular remodelling. *Cardiovasc. Res.* 113, 1433–1440. doi: 10.1093/cvr/cvx153

Becker, M. O., Kill, A., Kutsche, M., Guenther, J., Rose, A., Tabeling, C., et al. (2014). Vascular receptor autoantibodies in pulmonary arterial hypertension associated with systemic sclerosis. *Am. J. Respir. Crit. Care Med.* 190, 808–817.

doi: 10.1164/rccm.201403-0442OC

Bellisai, F., Morozzi, G., Scaccia, F., Chellini, F., Simpatico, A., Pecetti, G., et al. (2011). Evaluation of the effect of Bosentan treatment on proinflammatory cytokine serum levels in patients affected by Systemic Sclerosis. *Int. J. Immunopathol. Pharmacol.* 24, 261–264. doi: 10.1177/039463201102400134

Böhm, F., and Pernow, J. (2007). The importance of endothelin-1 for vascular dysfunction in cardiovascular disease. *Cardiovasc. Res.* 76, 8–18. doi: 10.1016/j.cardiores.2007.06.004

Bonderman, D., Turecek, P. L., Jakowitsch, J., Weltermann, A., Adlbrecht, C., Schneider, B., et al. (2003). High prevalence of elevated clotting factor VIII in chronic thromboembolic pulmonary hypertension. *Thromb. Haemost.* 90, 372–376. doi: 10.1160/TH03-02-0067

Cabral-Marques, O., and Riemekasten, G. (2016). Vascular hypothesis revisited: role of stimulating antibodies against angiotensin and endothelin receptors in the pathogenesis of systemic sclerosis. *Autoimmun. Rev.* 15, 690–694. doi: 10.1016/j.autrev.2016.03.005

Cavagna, L., Caporali, R., Klersy, C., Ghio, S., Albertini, R., Scelsi, L., et al. (2010). Comparison of brain natriuretic peptide (BNP) and NT-proBNP in screening for pulmonary arterial hypertension in patients with systemic sclerosis. *Rheumatol.* 37, 2064–2070. doi: 10.3899/jrheum.090997

Chaisson, N. F., and Hassoun, P. M. (2013). Systemic sclerosis-associated pulmonary hypertension. *Chest* 144, 1346–1356. doi: 10.1378/chest.12-2396

Choi, M. Y., and Fritzler, M. J. (2016). Progress in understanding the diagnostic and pathogenic role of autoantibodies associated with systemic sclerosis. *Curr. Opin. Rheumatol.* 28, 586–594. doi: 10.1097/BOR.0000000000000325

Christmann, R. B., Hayes, E., Pendergrass, S., Padilla, C., Farina, G., Affandi, A. J., et al. (2011). Interferon and alternative activation of monocyte/macrophages in systemic sclerosis-associated pulmonary arterial hypertension. *Arthritis Rheum.* 63, 1718–1728. doi: 10.1002/art.30318

Chung, L., Domsic, R. T., Lingala, B., Alkassab, F., Bolster, M., Csuka, M. E., et al. (2014a). Survival and predictors of mortality in systemic sclerosis-associated pulmonary arterial hypertension: outcomes from the pulmonary hypertension assessment and recognition of outcomes in scleroderma registry. *Arthritis Care Res.* 66, 489–495. doi: 10.1002/acr.22121

Chung, L., Farber, H. W., Benza, R., Miller, D. P., Parsons, L., Hassoun, P. M., et al. (2014b). Unique predictors of mortality in patients with pulmonary arterial hypertension associated with systemic sclerosis in the REVEAL registry. *Chest* 146, 1494–1504. doi: 10.1378/chest.13-3014

Chung, L., Liu, J., Parsons, L., Hassoun, P. M., McGoon, M., Badesch, D. B., et al. (2010). Characterization of connective tissue disease-associated pulmonary arterial hypertension from REVEAL. *Chest* 138, 1383–1394. doi: 10.1378/chest.10-0260

Ciurzynski, M., Bienias, P., Irzyk, K., Kostrubiec, M., Bartoszewicz, Z., Siwicka, M., et al. (2014). Serum endothelin-1 and NT-proBNP, but not ADMA, endoglin and TIMP-1 levels, reflect impaired right ventricular function in patients with systemic sclerosis. *Clin. Rheumatol.* 33, 83–89. doi: 10.1007/s10067-013-2354-8

Ciurzynski, M., Bienias, P., Lichodziejewska, B., Kurnicka, C., Szewczyk, A., Glinska-Wielochowska, M., et al. (2008). Non-invasive diagnostic and functional evaluation of cardiac involvement in patients with systemic sclerosis. *Clin. Rheumatol.* 27, 991–997. doi: 10.1007/s10067-008-0837-9

Coral-Alvarado, P., Quintana, G., Garces, M. F., Cepeda, L. A., Caminos, J. E., Rondon, F., et al. (2009). Potential biomarkers for detecting pulmonary arterial hypertension in patients with systemic sclerosis. *Rheumatol. Int.* 29, 1017–1024. doi: 10.1007/s00296-008-0829-8

Dag, S., Budulgan, M., Dilek, B., Batmaz, I., Aritürk, Z., Nas, K., et al. (2014). Relation of asymmetric dymethylarginine and cardiac involvement in systemic sclerosis. *Acta Rheumatol. Port.* 39, 228–235.

Damico, R., Kolb, T. M., Valera, L., Wang, L., Housten, T., Tedford, R. J., et al. (2015). Serum endostatin is a genetically determined predictor of survival in pulmonary arterial hypertension. *Am. J. Resp. Crit. Care Med.* 191, 208–218. doi: 10.1164/rccm.201409-1742OC

Deidda, M., Piras, C., Cadeddu Dessalvi, C., Locci, E., Barberini, L., Orofino, S., et al. (2017). Distinctive metabolomic fingerprint in scleroderma patients with pulmonary arterial hypertension. *Int. J. Cardiol.* 241, 401–406. doi: 10.1016/j.ijcard.2017.04.024

Del Papa, N., Colombo, G., Fracchiolla, N., Moronetti, L. M., Ingegnoli, F., Maglione, W., et al. (2004). Circulating endothelial cells as a marker of ongoing vascular disease in systemic sclerosis. *Arthritis Rheum.* 50, 1296–1304. doi: 10.1002/art.20116

Denton, C. P. (2015). Advances in pathogenesis and treatment of systemic sclerosis. *Clin. Med.* 15, s58–s63. doi: 10.7861/clinmedicine.15-6-s58

Denton, C. P., and Khanna, D. (2017). Systemic Sclerosis. *Lancet* 390, 1685–1699. doi: 10.1016/S0140-6736(17)30933-9

Dimitroulas, T., Giannakoulas, G., Karvounis, H., Gatzoulis, M. A., and Settas, L. (2010). Natriuretic peptides in systemic sclerosis-related pulmonary arterial hypertension. *Semin. Arthritis Rheum.* 39, 278–284. doi: 10.1016/j.semarthrit.2009.03.005

Dimitroulas, T., Giannakoulas, G., Sfetsios, T., Karvounis, H., Dimitroula, H., Koliakos, G., et al. (2008). Asymmetrical dimethylarginine in systemic sclerosis-related pulmonary arterial hypertension. *Rheumatology* 47, 1682–1685. doi: 10.1093/rheumatology/ken346

Dorfmüller, P., Humbert, M., Perros, F., Sanchez, O., Simmonneau, G., Müller, K. M., et al. (2007). Fibrous remodeling of the pulmonary venous system in pulmonary arterial hypertension associated with connective tissue diseases. *Hum. Pathol.* 38, 893–902. doi: 10.1016/j.humpath.2006.11.022

Eloranta, M. L., Franck-Larsson, K., Lövgren, T., Kalamajski, S., Rönnblom, A., Rubin, K., et al. (2010). Type I interferon system activation and association with disease manifestations insystemic sclerosis. *Ann. Rheum. Dis.* 69, 1396–1402. doi: 10.1136/ard.2009.121400

Foris, V., Kovacs, G., Marsh, L. M., Bálint, Z., Tötsch, M., Avian, A., et al. (2016). CD133+ cells in pulmonary arterial hypertension. *Eur. Respir. J.* 48, 459–469. doi: 10.1183/13993003.01523-2015

Foris, V., Kovacs, G., Tscherner, M., Olschewski, A., and Olschewski, H. (2013). Biomarkers in pulmonary hypertension. *Chest* 144, 274–283. doi: 10.1378/chest.12-1246

Galiè, N., Humbert, M., Vachiery, J. L., Gibbs, S., Lang, I., Torbicki, A., et al. (2015). 2015 ESC/ERS guidelines for the diagnosis and treatment of pulmonary hypertension: the Joint Task Force for the Diagnosis and Treatment of Pulmonary Hypertension of the European Society of Cardiology (ESC) and the European Respiratory Society (ERS). *Eur. Heart J.* 37, 67–119. doi: 10.1093/eurheartj/ehv317

George, P. M., Oliver, E., Dorfmuller, P., Dubois, O. D., Reed, D. M., Kirkby, N. S., et al. (2014). Evidence for the involvement of type I interferon in pulmonary arterial hypertension. *Circ. Res.* 114, 677–688. doi: 10.1161/CIRCRESAHA.114.302221

Gialafos, E. J., Moyssakis, I., Psaltopoulou, T., Papadopoulos, D. P., Perea, D., Vlasis, K., et al. (2008). Circulating tissue inhibitor of matrix metalloproteinase-4 (TIMP) in systemic sclerosis patients with elevated pulmonary arterial pressure. *Mediators Inflamm.* 2008:164134. doi: 10.1155/2008/164134

Groseanu, L., Bojinca, V., Gudu, T., Saulescu, I., Predeteanu, D., Balanescu, A., et al. (2016). Low vitamin D status in systemic sclerosis and impact on disease phenotype. *Eur. J. Rheumathol.* 3, 50–55. doi: 10.5152/eurjrheum.2015.0065

Gu, Y. S., Kong, J., Cheema, G. S., Keen, C. L., Wick, G., and Gershwin, M. E. (2008). The immunobiology of systemic sclerosis. *Semin. Arthritis Rheum.* 38, 132–160. doi: 10.1016/j.semarthrit.2007.10.010

Hamaguchi, Y., Sumida, T., Kawaguchi, Y., Ihn, H., Tanaka, S., Asano, Y., et al. (2017). Safety and tolrealibity of bosentan for digital ulcers in Japanese patients with systemic sclerosis: prospective, multicenter, open-label study. *J. Dermatol.* 44, 13–17. doi: 10.1111/1346-8138.13497

Hao, Y., Thakkar, V., Stevens, W., Morrisroe, K., Prior, D., Rabusa, C., et al. (2015). A comparison of the predictive accuracy of three screening models for pulmonary arterial hypertension in systemic sclerosis. *Arthritis Res. Ther.* 17, 7–18. doi: 10.1186/s13075-015-0517-5

Hasegawa, M., Asano, Y., Endo, H., Fujimoto, M., Goto, D., Ihn, H., et al. (2014). Serum adhesion molecule levels as prognostic markers in patients with early systemic sclerosis: a multicentre, prospective, observational study. *PLoS ONE* 9:e88150. doi: 10.1371/journal.pone.0088150

Hickey, K. A., Rubanyi, G., Paul, R. J., and Highsmith, R. F. (1985). Characterization of a coronary vasoconstrictor produced by cultured endothelial cells. *Am. J. Physiol.* 248, C550–C556. doi: 10.1152/ajpcell.1985.248.5.C550

Hinchliff, M., Khanna, S., Hsu, V. M., Lee, J., Almagor, O., Chang, R. W., et al. (2015). Survival in systemic sclerosis-pulmonary arterial hypertension by serum autoantibody status in the Pulmonary Hypertension Assessment and Recognition of Outcomes in Scleroderma (PHAROS) Registry. *Semin. Arthritis Rheum.* 45, 309–314. doi: 10.1016/j.semarthrit.2015.06.011

Hoffmann, J., Marsch, L. M., Pieper, M., Stacher, E., Ghanim, B., Kovacs, G., et al. (2015). Compartment-specific expression of collagens and their processing enzymes in intrapulmonary arteries of IPAH patients. *Am. J. Physiol. Lung Cell. Mol. Physiol.* 308, L1002–L1013. doi: 10.1152/ajplung.00383.2014

Hoffmann-Vold, A. M., Midtvedt, O., Tennoe, A. H., Garen, T., Lund, M.

B., Alolokken, T. M., et al. (2017). Cardiopulmonary disease development in anti-RNA polymerase III-positive systemic sclerosis: comparative analysis from an unselected, prospective patient cohort. *J. Rheumatol.* 44, 459–465. doi: 10.3899/jrheum.160867

Hudson, M., Mahler, M., Pope, J., You, D., Tatibouet, S., Steele, R., et al. (2012). Clinical correlates of CENP-A and CENP-B antibodies in a large cohort of patients with systemic sclerosis. *J. Rheumatol.* 39, 787–794. doi: 10.3899/rheum.111133

Huertas, A., Tu, L., Gambaryan, N., Girerd, B., Perros, F., Montani, D., et al. (2012). Leptin and regulatory T-lymphocytes in idiopathic pulmonary arterial hypertension. *Eur. Respir. J.* 40, 895–904. doi: 10.1183/09031936.00159911

Iannone, F., Riccardi, M. T., Guiducci, S., Bizzoca, R., Cinelli, M., Matucci-Cerinic, M., et al. (2008). Bosentan regulates the expression of adhesion molecules on circulating T cells and serum soluble adhesion molecules in systemic sclerosis-associated pulmonary arterial hypertension. *Ann. Rheum. Dis.* 67, 1121–1126. doi: 10.1136/ard.2007.080424

Iwamoto, N., Vettori, S., Maurer, B., Brock, M., Pachera, E., Jüngel, A., et al. (2016). Downregulation of miR-193b in systemic sclerosis regulates the proliferative vasculopathy by urokinase-type plasminogen activator expression. *Ann. Rheum. Dis.* 75, 303–310. doi: 10.1136/annrheumdis-2014-205326

Izumiya, Y., Jinnn, M., Kimura, Y., Wang, Z., Onoue, Y., Hanatani, S., et al. (2015). Expression of let-7 family microRNAs in skin correlates negatively with severity of pulmonary hypertension in patients with systemic scleroderma. *Int. J. Cardiol. Heart Vasc.* 8, 98–102. doi: 10.1016/j.ijcha.2015.06.006

Janda, S., and Swiston, J. (2010). Diagnostic accuracy of plural fluid NT-pro-BNP for pleural effusions of cardiac origin: a systematic review and meta-analysis. *BMC Pulm. Med.* 10:58. doi: 10.1186/1471-2466-10-58

Jasiewicz, M., Moniuszko, M., Pawlak, D., Knapp, M., Rusak, M., Kazimierczyk, R., et al. (2016). Activity of the kynurenine pathway and its interplay with immunity in patients with pulmonary arterial hypertension. *Heart* 102, 230–237. doi: 10.1136/heartjnl-2015-308581

Jordan, S., Maurer, B., Toniolo, M., Michel, B., and Distler, O. (2015). Performance of the new ACR/EULAR classification criteria for systemic sclerosis in clinical practice. *Rheumatology* 54, 1454–1458. doi: 10.1093/rheumatology/keu530

Kawashiri, S. Y., Ueki, Y., Terada, K., Yamasaki, S., Aoyagi, K., and Kawakami, A. (2014). Improvement of plasma endothelin-1 and nitric oxide in patients with systemic sclerosis by bosentan therapy. *Rheumatol. Int.* 34, 221–225. doi: 10.1007/s00296-013-2861-6

Kiatchoosakun, S., Unqkasekvinai, W., Wonvipaporn, C., Tatsanavivat, P., Foocharoen, C., Suwannaroj, S., et al. (2007). D-dimer and pulmonary arterial hypertension in systemic sclerosis. *J. Med. Assoc. Thai.* 90, 2024–2029.

Kill, A., Tabeling, C., Undeutsch, R., Kühl, A. A., Günther, J., Radic, M., et al. (2014). Autoantibodies to angiotensin and endothelin receptors in systemic sclerosis induce cellular and systemic events associated with disease pathogenesis. *Arthritis Res. Ther.* 16:R29. doi: 10.1186/ar4457

Kim, H. S., Park, M. K., Kim, H. Y., and Park, S. H. (2010). Capillary dimension measured by computer-based digitalized image correlated with plasma endothelin-1 levels in patients with systemic sclerosis. *Clin. Rheumatol.* 29, 247–254. doi: 10.1007/s10067-009-1288-7

Koch, A. E., Polverini, P. J., Kunkel, S. L., Harlow, L. A., DiPietro, L. A., Elner, V. M., et al. (1992). Interleukin-8 as a macrophage-derived mediator of angiogenesis. *Science* 258, 1798–1801. doi: 10.1126/science.1281554

Költo, G., Vuolteenaho, O., Szokodi, I., Faludi, R., Tornyos, A., Ruskoaho, H., et al. (2014). Prognostic value of N-terminal natriuretic peptides in systemic sclerosis: a single center study. *Clin. Exp. Rheumatol.* 32(6 Suppl. 86), S75–S81.

Korman, B. D., Marangoni, R. G., Hinchcliff, M., Shah, S. J., Carns, M., Hoffmann, A., et al. (2017). Brief report: association of elevated adipsin levels with pulmonary arterial hypertension in systemic sclerosis. *Arthritis Rheumatol.* 69, 2062–2068. doi: 10.1002/art.40193

Kovacs, G., Avian, A., N., Wutte, Hafner, F., Moazedi-Fürst, F., Kielhauser, S., et al. (2017). Changes in pulmonary hemodynamics in scleroderma: a 4-year prospective study. *Eur. Respir. J.* 50:1601708. doi: 10.1183/13993003.01708-2016

Kowal-Bielecka, O., Avouac, J., Pittrow, D., Huscher, D., Behrens, F., Denton, C. P., et al. (2010). Echocardiography as an outcome measure in scleroderma-related pulmonary arterial hypertension: a systematic literature analysis by the EPOSS group. *J. Rheumatol.* 37, 105–115. doi: 10.3899/jrheum.090661

Leroy, E. C., Black, C., Fleischmajer, R., Jablonska, S., Krieg, T., Medsger, T. A. Jr, et al. (1988). Scleroderma (systemic sclerosis): classification, subsets and pathogenesis. *J. Rheumatol.* 15, 202–205.

Lewis, G. D., Ngo, D., Hemnes, A. R., Farrell, L., Domos, C., Pappagianopoulos, P. P., et al. (2016). Metabolic profiling of right ventricular-pulmonary vascular function reveals circulating biomarkers of pulmonary hypertension. *J. Am. Coll. Cardiol.* 67, 174–189. doi: 10.1016/j.jacc.2015.10.072

Lip, G. Y., and Blann, A. (1997). Von Willebrand factor: a marker of endothelial dysfunction in vascular disorders? *Cardiovasc. Res.* 34, 255–265. doi: 10.1016/S0008-6363(97)00039-4

Lorenzen, J. M., Krämer, R., Meier, M., Werfel, T., Whichmann, K., Hoeper, M. M., et al. (2010). Osteopontin in the development of systemic sclerosis – relation to disease activity and organ manifestation. *Rheumatology* 49, 1989–1991. doi: 10.1093/rheumatology/keq223

Lorenzen, J. M., Nickel, N., Kramer, R., Golpon, H., Westerkamp, V., Olsson, K. M., et al. (2011). Osteopontin in patients with idiopathic pulmonary hypertension. *Chest* 139, 1010–1017. doi: 10.1378/chest.10-1146

Manetti, M., Guiducci, S., Romano, E., Bellando-Randone, S., Conforti, M. L., Ibba-Manneschi, L., et al. (2012). Increased serum levels and tissue expression of matrix metalloproteinase-12 in patients with systemic sclerosis: correlation with severity of skin and pulmonary fibrosis and vascular damage. *Ann. Rheum. Dis.* 71, 1064–1072. doi: 10.1136/annrheumdis-2011-200837

Marsh, L. M., Jandl, K., Grünig, G., Foris, V., Bashir, M., Ghanim, B., et al. (2018). The inflammatory cell landscape in the lungs of patients with idiopathic pulmonary arterial hypertension. *Eur. Respir. J.* 51:1701214. doi: 10.1183/13993003.01214-2017

Masui, Y., Asano, Y., Akamata, K., Aozasa, N., Noda, S., Taniguchi, T., et al. (2014). Serum resistin levels: a possible correlation with pulmonary vascular involvement in patients with systemic sclerosis. *Rheumatol. Int.* 34, 1165–1170. doi: 10.1007/s00296-013-2880-3

McMahan, Z., Schoenhoff, F., Van Eyk, J. E., Wigley, F. M., and Hummers, L. K. (2015). Biomarkers of pulmonary hypertension in patients with scleroderma: a case-control study. *Arthritis Res. Ther.* 17:201. doi: 10.1186/s13075-015-0712-4

Meadows, C. A., Risbano, M. G., Zhang, L., Geraci, M. W., Tuder, R. M., Collier, D. H., et al. (2011). Increased expression of growth differentiation factor-15 in systemic sclerosis-associated pulmonary arterial hypertension. *Chest* 139, 994–1002. doi: 10.1378/chest.10-0302

Michelakis, E. D., Gurtu, V., Webster, L., Barnes, G., Watson, G., Howard, L., et al. (2017). Inhibition of pyruvate dehydrogenase improves pulmonary arterial hypertension in genetically susceptible patients. *Sci. Transl. Med.* 9:eaao4583. doi: 10.1126/scitranslmed.aao4583

Miller, L., Chartrand, S., Koenig, M., Goulet, J. R., Rich, É., Chin, A. S., et al. (2014). Left heart disease: a frequent cause of early pulmonary hypertension in systemic sclerosis, unrelated to elevated NT-proBNP levels or overt cardiac fibrosis but associated with increased levels of MR-proANP and MR-proADM: retrospective analysis of a French Canadian cohort. *Scand. J. Rheumatol.* 43, 314–323. doi: 10.3109/03009742.2013.854407

Mitri, G. M., Lucas, M., Fertig, N., Steen, V. D., and Medsger, T. A. Jr. (2003). A comparison between anti-Th/To- and anticentromere antibody-positive systemic sclerosis patients with limited cutaneous involvement. *Arthritis Rheum.* 48, 203–209. doi: 10.1002/art.10760

Miura, S., Asano, Y., Saigusa, R., Yamashita, T., Taniguchi, T., Takahashi, T., et al. (2015). Serum omentin levels: a possible contribution to vascular involvement in patients with systemic sclerosis. *J. Dermatol.* 42, 461–466. doi: 10.1111/1346-8138.12824

Moinzadeh, P., Krieg, T., Hellmich, M., Brinckmann, J., Neumann, E., Müller-Ladner, U., et al. (2011). Elevated MMP-7 levels in patients with systemic sclerosis: correlation with pulmonary involvement. *Exp. Dermatol.* 20, 770–773. doi: 10.1111/j.1600-0625.2011.01321.x

Morrisroe, K., Stevens, W., Sahhar, J., Rabusa, C., Nikpour, M., Proudman, S., et al. (2017). Epidemiology and disease characteristics of systemic sclerosis-related pulmonary arterial hypertension: results from a real-life screening programme. *Arthritis Res. Ther.* 19:42. doi: 10.1186/s13075-017-1250-z

Morse, J., Barst, R., Horn, E., Cuervo, N., Deng, Z., and Knowles, J. (2002). Pulmonary hypertension in scleroderma spectrum of disease: lack of bone morphogenetic protein receptor 2 mutations. *J. Rheumatol.* 29, 2379–2381.

Mukerjee, D., Yap, L. B., Holmes, A. M., Nair, D., Ayrton, P., Black, C. M., et al. (2003). Significance of plasma N-terminal pro-brain natriuretic peptide in patients with systemic sclerosis-related pulmonary arterial hypertension. *Respir. Med.* 97, 1230–1236. doi: 10.1016/S0954-6111(03)00254-3

Nagase, H., Visse, R., and Murphy, G. (2006). Structure and function of matrix metalloproteases and TIMPs. *Cardiovasc. Res.* 69, 562–573. doi: 10.1016/j.cardiores.2005.12.002

Nagy, B. M., Nagaraj, C., Meinitzer, A., Sharma, N., Papp, R., Foris, V., et al. (2017).

Importance of kynurenine in pulmonary hypertension. *Am. J. Physiol. Lung Cell. Mol. Physiol.* 313, L741–L751. doi: 10.1152/ajplung.00517.2016

Nakamura, K., Asano, Y., Taniquchi, T., Minatsuki, S., Inaba, T., Maki, H., et al. (2016a). Serum levels of interleukin-18-binding protein isoform a: clinical association with inflammation and pulmonary hypertension in systemic sclerosis. *J. Dermatol.* 43, 912–918. doi: 10.1111/1346-8138.13252

Nakamura, K., Jinnin, M., Harada, M., Kudo, H., Nakayama, W., Inoue, K., et al. (2016b). Altered expressionof CD63 and exosomes in scleroderma dermal fibroblasts. *J. Dermal. Sci.* 84, 30–39. doi: 10.1016/j.jdermsci.2016.06.013

Nevskaya, T., Bykovskaia, S., Lyssuk, E., Shakhov, I., Zaprjagaeva, M., Mach, E., et al. (2008). Circulating endothelial progenitor cells in systemic sclerosis: relation to impaired angiogenesis and cardiovascular manifestations. *Clin. Exp. Rheumatol.* 26, 421–429.

Nickel, N., Joniqk, D., Kempf, T., Bockmeyer, C. L., Maegel, L., Rische, J., et al. (2011). GDF-15 is abundantly expressed in plexiform lesions in patients with pulmonary arterial hypertension and affects proliferation and apoptosis of pulmonary endothelial cells. *Respir. Res.* 12:62. doi: 10.1186/1465-9921-12-62

Nickel, N., Kempf, T., Tapken, H., Tongers, J., Laenger, F., Lehmann, U., et al. (2008). Growth differentiation factor-15 in idiopathic pulmonary arterial hypertension. *Am. J. Respir. Crit. Care Med.* 178, 534–541. doi: 10.1164/rccm.200802-235OC

Nihtyanova, S. I., Schreiber, B. E., Ong, V. H., Rosenberg, D., Moinzadeh, P., Coghlan, J. G., et al. (2014). Prediction of pulmonary complications and long-term survival in systemic sclerosis. *Arth. Rheumatol.* 66, 1625–1635. doi: 10.1002/art.38390

Nishimaki, T., Aotsuka, S., Kondo, H., Yamamoto, K., Takasaki, Y., Sumiya, M., et al. (1999). Immunological analysis of pulmonary hypertension in connective tissue diseases. *J. Rheumatol.* 26, 2357–2362.

Nordin, A., Svenungsson, E., Bjornadal, L., Elvin, K., Larsson, A., and Jensen-Urstad, K. (2017). Troponin, I., and echocardiography in patient with systemic sclerosis and matched population controls. *Scand. J. Rheumatol.* 46, 226–235. doi: 10.1080/03009742.2016.1192217

Okano, Y., Steen, V. D., and Medsger, T. A. Jr. (1992). Autoantibody to U3 nucleolar ribonucleoprotein (fibrillarin) in patients with systemic sclerosis. *Arthritis Rheum.* 35, 95–100. doi: 10.1002/art.1780350114

Papaioannou, A. I., Zakynthinos, E., Kostikas, K., Kiropoulos, T., Koutsokera, A., Ziogas, A., et al. (2009). Serum VEGF levels are related to the presence of pulmonary arterial hypertension in systemic sclerosis. *BMC Pulm. Med.* 9:18. doi: 10.1186/1471-2466-9-18

Paulin, R., and Michelakis, E. D. (2014). The metabolic theory of pulmonary arterial hypertension. *Circ. Res.* 115, 148–164. doi: 10.1161/CIRCRESAHA.115.301130

Pendergrass, S. A., Hayes, E., Farina, G., Lemaire, R., Farber, H. W., Whitfield, M. L., et al. (2010). Limited systemic sclerosis patients with pulmonary arterial hypertension show biomarkers of inflammation and vascular injury. *PLoS ONE* 5:e12106. doi: 10.1371/journal.pone.0012106

Qian, Z., Li, Y., Chen, J., Li, X., and Gou, D. (2017). miR-4632 mediates PDFG-BB-induced proliferation and apoptosis of human pulmonary artery smooth muscle cells via targeting cJUN. *Am. J. Physiol. Cell Physiol.* 313, C380–C391. doi: 10.1152/ajpcell.00061.2017

Rabquer, B. J., Tsou, P. S., Hou, Y., Thirunavukkarasu, E., Haines, G. K. III, Impens, A. J., et al. (2011). Dysregulated expression of MIG/CXCL9, IP-10/CXCL10 and CXCL16 and their receptors in systemic sclerosis. *Arthritis Res. Ther.* 13:R18. doi: 10.1186/ar3242

Reiseter, S., Molberg, O., Gunnarsson, R., Lund, M. B., Aalokken, T. M., Aukrust, P., et al. (2015). Associations between circulating endostatin levels and vascular organ damage in systemic sclerosis and mixed connective tissue disease: an observational study. *Arthritis Res. Ther.* 17:231. doi: 10.1186/s13075-015-0756-5

Riccieri, V., Stefanantoni, K., Vasile, M., Macrì, V., Sciarra, I., Iannace, N., et al. (2011). Abnormal plasma levels of different angiogenic molecules are associated with different clinical manifestations in patients withsystemic sclerosis. *Clin. Exp. Rheumatol.* 29, S46–S52.

Rotondo, C., Praino, E., Nivuori, M., di Serio, F., Lapadula, G., and Iannone, F. (2017). No changes in N-terminal pro-brain natriuretic peptide in a longitudinal cohort of patients with systemic sclerosis-associated pulmonary arterial hypertension on therapy with bosentan. *Int. J. Rheum. Dis.* 20, 90–96. doi: 10.1111/1756-185X.12721

Rubin, L. J. (2017). Targeting bone morphogenic protein receptor 2 (BMPR2) signalling to treat pulmonary arterial hypertension. *Eur. Respir. J.* 50:1701370. doi: 10.1183/13993003.01370-2017

Rusnati, M., Camozzi, M., Moroni, E., Bottazzi, B., Peri, G., Indracollo, S., et al. (2004). Selective recognition of fibroblast growth factor-2 by the long pentraxin PTX3 inhibits angiogenesis. *Blood* 104, 92–99. doi: 10.1182/blood-2003-10-3433

Shirai, Y., Okazaki, Y., Inoue, Y., Tamura, Y., Yasuoka, H., Takeuchi, T., et al. (2015). Elevated levels of Pentraxin 3 in systemic sclerosis: associations with vascular manifestations and defective vasculogenesis. *Arthritis Rheum.* 67, 498–507. doi: 10.1002/art.38953

Sobanski, V., Giovanelli, J., Lynch, B. M., Schreiber, B. E., Nihtyanova, S. I., Harvey, J., et al. (2016). Characteristics and survival of anti-U1 RNP antibody patients with connective disease-associated pulmonary arterial hypertension. *Arthritis Rheumatol.* 68, 484–493. doi: 10.1002/art.39432

Stefanantoni, K., Sciarra, I., Vasile, M., Badagliacca, R., Poscia, R., Pendolino, M., et al. (2015). Elevated serum levels of macrophage migration inhibitory factor and stem cell growth factor β in patients with idiopathic and systemic sclerosis associated pulmonary arterial hypertension. *Reumatismo* 66, 270–276. doi: 10.4081/reumatismo.2014.774

Stratton, R. J., Coghlan, J. G., Pearson, J. D., Burns, A., Sweny, P., Abraham, D. J., et al. (1998). Different patterns of endothelial cell activation in renal and pulmonary vascular disease in scleroderma. *QJM* 91, 561–566. doi: 10.1093/qjmed/91.8.561

Strieter, R. M., Polverini, P. J., Kunkel, S. L., Arenberg, D. A., Burdick, M. D., Kasper, J., et al. (1995). The functional role of the ELR motif in CXC chemokine-mediated angiogenesis. *J. Biol. Chem.* 270, 27348–27357. doi: 10.1074/jbc.270.45.27348

Sweiss, N. J., Hushaw, L., Thenappan, T., Sawaqed, R., Machado, R. F., Patel, A. R., et al. (2010). Diagnosis and management of pulmonary hypertension in systemic sclerosis. *Curr. Rheumatol. Rep.* 12, 8–18. doi: 10.1007/s11926-009-0078-1

Thakkar, V., Stevens, W., Prior, D., Rabusa, C., Sahhar, J., Walker, J. G., et al. (2016). The role of asymmetric dymethylarginine alone and in combination with N-terminal pro-B-type natriuretic peptide as a screening biomarker for systemic sclerosis-related pulmonary arterial hypertension: a case control study. *Clin. Exp. Rheumatol.* 100, 129–136.

Thenappan, T., Ormiston, M. L., Ryan, J. J., and Archer, S. L. (2018). Pulmonary arterial hypertension: pathogenesis and clinical management. *BMJ* 360:j5492. doi: 10.1136/bmj.j5492

Tiede, S. L., Wassenberg, M., Christ, K., Schermuly, R. T., Seeger, W., Grimminger, F., et al. (2016). Biomarkers of tissue remodeling predict survival in patients with pulmonary hypertension. *Int. J. Cardiol.* 223, 821–826. doi: 10.1016/j.ijcard.2016.08.240

Tilg, H., and Moschen, A. R. (2006). Adipocytokines: mediators linking adipose tissue, inflammation and immunity. *Nat. Rev. Immun.* 6, 772–783. doi: 10.1038/nri1937

Toshner, M., Voswinckel, R., Southwood, M., Al-Lamki, R., Howard, L. S., Marchesan, D., et al. (2009). Evidence of dysfunction of endothelial progenitors in pulmonary arterial hypertension. *Am. J. Resp. Crit. Care Med.* 180, 780–787. doi: 10.1164/rccm.200810-1662OC

Tyndall, A. J., Bannert, B., Vonk, M., Airò, P., Cozzi, F., Carreira, P. E., et al. (2010). Causes and risk factors for death in systemic sclerosis: a study from the EULAR Scleroderma Trials and Research (EUSTAR) database. *Ann. Rheum. Dis.* 69, 1809–1815. doi: 10.1136/ard.2009.114264

Ueda-Hayakawa, I., Hasegawa, M., Hamaguchi, Y., Takehara, K., and Fujimoto, M. (2013). Circulating γ/δ T cells in systemic sclerosis exhibit activated phenotype and enhance gene expression of proalpha2(I) collagen of fibroblasts. *J. Dermatol. Sci.* 69, 54–60. doi: 10.1016/j.jdermsci.2012.10.003

van Bon, L., Affandi, A. J., Broen, J., Christmann, R. B., Marijnissen, R. J., Stawski, L., et al. (2014). Proteome-wide analysis and CXCL4 as a biomarker in systemic sclerosis. *N. Eng. J. Med.* 370, 433–443. doi: 10.1056/NEJMoa1114576

van den Hoogen, F., Khanna, D., Fransen, J., Johnson, S. R., Baron, M., Tyndall, A., et al. (2013). 2013 Classification criteria for systemic sclerosis: an American College of Rheumatology/European League against Rheumatism collaborative initiative. *Ann. Rheum. Dis.* 72, 1747–1755. doi: 10.1136/annrheumdis-2013-20442.

Varga, J., and Abraham, D. (2007). Systemic sclerosis: a prototypic multisystem fibrotic disorder. *J. Clin. Invest.* 117, 557–567. doi: 10.1172/JCI31139

Vegh, J., Szodoray, P., Kappelmayer, J., Csipo, I., Udvardy, M., Lakos, G., et al. (2006). Clinical and immunoserological characteristics of mixed connective tissue disease associated with pulmonary arterial hypertension. *Scand. J.*

Immunol. 64, 69–76. doi: 10.1111/j.1365-3083.2006.01770.x

Wei, C., Henderson, H., Spradley, C., Li, L., Kim, I. K., and Kumar, S. (2013). Circulating miRNAs as potential marker for pulmonary hypertension. *PLoS ONE* 8:e64396. doi: 10.1371/journal.pone.0064396

Wermuth, P. J., Piera-Velazquez, S., and Jimenez, S. A. (2017). Exosomes isolated from serum of systemic scelorsis patients display alteration in their content of profibrotic and antifibrotic microRNA and induce a profibrotic phenotype in cultured normal dermal fibroblasts. *Clin. Exp. Rheumatol.* 106, 21–30.

Wiedemann, R., Ghofrani, H. A., Weissmann, N., Schermuly, R., Quanz, K., Grimminger, F., et al. (2001). Atrial natriuretic peptide in severe primary and nonprimary pulmonary hypertension: response to iloprost inhalation. *J. Am. Coll. Cardiol.* 38, 1130–1136. doi: 10.1016/S0735-1097(01)01490-5

Williams, M. H., Handler, C. E., Akram, R., Smith, C. J., Das, C., Smee, J., et al. (2006). Role of N-terminal brain natriuretic peptide (N-TproBNP) in scleroderma-associated pulmonary arterial hypertension. *Eur. Heart J.* 27, 1485–1494. doi: 10.1093/eurheartj/ehi891

Yamane, K., Kashiwagi, H., Suzuki, N., Miyauchi, T., Yanagisawa, M., Goto, K., et al. (1991). Elevated plasma levels of endothelin-1 in systemic sclerosis. *Arthritis Rheum.* 34, 243–244. doi: 10.1002/art.17803 40220

Zhao, Y., Ponnusamy, M., Zhang, L., Zhang, Y., Liu, C., Yu, W., et al. (2017). The role of miR-214 in cardiovascular diseases. *Eur. J. Pharmacol.* 816, 138–145. doi: 10.1016/j.ejphar.2017.08.009

18

Circulating Protein Biomarkers in Systemic Sclerosis Related Pulmonary Arterial Hypertension

*Peter M. Hickey [1,2], Allan Lawrie [1] and Robin Condliffe [2]**

[1] Department of Infection, Immunity and Cardiovascular Disease, University of Sheffield, Sheffield, United Kingdom,
[2] Pulmonary Vascular Diseases Unit, Royal Hallamshire Hospital, Sheffield, United Kingdom

***Correspondence:**
Robin Condliffe
robin.condliffe@sth.nhs.uk

Pulmonary arterial hypertension (PAH) develops in 7–12% of patients with systemic sclerosis (SSc) and is associated with a 3 year survival of 52%. Early detection by screening is therefore recommended for all patients with SSc. Historically, screening has been performed using echocardiography and measurement of gas transfer. More recently the DETECT protocol, using a combination of biomarkers (including N-terminal pro-brain natriuretic peptide) and clinical parameters, has been developed. The optimal method of screening for PAH with high sensitivity and specificity is, however, not clear. Protein expression differences between different SSc disease phenotypes have been reported, and include alterations in concentration of NT-proBNP, endoglin, soluble vascular endothelial growth factor receptor 1, placenta growth factor, growth differentiation factor-15, vascular endothelial growth factor alpha, resistin-like molecule beta, and soluble thrombomodulin. This review summarizes the current knowledge of these protein changes in patients with SSc and PAH.

Keywords: systemic sclerosis, pulmonary arterial hypertension, protein, biomarkers, diagnosis

INTRODUCTION

Pulmonary arterial hypertension (PAH) is a rare disease characterized by a progressive vasculopathy of the small pulmonary arteries leading to increased pulmonary vascular resistance and right ventricular afterload. This results in right ventricular failure and premature death. PAH may be idiopathic, heritable, related to various drugs and toxins or may be associated with a number of medical conditions including congenital systemic to pulmonary shunts, portal hypertension, HIV and connective tissue disease, most notably systemic sclerosis (SSc). Although these forms of PAH have similarities in underlying pathophysiology and treatment regime, it is increasingly recognized that there are differences in pathobiology, response to treatment and prognosis.

Between 7 and 12% of patients with SSc develop PAH (SSc-PAH) at some point in their disease course (1–4). Compared to idiopathic pulmonary arterial hypertension (IPAH), histological patterns in SSc-PAH show greater intra-individual variability, a relative absence of plexiform lesions, more prominence of intimal fibrosis and a much greater involvement of pulmonary venules (5). Prognosis is significantly worse than in other forms of PAH with median survival of 3 and 7.8 years in SSc-PAH and IPAH cohorts respectively (6). Response to treatment is generally felt to be worse in SSc-PAH than in IPAH (7).

The diagnosis of PAH can be challenging, due in part to the relatively low incidence of this condition, and in part due to the non-specific nature of the early symptoms. As a result, the diagnosis of PAH is often made at an advanced stage after a large proportion of the pulmonary vascular bed has been irreversibly obliterated by pathological vascular remodeling.

Given the progressive nature of vascular remodeling in PAH, interest in the outcome of patients detected early has led to investigation of alternative screening methods in patients with systemic sclerosis. It is thought that early diagnosis and treatment leads to a favorable prognosis (8, 9). Historically, screening for PAH in SSc has involved estimating systolic pulmonary arterial pressure at annual echocardiography ± the measurement of diffusion capacity of the lung for carbon monoxide (DL_{CO}). The DETECT protocol was developed to provide an evidence-based multi-modality approach to screening patients with SSc for the presence of PAH. It combines variables from clinical examination, echocardiography, electrocardiography, pulmonary function tests and blood tests [uric acid and N-terminal pro-brain type natriuretic peptide (NT-proBNP)] to produce a score with high sensitivity (95%), but relatively low specificity (48%) for the presence of PAH (10). The DETECT protocol involves several steps which add complexity and in real-life clinical practice, may prove significantly more expensive and can lead to delay and even failure to refer for definitive investigations (11).

Abnormal concentrations of many candidate proteins have been shown in both the tissue and circulating compartments in patients with PAH. These proteins may reflect the underlying pulmonary vascular disease as well as the response of the right ventricle to the increased afterload. They may also reflect the underlying SSc rather than PAH. It is conceivable that a panel of protein biomarkers may have utility in identifying PAH in still asymptomatic patients with systemic sclerosis. This paper reviews the current published evidence base for altered protein biomarker concentrations in SSc-PAH.

METHODS

To identify suitable primary research articles on this topic, a literature search was conducted using Ovid Medline and PubMed. Keywords used were "Systemic sclerosis," "Scleroderma," "Pulmonary hypertension," "PAH," "Protein," and "Biomarker." Date of publication was limited from 1990 to present day. One hundred and forty eight publications were returned from this search.

We included studies identifying a cohort of patients diagnosed with systemic sclerosis with PAH with comparator groups including healthy volunteers (HV), systemic sclerosis without pulmonary hypertension (SSc-no PAH) and/or idiopathic PAH.

Studies were included if they reported data on differential protein expression between subgroups which were related to objective measurements of pulmonary hypertension.

Protein Biomarkers in SSc-PAH

The circulating protein biomarkers identified by the literature search are summarized in **Table 1** and **Figure 1**.

N-Terminal Pro-Brain Natriuretic Peptide (NT-proBNP)

NT-proBNP is a marker of myocardial stress and therefore a non-specific marker for pulmonary hypertension (PH). Brain type natriuretic peptide (BNP) and NT-proBNP remain the only blood-based biomarkers suggested by guidelines for routine clinical use (21). NT-proBNP is an inactive cleavage product released during the activation of BNP from its prohormone. BNP is released in response to ventricular stretch and stimulates natriuresis and diuresis via the kidney in order to reduce ventricular preload. NT-proBNP is elevated in PH of any cause (22) and correlates with echocardiographic, hemodynamic and functional measurements (23–25).

NT-proBNP may be elevated in systemic sclerosis in the absence of pulmonary hypertension as a result of left ventricular disease and primary myocardial involvement (26).

In a prospective observational study of 109 patients with systemic sclerosis, including 68 with PH and 41 without PH at right heart catheter, Williams et al. set out to evaluate the utility of NT-proBNP concentrations as a screening tool for PAH. NT-proBNP concentration was significantly higher in patients with PAH than without (1474 pg/ml vs. 139 pg/ml respectively, $p = 0.0002$). The authors also reported a significant correlation between NT-proBNP concentration and mean pulmonary arterial pressure (mPAP) ($r = 0.62, p < 0.0001$), pulmonary vascular resistance (PVR) ($r = 0.81$, $p < 0.0001$) and right atrial pressure (RAP) ($r = 0.53$, $p < 0.0001$) at right heart catheterization (RHC). For the ability to accurately diagnose PAH a threshold of 395 pg/ml was selected, returning a sensitivity 55.9%, specificity 95.1%, PPV 95.1% and NPV 56.5%. Longitudinal analysis of baseline and change in serial NT-proBNP measurements both demonstrated significant prognostic utility (27). More recent work has provided validation, with Chung et al. reporting a sensitivity and specificity of 73 and 78% respectively for NT-proBNP at a threshold of 210 pg/ml, slightly superior to that of BNP at 71 and 59% respectively at a threshold concentration of 64 pg/ml (13).

Comparing between PAH phenotypes in a study of 98 prevalent PAH patients (SSc-PAH $n = 55$; IPAH $n = 38$; Anorexigen $n = 5$), Mathai et al. found that NT-proBNP levels were significantly higher in the SSc-PAH group vs. IPAH group (1846 pg/ml vs. 808.5 pg/ml respectively, $p < 0.01$), and this was despite a significantly higher mPAP in the patients with IPAH (41 mmHg vs. 48 mmHg, SSc vs. IPAH respectively, $p < 0.01$). The authors also noted stronger correlations between NT-proBNP concentrations and hemodynamic measures of PAH for patients with SSc-PAH than for those with IPAH; cardiac index (CI) ($r = -0.58$, $p < 0.01$ vs. $r = -0.46$, $p < 0.01$ respectively); PVR ($r = 0.54$, $p < 0.01$ vs. $r = 0.41$, $p < 0.01$ respectively). When serial protein measurements were analyzed in each subgroup, the prognostic value of NT-proBNP for predicting death remained only in the group with SSc-PAH (SSc-PAH: hazard ratio (HR) 3.07, $p < 0.01$; IPAH: HR 2.02, $p = 0.29$) (14).

The DETECT study investigated a population of SSc patients who were enriched for the presence of PAH by the inclusion of patients with a DL_{CO} <60% predicted (10). NT-proBNP

TABLE 1 | Summary of potential protein biomarkers in SSc-PAH.

Protein	Comparison Groups	Number of Patients	Outcome	Correlations in SSc-PAH	Reference
NT-proBNP	SSc-PAH vs. SSc SSc-PAH vs. SSc SSc-PAH vs. IPAH	109 329 98	Significantly higher in SSc-PAH vs. SSc. Sens 55.9%, Spec 95.1%. Correlated with invasive hemodynamics NT-proBNP superior to BNP for detection of PAH in SSc Significantly higher in SSc-PAH, correlated with hemodynamics and predicted survival in SSc-PAH group.	mPAP ($r = 0.62$; $p < 0.0001$) PVR ($r = 0.81$; $p < 0.0001$) CI ($r = -0.58$; $p < 0.01$) PVR ($r = 0.54$; $p < 0.01$)	(12) (13) (14)
Endoglin	SSc-PAH vs. SSc vs. HV	60	Serum levels significantly higher in SSc-PAH than control		(15)
sFLT-1	SSc-PAH vs. SSc	77	Plasma levels significantly higher in SSc-PAH and correlate with RVSP and inversely with DL_{CO}. Possible predictor of PH progression.	RVSP ($r = 0.32$; $p = 0.01$) DL_{CO} (−0.29; $p = 0.01$)	(16)
PIGF	SSc-PAH vs. SSc	77	Plasma levels significantly higher in SSc-PAH. Correlates with severity of Raynaud's phenomenon and inversely with DL_{CO}.	DL_{CO} ($r = -0.031$; $p = 0.01$)	(16)
VEGF-A	SSC-PAH vs. SSc vs. HV	53	Serum levels significantly higher in SSc-PAH than either SSc or HV. Levels correlate with echocardiographic sPAP, dyspnoea score and DL_{CO}.	sPAP ($r = 0.58$; $p < 0.01$) DL_{CO} ($r = -0.47$; $p < 0.01$)	(17)
GDF-15	SSc-PAH vs. SSc	54	Plasma levels significantly higher in SSc-PAH, correlate with echocardiographic RVSP and circulating NT-proBNP. Discriminates between PH and non-PH.	RVSP ($r = 0.56$; $p < 0.001$)	(18)
RELM-ß	SSc-PAH vs. IPAH vs. HV	26	Tissue concentrations significantly higher in SSc-PAH than in IPAH or HV.		(19)
sThrombomodulin	SSc-PAH vs. SSc vs. HV	92	Significantly higher plasma levels in SSc-PAH compared to either SSc or HV.		(20)

NT-proBNP, N-terminal pro-brain type natriuretic protein; sFLT-1, soluble vascular endothelial growth factor receptor 1; PIGF, placenta growth factor; VEGF-A, vascular endothelial growth factor A; GDF-15, growth differentiation factor-15; RELM-ß, resistin like molecule-ß; sThrombomodulin, soluble thrombomodulin; SSc-PAH, systemic sclerosis related pulmonary arterial hypertension; SSc, systemic sclerosis; IPAH, idiopathic pulmonary arterial hypertension; HV, healthy volunteer; Sens, sensitivity; PH, pulmonary hypertension; Spec, specificity; mPAP, mean pulmonary artery pressure; PVR, pulmonary vascular resistance; CI, cardiac index; RVSP, right ventricular systolic pressure; DL_{CO}, diffusing capacity for carbon monoxide; sPAP, systolic pulmonary artery pressure; EC, endothelial cells.

was included in a final 2-step algorithm which also included electrocardiography and echocardiography to select patients to proceed to RHC. Sensitivity for the detection of PAH was high (96%) but specificity was only 48%.

Both BNP and NT-proBNP levels have been demonstrated to be important prognostic predictors at baseline in PAH (28, 29). Subsequently, the change in NT-proBNP level after therapy was shown to be a powerful independent predictor of survival (30). More recently three large studies have confirmed the importance of changes in NT-proBNP in the risk stratification of patients with PAH during follow-up. (12, 31, 32).

Endoglin

Transforming growth factor beta (TGF-ß) signaling has been strongly implicated in the pathogenesis of PAH, and extensively studied, particularly with regard to bone morphogenetic protein receptor type-2 mutations (26). TGF-ß signaling regulates several processes including cellular proliferation and angiogenesis. Endoglin (Eng) is a transmembrane protein expressed in endothelial cells which acts as a TGF-ß signaling complex component (33).

Both TGF-ß serum concentration and Eng level are raised in IPAH patients, with Eng localized to endothelial cells in tissue samples (34). Germline Eng mutation have shown a protective effect against the development of pulmonary hypertension in heterozygous models exposed to chronic hypoxia (34).

Coral-Alvarado et al. investigated circulating Eng concentration in 60 patients (20 SSc-PAH; 20 SSc-no PAH; 20 HV). PH was diagnosed by estimation of systolic pulmonary artery pressure >35 mmHg, or tricuspid regurgitant jet velocity >3 m/s. The authors report higher Eng concentrations in the SSc-PAH group, however possibly due to small study numbers, the difference is only statistically significant between SSc-PAH vs. healthy volunteer (HV) groups (SSc-PAH: 6.89 ng/ml, SSc-no PAH: 6.2 ng/ml, HV: 5.42 ng/ml; SSc-PAH vs. SSc-no PAH $p = 0.2447$, SSc-PAH vs. HV $p = 0.0006$, SSc-no PAH vs. HV $p = 0.057$). There was no correlation noted between Eng concentration and echocardiographic measurements of PH (15).

There is some evidence for altered Eng expression in PAH, however in SSc specifically, this evidence is weak in part due to small study sizes and study design. Given the potential role of Eng in TGF-ß signaling, a role in the pathogenesis of PAH

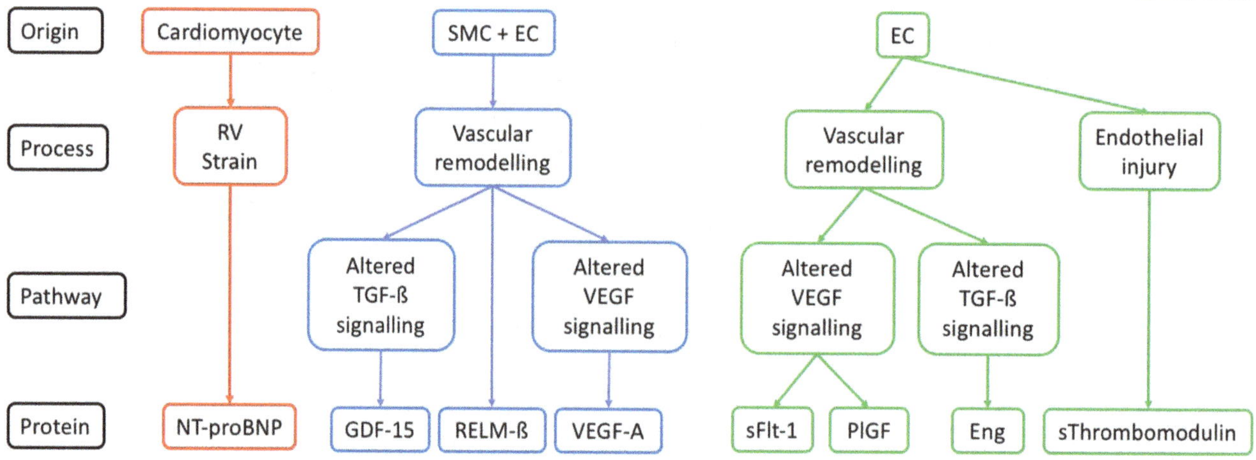

FIGURE 1 | Cellular origin and pathways for each protein described in the context of SSc-PAH. Description of the likely origin of each protein, along with the pathophysiological process it has a role in. If a component of one of the pathways known to be relevant to pathogenesis of PAH then this is also given. SMC, vascular smooth muscle cell; EC, vascular endothelial cell; RV, right ventricle; TGF-ß, transforming growth factor beta; VEGF, vascular endothelial growth factor; NT-proBNP, N-terminal pro-brain natriuretic peptide; GDF-15, growth differentiation factor-15; RELM-ß, resistin-like molecule beta; VEGF-A, vascular endothelial growth factor A; sFLT-1, soluble vascular endothelial growth factor receptor 1; PlGF, placenta growth factor; Eng, endoglin; sThrombomodulin, soluble thrombomodulin.

remains reasonable, however further work in this area is needed to establish its role.

VEGF-A

Vascular Endothelial Growth Factor-A (VEGF-A) is a member of the PDGF superfamily of growth factors. It is one of the most potent regulators of angiogenesis, and acts on vascular endothelial cells through stimulation of KDR (VEGF receptor 2) and FLT-1 (VEGF receptor 1) to promote angiogenesis, increase vascular permeability and stimulate endothelial cell migration (35, 36).

Serum VEGF-A concentrations are known to be elevated in patients with PAH and have been demonstrated within plexiform lesions of remodeled vasculature (17, 37).

In a study including 53 participants (SSc-PAH $n = 20$, SSc-no PAH $n = 20$, HV $n = 13$) Papaioannou et al. examined the relationship of serum VEGF-A concentration to echocardiographic markers of pulmonary hypertension. In this study, participants were treatment naive, and any patients with pulmonary fibrosis were excluded. Estimated sPAP >35 mmHg was used to define patients with SSc-PAH. The authors found significantly higher VEGF-A concentrations in all patients with SSc as compared to HV (267 pg/ml vs. 192 pg/ml respectively, $p < 0.01$), and further found that those with SSc-PAH had higher levels than those with SSc-no PAH (352 pg/ml vs. 240 pg/ml respectively, $p < 0.01$). In patients with SSc, significant correlations were found between serum VEGF-A concentration and systolic pulmonary arterial pressure (sPAP) ($r = 0.58$, $p < 0.01$); MRC dyspnoea score ($r = 0.34$, $p = 0.031$); and DLco ($r = -0.47$, $p < 0.01$). In multivariate modeling of sPAP as the dependent variable, VEGF-A concentration remained a significant predictor when adjusted for age and gender (17).

VEGF-A expression is known to be upregulated in both patients PAH, and with systemic sclerosis, both conditions characterized by pathologically excessive endothelial activation. In patients with SSc-PAH the VEGF pathway is upregulated, however baseline levels have not been assessed for utility as diagnostic biomarkers.

Placenta Growth Factor (PlGF) and Soluble Vascular Endothelial Growth Factor (VEGF) Receptor 1 (sFLT-1)

Placenta growth factor is a member of the vascular endothelial growth factor family of proteins which binds with high affinity for VEGF receptor 1 (FLT-1/ VEGF-R1), but not for VEGF receptor 2 (KDR/ VEGFR2)—regarded as the main effector protein of VEGF signaling (38). PlGF alone does not stimulate tyrosine kinase phosphorylation or proliferation in human endothelial cell lines, however the addition of PlGF potentiates the effect of VEGF-A in stimulating proliferation of cultured endothelial cells (38).

sFLT-1 is a variant of VEGF receptor 1 (FLT-1) which can bind VEGF-A, VEGF-B, and Placenta growth factor (PlGF). It functions as a decoy receptor, downregulating free ligand and therefore thought to control excessive endothelial activity (39).

Recognizing the need for further study into diagnostic biomarkers for patients with SSc-PAH, McMahan et al. designed a case-control study of 77 patients with SSc (37 with PH, 40 without PH). The groups were unbalanced for age (64.9 vs. 55.9 respectively, $p < 0.01$) and lung volumes (FVC% 67.5 vs. 88.1 respectively, $p < 0.01$). Diagnosis of PH was based on mPAP $\geq$ 25 mmHg at right heart catheterization. The authors report that both PlGF (24.8 pg/ml vs. 19.1 pg/ml, $p = 0.02$) and sFLT-1 (101.8 pg/ml vs. 89.7 pg/ml, $p = 0.02$) are significantly upregulated in patients with PH that in those without. Both proteins were significantly inversely correlated to DLco (PlGF: $r = -0.31$,

$p = 0.01$ and sFLT-1: $r = -0.29$, $p = 0.01$). sFLT-1 was also correlated to RVSP ($r = 0.32$, $p = 0.01$) (16).

This study was designed to evaluate potential biomarkers of pulmonary hypertension in systemic sclerosis. No comment is made about extent of pulmonary fibrosis, so it remains conceivable that these are imbalanced given the difference in baseline pulmonary function tests, and it is not clear why no comparisons were given for protein concentration and invasive right heart catheter measurements. Although protein concentration changes are noted, no statistics have been given for the performance of these proteins as diagnostic markers.

GDF-15

Growth Differentiation Factor-15 (GDF-15) is a member of the TGF-ß superfamily of cytokines playing an important role in cell growth and differentiation. It is a stress responsive cytokine associated with tissue damage and inflammation. Increased levels have been reported in heart failure, atherosclerosis, endothelial dysfunction and diabetes and have been linked to disease progression and prognosis (40).

In treatment naïve IPAH, serum GDF-15 is increased and is a significant predictor of survival (41). In a mixed cohort of PAH patients, tissue levels of GDF-15 are increased—localizing to the pulmonary endothelium, and in remodeled vessels strong signals are identified in plexiform lesions (42). *In-vitro* studies using pulmonary endothelial cells and varying concentrations of GDF-15 resulted in reduction in hypoxia induced apoptosis suggesting a potential pathological mechanism in PAH (42).

Meadows et al. studied a cohort of 111 patients (SSc-PAH $n = 30$, SSc-no PAH $n = 24$, IPAH $n = 44$, HV $n = 13$) for circulating GDF-15 concentrations. PH was defined at right heart catheterization. Patients with PAH were already established on PH specific therapy at the time of entry to study. Both plasma and tissue levels of GDF-15 were elevated in SSc-PAH (442 pg/ml), and differentiated it from SSc without PAH (108 pg/ml, $p = 0.0004$), IPAH (173 pg/ml, $p = 0.0003$) and HV (66 pg/ml, $p = 0.0013$). Within the SSc subgroup, GDF-15 levels correlated with echocardiographic RVSP ($r = 0.556$, $p < 0.001$), and with NT-proBNP concentration ($r = 0.484$, $p < 0.001$), but not with other invasive hemodynamics. On diagnostic ROC analysis, GDF-15 has been shown to have good discriminative power with area under curve (AUC) 0.91 for differentiation of SSc-PAH from SSc without PH with an optimal threshold for GDF-15 of 125 pg/ml demonstrating 93% sensitivity and 88% specificity for the presence of SSc-PAH. Furthermore, patients below this threshold were found to have significantly improved survival (18).

Resistin-Like Molecule-ß (RELM-ß)

RELM-ß is a member of a relatively newly described resistin family. Largely studied through their effects on animal models, these proteins have been shown to induce angiogenesis and vascular remodeling (19).

Following the identification that hypoxia induced mitogenic factor(HIMF) is upregulated in animal models of PH, Angelini et al. sought to evaluate this in human tissues. In a small study involving 26 prevalent patients (SSc-PAH $n = 9$, IPAH $n = 11$, HV $n = 6$), the authors found that in human lung tissue samples, RELM-ß (a close human homolog to HIMF) is upregulated in patients with SSc-PAH as compared to healthy control ($p < 0.01$, measured by relative intensity on western blot) and localizes to remodeled vasculature. In comparison, although some expression of RELM-ß was noted in remodeled vessels of patients with IPAH, this was inconsistent, and relative quantification showed no difference between IPAH and HV concentrations. Additional *in-vitro* study showed mitogenic activity of RELM-ß on both human lung microvascular endothelial cells and human pulmonary artery smooth muscle cells (19).

This is a relatively novel candidate protein, which appears to show higher expression in SSc-PAH, however more work is needed to assess its concentration in the circulating compartment if it is to be considered further as a biomarker as lung tissue samples are not practical for this purpose.

Soluble Thrombomodulin (sThrombomodulin)

Thrombomodulin is a glycoprotein expressed on endothelial cells. Its physiological function is to bind thrombin and alter its activity, to subsequently activate protein C (15). The pathogenesis of both systemic sclerosis and PAH involves and injury to and activation of the vascular endothelium. Soluble thrombomodulin is increased in conditions associated with endothelial damage (43).

Stratton et al. studied 92 patients (SSc-PAH $n = 34$, SSc-no PAH $n = 38$, HV $n = 20$) and found that sThrombomodulin was increased plasma of patients with SSc-PAH (65.4 ng/ml) compared to SSc without PH (43.3 ng/ml, $p < 0.05$), and healthy controls (38.1 ng/ml, $p < 0.05$). There was no difference in circulating concentration between SSc without PH and healthy control (20). This is in contrast to previous studies which have shown a significant decrease in circulating sThrombomodulin concentration in patients with PAH (IPAH and PAH due to Eisenmenger's' syndrome) compared to healthy controls (26 vs. 44 ng/ml respectively, $p = 0.0001$) (44).

DISCUSSION

A biomarker has been defined by the NIH as "a characteristic that is objectively measured and evaluated as an indicator of normal biological processes, pathogenic processes, or pharmacologic responses to a therapeutic intervention." Strimbu, et al. (45) NT-proBNP is the most widely studied circulating biomarker in clinical use in patients with suspected or known PAH. Elevations in NT-proBNP result from right ventricular (RV) strain as a result of increased RV afterload. As it does not reflect the underlying pathophysiology of the pulmonary arterial vasculopathy resulting in increased RV afterload in PAH, NT-proBNP levels can be elevated due to other pathophysiological processes including increased RV afterload due to PH arising from left heart disease and from disease processes directly affecting the myocardium. As such, the specificity of NT-proBNP in the diagnosis of SSc-PAH tends to be rather low resulting in a significant number of RHCs being performed in patients who do not in the end have PAH (10). Furthermore, given the dismal prognosis in SSc-PAH, identifying patients early in their disease process before the development of RV strain is desirable (46, 47). The identification of a biomarker or panel of biomarkers which more reflect the underlying pulmonary vasculopathy in SSc-PAH prior to the development of RV strain is therefore of interest.

The data described in the current manuscript summaries the current evidence for various candidate circulating diagnostic biomarkers for SSc-PAH, several of which do relate known pathways known to be important in PAH pathogenesis, especially the TGF-ß and VEGF pathways. Further study within well phenotyped cohorts of patients to compare the performance of these candidate circulating biomarkers against NT-proBNP and the DETECT protocol are clearly warranted.

AUTHOR CONTRIBUTIONS

PH wrote and reviewed manuscript. AL supervised, and reviewed manuscript making comments and alterations. RC supervised writing and manuscript, reviewed and made significant alterations and changes.

REFERENCES

1. Tyndall AJ, Bannert B, Vonk M, Airò P, Cozzi F, Carreira PE, et al. Causes and risk factors for death in systemic sclerosis: a study from the EULAR Scleroderma Trials and Research (EUSTAR) database. *Ann Rheum Dis.* (2010) **69**:1809–15. doi: 10.1136/ard.2009.114264
2. Hachulla E, Gressin V, Guillevin L, Carpentier P, Diot E, Sibilia J, et al. Early detection of pulmonary arterial hypertension in systemic sclerosis: a French nationwide prospective multicenter study. *Arthritis Rheum.* (2005) **52**:3792–800. doi: 10.1002/art.21433
3. Mukerjee D, St George D, Coleiro B, Knight C, Denton CP, Davar J, et al. Prevalence and outcome in systemic sclerosis associated pulmonary arterial hypertension: application of a registry approach. *Ann Rheum Dis.* (2003) **62**:1088–93. doi: 10.1136/ard.62.11.1088
4. Lefèvre G, Dauchet L, Hachulla E, Montani D, Sobanski V, Lambert M, et al. Survival and prognostic factors in systemic sclerosis–associated pulmonary hypertension: a systematic review and meta–analysis. *Arthritis Rheum.* (2013) **65**:2412–23.doi: 10.1002/art.38029
5. Overbeek MJ, Vonk MC, Boonstra A, Voskuyl AE, Vonk-Noordegraaf A, Smit EF, et al. Pulmonary arterial hypertension in limited cutaneous systemic sclerosis: a distinctive vasculopathy. *Eur Respir J.* (2009) **34**:371–9. doi: 10.1183/09031936.00106008
6. Ramjug S, Hussain N, Hurdman J, Billings C, Charalampopoulos A, Elliot CA, et al. Idiopathic and systemic sclerosis-associated pulmonary arterial hypertension: a comparison of demographic, hemodynamic, and mri characteristics and outcomes. *Chest* (2017) **152**:92–102. doi: 10.1016/j.chest.2017.02.010
7. Rhee RL, Gabler NB, Sangani S, Praestgaard A, Merkel PA, Kawut SM. Comparison of treatment response in idiopathic and connective tissue disease–associated pulmonary arterial hypertension. *Am J Respir Crit Care Med.* (2015) **192**:1111–7. doi: 10.1164/rccm.201507-1456OC
8. Humbert M, Gerry Coghlan J, Khanna D. Early detection and management of pulmonary arterial hypertension. *Eur Respir J.* (2012) **21**:306–12. doi: 10.1183/09059180.00005112
9. Lau EMT, Humbert M, Celermajer DS. Early detection of pulmonary arterial hypertension. *Nat Rev Cardiol.* (2015) **12**:143–55. doi: 10.1038/nrcardio.2014.191
10. Coghlan JG, Denton CP, Grünig E, Bonderman D, Distler O, Khanna D, et al. Evidence-based detection of pulmonary arterial hypertension in systemic sclerosis: the DETECT study. *Ann Rheum Dis.* (2014) **73**:1340–9. doi: 10.1136/annrheumdis-2013-203301
11. Vandecasteele E, Drieghe B, Melsens K, Thevissen K, De Pauw M, Deschepper E, et al. Screening for pulmonary arterial hypertension in an unselected prospective systemic sclerosis cohort. *Eur Respir J.* (2017) **49**:1602275. doi: 10.1183/13993003.02275-2016
12. Hoeper MM, Kramer T, Pan Z, Eichstaedt CA, Spiesshoefer J, Benjamin N, et al. Mortality in pulmonary arterial hypertension: prediction by the 2015 European pulmonary hypertension guidelines risk stratification model. *Eur Respir J.* (2017) **50**:1700740. doi: 10.1183/13993003.00740-2017
13. Chung L, Fairchild RM, Furst DE, Li S, Alkassab F, Bolster MB, et al., (2017). Utility of B-type natriuretic peptides in the assessment of patients with systemic sclerosis-associated pulmonary hypertension in the PHAROS registry. *Clin Exp Rheumatol.* **35**(Suppl. 106):106–13.
14. Mathai SC, Bueso M, Hummers LK, Boyce D, Lechtzin N, Le Pavec J, et al. Disproportionate elevation of N-terminal pro-brain natriuretic peptide in scleroderma-related pulmonary hypertension. *Eur Respir J.* (2010) **35**:95–104. doi: 10.1183/09031936.00074309
15. Coral-Alvarado PX, Garces MF, Caminos JE, Iglesias-Gamarra A, Restrepo JF, Quintana G. Serum endoglin levels in patients suffering from systemic sclerosis and elevated systolic pulmonary arterial pressure. *Int J Rheumatol.* (2010) **2010**:969383. doi: 10.1155/2010/969383
16. McMahan Z, Schoenhoff F, Van Eyk J. E, Wigley F. M, Hummers L. K (2015). Biomarkers of pulmonary hypertension in patients with scleroderma: a case-control study. *Arthritis Res Ther.* **17**:201. doi: 10.1186/s13075-015-0712-4
17. Papaioannou AI, Zakynthinos E, Kostikas K, Kiropoulos T, Koutsokera A, Ziogas A, et al. Serum VEGF levels are related to the presence of pulmonary arterial hypertension in systemic sclerosis. *BMC Pulm. Med.* (2009) **9**:18. doi: 10.1186/1471-2466-9-18
18. Meadows CA, Risbano MG, Zhang L, Geraci MW, Tuder RM, Collier DH, et al. Increased expression of growth differentiation factor-15 in systemic sclerosis-associated pulmonary arterial hypertension. *Chest* (2011) **139**:994–1002. doi: 10.1378/chest.10-0302
19. Angelini DJ, Su Q, Yamaji-Kegan K, Fan C, Teng X, Hassoun PM, et al. Resistin-like molecule-beta in scleroderma-associated pulmonary hypertension. *Am J Respir Cell Mol. Biol.* (2009) **41**:553–61. doi: 10.1165/rcmb.2008-0271OC
20. Stratton RJ, Pompon L, Coghlan JG, Pearson JD, Black CM. (2000). Soluble thrombomodulin concentration is raised in scleroderma associated pulmonary hypertension. *Ann Rheum Dis.* (1997) **59**:132–4. doi: 10.1136/ard.59.2.132
21. Galiè N, Humbert M, Vachiery JL, Gibbs S, Lang I, Torbicki A et al. *2015 ESC/ERS Guidelines for the Diagnosis and Treatment of Pulmonary Hypertension: the Joint Task Force for the Diagnosis and Treatment of Pulmonary.* (2015). Available online at: https://academic.oup.com/eurheartj/article-abstract/37/1/67/2887599
22. Warwick G, Thomas PS, Yates DH. Biomarkers in pulmonary hypertension. *Eur Respir J.* (2008) **32**:503–12. doi: 10.1183/09031936.00160307
23. Leuchte HH, Holzapfel M, Baumgartner RA, Ding I, Neurohr C, Vogeser M, et al. Clinical significance of brain natriuretic peptide in primary pulmonary hypertension. *J Am Coll Cardiol* (2004) **43**:764–70. doi: 10.1016/j.jacc.2003.09.051
24. Fijalkowska A, Kurzyna M, Torbicki A, Szewczyk G, Florczyk M, Pruszczyk P, et al. Serum N-terminal brain natriuretic peptide as a prognostic parameter in patients with pulmonary hypertension. *Chest* (2006) **129**:1313–21. doi: 10.1378/chest.129.5.1313
25. Avouac J, Meune C, Chenevier-Gobeaux C, Borderie D, Lefevre G, Kahan A, et al. Cardiac biomarkers in systemic sclerosis: contribution of high-sensitivity cardiac troponin in addition to N-terminal pro-brain natriuretic peptide. *Arthritis Care Res.* (2015) **67**:1022–30. doi: 10.1002/acr.22547
26. Machado RD, Southgate L, Eichstaedt CA, Aldred MA, Austin ED, Best DH, et al. Pulmonary arterial hypertension: a current perspective on established and emerging molecular genetic defects. *Hum Mutat.* (2015) **36**:1113–27. doi: 10.1002/humu.22904
27. Williams MH, Handler CE, Akram R, Smith CJ, Das C, Smee J, et al. Role of N-terminal brain natriuretic peptide (N-TproBNP) in scleroderma-associated pulmonary arterial hypertension. *Eur Heart J.* (2006) **27**:1485–94. doi: 10.1093/eurheartj/ehi891
28. Nagaya N, Nishikimi T, Uematsu M, Satoh T, Kyotani S, Sakamaki F, et al. Plasma brain natriuretic peptide as a prognostic indicator in patients

with primary pulmonary hypertension. *Circulation* (2000) **102**:865–70. doi: 10.1161/01.CIR.102.8.865

29. Andreassen AK, Wergeland R, Simonsen S, Geiran O, Guevara C, Ueland T. N-terminal pro-B-type natriuretic peptide as an indicator of disease severity in a heterogeneous group of patients with chronic precapillary pulmonary hypertension. *Am J Cardiol.* (2006) **98**:525–9. doi: 10.1016/j.amjcard.2006.02.061
30. Nickel N, Golpon H, Greer M, Knudsen L, Olsson K, Westerkamp V, et al. The prognostic impact of follow-up assessments in patients with idiopathic pulmonary arterial hypertension. *Eur Respir J.* (2012) **39**:589–96. doi: 10.1183/09031936.00092311
31. Kylhammar D, Kjellström B, Hjalmarsson C, Jansson K, Nisell M, Söderberg S, et al. A comprehensive risk stratification at early follow-up determines prognosis in pulmonary arterial hypertension. *Eur Heart J.* (2017). doi: 10.1093/eurheartj/ehx257
32. Boucly A, Weatherald J, Savale L, Jaïs X, Cottin V, Prevot G, et al. Risk assessment, prognosis and guideline implementation in pulmonary arterial hypertension. *Eur Respir J.* (2017) **50**:1700889. doi: 10.1183/13993003.00889-2017
33. Conley BA, Smith JD, Guerrero-Esteo M, Bernabeu C, Vary CP. Endoglin, a TGF-β receptor-associated protein, is expressed by smooth muscle cells in human atherosclerotic plaques. *Atherosclerosis* (2000) **153**:323–35. doi: 10.1016/S0021-9150(00)00422-6
34. Gore B, Izikki M, Mercier O, Dewachter L, Fadel E, Humbert M et al. Key role of the endothelial TGF-β/ALK1/endoglin signaling pathway in humans and rodents pulmonary hypertension. *PLoS ONE* (2014) **9**:e100310. doi: 10.1371/journal.pone.0100310
35. Shibuya M. (2011). Vascular Endothelial Growth Factor (VEGF) and its receptor (VEGFR) signaling in angiogenesis: a crucial target for anti- and pro-angiogenic therapies. *Genes Cancer* (2010) **2**:1097–105. doi: 10.1177/1947601911423031
36. Voelkel NF, Gomez-Arroyo J. The role of vascular endothelial growth factor in pulmonary arterial hypertension. *Am J Respir Cell Mol Biol.* (2014) **51**:474–84. doi: 10.1165/rcmb.2014-0045TR
37. Eddahibi S, Humbert M, Sediame S, Chouaid C, Partovian C, Maître B et al., (2000). Imbalance between platelet vascular endothelial growth factor and platelet-derived growth factor in pulmonary hypertension. Effect of prostacyclin therapy. *Am J Respir Crit Care Med.* **162**(4 Pt 1):1493–9. doi: 10.1164/ajrccm.162.4.2003124
38. Park JE, Chen HH, Winer J, Houck KA, Ferrara N. Placenta growth factor. Potentiation of vascular endothelial growth factor bioactivity, *in vitro* and *in vivo*, and high affinity binding to Flt-1 but not to Flk-1/KDR. *J Biol Chem.* (1994) **269**:25646–54.
39. Olsson AK, Dimberg A, Kreuger J, Claesson-Welsh L. VEGF receptor signalling - in control of vascular function. *Nat Rev Mol Cell Biol.* (2006) **7**:359–71. doi: 10.1038/nrm1911
40. Adela R, Banerjee SK. GDF-15 as a target and biomarker for diabetes and cardiovascular diseases: a translational prospective. *J Diabetes Res.* (2015) **2015**:490842. doi: 10.1155/2015/490842
41. Nickel N, Kempf T, Tapken H, Tongers J, Laenger F, Lehmann U, et al. Growth differentiation factor-15 in idiopathic pulmonary arterial hypertension. *Am J Respir Crit Care Med.* (2008) **178**:534–41. doi: 10.1164/rccm.200802-235OC
42. Nickel N, Jonigk D, Kempf T, Bockmeyer CL, Maegel L, Rische J, et al. GDF-15 is abundantly expressed in plexiform lesions in patients with pulmonary arterial hypertension and affects proliferation and apoptosis of pulmonary endothelial cells. *Respir Res.* (2011) **12**:62. doi: 10.1186/1465-9921-12-62
43. Mercié, P., Seigneur M, Constans J, Boisseau M, Conri C. Assay of plasma thrombomodulin in systemic diseases. *La Revue de.* (1997) **18**:126–31.
44. Cacoub P, Karmochkine M, Dorent R, Nataf P, Piette JC, Godeau P, et al. Plasma levels of thrombomodulin in pulmonary hypertension. *Am J Med.* (1996) **101**:160–4. doi: 10.1016/S0002-9343(96)80070-2
45. Strimbu K, Tavel JA. What are biomarkers? *Curr Opin HIV AIDS* (2010) **5**:463–6. doi: 10.1097/COH.0b013e32833ed177
46. Coghlan JG, Wolf M, Distler O, Denton CP, Doelberg M, Harutyunova S, et al. Incidence of pulmonary hypertension and determining factors in patients with systemic sclerosis. *Eur Respir J.* (2018) **51**:1701197. doi: 10.1183/13993003.01197-2017
47. Condliffe R, Kovacs G. Identifying early pulmonary arterial hypertension in patients with systemic sclerosis. *Eur Respir J.* (2018) **51**:1800495. doi: 10.1183/13993003.00495-2018

19

rhACE2 Therapy Modifies Bleomycin-Induced Pulmonary Hypertension via Rescue of Vascular Remodeling

*Anandharajan Rathinasabapathy[1], Andrew J. Bryant[2], Toshio Suzuki[1], Christy Moore[1], Sheila Shay[1], Santhi Gladson[1], James D. West[1] and Erica J. Carrier[1]**

[1] *Allergy, Pulmonary and Critical Care Medicine, Vanderbilt University Medical Center, Nashville, TN, United States,*
[2] *Pulmonary, Critical Care, and Sleep Medicine, College of Medicine, University of Florida, Gainesville, FL, United States*

Correspondence:
Erica J. Carrier
erica.carrier@vanderbilt.edu

Background: Pulmonary hypertension (PH) is a progressive cardiovascular disease, characterized by endothelial and smooth muscle dysfunction and vascular remodeling, followed by right heart failure. Group III PH develops secondarily to chronic lung disease such as idiopathic pulmonary fibrosis (IPF), and both hastens and predicts mortality despite of all known pharmacological interventions. Thus, there is urgent need for development of newer treatment strategies.

Objective: Angiotensin converting enzyme 2 (ACE2), a member of the renin angiotensin family, is therapeutically beneficial in animal models of pulmonary vascular diseases and is currently in human clinical trials for primary PH. Although previous studies suggest that administration of ACE2 prevents PH secondary to bleomycin-induced murine IPF, it is unknown whether ACE2 can reverse or treat existing disease. Therefore, in the present study, we tested the efficacy of ACE2 in arresting the progression of group 3 PH.

Methods: To establish pulmonary fibrosis, we administered 0.018 U/g bleomycin 2x/week for 4 weeks in adult FVB/N mice, and sacrificed 5 weeks following the first injection. ACE2 or vehicle was administered via osmotic pump for the final 2 weeks, beginning 3 weeks after bleomycin. Echocardiography and hemodynamic assessment was performed prior to sacrifice and tissue collection.

Results: Administration of bleomycin significantly increased lung collagen expression, pulmonary vascular remodeling, and pulmonary arterial pressure, and led to mild right ventricular hypertrophy. Acute treatment with ACE2 significantly attenuated vascular remodeling and increased pulmonary SOD2 expression without measurable effects on pulmonary fibrosis. This was associated with nonsignificant positive effects on pulmonary arterial pressure and cardiac function.

Conclusion: Collectively, our findings enumerate that ACE2 treatment improved pulmonary vascular muscularization following bleomycin exposure, concomitant with increased SOD2 expression. Although it may not alter the pulmonary disease course of IPF, ACE2 could be an effective therapeutic strategy for the treatment of group 3 PH.

Keywords: pulmonary hypertension, pulmonary fibrosis, ACE2, bleomycin, mice

INTRODUCTION

Pulmonary hypertension (PH) is a progressive, rare lung disease, which results in right heart malfunction and is fatal when untreated. The pathogenesis of PH often begins with elevated resistance in the pulmonary circulation due to endothelial dysfunction and underlying vascular remodeling, which eventually leads to increased pulmonary arterial pressure (Schermuly et al., 2011). This increased pulmonary pressure increases the right ventricular (RV) work load and maladaptive RV remodeling, and culminates in right heart failure (Schermuly et al., 2011). The median survival of a PH patient is <3 years. As per the most recent WHO guidelines, PH is classified into 5 groups, by origin: idiopathic, heritable, or drug/toxin-induced in group I, left heart disease in group 2, chronic lung disease in group 3, chronic thromboembolic pulmonary hypertension in group 4, and hematologic, systemic, or metabolic disorders in group 5 (Oudiz, 2016).

The present study focuses on chronic lung disease associated PH. The Global Burden of Disease Study on global life expectancy in 2013 (Mortality and Causes of Death, 2015) summarized that the death rate of interstitial lung disease grew more than 50% between 1990 and 2013, while its global ranking escalated from 64 (1990) to 40 (2013). Idiopathic pulmonary fibrosis (IPF) is a chronic, fatal interstitial lung disease associated with recurrent pulmonary epithelial injury and maladaptive repair, which results in a progressive interstitial fibrosis and compromised gaseous exchange (Richeldi et al., 2017). These pathological symptoms in conjunction with a concomitant endothelial dysfunction, and vascular remodeling results in group 3 PH (PH associated with IPF). PH develops in more than 32–50% of advanced IPF patients (Patel et al., 2007; Shorr et al., 2007), where it significantly impacts survival, with an increased mortality rate of 2.2–4.85-fold compared to IPF patients with no PH (Hamada et al., 2007). Despite pharmacological interventions including phosphodiesterase or endothelin receptor inhibition, or activation of prostacyclin or guanylate cyclase pathways, there has been little improvement in the mortality of IPF-associated PH (Klinger, 2016). Thus, there is great need for the development of newer therapeutic strategies to treat group 3 PH.

One promising new PH therapy is a modulator of the renin-angiotensin system (RAS). The RAS is a hormonal system of enzymes, ligands, and receptors that regulates pathophysiological events in the lung, heart, kidney, and other organs (Ferreira et al., 2010; Hsueh and Wyne, 2011; Kalra et al., 2015; Passos-Silva et al., 2015). The RAS can be categorized into two divergent axes: either the angiotensin converting enzyme (ACE), its product angiotensin II (Ang II), and the angiotensin receptor type 1 (AT1), or the angiotensin converting enzyme-2 (ACE2), the ACE2 product angiotensin-(1-7) [Ang-(1-7)], and the Ang-(1-7) receptor, Mas1 (Passos-Silva et al., 2015). Activation of the ACE2/Ang-(1-7)/Mas1 axis with administration of either rhACE2 or Ang-(1-7) also improves the cardio-pulmonary defects associated with experimental PH and PF (Shenoy et al., 2010, 2013; Meng et al., 2015). ACE2 treatment is also one of the only therapies to reverse murine BMPR2-related PAH, the cause of most heritable PH (Johnson et al., 2012), and improves right ventricular function under stress (Johnson et al., 2011).

The primary rodent model of pulmonary fibrosis and group 3 PH is a single intratracheal installation of bleomycin, which after 2 weeks recapitulates many of the functional, molecular and pathological defects associated with IPF (Mouratis and Aidinis, 2011; Meng et al., 2015), including cardiac and pulmonary vascular remodeling (Shenoy et al., 2013; Rathinasabapathy et al., 2016). A repeated low dose bleomycin insult in mice, over a period of 5 weeks, results in cardio and pulmonary vascular remodeling in addition to extensive lung fibrosis (Bryant et al., 2015; Chen et al., 2016).

The therapeutic benefits of ACE2 in prevention have been assessed in multiple bleomycin studies (Shenoy et al., 2010, 2013; Rey-Parra et al., 2012; Meng et al., 2015). These prevention studies all relied on a single dose of bleomycin, rather than repeated low doses, and the ACE2 treatment regimen was initiated either concurrent with or prior to bleomycin instillation, while development of PH/PF was acute and robust. To date, no treatment studies have assessed the therapeutic effect of ACE2 in arresting or reversing the progression of bleomycin-induced damages (treatment), over a longer course of time. Potential translation of ACE2 to human studies requires identification of potential to reverse, not just treat, IPF and IPF-associated PH, using the more human disease relevant repeated dosing model of IPF. The goal of these studies was to fill this gap in our knowledge.

MATERIALS AND METHODS

Reagents and Chemicals

Bleomycin (bleomycin sulfate, Cipla, Goa, India) was purchased from the Vanderbilt University Medical Center pharmacy. Recombinant human angiotensin converting enzyme 2 (rhACE2) was a kind gift from GlaxoSmithKline, UK. α-smooth muscle actin (α-SMA), SOD2, and β-actin antibodies were purchased from Abcam (Cambridge, MA, USA) and CD68 antibody purchased from Dako (Santa Clara, CA, USA).

Animals

All the mice utilized in this study were housed at Vanderbilt University Medical Center animal care facility, which is certified by the Association for Assessment and Accreditation of Laboratory Animal Care International. All animal protocols were approved by the Institutional Animal Care and Use Committee at Vanderbilt University Medical Center (Approval number-M12/110) in compliance with National Institute of Health

Abbreviations: α-SMA, alpha smooth muscle actin; ACE, angiotensin converting enzyme; Argl, arginase 1; AT1, angiotensin type 1 receptor; Bleo, bleomycin; Col1, collagen, type 1; Col3, collagen, type 3; echo, echocardiography; EF, ejection fraction; IPF, idiopathic pulmonary fibrosis; LV, left ventricle; Mas1, Mas receptor; MRC1, mannose receptor C-type 1; PH, pulmonary hypertension; rhACE2, recombinant human angiotensin converting enzyme 2; RAS, renin angiotensin system; Retnla, Resistin like alpha; RV, right ventricle; RVH, right ventricular hypertrophy; RVSP, right ventricular systolic pressure; SOD2-superoxide dismutase-2 (manganese superoxide dismutase); WBC, white blood cell.

guidelines. Animals housed in the conventional cages were exposed to 12:12 h, day:night cycle with free access to food (normal chow) and water. One week prior to the start of the study, animals were fed with 60% high-fat, high-calorie diet (Bio-Serv, Flemington, NJ, USA) to assist in weight maintenance, and this diet was continued until the termination of the study.

Study Design

Eighteen to 26 week old inbred male and female FVBN mice were used in this 5-week study. For the first 4 weeks, animals were challenged with bleomycin (0.018 U/g, injected i.p.), every 4 days, for a total of eight doses. Bleomycin was aseptically dissolved in saline, and the control animals for the bleomycin group were administered saline. Eighteen days following the first bleomycin injection (immediately after 6th dose), rhACE2 (1.2 mg/kg/day) was administered through mini-osmotic pumps (Durect Corporation, Cupertino, CA, USA), and the pumps were continued for 2 weeks, 1 week past the final administration of bleomycin. rhACE2 was solubilized in a buffer containing 100 mM glycine, 150 mM NaCl, 50 mM $ZnCl_2$, pH 7.5. This buffer without rhACE2 was implanted in the vehicle group. Original $n = 17$ for each bleomycin group and $n = 7$ for each control group; two animals from each Bleo+vehicle and Bleo+ACE2 group died prior to obtaining invasive hemodynamics. All of these deaths occurred in the last 2 days of the study, either during or just following isoflurane anesthesia.

Transthoracic Echocardiography, Hemodynamic Measurements, and Right Ventricular Hypertrophy

One day prior to the end of study, transthoracic echocardiography was performed using the Vivo 770 high-resolution image systems (VisualSonics, Toronto, Canada). On day 33, invasive hemodynamics were conducted to measure the right ventricular systolic pressure (RVSP) as described in Bryant et al. (2015). Right ventricular hypertrophy (RVH or Fulton's index) was assessed at sacrifice, and blood and tissues collected for RNA and histology. A complete blood count (CBC) analysis was performed by the Vanderbilt University Medical Center pathology core.

Real Time Quantitative RT-PCR Analysis

Real time RT-PCR was used to study the transcript expression of collagen type 1 (Col1), collagen type 3 (Col3), resistin like alpha (Retnla/Fizz1), mannose receptor C-type 1 (Mrc1), and arginase 1 (Arg1). In brief, total RNA was isolated from the frozen lung using RNeasy (Qiagen, Valencia, CA, USA) as per the supplier's instruction. 1 μg of total RNA was utilized to synthesis the first strand cDNA using QuantiTect reverse transcription kit (Qiagen, Valencia, CA, USA). Real-time RT-PCR was performed in a 96-well format using Power SYBR green mastermix on Applied Biosystems platform (Applied Biosystems Corporation, Foster City, CA, USA). The expression of target gene transcripts was normalized against the internal control Hprt (hypoxanthine-guanine phosphoribosyltransferase) using the comparative ΔΔCT method ($2^{-\Delta\Delta}$Ct). Mouse primers are listed in **Table 1**.

Western Blotting

A portion of the right lung lobe was homogenized in RIPA buffer with protease inhibitors for protein isolation and debris cleared by centrifugation. Proteins were resolved on a 4–12% SDS-PAGE gel (Thermo Fisher Scientific, Waltham, MA, USA), transferred to PVDF, and visualized on the ChemiDoc MP imaging system (Bio-Rad Laboratories, Hercules, CA, USA). Antibodies were diluted in 2% milk/TBST.

Immunohistochemical Analysis (IHC)

The left lung lobe was perfused with PBS, inflated with 0.8% agarose solution and stored in 10% neutral buffered formalin overnight. The following day, the fixed tissues were rinsed in 70% alcohol and subsequently processed for paraffin embedding. Paraffin-embedded tissue samples were sectioned (5 micron), de-paraffined and stained with either CD68 at 1:100, or α-SMA at 1:200. For muscularized vessel wall analysis, the total number of vessels and vessels per size group were counted at 10X (10 fields/lung; 4 animals/group). Similarly, the CD68-stained macrophages were also analyzed and counted at 10X (10 fields/lung; 4 animals/group). To analyze lung remodeling, lung sections were stained with Masson's trichrome (Sigma, St. Louis, MO, USA) and the scoring was performed in a blinded fashion as previously described (Lawson et al., 2005). 10 non-overlapping randomly photographed images were analyzed from multiple slices per animal, and the results from each animal were averaged.

Statistics

JMP (SAS, Cary, NC) was used for statistical analysis. A two-way ANOVA with Holm-Sidak multiple comparison post-test was use to compare groups. Values are represented as mean ± SEM, and $p \leq 0.05$ considered statistically significant.

TABLE 1 | Mouse primers used for RT-PCR.

No	Gene		Sequence
1.	Col1	F	ACG CAT GAG CCG AAG CTA AC
		R	ACT TCA GGG ATG TCT TCT TGG C
2.	Col3	F	CCT GGA AGG GAT GGA AAC CC
		R	CAG GGC CAG TTT CTC CTC TG
3.	Retnla/Fizz1	F	CCT GCT GGG ATG ACT GCT AC
		R	CGA GTA AGC ACA GGC AGT TG
4.	Mrc1	F	AAC AAG AAT GGT GGG CAG TC
		R	TTT GCA AAG TTG GGT TCT CC
5.	Arg1	F	GAC AGG GCT CCT TTC AGG AC
		R	GCC AAG GTT AAA GCC ACT GC
6.	Hprt	F	TGC TCG AGA TGT CAT GAA GGA G
		R	TTT AAT GTA ATC CAG CAG GTC AGC

RESULTS

rhACE2 Does Not Slow or Reverse the Progression of Lung Fibrosis in the Bleomycin Model of Group 3 PH

A near-infrared blood pool imaging agent (Angiosense-750 EX, Perkin-Elmer) was used to measure pulmonary vascular leak on Day 18 after the onset of the first bleomycin injection and just prior to ACE2 pump installation. This non-invasive proxy measurement was utilized to confirm the development of pulmonary fibrosis (Supplementary Figure). Animals were then treated with ACE2 or vehicle for 2 weeks; during this time, they were exposed to bleomycin for a week and allowed a recovery period of a week before sacrifice. Administration of repeated bleomycin over the period of 4 weeks resulted in significant alteration of lung tissue architecture. Blinded scoring of Masson's trichrome-stained lung sections demonstrated a significant deposition of collagen fibers ($p < 0.0001$ by two-way ANOVA) in bleomycin-treated animals (**Figures 1A,B**), matched to increased hydroxyproline (**Figure 1C**). RT-PCR analysis demonstrated a significant increase in Col1 and Col3 expression in the lung (**Figures 1D,E**). Treatment of the Bleo animals with recombinant human ACE2 in weeks 4 and 5 had no significant effect on histology ($p = 0.62$, **Figures 1A,B**), hydroxyproline (**Figure 1C**), or expression of Col1 and Col3 (**Figures 1D,E**), compared with vehicle-treated animals.

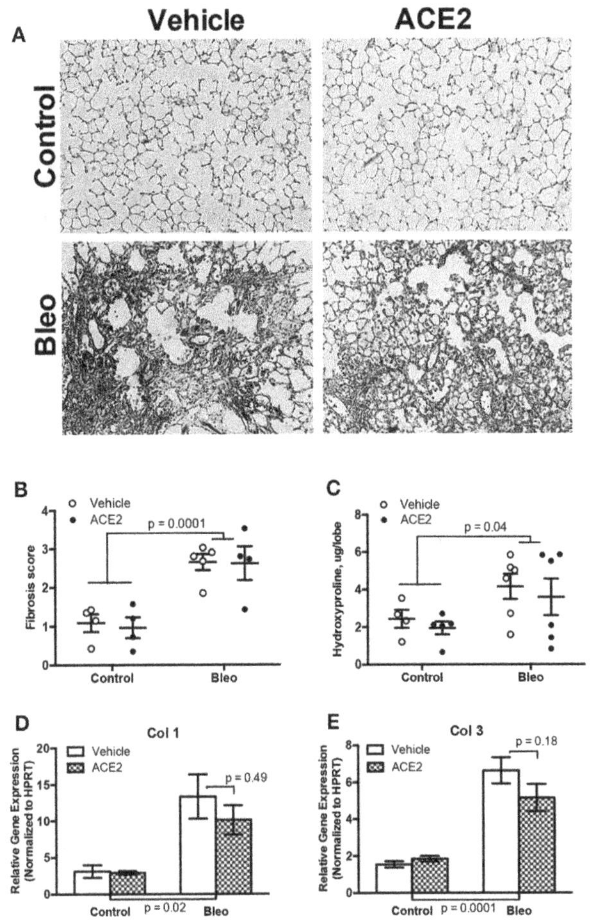

FIGURE 1 | Effect of rhACE2 treatment on bleomycin-induced pulmonary fibrosis. Lung sections were stained with Masson's trichrome, visualized at 10X **(A)** and scored for parenchymal remodeling and fibrosis **(B)**. Lung collagen was estimated from tissue by hydroxyproline assay **(C)**, and expression of collagens Col1 **(D)** and Col3 **(E)** were estimated by RT-PCR. Data presented in **(D,E)** are ± SEM mean, $n = 4$, 5, 6, and 6 for the control, ACE2, Bleo and Bleo+ACE2 groups respectively. *P*-values are the result of two-way ANOVA followed by Holm-Sidak's multiple comparison post-test; in each case, bleomycin groups were significantly different from control, and ACE2-treated not significantly from vehicle.

RV Dynamics and Cardiac Function Associated With Group 3 PH Animals

As expected (**Figures 2A,B**), bleomycin insult resulted a significant increase in RVSP (Con; 21.8 ± 0.7 *vs.* Bleo; 30.6 ± 1.7, mmHg, $p < 0.0001$ by two-way ANOVA) with a concomitant change in Fulton's index (Con; 0.28 ± 0.006 *vs.* Bleo; 0.31 ± 0.01, $p = 0.03$). ACE2 reduced the RVSP variance ($p = 0.028$ by *F*-test) but failed to overall significantly decrease RVSP in response to bleomycin ($p = 0.19$ by two-way ANOVA/Holm-Sidak). We performed transthoracic echocardiography (echo) to determine cardiac function in these animals. Bleomycin-treated animals showed only a trend toward decreased LV ejection fraction and fractional shortening, which were reversed with ACE2 treatment (**Figures 2C,D**). There was no overall change in cardiac index with bleomycin (**Figure 2E**), and so ACE2 had no impact. Cardiac index (cardiac output normalized to body surface area) rather than cardiac output is displayed because of the large differences in weight between control and bleomycin treated animals (**Figure 2F**), also not impacted by ACE2 treatment.

rhACE2 Does Not Alter Lung Inflammation in Group 3 PH Animals

Because remodeling is often caused by inflammation, we assessed inflammatory cells in the lungs and circulation. In the peripheral circulation, bleomycin slightly increased white blood count, circulating neutrophil numbers, red cell distribution width, and platelet count (**Table 2**). ACE2 treatment had no impact on any of these parameters, but did cause a slight increase in mean platelet volume, likely not functionally meaningful.

To assess the status of inflammatory cells in the lung, we stained sections for CD68, a marker for monocytes/macrophages, and found that macrophage presence was significantly increased in the Bleo lungs (**Figures 3A,B**), with an approximately 4-fold increase in pulmonary macrophages. Because IPF patients predominantly have M2 macrophage lung infiltrates (He et al., 2013), we used RT-PCR to more closely examine macrophage polarization following bleomycin administration. Expression of the M2 macrophage markers Retnla (Fizz1), Mrc1, and Arg1 were all significantly elevated in the Bleo lung (**Figures 3C–E**), with Fizz1

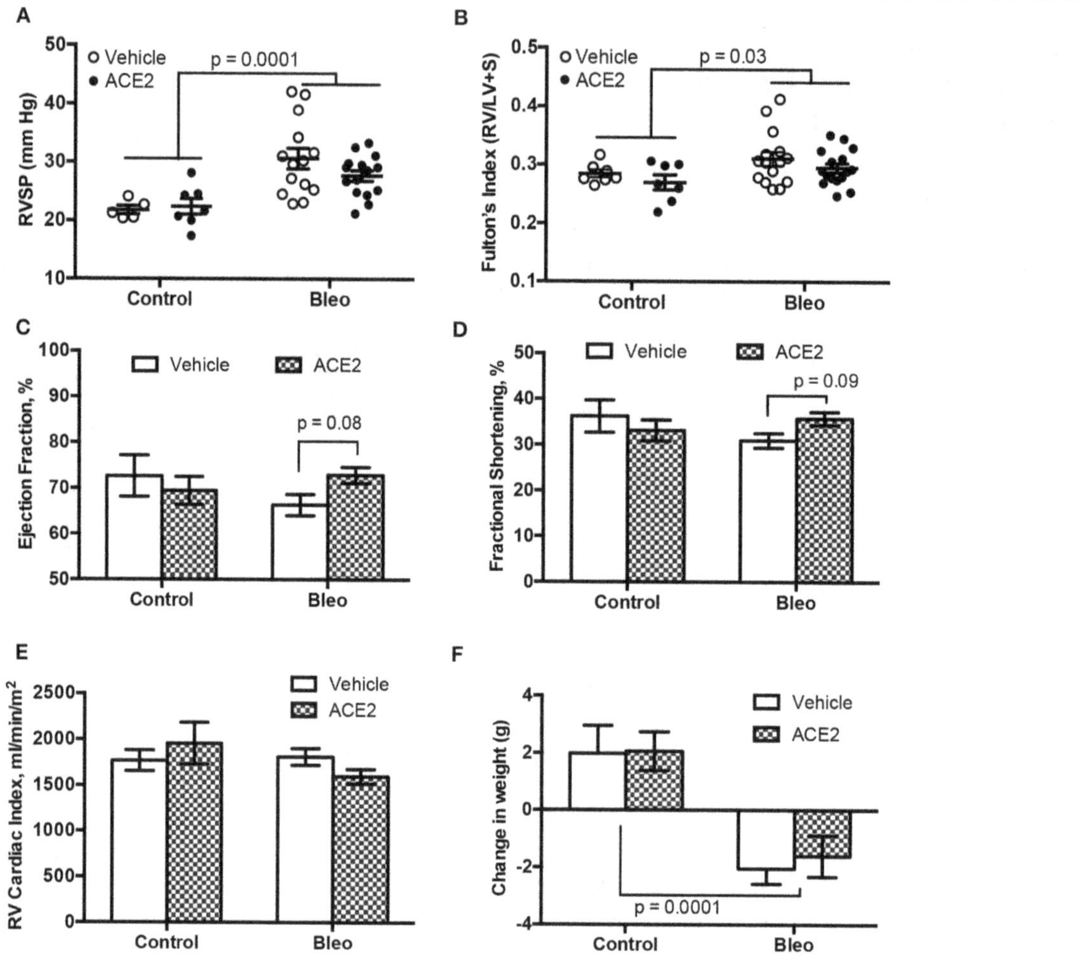

FIGURE 2 | RVSP and cardiac function in group 3 PH animals. RVSP, measured by RV catheterization, and hypertrophy, measured by Fulton's index, both increase with bleomycin treatment **(A,B)**. ACE2 significantly improved the fractional shortening and ejection fraction in bleomycin-treated animals, compared with vehicle **(C,D)**, while there was no change in RV cardiac output normalized for weight across groups **(E)**. ACE2 did not significantly decrease the weight loss associated with Bleo treatment **(F)**. Data are mean ± SEM; $n = 7, 7, 15$, and 16 for the control, ACE2, Bleo and Bleo+ACE2 groups respectively in **(B–F)**, and $n = 5, 7, 14$, and 15 in **(A)**. Comparisons shown are the result of two-way ANOVA followed by Holm-Sidak's post-test.

increased 10-fold (greater than the increase in macrophages). However, ACE2 did not reduce this increase in M2 markers.

rhACE2 Treatment Improves the Pulmonary Vascular Remodeling in Group 3 PH Animals

To assess pulmonary vascular remodeling, we stained lung sections with α-SMA. Scoring of non-overlapping images at 10x demonstrated a significant muscularization of pulmonary vessel wall in the Bleo animals (**Figures 4A–E**). A vessel was considered to have total muscularization when ≥70% of the vessel perimeter stained positive for α-SMA. Muscularization was further characterized based on vessel diameter. There was pronounced remodeling in the smaller ($p = 0.0001$, **Figure 4C**) and larger vessels ($p = 0.03$, **Figure 4E**) following Bleo administration. In agreement with the trends in RVSP and cardiac function, rhACE2 treatment attenuated muscularization (**Figures 4A–E**), in Bleo animals, particularly in vessels <25 microns in size (**Figure 4C**). Similarly, mice treated with ACE2 had fewer vessels of any size that were partially (<70%) muscularized (**Figure 4F**). We have recently investigated the effects of short-term ACE2 infusion in human PAH patients, and found reduced oxidant stress and increased plasma superoxide dismutase-2 (SOD2) with ACE2; in parallel, we have found that application of a synthetic agonist for Mas receptor increases SOD2 expression in porcine pulmonary vessels (Carrier et al., 2016). Because Mas receptor activation or ACE2 treatment can increase SOD2 protein levels, and SOD2 has been shown to decrease vascular smooth muscle proliferation and neointimal formation, we examined the effects of ACE2 on pulmonary SOD2 expression in Bleo-treated mice. Bleomycin instillation reduced SOD2 expression, but was normalized in Bleo animals treated with ACE2 (**Figures 4G,H**). Taken in combination, these data suggest

TABLE 2 | Results of complete blood count.

	Control		Bleomycin-treated		Significance	
	Vehicle	ACE2	Vehicle	ACE2	Bleo:	ACE2:
White blood count (10^9/L)	1.7	2.2	2.6	2.5	0.037	
Neutrophil # (10^9/L)	0.6	0.9	1.2	1.2	0.009	
Lymphocyte # (10^9/L)	1.1	1.2	1.3	1.2		
Monocyte # (10^9/L)	0.08	0.10	0.10	0.12		
Hematocrit (%)	49.3	52.2	51.8	54.1		
Red cell distribution width (%)	13.8	13.9	14.2	14.3	0.015	
Platelet count (10^9/L)	837.1	717.7	1005.6	941.9	0.013	
Mean platelet volume (fL)	5.23	5.37	5.33	5.39		0.027

Data are mean ± SEM, $n = 7, 7, 14$, and 15 for the control, ACE2, Bleo and Bleo+ACE2 groups respectively; comparisons between groups were made with two-way ANOVA followed by Holm-Sidak's multiple comparison post-test.

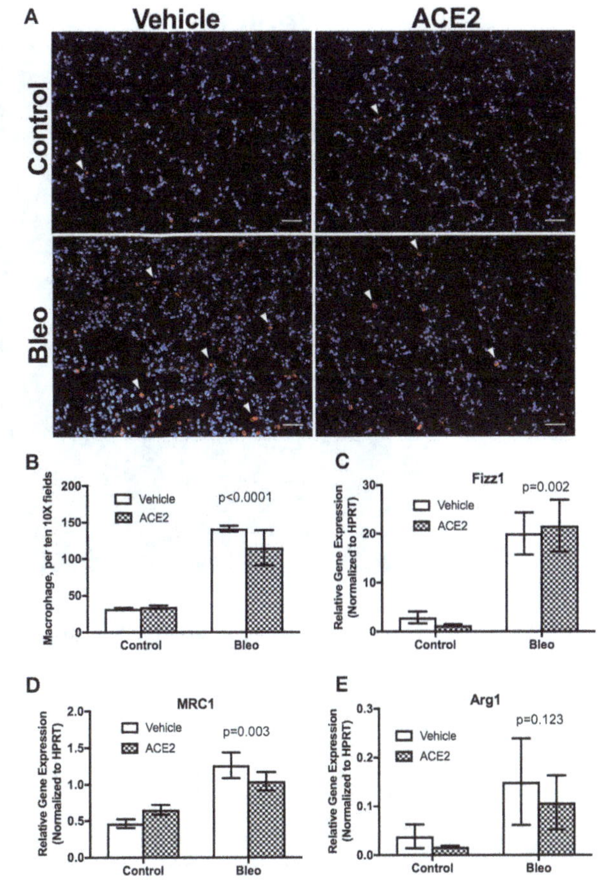

FIGURE 3 | Pulmonary macrophage dynamics in group 3 PH animals. Lung sections were stained for CD68 and random fields photographed at 10X and $CD68^+$ cells counted **(A,B,** $n = 4$**)**. RNA was isolated from frozen lungs and RT-PCR used to assess the expression of markers of macrophage polarization. **(C)** Retnla (Fizz1), **(D)** MRC1, **(E)** Arg1. Data presented in **(C–E)** are mean ± SEM, $n = 4, 5, 6$, and 6 for the control, ACE2, Bleo and Bleo+ACE2 groups respectively. Bleomycin-treated groups significantly differed from control groups by two-way ANOVA followed by Holm-Sidak's post-test, $p < 0.0001$ in **(B–E)**. Scale bars shown are 50 microns.

that the significant reduction in vessel muscularization with ACE2 in bleomycin treated mice was not the result of altered inflammatory cell numbers but possibly due to improved SOD2 expression.

DISCUSSION

Although the body of existing literature suggests a beneficial effect of ACE2 in various animal models of PH and PF (Shenoy et al., 2010, 2013; Meng et al., 2015), our study would be the first to examine recombinant human ACE2 as treatment for previously established pulmonary fibrosis, and against the development of group 3 PH and the associated cardiac abnormalities in animals following extended Bleo exposure. Our data suggest that rhACE2 treatment does not significantly alter PF in these animals, but prevents the vascular remodeling that may lead to PH, and improves some markers of cardiac function.

Although the onset of fibrotic scar in the IPF lung is idiopathic, this chronic lung disease is promoted by repeated parenchymal injury, vascular leak, recruitment and differentiation of fibroblasts, and pathologic remodeling in pulmonary circulation that culminates in *cor pulmonale* (Fernandez and Eickelberg, 2012). Bleomycin insult in rodents recreates these cascades of events with a significant disruption in the expression pattern of RAS components (Meng et al., 2015). A single injection of bleomycin in rodents causes the robust development of lung fibrosis and symptoms of PH, including elevated RVSP and RV dysfunction (Shenoy et al., 2010, 2013). To better mimic the slower progression of group 3 PH, in this study we utilized an animal model with repeated Bleo insult. The advantage of repeated Bleo administration is that it better mimics the sustained alveolar epithelial injury of IPF (Fernandez and Eickelberg, 2012), and pulmonary recovery, which limits the usefulness of the single-administration mouse model, is prevented. Functionally, these animals exhibited severe alteration in the lung architecture in addition to cardio-pulmonary vascular remodeling and elevated pulmonary arterial pressure. Recently, Bryant et al. demonstrated that vascular leak and interaction between vascular smooth muscle and endothelial cells in animals given repeated bleomycin results in vascular remodeling, independent of the severity of PF (Bryant et al., 2016). Clinically, IPF-PH results in a progressive, irreversible lung damage; therefore, the treatment regimen for those patients are aimed at improving the pulmonary vascular rather than the fibrotic symptoms (Klinger, 2016). One weakness of the bleomycin rodent IPF model is that it depends on an initial inflammatory reaction, and compounds that prevent this inflammatory phase can show false promise for IPF treatment (Moeller et al., 2008). Thus, although multiple studies describe the preventive effect of ACE2 and Ang-(1-7) in bleomycin-induced PF, for better translation to human disease it is imperative to assess post-induction treatment. Here, we demonstrate that rhACE2 treatment after induction of IPF with repeated Bleo does not affect pulmonary fibrogenesis,

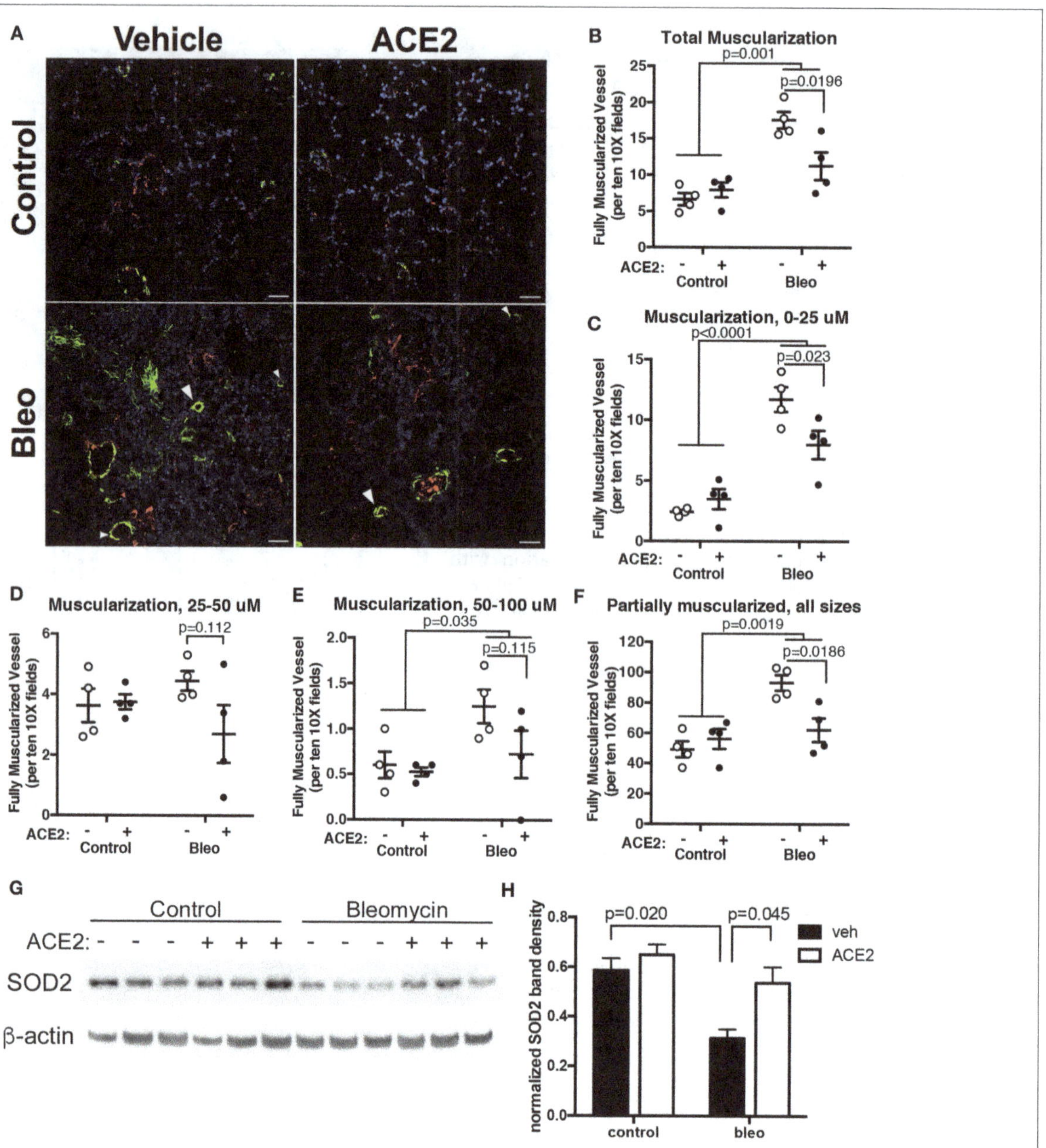

FIGURE 4 | rhACE2 treatment improves the pulmonary vascular remodeling in group 3 PH animals, while increasing pulmonary SOD2 expression. Lung sections were stained for α-SMA and von Willebrand factor, and random fields photographed at 10X. **(A)** Representative images of α-SMA-positive muscularized vessels (arrowheads). **(B–E)** ACE2 treatment decreased per field complete vessel muscularization regardless of vessel size: total (B), 0–25 μm **(C)**, 25–50 μm **(D)**, and 50–100 μm **(E)**, as well as partial muscularization of all vessels (**F**; mean ± SEM, $n = 4$ for all experimental groups). The results of two-way ANOVA followed by Holm-Sidak's post-test are shown; scale bars are 50 microns. **(G–H)** Bleomycin decreased SOD2 expression in mouse lung, which was normalized in mice treated with ACE2. Bands were quantified in ImageJ and normalized to β-actin. Shown are the results of a two-way ANOVA comparison followed by Holm-Sidek test ($n = 3$).

collagen expression, and extracellular remodeling, yet still decreases vascular remodeling. Similar to previous studies from our lab, using different models of pulmonary arterial hypertension (West et al., 2016a,b), the modest increase in RVSP was not enough to cause cardiac dysfunction as measured by echo. Thus, we are unable to conclusively comment on any rescue effects of ACE2 on RV function in this model. However, our observations are in line with our findings that rhACE2 treatment primarily improved the PH symptoms in the present study.

The RAS is dysregulated in IPF, animal models of PF, PH, and in the animal PH model of RV pressure overload (Johnson et al., 2011; Shenoy et al., 2013; Meng et al., 2015). In IPF and bleomycin lungs, there is attenuated expression and activity of ACE2 (Li et al., 2008). Similarly, a number of groups have demonstrated the dominant expression pattern of ACE and AT_1 receptor over ACE2 and Mas1 receptor in pulmonary and cardiovascular diseases (Qi et al., 2011; Shenoy et al., 2013; Meng et al., 2015). Activation of the ACE2/Ang-(1-7)/Mas1 axis by the administration of ACE2 or Ang-(1-7) results in enhanced ACE2 activity and promotes expression of ACE2/Mas1 over ACE/AT_1 in PF and PH; furthermore, augmentation of the ACE2/Ang-(1-7)/Mas1 axis improved the pathological symptoms associated with these heart and lung tissues (Shenoy et al., 2013; Meng et al., 2014, 2015). While ACE2 can also hydrolyze AngI to produce the bioactive peptide Ang-(1-9), its affinity for AngII is approximately 400x greater (Vickers et al., 2002); thus, the effects seen with ACE2 administration are more likely to be mediated by Ang-(1-7). Our group recently conducted an open-label phase IIa pilot study of rhACE2, and found that even an acute 4 h infusion of rhACE2 greatly improved the Ang II/Ang-(1-7) ratio, with a concomitant increase in the cardiac output (Hemnes et al., 2017). In the present study, we used continuously infused rhACE2 to activate the ACE2/Ang-(1-7)/Mas1 axis following induction of PF in mice with repeated Bleo injection. Although we did not quantify the expression pattern or the peptide levels of RAS members pre- and post-rhACE2 treatment, we have previously found that administration of rhACE2 for 2 weeks increases RV Mas1 expression in a mouse model of PAH (Johnson et al., 2011). To support the involvement of the Ang-(1-7)/Mas1 axis in this study, we have found that ACE2 treatment normalized pulmonary expression of SOD2 in Bleo mice; this complements our previous finding that synthetic agonist of the Mas receptor increases SOD2 expression in porcine pulmonary vessels (Carrier et al., 2016).

In our study, ACE2 treatment reduced muscularization of pulmonary vessels following bleomycin. We also observed an extensive lung tissue remodeling in conjunction with an accumulation of macrophages after repeated bleomycin. Numerous studies on PH have implicated that inflammatory signals produced at the site of injury due to infiltration of monocytes, macrophages, dendritic or natural killer cells or any other immune cells compliment disease progression by directly promoting pulmonary vascular remodeling (El Chami and Hassoun, 2012; Rabinovitch et al., 2014). In this study, the increased $CD68^{+}$ macrophages and expression of M2 macrophage markers in the bleomycin lung were not significantly diminished with ACE2 treatment, suggesting that reduced macrophage infiltration was not responsible for the reduction in vessel muscularization with ACE2 in bleomycin treated mice. Ang-(1-7) does reduce vascular smooth muscle proliferation *in vitro* (Freeman et al., 1996), and following vascular injury (Strawn et al., 1999) suggesting a possible direct effect on vascular smooth muscle. Short-term ACE2 treatment increases SOD2 expression in PH patients (Carrier et al., 2016), and SOD2 overexpression decreases proliferation and migration of vascular SMC while normalizing apoptosis (Archer et al., 2010; Wang et al., 2012). Because SOD2 is known to be reduced in PH patients (Bowers et al., 2004; Archer et al., 2010), and SOD2 siRNA creates a PAH phenotype in vascular SMC (Archer et al., 2010), this suggests that ACE2 treatment could fill a necessary void in PH treatment by decreasing vascular remodeling.

Noticeable shortcomings of our study are the modest effects of bleomycin-induced PH on cardiac function, and the variable and limited rescue of PF and PH symptoms by rhACE2. The length of our rhACE2 treatment, and thus the study length, was limited by the potential immune response of mice to a recombinant human protein. Therefore, a follow-up study that used murine ACE2 to extend bleomycin exposure and mACE2 treatment time may find more significant effects both of Bleo-induced PF as well as mACE2 rescue and strengthen the case for the therapeutic benefits of rhACE2 in group 3 PH. However, our investigation is the first attempt to demonstrate that the rhACE2 limited the progression of group 3 PH in animal model, by improving vascular remodeling and normalizing SOD2 expression. Limiting vascular muscularization and possibly improving RV function would dramatically improve patient quality of life, since the available pharmacologically agents marginally benefit the irreversible chronic lung conditions in group 3 PH, and one study of lungs from 62 mixed-origin PH patients demonstrated that prostacyclin treatment does not reduce the pathology of vascular remodeling (Stacher et al., 2012). Although triple-combination therapy including synthetic prostacyclin may reduce pulmonary arterial pressure in group 1 PAH patients (Sitbon et al., 2014), it is yet unknown whether this will benefit IPF-associated PAH though the TRITON clinical trial investigating the efficacy of triple-combination therapy is currently including group 3 PAH patients (clinicaltrials.gov study NCT02558231). Despite the limitations of this investigation, the outcome of rhACE2 treatment in bleomycin animals contributes to a growing body of evidence that warrants further consideration of rhACE2 or promoters of the ACE2/Ang-(1-7)/Mas axis for treatment of group 3 PH.

AUTHOR CONTRIBUTIONS

AR, AB, JW, and EC conceived and designed the experiment. AR, AB, EC, TS, CM, SS, and SG performed the experiment. AR, JW, and EC analyzed the data. AR, JW, and EC wrote the paper.

ACKNOWLEDGMENTS

We thank GlaxoSmithKline Inc for providing recombinant human ACE2.

REFERENCES

Archer, S. L., Marsboom, G., Kim, G. H., Zhang, H. J., Toth, P. T., Svensson, E. C., et al. (2010). Epigenetic attenuation of mitochondrial superoxide dismutase 2 in pulmonary arterial hypertension: a basis for excessive cell proliferation and a new therapeutic target. *Circulation* 121, 2661–2671. doi: 10.1161/CIRCULATIONAHA.109.916098

Bowers, R., Cool, C., Murphy, R. C., Tuder, R. M., Hopken, M. W., Flores, S. C., et al. (2004). Oxidative stress in severe pulmonary hypertension. *Am. J. Respir. Crit. Care Med.* 169, 764–769. doi: 10.1164/rccm.200301-147OC.

Bryant, A. J., Carrick, R. P., McConaha, M. E., Jones, B. R., Shay, S. D., Moore, C. S., et al. (2016). Endothelial HIF signaling regulates pulmonary fibrosis-associated pulmonary hypertension. *Am. J. Physiol. Lung Cell. Mol. Physiol.* 310, L249–L262. doi: 10.1152/ajplung.00258.2015

Bryant, A. J., Robinson, L. J., Moore, C. S., Blackwell, T. R., Gladson, S., Penner, N. L., et al. (2015). Expression of mutant bone morphogenetic protein receptor II worsens pulmonary hypertension secondary to pulmonary fibrosis. *Pulm. Circ.* 5, 681–690. doi: 10.1086/683811

Carrier, E. J., Rathinasabapathy, A., Menon, S., Kaplowitz, M. R., Fike, C. D., and West, J. D. (2016). Mas receptor activation increases Sod2 expression in pulmonary vessels and decreases endothelial dysfunction. *Am. J. Respir. Crit. Care Med.* 193:A2234. Available online at: https://www.atsjournals.org/doi/pdf/10.1164/ajrccm-conference.2016.193.1_MeetingAbstracts.A2234

Chen, N. Y., D Collum, S., Luo, F., Weng, T., Le, T. T., M Hernandez, A., et al. (2016). Macrophage bone morphogenic protein receptor 2 depletion in idiopathic pulmonary fibrosis and Group III pulmonary hypertension. *Am. J. Physiol. Lung Cell. Mol. Physiol.* 311, L238–L254. doi: 10.1152/ajplung.00142.2016

El Chami, H., and Hassoun, P. M. (2012). Immune and inflammatory mechanisms in pulmonary arterial hypertension. *Prog. Cardiovasc. Dis.* 55, 218–228. doi: 10.1016/j.pcad.2012.07.006

Fernandez, I. E., and Eickelberg, O. (2012). New cellular and molecular mechanisms of lung injury and fibrosis in idiopathic pulmonary fibrosis. *Lancet* 380, 680–688. doi: 10.1016/S0140-6736(12)61144-1.

Ferreira, A. J., Santos, R. A., Bradford, C. N., Mecca, A. P., Sumners, C., Katovich, M. J., et al. (2010). Therapeutic implications of the vasoprotective axis of the renin-angiotensin system in cardiovascular diseases. *Hypertension* 55, 207–213. doi: 10.1161/HYPERTENSIONAHA.109.140145

Freeman, E. J., Chisolm, G. M., Ferrario, C. M., and Tallant, E. A. (1996). Angiotensin-(1-7) inhibits vascular smooth muscle cell growth. *Hypertension* 28, 104–108. doi: 10.1161/01.HYP.28.1.104

Hamada, K., Nagai, S., Tanaka, S., Handa, T., Shigematsu, M., Nagao, T., et al. (2007). Significance of pulmonary arterial pressure and diffusion capacity of the lung as prognosticator in patients with idiopathic pulmonary fibrosis. *Chest* 131, 650–656. doi: 10.1378/chest.06-1466

He, C., Ryan, A. J., Murthy, S., and Carter, A. B. (2013). Accelerated development of pulmonary fibrosis via Cu, Zn-superoxide dismutase-induced alternative activation of macrophages. *J. Biol. Chem.* 288, 20745–20757. doi: 10.1074/jbc.M112.410720

Hemnes, A. R., Robbins, I. M., Pugh, M. E., Brittain, E. L., Piana, R., Fong, P., et al. (2017). Preliminary safety and acute hemodynamic effects of rhACE2 in human pulmonary arterial hypertension. *Am. J. Respir. Crit. Care Med.* 195:A7688. Available online at: https://www.atsjournals.org/doi/pdf/10.1164/ajrccm-conference.2017.195.1_MeetingAbstracts.A7688

Hsueh, W. A., and Wyne, K. (2011). Renin-Angiotensin-aldosterone system in diabetes and hypertension. *J. Clin. Hypertens.* 13, 224–237. doi: 10.1111/j.1751-7176.2011.00449.x

Johnson, J. A., Hemnes, A. R., Perrien, D. S., Schuster, M., Robinson, L. J., Gladson, S., et al. (2012). Cytoskeletal defects in Bmpr2-associated pulmonary arterial hypertension. *Am. J. Physiol. Lung Cell. Mol. Physiol.* 302, L474–L484. doi: 10.1152/ajplung.00202.2011

Johnson, J. A., West, J., Maynard, K. B., and Hemnes, A. R. (2011). ACE2 improves right ventricular function in a pressure overload model. *PLoS ONE* 6:e20828. doi: 10.1371/journal.pone.0020828

Kalra, J., Prakash, A., Kumar, P., and Majeed, A. B. (2015). Cerebroprotective effects of RAS inhibitors: beyond their cardio-renal actions. *J. Renin Angiotensin Aldosterone Syst.* 16, 459–468. doi: 10.1177/1470320315583582

Klinger, J. R. (2016). Group III pulmonary hypertension: pulmonary hypertension associated with lung disease: epidemiology, pathophysiology, and treatments. *Cardiol. Clin.* 34, 413–433. doi: 10.1016/j.ccl.2016.04.003

Lawson, W. E., Polosukhin, V. V., Stathopoulos, G. T., Zoia, O., Han, W., Lane, K. B., et al. (2005). Increased and prolonged pulmonary fibrosis in surfactant protein C-deficient mice following intratracheal bleomycin. *Am. J. Pathol.* 167, 1267–1277. doi: 10.1016/S0002-9440(10)61214-X.

Li, X., Molina-Molina, M., Abdul-Hafez, A., Uhal, V., Xaubet, A., and Uhal, B. D. (2008). Angiotensin converting enzyme-2 is protective but downregulated in human and experimental lung fibrosis. *Am. J. Physiol. Lung Cell. Mol. Physiol.* 295, L178–L185. doi: 10.1152/ajplung.00009.2008.

Meng, Y., Li, T., Zhou, G. S., Chen, Y., Yu, C. H., Pang, M. X., et al. (2015). The angiotensin-converting enzyme 2/angiotensin (1-7)/Mas axis protects against lung fibroblast migration and lung fibrosis by inhibiting the NOX4-derived ROS-mediated RhoA/Rho kinase pathway. *Antioxid. Redox Signal.* 22, 241–258. doi: 10.1089/ars.2013.5818

Meng, Y., Yu, C. H., Li, W., Li, T., Luo, W., Huang, S., et al. (2014). Angiotensin-converting enzyme 2/angiotensin-(1-7)/Mas axis protects against lung fibrosis by inhibiting the MAPK/NF-kappaB pathway. *Am. J. Respir. Cell Mol. Biol.* 50, 723–736. doi: 10.1165/rcmb.2012-0451OC

Moeller, A., Ask, K., Warburton, D., Gauldie, J., and Kolb, M. (2008). The bleomycin animal model: a useful tool to investigate treatment options for idiopathic pulmonary fibrosis? *Int. J. Biochem. Cell Biol.* 40, 362–382. doi: 10.1016/j.biocel.2007.08.011

Mortality, G. B. D., and Causes of Death, C. (2015). Global, regional, and national age-sex specific all-cause and cause-specific mortality for 240 causes of death, 1990-2013: a systematic analysis for the global burden of disease study 2013. *Lancet* 385, 117–171. doi: 10.1016/S0140-6736(14)61682-2

Mouratis, M. A., and Aidinis, V. (2011). Modeling pulmonary fibrosis with bleomycin. *Curr. Opin. Pulm. Med.* 17, 355–361. doi: 10.1097/MCP.0b013e328349ac2b

Oudiz, R. J. (2016). Classification of pulmonary hypertension. *Cardiol. Clin.* 34, 359–361. doi: 10.1016/j.ccl.2016.04.009

Passos-Silva, D. G., Brandan, E., and Santos, R. A. (2015). Angiotensins as therapeutic targets beyond heart disease. *Trends Pharmacol. Sci.* 36, 310–320. doi: 10.1016/j.tips.2015.03.001

Patel, N. M., Lederer, D. J., Borczuk, A. C., and Kawut, S. M. (2007). Pulmonary hypertension in idiopathic pulmonary fibrosis. *Chest* 132, 998–1006. doi: 10.1378/chest.06-3087

Qi, Y., Shenoy, V., Wong, F., Li, H., Afzal, A., Mocco, J., et al. (2011). Lentivirus-mediated overexpression of angiotensin-(1-7) attenuated ischaemia-induced cardiac pathophysiology. *Exp. Physiol.* 96, 863–874. doi: 10.1113/expphysiol.2011.056994

Rabinovitch, M., Guignabert, C., Humbert, M., and Nicolls, M. R. (2014). Inflammation and immunity in the pathogenesis of pulmonary arterial hypertension. *Circ. Res.* 115, 165–175. doi: 10.1161/CIRCRESAHA.113.301141

Rathinasabapathy, A., Bruce, E., Espejo, A., Horowitz, A., Sudhan, D. R., Nair, A., et al. (2016). Therapeutic potential of adipose stem cell-derived conditioned medium against pulmonary hypertension and lung fibrosis. *Br. J. Pharmacol.* 173, 2859–2879. doi: 10.1111/bph.13562

Rey-Parra, G. J., Vadivel, A., Coltan, L., Hall, A., Eaton, F., Schuster, M., et al. (2012). Angiotensin converting enzyme 2 abrogates bleomycin-induced lung injury. *J. Mol. Med.* 90, 637–647. doi: 10.1007/s00109-012-0859-2

Richeldi, L., Collard, H. R., and Jones, M. G. (2017). Idiopathic pulmonary fibrosis. *Lancet* 389, 1941–1952. doi: 10.1016/S0140-6736(17)30866-8

Schermuly, R. T., Ghofrani, H. A., Wilkins, M. R., and Grimminger, F. (2011). Mechanisms of disease: pulmonary arterial hypertension. *Nat. Rev. Cardiol.* 8, 443–455. doi: 10.1038/nrcardio.2011.87

Shenoy, V., Ferreira, A. J., Qi, Y., Fraga-Silva, R. A., Díez-Freire, C., Dooies, A., et al. (2010). The angiotensin-converting enzyme 2/angiogenesis-(1-7)/Mas axis confers cardiopulmonary protection against lung fibrosis and pulmonary hypertension. *Am. J. Respir. Crit. Care Med.* 182, 1065–1072. doi: 10.1164/rccm.200912-1840OC

Shenoy, V., Gjymishka, A., Jarajapu, Y. P., Qi, Y., Afzal, A., Rigatto, K., et al. (2013). Diminazene attenuates pulmonary hypertension and improves angiogenic progenitor cell functions in experimental models. *Am. J. Respir. Crit. Care Med.* 187, 648–657. doi: 10.1164/rccm.201205-0880OC

Shorr, A. F., Wainright, J. L., Cors, C. S., Lettieri, C. J., and Nathan, S. D. (2007). Pulmonary hypertension in patients with pulmonary fibrosis awaiting lung transplant. *Eur. Respir. J.* 30, 715–721. doi: 10.1183/09031936.00107206

Sitbon, O., Jaïs, X., Savale, L., Cottin, V., Bergot, E., Macari, E. A., et al. (2014). Upfront triple combination therapy in pulmonary arterial hypertension: a pilot study. *Eur. Respir. J.* 43, 1691–1697. doi: 10.1183/09031936.00116313

Stacher, E., Graham, B. B., Hunt, J. M., Gandjeva, A., Groshong, S. D., McLaughlin, V. V., et al. (2012). Modern age pathology of pulmonary arterial hypertension. *Am. J. Respir. Crit. Care Med.* 186, 261–272. doi: 10.1164/rccm.201201-0164OC

Strawn, W. B., Ferrario, C. M., and Tallant, E. A. (1999). Angiotensin-(1-7) reduces smooth muscle growth after vascular injury. *Hypertension* 33(1 Pt 2), 207–211. doi: 10.1161/01.HYP.33.1.207

Vickers, C., Hales, P., Kaushik, V., Dick, L., Gavin, J., Tang, J., et al. (2002). Hydrolysis of biological peptides by human angiotensin-converting enzyme-related carboxypeptidase. *J. Biol. Chem.* 277, 14838–14843. doi: 10.1074/jbc.M200581200.

Wang, J. N., Shi, N., and Chen, S. Y. (2012). Manganese superoxide dismutase inhibits neointima formation through attenuation of migration and proliferation of vascular smooth muscle cells. *Free Radic. Biol. Med.* 52, 173–181. doi: 10.1016/j.freeradbiomed.2011.10.442.

West, J. D., Carrier, E. J., Bloodworth, N. C., Schroer, A. K., Chen, P., Ryzhova, L. M., et al. (2016a). Serotonin 2B receptor antagonism prevents heritable pulmonary arterial hypertension. *PLoS ONE* 11:e0148657. doi: 10.1371/journal.pone.0148657

West, J. D., Voss, B. M., Pavliv, L., de Caestecker, M., Hemnes, A. R., and Carrier, E. J. (2016b). Antagonism of the thromboxane-prostanoid receptor is cardioprotective against right ventricular pressure overload. *Pulm. Circ.* 6, 211–223. doi: 10.1086/686140

20

The Role of Neutrophils and Neutrophil Elastase in Pulmonary Arterial Hypertension

Shalina Taylor[1,2†], *Omar Dirir*[3†], *Roham T. Zamanian*[2,4], *Marlene Rabinovitch*[1,2] *and A. A. Roger Thompson*[3*]

[1] *Department of Pediatrics, Stanford University School of Medicine, Stanford, CA, United States,* [2] *Vera Moulton Wall Center for Pulmonary Vascular Disease, Stanford University, Stanford, CA, United States,* [3] *Infection, Immunity, and Cardiovascular Disease, University of Sheffield, Sheffield, United Kingdom,* [4] *Division of Pulmonary and Critical Care Medicine, Stanford University School of Medicine, Stanford, CA, United States*

Correspondence:
A. A. Roger Thompson
r.thompson@sheffield.ac.uk

† *These authors have contributed equally to this work.*

Pulmonary arterial hypertension (PAH) is a severe vasculopathy characterized by the presence of fibrotic lesions in the arterial wall and the loss of small distal pulmonary arteries. The vasculopathy is accompanied by perivascular inflammation and increased protease levels, with neutrophil elastase notably implicated in aberrant vascular remodeling. However, the source of elevated elastase levels in PAH remains unclear. A major source of neutrophil elastase is the neutrophil, an understudied cell population in PAH. The principal function of neutrophils is to destroy invading pathogens by means of phagocytosis and NET formation, but proteases, chemokines, and cytokines implicated in PAH can be released by and/or prime and activate neutrophils. This review focuses on the contribution of inflammation to the development and progression of the disease, highlighting studies implicating neutrophils, neutrophil elastase, and other neutrophil proteases in PAH. The roles of cytokines, chemokines, and neutrophil elastase in the disease are discussed and we describe new insight into the role neutrophils potentially play in the pathogenesis of PAH.

Keywords: neutrophils, neutrophil elastase, pulmonary hypertension, pulmonary arterial hypertension, vascular remodeling

PULMONARY ARTERIAL HYPERTENSION AND INFLAMMATION

Pulmonary arterial hypertension (PAH) is a progressive disease characterized by thickening, and progressive occlusion of distal arteries in the lung related to vascular cell dysfunction, and perivascular inflammation. As a consequence of elevation in pulmonary arterial pressure, the right ventricle hypertrophies and later becomes dysfunctional leading to right heart failure (1, 2). Perivascular inflammation has been observed in all subsets of PAH and correlates with clinical markers of disease progression such as an increase in pulmonary vascular resistance and a decrease in the 6-min walk test (3, 4). The consequences of perivascular inflammation include cytokine production by vascular and inflammatory cells, and degradation of the extracellular matrix (ECM) by proteases (5, 6). Both the increased cytokine production and the peptides that are released as a result of ECM degradation cause activation and recruitment of circulating immune cells (6, 7). Neutrophils are among the cells that are recruited, and these cells release proteolytic enzymes, including neutrophil elastase (NE), that cause vascular injury (8). Although many aspects of perivascular inflammation can cause progressive PAH, this review will focus on neutrophils and NE. We will review evidence of neutrophil accumulation in PAH, discuss the role of NE and other proteases in driving vascular remodeling and highlight potential interactions between neutrophils, NE and the key genetic driver of PAH, bone morphogenetic protein receptor type 2 (BMPR2).

NEUTROPHILS AND PAH

Neutrophils are the predominant circulating leukocyte population and are important in modulating innate and adaptive immunity. They are early responders and are recruited to sites of sterile inflammation and infection by environmental cues.

Relatively little attention has been given to the role of neutrophils in the pathogenesis of PAH. Neutrophil and macrophage perivascular accumulation has been observed in murine lungs in association with hypoxic pulmonary hypertension (PH) and in monocrotaline-induced PH in rats (9, 10). It has also been established that the neutrophil to lymphocyte ratio is increased in PAH patients when compared to healthy controls (11) and that increased neutrophil to lymphocyte ratio positively correlates with New York Heart Association (NYHA) functional class (FC) and predicts event free survival (12, 13). It is not clear why this relative increase in circulating neutrophils is associated with PAH progression. However, neutrophils produce a wide range of substances that could contribute to vascular remodeling and promote inflammation in PAH. For example, myeloperoxidase (MPO), a catalyst for reactive oxygen species (ROS) formation, has recently been implicated in the pathophysiology of PAH (14). Two independent cohorts of PAH patients had increased plasma MPO relative to healthy controls and $Mpo^{-/-}$ mice displayed reduced right ventricular pressures following hypoxic exposure (14). Interestingly, although MPO can reduce nitric oxide (NO) bioavailability in other vascular beds (15), there was no evidence supporting a difference in NO availability between wild-type and MPO-deficient mice (14). Instead, activation of a Rho kinase pathway by MPO was found to drive pulmonary vasoconstriction and SMC proliferation (14).

In addition to MPO and ROS, neutrophils produce proteolytic enzymes. Activity of these enzymes is tightly controlled by endogenous inhibitors, but excessive protease activity has the potential to destroy tissue and cause extensive fibrotic remodeling, leading to organ failure (16). Indeed neutrophil proteases are implicated in airway and parenchymal lung diseases [reviewed by Taggart et al. (17)] and are known to have roles in systemic vascular pathology (18, 19).

Neutrophil granule proteases include members of the serine protease family (NE, cathepsin G, proteinase 3) and matrix metalloproteinases [neutrophil collagenase (MMP-8) and gelatinase (MMP-9)] (20). Of these proteases, NE has been most heavily implicated in the pathogenesis of PAH, as described below.

SOURCES OF NEUTROPHIL ELASTASE IN PAH

Neutrophils are the dominant cellular source of NE but it is also produced by macrophages and smooth muscle cells (SMC) (21–24). There is evidence of both augmented NE release from neutrophils isolated from PAH patients (25) and upregulation of endogenous NE in PAH patient SMCs and in experimental animal models of PH (23, 26, 27). Macrophages are observed in the plexiform lesions of PAH patient lungs and activated macrophages release leukotriene B4, which induces endothelial cell (EC) injury and results in EC apoptosis, but could also promote neutrophil recruitment (28). Moreover, *in vitro* work suggests that human alveolar macrophages internalize NE through ingestion of apoptotic neutrophils, and act as a vehicle for the enzyme, transporting it to the tissues and subsequently releasing the active form (29). However, further work is required to show conservation of this mechanism in perivascular or interstitial lung macrophages.

NE is dispensed by neutrophils during degranulation and upon release of neutrophil extracellular traps (NETs). NETs consist of decondensed chromatin decorated with NE and other antimicrobial proteases. NE plays an important role in NET release, evidenced by reduced NET formation in the presence of NE inhibitors and in NE knockout mice (30). Upon stimulation, NE is discharged from azurophilic granules and translocates to the nucleus where it contributes to histone degradation, facilitating chromatin decondensation (30). Depending on the stimulus, chromatin is then expelled via vesicles (31) or suicidal NETosis (32), reviewed by Jorch et al. (33).

NETs assist in microbial trapping and killing (32), but non-infectious roles for NETs are emerging and NETs have been identified in vascular pathologies such as atherosclerosis and PAH (34, 35). Detrimental consequences attributed to NETs include nuclear factor kappa-light-chain-enhancer of activated B cells-dependent PA EC pathological angiogenesis, release of the vasoactive agent endothelin-1, and promotion of SMC proliferation (34). NETs can also directly induce EC cell death (36) and promote thrombus formation (37). In PAH lung tissue, markers of NET formation (DNA, myeloperoxidase, and citrullinated histone H3) have been identified in proximity to plexiform lesions and circulating DNA levels were elevated in IPAH patient plasma (34), although this study did not investigate whether IPAH patient neutrophils are more prone to releasing NETs.

Studies prior to the identification of NETs had suggested that binding of NE to DNA inhibited the activity of the protease (38). However, Kolaczkowska et al. used an *in vivo* zymography assay to demonstrate that NE associated with NETs remains proteolytically active (39). This implies that NE attached to NETs is shielded from endogenous anti-protease activity and thus high NET levels in PAH may represent an important source of active NE.

NEUTROPHIL ELASTASE IN THE PATHOLOGY OF PAH

Elastolytic activity has been implicated in the pathogenesis of PAH for over three decades, with evidence of fragmented internal elastic laminae in the pulmonary arteries of children with congenital heart defects (40). There is a clear temporal relationship between increased NE activity and vascular changes in PAH experimental rat models (41). Furthermore, inhibition of NE enzymatic activity not only attenuates the progression of PAH but can also reverse the disease process in experimental models. This was first shown in the monocrotaline model where a progressive and fatal form of PH was reversed by elastase inhibitors in association with normalization of hemodynamic changes of PH and structural abnormalities that included extensive occlusive muscularization (26). Nickel et al. also demonstrated reversal of hemodynamic and histological measures of PH in the Sugen/Hypoxia rat model following treatment with recombinant human elafin (42). Increased NE activity was demonstrated in the lungs of rats with Sugen/Hypoxia-induced PH and this was attenuated by elafin (42). Importantly, relevance to human disease was confirmed through use of a human pulmonary artery explant model. Tissue sections containing pulmonary arteries were isolated from the explanted lungs of PAH patients and treatment with elafin induced regression of neointimal changes and improved measures of vessel lumen size (42).

Release of NE can stimulate adverse remodeling by degrading virtually all the components of the ECM in addition to elastin, and including collagen, fibronectin, and laminin (43). As a consequence, degraded ECM releases bioactive peptides and growth factors such as epidermal growth factor (EGF) and fibroblast growth factor (FGF), which have both mitogenic and motogenic effects on SMCs and fibroblasts (44–47). Additionally, heightened NE activity leads to the activation of matrix metalloproteinases (MMPs), which could potentiate ECM degradation, and induction of tenascin C, a glycoprotein associated with the upregulation of growth factor receptors and proliferation of SMCs (48). The sub-endothelial deposition of tenascin C and fibronectin appears to be a chemotactic factor for PA SMCs, facilitating their migration and the formation of neointimal lesions (48, 49). Conversely, inhibition of NE leads to reduced tenascin C, induction of SMC apoptosis, and regression of pulmonary artery (PA) medial hypertrophy (26).

The role of elastase in vascular remodeling was further explored using transgenic mice that over-express the S100A4 protein (23, 27). Following infection with the murine herpes virus, MHV-68, S100A4 mice develop histological features of human PAH including neointima formation (27). These vascular lesions display fragmented elastic laminae associated with heightened lung elastase activity (27). Infusion of recombinant human elafin, an endogenous elastase inhibitor, reduced the number and severity of neointimal lesions in this model (23). Furthermore, using FLAG-tagged elafin, NE was identified as the serine elastase responsible for the elevation in elastase activity in the S100A4 lungs (23). While this finding implies that NE is the dominant target in this model, the relative importance of NE above other proteases in human disease has not been confirmed and the potential roles of other proteases will be discussed below.

The source of NE in the S100A4 lungs was localized not only to neutrophils but also to PA SMCs and, as indicated above, this finding was conserved in human disease, evidenced by cultured PA SMCs from IPAH patients expressing higher levels of NE than cells from control donor lungs (23). Interestingly, *ex vivo* perfusion of S100A4 lungs with porcine pancreatic elastase suggested that the elastin fibers in these mice were more prone to degradation (23). This implies that certain viral infections, and potentially other inflammatory stimuli, may predispose the vasculature to pathological remodeling upon exposure to elastase.

NEUTROPHIL ELASTASE AND PERPETUATION OF INFLAMMATION IN PAH

In addition to the impact of NE on SMC migration and proliferation, this enzyme contributes to PAH pathogenesis by proteolytic modification of cytokines. For example, NE promotes IL-1β activity by cleaving the pro-isoform of IL-1β in human coronary ECs, thereby increasing the secretion of the bioactive form in extracellular vesicles (50). Notably, secretion of active IL-1β could promote neutrophil survival, an example of positive regulation of neutrophil activity by cytokines (51).

NE also cleaves CXCL12 (SDF-1 alpha), a chemokine involved in the regulated release of neutrophils from the bone marrow (52–54). CXCL12 inactivation would promote mobilization of neutrophils into the circulation, particularly in the context of elevated plasma IL-8 levels, as observed in PAH patients (4, 54). On the other hand, NE can inactivate tumor-necrosis factor (55) and IL-6 (56), suggesting that there is a balance that must be maintained between elastase and anti-elastase activity. The chronic perivascular inflammatory phenotype of PAH patients characterized by elevated levels of circulating and tissue cytokines, is consistent with persistent neutrophil activation. Indeed, many of the cytokines elevated in PAH are known to enhance neutrophil function and survival and may thus perpetuate neutrophil-mediated inflammation (**Table 1**).

OTHER PROTEASES IMPLICATED IN TISSUE REMODELING IN PAH

As mentioned above, other neutrophil proteases may contribute to the vascular remodeling observed in PAH. For example, MMP-9 expression is upregulated in human plexiform pulmonary arterial lesions (61) and in lungs isolated from rats with monocrotaline-induced pulmonary hypertension (62). Furthermore, transgenic overexpression of human MMP-9 exacerbated monocrotaline-induced pulmonary hypertension in mice (63). The role of other MMPs and MMP inhibitors in PAH has been reviewed by Chelladuri et al. (64).

This review has focused mainly on neutrophil proteases, but it should be noted that many other cells release proteases. For example, upregulation of MMP-9 has been detected in natural killer cells from patients with PAH (65) and it is also released by monocytes and macrophages (66). Further examples of important non-neutrophil proteases are chymase and tryptase, the main proteases released by mast cells. Heath and Yacoub (67) noted increased perivascular mast cell numbers in both primary and secondary forms of pulmonary hypertension compared to controls, an observation confirmed more recently by others (68,

TABLE 1 | Cytokines elevated in PAH and known to alter neutrophil function.

Cytokine	Release	Priming	Adhesion	Chemotaxis	ROS	Survival	References
CCL2	x		x	x		x	(57)
IL-1α	x						(58)
IL-1β	x	x	x	x	x	x	(4, 58, 59)
IL-4	x						(4)
IL-6	x		x	x			(4, 58–60)
IL-8	x	x	x	x			(4)
IL-10	x						(4)
IL-12	x						(4)
Interferon- γ	x	x				x	(4)
TNF-α	x	x	x	x	x	x	(4, 58)

The x symbols indicate which functions are altered by each cytokine. ROS, reactive oxygen species generation; CCL2, C-C Motif Chemokine Ligand 2, also known as monocyte chemoattractant protein 1; IL, interleukin; TNF, tumor necrosis factor.

69). Circulating tryptase levels were elevated in PAH patients compared to controls and correlated with disease severity as assessed by brain natriuretic peptide level (68). In this study a small number of patients were treated with mast cell stabilizers, but there were no changes in clinical endpoints such as 6-min walk distance or BNP level.

A key question about protease activity in any disease process is how the protease evades suppression by endogenous inhibitors. NE is inhibited by several anti-proteases including α1-antitrypsin, secretory leucocyte peptidase inhibitor (SLPI) and elafin. On the one hand it is possible that localized release of the protease simply overcomes anti-protease activity in the immediate microenvironment. Indeed, markers of pre-inhibited elastase activity have been reported including the cleaved fibrinogen product, Aα-Val^{360} (70). On the other hand, proteases may be shielded from their inhibitors by attachment to NETS (discussed above), or via transport in exosomes. Neutrophil-derived exosomes degrade NE substrates and induce emphysematous changes in murine lungs following intra-tracheal administration (71). It is also possible that proteases have enzyme-independent functions but the beneficial consequences of elafin treatment in animal models of PH and in lung explant models (23, 42) would favor the hypothesis that there is an excess of protease activity. Interestingly, however, elafin may exert protective effects independently of protease inhibition as described below.

NEUTROPHILS AND PAH RELATED TO BMPR2 DEFICIENCY

The bone morphogenetic protein receptor 2 (BMPR2) signaling pathway has become a key focus of investigation since *BMPR2* gene mutations were identified as the main predisposing risk factor in the heritable forms of PAH (HPAH) (72), with dysfunction in the signaling pathway present in all subtypes of PAH (73). However, although present in a high proportion of HPAH cases—identified in 70% of familial PAH cases (74)—the autosomal dominant *BMPR2* mutation exhibits low penetrance with 70–80% of those carrying the mutation never developing PAH (75). This, and the lack of spontaneous PAH in most heterozygous *BMPR2* animal models, implies that a second insult or background genetic variants are needed for predisposed individuals to develop PAH. Inflammation has been proposed as a second hit which promotes adverse remodeling when there is a loss of BMPR2.

BMPR2 is expressed by all cells in the arterial wall but by far the highest level of expression is present in endothelial cells (73). Reduced BMPR2 signaling is related both to excessive vascular smooth muscle proliferation (76) and exaggerated PA EC apoptosis (77). A study by Burton et al. (78) investigated the role of BMPR2 in maintaining the barrier function of PA ECs and in suppressing inflammation within the pulmonary vasculature. Using static and flow-based *in vitro* systems, they were able to demonstrate that a reduction in BMPR2 expression facilitated neutrophil transmigration across the PA EC monolayer and reported that a lack of BMPR2 led to overexpression of IL-8, which in turn led to the recruitment of neutrophils. Similarly, loss of BMPR2 can lead to heightened expression of IL-6, an inducer of SMC proliferation (79). Taken together, BMPR2 plays a role in dampening inflammatory signals in the pulmonary vasculature that could influence neutrophil recruitment and elastase activity.

Conversely, neutrophils may also impact BMPR2 function by releasing NE and degrading BMP9, an anti-angiogenic ligand for the BMPR2/ALK1 heterodimer present on PA ECs (80). BMP9 has been shown to circulate in humans at biologically active levels (81), maintaining vascular quiescence. Li et al. showed that BMP9 is readily cleaved by NE, released by activated neutrophils (80). Further work by this group demonstrated that the administration of recombinant BMP9 reversed established PH in *BMPR2*-deficient mice, overcoming reduced BMPR2 levels, and preventing lung vascular leakage (82). Paradoxically, Appleby et al. demonstrated that BMP9 could have a pro-inflammatory role and, in fact, facilitate neutrophil recruitment to the pulmonary vasculature by activated endothelial cells (83). However, the mouse model used in that study was acute endotoxemia, so this may not relate directly to PAH pathogenesis.

Overall, it appears that inflammation-driven release of NE can suppress BMPR2 signaling. Nickel and colleagues investigated the impact of the NE inhibitor elafin on BMPR2 signaling in PAH (42). In the Sugen/Hypoxia rat model of PH, elafin improved pulmonary endothelial expression of apelin, a BMPR2 target gene. Loss of apelin expression in the pulmonary endothelium during PAH is associated with the failure to repress the release of fibroblast growth factor-2 (FGF2) (84). Nickel et al. also found that in human cells, elafin augmented BMPR2 interactions with caveolin-1, another downstream target of BMPR2 signaling (42). Unfortunately, changes in BMP9 levels following elafin administration were not measured. Nonetheless, the findings suggest that improving BMPR2 signaling in addition to the beneficial sequelae of inhibiting NE, described earlier in this review, could reverse the vascular remodeling observed in PAH. Interestingly, targeting NE activity may be of particular importance in patients with BMPR2 mutations, as histological assessment of pulmonary vessels in such patients demonstrates a reduction in elastin and fibrillin-1, the two major constituents of elastic fibers (85). Furthermore, pulmonary artery elastic fibers from mice with compound *Bmpr2/1a* mutations were more susceptible to elastase-mediated degradation of elastic fibers compared to wild-type mice (85).

SUMMARY

Collectively the studies discussed above implicate the neutrophil and neutrophil products such as MPO, proteases and NETs in the pathogenesis of PAH. Neutrophils are attractive candidates in contributing to vascular changes seen in PAH because they are among the first cells to arrive at sites of inflammation. The evidence of increased circulating elastase in PAH patients and fragmented elastic lamina in PAH vessels, highlights a key pathogenic role for proteolytic enzymes and in particular NE. NE has a wide range of targets, but we describe evidence for how it could contribute to PAH pathogenesis by modulating the activity of cytokines and degrading ECM releasing growth factors that promote remodeling. Moreover, the release of NE and NETs is likely to alter the local inflammatory environment, augmenting leukocyte responses and further driving inflammation in PAH. It is also evident that reduced BMPR2 receptor signaling cooperatively interacts with the sequelae of inflammation and neutrophil activation in contributing to adverse vascular remodeling. **Figure 1** provides a summary of the role of neutrophils, NE and NETs in PAH.

While increases in NE activity coincide with changes in vascular remodeling in animal models, it remains unclear whether intrinsic neutrophil abnormalities are necessary to initiate aberrant remodeling in human lungs or whether alterations in NET and NE release by neutrophils are a consequence of other features of the disease. To better understand the role of neutrophils at different stages of PAH pathogenesis, a longitudinal study to evaluate how they become increased and activated would be important. However,

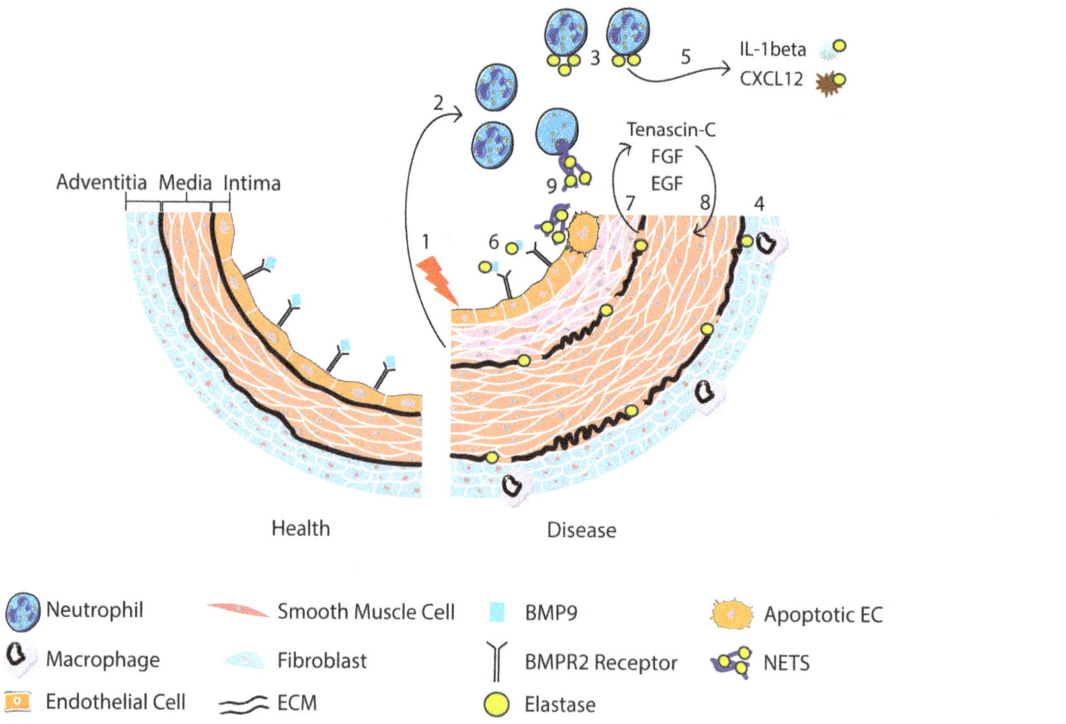

FIGURE 1 | Following vascular injury (1), the release of chemokines and chemotactic peptides from surrounding tissue recruits and activates neutrophils (2). Neutrophils release elastase (3) although it can also be released from activated macrophages that engulf neutrophil elastase (4) and from smooth muscle cells. Release of neutrophil elastase leads to cleavage of cytokines resulting in the conversion of the pro-to active form of IL-1b, promoting neutrophil survival, and degradation of CXCL12, favoring release of neutrophils from the bone marrow (5). BMP9 is also cleaved, impacting upon BMPR2 receptor signaling (6). Degradation of the ECM by elastase (7) releases SMC mitogenic growth factors promoting SMC proliferation (8). Neutrophil elastase is also involved in the release of NETs, which may induce EC apoptosis (9) and therefore contribute to endothelial dysfunction.

directly targeting neutrophils as a therapeutic strategy would be challenging given their vital role in host defense and as mentioned above, cells other than neutrophils can produce damaging proteases. Of these proteases, NE provides an attractive target as evidence from animal models suggests that NE inhibition has the potential to inhibit aberrant remodeling of the pulmonary vessels and indirectly dampen persistent inflammation in PAH. These findings have encouraged initiation of clinical trials of elastase inhibitors such as elafin for PAH (NCT03522935). Further, the potential for NE inhibitors such as elafin to enhance BMPR2 signaling and target pathology driven by BMPR2 deficiency, identifies these drugs as promising novel therapies for PAH.

AUTHOR CONTRIBUTIONS

ST and OD wrote sections of the manuscript; AT initiated the work and drafted sections of the manuscript; AT, MR and RZ revised the manuscript critically for important intellectual content.

REFERENCES

1. Rabinovitch M. Molecular pathogenesis of pulmonary arterial hypertension. *J Clin Invest.* (2008) 118:2372–9. doi: 10.1172/JCI33452
2. Rabinovitch M. Molecular pathogenesis of pulmonary arterial hypertension. *J Clin Invest.* (2012) 122:4306–13. doi: 10.1172/JCI60658
3. Stacher E, Graham BB, Hunt JM, Gandjeva A, Groshong SD, McLaughlin VV, et al. Modern age pathology of pulmonary arterial hypertension. *Am J Respir Crit Care Med.* (2012) 186:261–72. doi: 10.1164/rccm.201201-0164OC
4. Soon E, Holmes AM, Treacy CM, Doughty NJ, Southgate L, Machado RD, et al. Elevated levels of inflammatory cytokines predict survival in idiopathic and familial pulmonary arterial hypertension. *Circulation* (2010) 122:920–7. doi: 10.1161/CIRCULATIONAHA.109.933762
5. Humbert M, Morrell NW, Archer SL, Stenmark KR, MacLean MR, Lang IM, et al. Cellular and molecular pathobiology of pulmonary arterial hypertension. *J Am Coll Cardiol.* (2004) 43(12 Suppl. S):13S–24. doi: 10.1016/j.jacc.2004.02.029
6. Rabinovitch M, Guignabert C, Humbert M, Nicolls MR. Inflammation and immunity in the pathogenesis of pulmonary arterial hypertension. *Circ Res.* (2014) 115:165–75. doi: 10.1161/CIRCRESAHA.113.301141
7. Senior RM, Griffin GL, Mecham RP. Chemotactic activity of elastin-derived peptides. *J Clin Invest.* (1980) 66:859–62. doi: 10.1172/JCI109926
8. Korkmaz B, Horwitz MS, Jenne DE, Gauthier F. Neutrophil elastase, proteinase 3, and cathepsin G as therapeutic targets in human diseases. *Pharmacol Rev.* (2010) 62:726–59. doi: 10.1124/pr.110.002733
9. Frid MG, Brunetti JA, Burke DL, Carpenter TC, Davie NJ, Reeves JT, et al. Hypoxia-induced pulmonary vascular remodeling requires recruitment of circulating mesenchymal precursors of a monocyte/macrophage lineage. *Am J Pathol.* (2006) 168:659–69. doi: 10.2353/ajpath.2006.050599
10. Schultze AE, Wagner JG, White SM, Roth RA. Early indications of monocrotaline pyrrole-induced lung injury in rats. *Toxicol Appl Pharmacol.* (1991) 109:41–50.
11. Yildiz A, Kaya H, Ertas F, Oylumlu M, Bilik MZ, Yuksel M, et al. Association between neutrophil to lymphocyte ratio and pulmonary arterial hypertension. *Turk Kardiyol Dern Ars.* (2013) 41:604–9. doi: 10.5543/tkda.2013.93385
12. Ozpelit E, Akdeniz B, Ozpelit ME, Tas S, Bozkurt S, Tertemiz KC, et al. Prognostic value of neutrophil-to-lymphocyte ratio in pulmonary arterial hypertension. *J Int Med Res.* (2015) 43:661–71. doi: 10.1177/0300060515589394
13. Harbaum L, Baaske KM, Simon M, Oqueka T, Sinning C, Glatzel A, et al. Exploratory analysis of the neutrophil to lymphocyte ratio in patients with pulmonary arterial hypertension. *BMC Pulm Med.* (2017) 17:72. doi: 10.1186/s12890-017-040
14. Klinke A, Berghausen E, Fr7-5iedrichs K, Molz S, Lau D, Remane L, et al. Myeloperoxidase aggravates pulmonary arterial hypertension by activation of vascular Rho-kinase. *JCI Insight* (2018) 3:530. doi: 10.1172/jci.insight.97530
15. Eiserich JP, Baldus S, Brennan ML, Ma W, Zhang C, Tousson A, et al. Myeloperoxidase, a leukocyte-derived vascular NO oxidase. *Science* (2002) 296:2391–4. doi: 10.1126/science.1106830
16. Segal AW. How neutrophils kill microbes. *Annu Rev Immunol.* (2005) 23:197–223. doi: 10.1146/annurev.immunol.23.021704.115653
17. Taggart C, Mall MA, Lalmanach G, Cataldo D, Ludwig A, Janciauskiene S, et al. Protean proteases: at the cutting edge of lung diseases. *Eur Respir J.* (2017) 49:2015. doi: 10.1183/13993003.01200-2015
18. Yan H, Zhou HF, Akk A, Hu Y, Springer LE, Ennis TL, et al. Neutrophil proteases promote experimental abdominal aortic aneurysm via extracellular trap release and plasmacytoid dendritic cell activation. *Arterioscler Thromb Vasc Biol.* (2016) 36:1660–9. doi: 10.1161/ATVBAHA.116.307786
19. Soehnlein O. Multiple roles for neutrophils in atherosclerosis. *Circ Res.* (2012) 110:875–88. doi: 10.1161/CIRCRESAHA.111.257535
20. Cowland JB, Borregaard N. Granulopoiesis and granules of human neutrophils. *Immunol Rev.* (2016) 273:11–28. doi: 10.1111/imr.12440
21. Belaaouaj A, Kim KS, Shapiro SD. Degradation of outer membrane protein A in *Escherichia coli* killing by neutrophil elastase. *Science* (2000) 289:1185–8. doi: 10.1126/science.289.5482.1185
22. Dollery CM, Owen CA, Sukhova GK, Krettek A, Shapiro SD, Libby P. Neutrophil elastase in human atherosclerotic plaques: production by macrophages. *Circulation* (2003) 107:2829–36. doi: 10.1161/01.CIR.0000072792.65250.4A
23. Kim YM, Haghighat L, Spiekerkoetter E, Sawada H, Alvira CM, Wang L, et al. Neutrophil elastase is produced by pulmonary artery smooth muscle cells and is linked to neointimal lesions. *Am J Pathol.* (2011) 179:1560–72. doi: 10.1016/j.ajpath.2011.05.051
24. Kobayashi J, Wigle D, Childs T, Zhu L, Keeley FW, Rabinovitch M. Serum-induced vascular smooth muscle cell elastolytic activity through tyrosine kinase intracellular signalling. *J Cell Physiol.* (1994) 160:121–31. doi: 10.1002/jcp.1041600115
25. Rose F, Hattar K, Gakisch S, Grimminger F, Olschewski H, Seeger W, et al. Increased neutrophil mediator release in patients with pulmonary hypertension–suppression by inhaled iloprost. *Thromb Haemost.* (2003) 90:1141–9. doi: 10.1160/TH03-03-0173
26. Cowan KN, Heilbut A, Humpl T, Lam C, Ito S, Rabinovitch M. Complete reversal of fatal pulmonary hypertension in rats by a serine elastase inhibitor. *Nat Med* (2000) 6:698–702. doi: 10.1038/76282
27. Spiekerkoetter E, Alvira CM, Kim YM, Bruneau A, Pricola KL, Wang L, et al. Reactivation of gammaHV68 induces neointimal lesions in pulmonary arteries of S100A4/Mts1-overexpressing mice in association with degradation of elastin. *Am J Physiol Lung Cell Mol Physiol.* (2008) 294:L276–89. doi: 10.1152/ajplung.00414.2007
28. Tian W, Jiang X, Tamosiuniene R, Sung YK, Qian J, Dhillon G, et al. Blocking macrophage leukotriene b4 prevents endothelial injury and reverses pulmonary hypertension. *Sci Transl Med.* (2013) 5:200ra117. doi: 10.1126/scitranslmed.3006674
29. Campbell EJ, Wald MS. Hypoxic injury to human alveolar macrophages accelerates release of previously bound neutrophil elastase. Implications for lung connective tissue injury including pulmonary emphysema. *Am Rev Respir Dis.* (1983) 127:631–5. doi: 10.1164/arrd.1983.127.5.631
30. Papayannopoulos V, Metzler KD, Hakkim A, Zychlinsky A. Neutrophil elastase and myeloperoxidase regulate the formation of neutrophil extracellular traps. *J Cell Biol.* (2010) 191:677–91. doi: 10.1083/jcb.201006052
31. Pilsczek FH, Salina D, Poon KK, Fahey C, Yipp BG, Sibley CD, et al. A novel mechanism of rapid nuclear neutrophil extracellular trap formation in response to Staphylococcus aureus. *J Immunol.* (2010) 185:7413–25. doi: 10.4049/jimmunol.1000675
32. Brinkmann V, Reichard U, Goosmann C, Fauler B, Uhlemann Y, Weiss DS, et al. Neutrophil extracellular traps kill bacteria. *Science* (2004) 303:1532–5. doi: 10.1126/science.1092385
33. Jorch SK, Kubes P. An emerging role for neutrophil extracellular traps in noninfectious disease. *Nat Med.* (2017) 23:279–87. doi: 10.1038/nm.4294
34. Aldabbous L, Abdul-Salam V, McKinnon T, Duluc L, Pepke-Zaba J, Southwood M, et al. Neutrophil extracellular traps promote angiogenesis: evidence from vascular pathology in pulmonary hypertension. *Arterioscler*

Thromb Vasc Biol. (2016) 36:2078–87. doi: 10.1161/ATVBAHA.116.307634
35. Borissoff JI, Joosen IA, Versteylen MO, Brill A, Fuchs TA, Savchenko AS, et al. Elevated levels of circulating DNA and chromatin are independently associated with severe coronary atherosclerosis and a prothrombotic state. *Arterioscler Thromb Vasc Biol.* (2013) 33:2032–40. doi: 10.1161/ATVBAHA.113.301627
36. Saffarzadeh M, Juenemann C, Queisser MA, Lochnit G, Barreto G, Galuska SP, et al. Neutrophil extracellular traps directly induce epithelial and endothelial cell death: a predominant role of histones. *PLoS ONE* (2012) 7:e32366. doi: 10.1371/journal.pone.0032366
37. Fuchs TA, Brill A, Duerschmied D, Schatzberg D, Monestier M, Myers DD Jr., et al. Extracellular DNA traps promote thrombosis. *Proc Natl Acad Sci USA.* (2010) 107:15880–5. doi: 10.1073/pnas.1005743107
38. Belorgey D, Bieth JG. DNA binds neutrophil elastase and mucus proteinase inhibitor and impairs their functional activity. *FEBS Lett.* (1995) 361:265–8.
39. Kolaczkowska E, Jenne CN, Surewaard BG, Thanabalasuriar A, Lee WY, Sanz MJ, et al. Molecular mechanisms of NET formation and degradation revealed by intravital imaging in the liver vasculature. *Nat Commun.* (2015) 6:6673. doi: 10.1038/ncomms7673
40. Rabinovitch M, Bothwell T, Hayakawa BN, Williams WG, Trusler GA, Rowe RD, et al. Pulmonary artery endothelial abnormalities in patients with congenital heart defects and pulmonary hypertension. A correlation of light with scanning electron microscopy and transmission electron microscopy. *Lab Invest.* (1986) 55:632–53.
41. Zhu L, Wigle D, Hinek A, Kobayashi J, Ye C, Zuker M, et al. The endogenous vascular elastase that governs development and progression of monocrotaline-induced pulmonary hypertension in rats is a novel enzyme related to the serine proteinase adipsin. *J Clin Invest.* (1994) 94:1163–71. doi: 10.1172/JCI117432
42. Nickel NP, Spiekerkoetter E, Gu M, Li CG, Li H, Kaschwich M, et al. Elafin reverses pulmonary hypertension via caveolin-1-dependent bone morphogenetic protein signaling. *Am J Respir Crit Care Med.* (2015) 191:1273–86. doi: 10.1164/rccm.201412-2291OC
43. Lee KM, Tsai KY, Wang N, Ingber DE. Extracellular matrix and pulmonary hypertension: control of vascular smooth muscle cell contractility. *Am J Physiol.* (1998) 274(1 Pt 2):H76–82.
44. Tsukamoto Y, Helsel WE, Wahl SM. Macrophage production of fibronectin, a chemoattractant for fibroblasts. *J Immunol.* (1981) 127:673–8.
45. Thompson K, Rabinovitch M. Exogenous leukocyte and endogenous elastases can mediate mitogenic activity in pulmonary artery smooth muscle cells by release of extracellular-matrix bound basic fibroblast growth factor. *J Cell Physiol.* (1996) 166:495–505. doi: 10.1002/(SICI)1097-4652(199603)166:3<495::AID-JCP4>3.0.CO;2-K
46. Tu L, Dewachter L, Gore B, Fadel E, Dartevelle P, Simonneau G, et al. Autocrine fibroblast growth factor-2 signaling contributes to altered endothelial phenotype in pulmonary hypertension. *Am J Respir Cell Mol Biol.* (2011) 45:311–22. doi: 10.1165/rcmb.2010-0317OC
47. Chen PY, Qin L, Li G, Tellides G, Simons M. Fibroblast growth factor (FGF) signaling regulates transforming growth factor beta (TGFbeta)-dependent smooth muscle cell phenotype modulation. *Sci Rep.* (2016) 6:33407. doi: 10.1038/srep33407
48. Jones PL, Cowan KN, Rabinovitch M. Tenascin-C, proliferation and subendothelial fibronectin in progressive pulmonary vascular disease. *Am J Pathol.* (1997) 150:1349–60.
49. Cowan KN, Jones PL, Rabinovitch M. Elastase and matrix metalloproteinase inhibitors induce regression, and tenascin-C antisense prevents progression, of vascular disease. *J Clin Invest.* (2000) 105:21–34. doi: 10.1172/JCI6539
50. Alfaidi M, Wilson H, Daigneault M, Burnett A, Ridger V, Chamberlain J, et al. Neutrophil elastase promotes interleukin-1beta secretion from human coronary endothelium. *J Biol Chem.* (2015) 290:24067–78. doi: 10.1074/jbc.M115.659029
51. Prince LR, Allen L, Jones EC, Hellewell PG, Dower SK, Whyte MK, et al. The role of interleukin-1beta in direct and toll-like receptor 4-mediated neutrophil activation and survival. *Am J Pathol.* (2004) 165:1819–26. doi: 10.1016/S0002-9440(10)63437-2
52. Valenzuela-Fernandez A, Planchenault T, Baleux F, Staropoli I, Le-Barillec K, Leduc D, et al. Leukocyte elastase negatively regulates Stromal cell-derived factor-1 (SDF-1)/CXCR4 binding and functions by amino-terminal processing of SDF-1 and CXCR4. *J Biol Chem.* (2002) 277:15677–89. doi: 10.1074/jbc.M111388200
53. Eash KJ, Greenbaum AM, Gopalan PK, Link DC. CXCR2 and CXCR4 antagonistically regulate neutrophil trafficking from murine bone marrow. *J Clin Invest.* (2010) 120:2423–31. doi: 10.1172/JCI41649
54. Martin C, Burdon PC, Bridger G, Gutierrez-Ramos JC, Williams TJ, Rankin SM. Chemokines acting via CXCR2 and CXCR4 control the release of neutrophils from the bone marrow and their return following senescence. *Immunity* (2003) 19:583–93. doi: 10.1016/S1074-7613(03)00263-2
55. Scuderi P, Nez PA, Duerr ML, Wong BJ, Valdez CM. Cathepsin-G and leukocyte elastase inactivate human tumor necrosis factor and lymphotoxin. *Cell Immunol.* (1991) 135:299–313.
56. Bank U, Kupper B, Reinhold D, Hoffmann T, Ansorge S. Evidence for a crucial role of neutrophil-derived serine proteases in the inactivation of interleukin-6 at sites of inflammation. *FEBS Lett.* (1999) 461:235–40.
57. Sanchez O, Marcos E, Perros F, Fadel E, Tu L, Humbert M, et al. Role of endothelium-derived CC chemokine ligand 2 in idiopathic pulmonary arterial hypertension. *Am J Respir Crit Care Med.* (2007) 176:1041–7. doi: 10.1164/rccm.200610-1559OC
58. Cracowski JL, Chabot F, Labarere J, Faure P, Degano B, Schwebel C, et al. Proinflammatory cytokine levels are linked to death in pulmonary arterial hypertension. *Eur Respir J.* (2014) 43:915–7. doi: 10.1183/09031936.00151313
59. Humbert M, Monti G, Brenot F, Sitbon O, Portier A, Grangeot-Keros L, et al. Increased interleukin-1 and interleukin-6 serum concentrations in severe primary pulmonary hypertension. *Am J Respir Crit Care Med.* (1995) 151:1628–31. doi: 10.1164/ajrccm.151.5.7735624
60. Heresi GA, Aytekin M, Hammel JP, Wang S, Chatterjee S, Dweik RA. Plasma interleukin-6 adds prognostic information in pulmonary arterial hypertension. *Eur Respir J.* (2014) 43:912–4. doi: 10.1183/09031936.00164713
61. Jonigk D, Golpon H, Bockmeyer CL, Maegel L, Hoeper MM, Gottlieb J, et al. Plexiform lesions in pulmonary arterial hypertension composition, architecture, and microenvironment. *Am J Pathol.* (2011) 179:167–79. doi: 10.1016/j.ajpath.2011.03.040
62. Schermuly RT, Yilmaz H, Ghofrani HA, Woyda K, Pullamsetti S, Schulz A, et al. Inhaled iloprost reverses vascular remodeling in chronic experimental pulmonary hypertension. *Am J Respir Crit Care Med.* (2005) 172:358–63. doi: 10.1164/rccm.200502-296OC
63. George J, D'Armiento J. Transgenic expression of human matrix metalloproteinase-9 augments monocrotaline-induced pulmonary arterial hypertension in mice. *J Hypertens.* (2011) 29:299–308. doi: 10.1097/HJH.0b013e328340a0e4
64. Chelladurai P, Seeger W, Pullamsetti SS. Matrix metalloproteinases and their inhibitors in pulmonary hypertension. *Eur Respir J.* (2012) 40:766–82. doi: 10.1183/09031936.00209911
65. Ormiston ML, Chang C, Long LL, Soon E, Jones D, Machado R, et al. Impaired natural killer cell phenotype and function in idiopathic and heritable pulmonary arterial hypertension. *Circulation* (2012) 126:1099–109. doi: 10.1161/CIRCULATIONAHA.112.110619
66. Goetzl EJ, Banda MJ, Leppert D. Matrix metalloproteinases in immunity. *J Immunol.* (1996) 156:1–4.
67. Heath D, Yacoub M. Lung mast cells in plexogenic pulmonary arteriopathy. *J Clin Pathol.* (1991) 44:1003–6.
68. Farha S, Sharp J, Asosingh K, Park M, Comhair SA, Tang WH, et al. Mast cell number, phenotype, and function in human pulmonary arterial hypertension. *Pulm Circ.* (2012) 2:220–8. doi: 10.4103/2045-8932.97609
69. Kosanovic D, Dahal BK, Peters DM, Seimetz M, Wygrecka M, Hoffmann K, et al. Histological characterization of mast cell chymase in patients with pulmonary hypertension and chronic obstructive pulmonary disease. *Pulm Circ.* (2014) 4:128–36. doi: 10.1086/675642
70. Carter RI, Mumford RA, Treonze KM, Finke PE, Davies P, Si Q, et al. The fibrinogen cleavage product Aalpha-Val360, a specific marker of neutrophil elastase activity *in vivo*. *Thorax* (2011) 66:686–91. doi: 10.1136/thx.2010.154690
71. Russell D, Genschmer KR, Szul T, Noerager B, Xu X, Viera L, et al. Neutrophil-derived exosomes purified from COPD patient bronchoalveolar fluid cause a COPD like phenotype in a mouse model via a neutrophil elastase dependent mechanism. *Am J Respir Crit Care Med.* (2018) 197:A2701-A. doi: 10.1164/ajrccm-conference.2018.197.1_MeetingAbstracts.A2701.
72. Deng Z, Morse JH, Slager SL, Cuervo N, Moore KJ, Venetos G, et al. Familial primary pulmonary hypertension (gene PPH1) is caused by mutations in the bone morphogenetic protein receptor-II gene. *Am J Hum Genet.* (2000) 67:737–44. doi: 10.1086/303059

73. Atkinson C, Stewart S, Upton PD, Machado R, Thomson JR, Trembath RC, et al. Primary pulmonary hypertension is associated with reduced pulmonary vascular expression of type II bone morphogenetic protein receptor. *Circulation* (2002) 105:1672–8. doi: 10.1161/01.Cir.0000012754.72951.3d
74. Cogan JD, Pauciulo MW, Batchman AP, Prince MA, Robbins IM, Hedges LK, et al. High frequency of BMPR2 exonic deletions/duplications in familial pulmonary arterial hypertension. *Am J Respir Crit Care Med.* (2006) 174:590–8. doi: 10.1164/rccm.200602-165OC
75. Hamid R, Cogan JD, Hedges LK, Austin E, Phillips JA, 3rd, Newman JH, et al. Penetrance of pulmonary arterial hypertension is modulated by the expression of normal BMPR2 allele. *Hum Mutat.* (2009) 30:649–54. doi: 10.1002/humu.20922
76. Morrell NW, Yang X, Upton PD, Jourdan KB, Morgan N, Sheares KK, et al. Altered growth responses of pulmonary artery smooth muscle cells from patients with primary pulmonary hypertension to transforming growth factor-beta(1) and bone morphogenetic proteins. *Circulation* (2001) 104:790–5. doi: 10.1161/hc3201.094152
77. Teichert-Kuliszewska K, Kutryk MJ, Kuliszewski MA, Karoubi G, Courtman DW, Zucco L, et al. Bone morphogenetic protein receptor-2 signaling promotes pulmonary arterial endothelial cell survival: implications for loss-of-function mutations in the pathogenesis of pulmonary hypertension. *Circ Res.* (2006) 98:209–17. doi: 10.1161/01.RES.0000200180.01710.e6
78. Burton VJ, Ciuclan LI, Holmes AM, Rodman DM, Walker C, Budd DC. Bone morphogenetic protein receptor II regulates pulmonary artery endothelial cell barrier function. *Blood* (2011) 117:333–41. doi: 10.1182/blood-2010-05-285973
79. Steiner MK, Syrkina OL, Kolliputi N, Mark EJ, Hales CA, Waxman AB. Interleukin-6 overexpression induces pulmonary hypertension. *Circ Res.* (2009) 104:236–44. doi: 10.1161/CIRCRESAHA.108.182014
80. Li W, Hoenderdos K, Salmon RM, Upton PD, Condliffe AM, Chilvers ER, et al. Neutrophil and redox dependent proteolysis of bone morphogenetic protein 9: potential role in the pathogenesis of pulmonary arterial hypertension. *Thorax* (2013) 68:A146-A. doi: 10.1136/thoraxjnl-2013-204457.307
81. David L, Mallet C, Keramidas M, Lamande N, Gasc JM, Dupuis-Girod S, et al. Bone morphogenetic protein-9 is a circulating vascular quiescence factor. *Circ Res.* (2008) 102:914–22. doi: 10.1161/CIRCRESAHA.107.165530
82. Long L, Ormiston ML, Yang X, Southwood M, Graf S, Machado RD, et al. Selective enhancement of endothelial BMPR-II with BMP9 reverses pulmonary arterial hypertension. *Nat Med.* (2015) 21:777–85. doi: 10.1038/nm.3877
83. Appleby SL, Mitrofan CG, Crosby A, Hoenderdos K, Lodge K, Upton PD, et al. Bone morphogenetic protein 9 enhances lipopolysaccharide-induced leukocyte recruitment to the vascular endothelium. *J Immunol.* (2016) 197:3302–14. doi: 10.4049/jimmunol.16 01219
84. Alastalo TP, Li M, Perez Vde J, Pham D, Sawada H, Wang JK, et al. Disruption of PPARgamma/beta-catenin-mediated regulation of apelin impairs BMP-induced mouse and human pulmonary arterial EC survival. *J Clin Invest.* (2011) 121:3735–46. doi: 10.1172/JCI43382
85. Tojais NF, Cao A, Lai YJ, Wang L, Chen PI, Alcazar MAA, et al. Codependence of bone morphogenetic protein receptor 2 and transforming growth factor-beta in elastic fiber assembly and its perturbation in pulmonary arterial hypertension. *Arterioscler Thromb Vasc Biol.* (2017) 37:1559–69. doi: 10.1161/ATVBAHA.117.309696

21

Inflammation in Right Ventricular Failure: Does it Matter?

Laurence Dewachter[1]* and *Céline Dewachter*[1,2]

[1] Laboratory of Physiology and Pharmacology, Faculty of Medicine, Université Libre de Bruxelles, Brussels, Belgium,
[2] Department of Cardiology, Erasmus Academic Hospital, Brussels, Belgium

Correspondence:
Laurence Dewachter
ldewacht@ulb.ac.be

Right ventricular (RV) failure is a common consequence of acute and chronic RV overload of pressure, such as after pulmonary embolism and pulmonary hypertension. It has been recently realized that symptomatology and survival of patients with pulmonary hypertension are essentially determined by RV function adaptation to increased afterload. Therefore, improvement of RV function and reversal of RV failure are treatment goals. Currently, the pathophysiology and the pathobiology underlying RV failure remain largely unknown. A better understanding of the pathophysiological processes involved in RV failure is needed, as there is no proven treatment for this disease at the moment. The present review aims to summarize the current understanding of the pathogenesis of RV failure, focusing on inflammation. We attempt to formally emphasize the importance of inflammation and associated representative inflammatory molecules and cells in the *primum movens* and development of RV failure in humans and in experimental models. We present inflammatory biomarkers and immune mediators involved in RV failure. We focus on inflammatory mediators and cells which seem to correlate with the deterioration of RV function and also explain how all these inflammatory mediators and cells might impact RV function adaptation to increased afterload. Finally, we also discuss the evidence on potential beneficial effects of targeted anti-inflammatory agents in the setting of acute and chronic RV failure.

Keywords: right ventricular failure, coupling, pulmonary hypertension, inflammation, cytokines, chemokines, immune cells

INTRODUCTION

Although the initial insult involves the pulmonary circulation, it has been better realized recently that symptomatology and poor clinical outcome in patients with pulmonary arterial hypertension (PAH), are essentially determined by the adaptation of right ventricular (RV) function to increased afterload (Galiè et al., 2010; Vonk-Noordegraaf et al., 2013; Vonk Noordegraaf et al., 2017; Friedberg and Redington, 2014), showing the importance to consider the coupling of the RV to the pulmonary circulation, as a sole functional unit (Naeije et al., 2014). Similarly, after pulmonary embolism, mortality and morbidity increase dramatically in patients, in presence of RV dysfunction (Kasper et al., 1997; Ribeiro et al., 1997; Kreit, 2004; Schoepf et al., 2004). We know that the RV initially adapts to an increase in afterload observed in pulmonary hypertension (PH) by an increased contractility with preserved dimensions and stroke volume (called Anrep's homeometric adaptation). This systolic function adaptation eventually fails, resulting in increased RV dimensions (called Starling's heterometric adaptation) and decreased stroke volume (Galiè et al., 2010; Vonk-Noordegraaf et al., 2013; Vonk Noordegraaf et al., 2017; Friedberg and Redington, 2014). Cellular and molecular mechanisms underlying the development of RV dysfunction (from adaptive to maladaptive processes) remains insufficiently understood (**Figure 1**). Moreover, specific pharmacologic therapy that can reverse RV failure is not yet available and the effects on RV function of available PAH therapies remain largely elusive.

In recent years, activation of inflammatory processes has been identified as one of the major pathogenic components of pulmonary vascular remodeling, contributing to the development of various forms of pulmonary PH (Humbert et al., 2004; Rabinovitch, 2012; Voelkel et al., 2016). Additionally, circulating levels of inflammatory mediators, such as interleukin (IL)-6, IL-1β, tumor necrosis factor (TNF)-α, and monocyte chemoattractant protein (MCP)-1, have been shown to be elevated in PAH and correlated to the severity of the disease (Humbert et al., 1995; Dolenc et al., 2014). However, the role of inflammation in the transition from RV adaptation to RV failure is still poorly understood.

Described in many different cardiovascular diseases (other than PAH) (Mann, 2002; Frangogiannis, 2014), myocardial inflammation has progressively emerged as a pathophysiologic process contributing to cardiac hypertrophy, fibrosis and dysfunction in heart failure (Frieler and Mortensen, 2015; Mann, 2015). In patients with idiopathic PAH (Overbeek et al., 2008; Condliffe et al., 2009) or selected forms of congenital heart diseases, such as Eisenmenger syndrome (Kuhn et al., 2003), RV failure is less prevalent and occurs later compared to patients with PAH associated to inflammatory diseases such as systemic sclerosis (Kawut et al., 2003; Kuhn et al., 2003; Overbeek et al., 2008; Condliffe et al., 2009). In these patients, RV inflammatory infiltrates were denser than in patients with idiopathic PAH, while interstitial fibrosis was similarly present in all the RV (Overbeek et al., 2010). This strongly suggests that RV failure is predominant in patients with PH presenting an inflammatory background. However, the implication of inflammation to RV dysfunction is suspected in all forms of PH, including both chronic and acute increase in RV afterload (Iwadate et al., 2003; Begieneman et al., 2008; Overbeek et al., 2010). In experimental models of RV failure, myocardial inflammation has also been described, with increased infiltration of inflammatory cells and expression of various cytokines and chemokines (Campian et al., 2010; Rondelet et al., 2012). We also know that, in the heart, inflammatory processes are inextricably linked to cell death, oxidative stress, altered cell metabolism and extracellular matrix remodeling, which all have been incriminated in the pathogenesis of RV failure (**Figures 1, 2**; Bogaard et al., 2009a).

In the present review article, we propose an overview of the multiple players involved in the complex inflammatory response to acute or chronic increased afterload and its contribution to subsequent (mal)adaptive remodeling of the RV leading to RV dysfunction, regarding what's already known in the left ventricle (LV) and in heart failure in general.

INFLAMMATION AND RV FAILURE

Inflammation is an essential biological stimulation-response system provided by the immune system to ensure the survival after noxious stimuli, such as infection or tissue injury. Inflammatory responses may, therefore, be considered as a classic homeostatic system, functioning to maintain normal organ function. In the heart, activation of inflammatory processes induced by sterile stressors is largely similar to that observed during infection, including the release of vasoactive peptides, the expression of adhesion molecules [e.g., vascular cell adhesion molecule (VCAM)-1, intercellular adhesion molecule (ICAM)-1] in cardiac cells (e.g., cardiomyocytes, fibroblasts, endothelial cells) that promote myocardial recruitment of inflammatory cells (e.g., neutrophils, macrophages, lymphocytes), the release of inflammatory cytokines and chemokines, and the activation of T cell-mediated adaptive immune responses (Chen and Nuñez, 2010; Frieler and Mortensen, 2015; Mann, 2015; Prabhu and Frangogiannis, 2016). This initial response to harmful stimuli represent *acute inflammation*, which probably evolves as an adaptive response to restore tissue homeostasis and function.

However, when this harmful inflammatory trigger persists, it can cause dramatic tissue damage eventually leading to cardiac loss of function (Libby, 2007). This prolonged dysregulated and maladaptive response of the body is *chronic inflammation*, which involves myocardial inflammation, tissue destruction and attempts to repair tissue damages, leading to altered myocardial function.

Accumulating evidence suggests that all cardiac cell types could participate to this inflammatory response by their own and therefore playing a central vicious role in the maintenance of these maladaptive processes associated to chronic inflammation (Van Linthout et al., 2014), leading to heart failure. RV activation of inflammatory processes is associated with and contributes to RV adverse remodeling and dysfunction (Campian et al., 2010; Rondelet et al., 2012; Dewachter et al., 2015). In RV failure, an elevated expression of cytokines and chemokines modulate various intracellular signaling pathways in cardiac cells, leading to cardiomyocyte hypertrophy and death, mitochondrial dysfunction, endoplasmic reticulum stress, and cardiac fibrosis characterized by fibroblast proliferation and differentiation and collagen deposition (**Figure 3**; Frieler and Mortensen, 2015; Mann, 2015; Prabhu and Frangogiannis, 2016). In addition, these inflammatory mediators also alter myocardial metabolic processes and cardiomyocyte contractile properties.

MEDIATORS AND EFFECTORS OF INFLAMMATION—CYTOKINES AND CHEMOKINES

Cytokines play a crucial role in inflammatory response to acute myocardial injury, mediating the recruitment of inflammatory and immune cells into the injured area (Seta et al., 1996) and exerting direct detrimental effects on the heart (Seta et al., 1996). Released directly by the heart itself (Shimano et al., 2012), cytokines can also be produced by cardiomyocytes

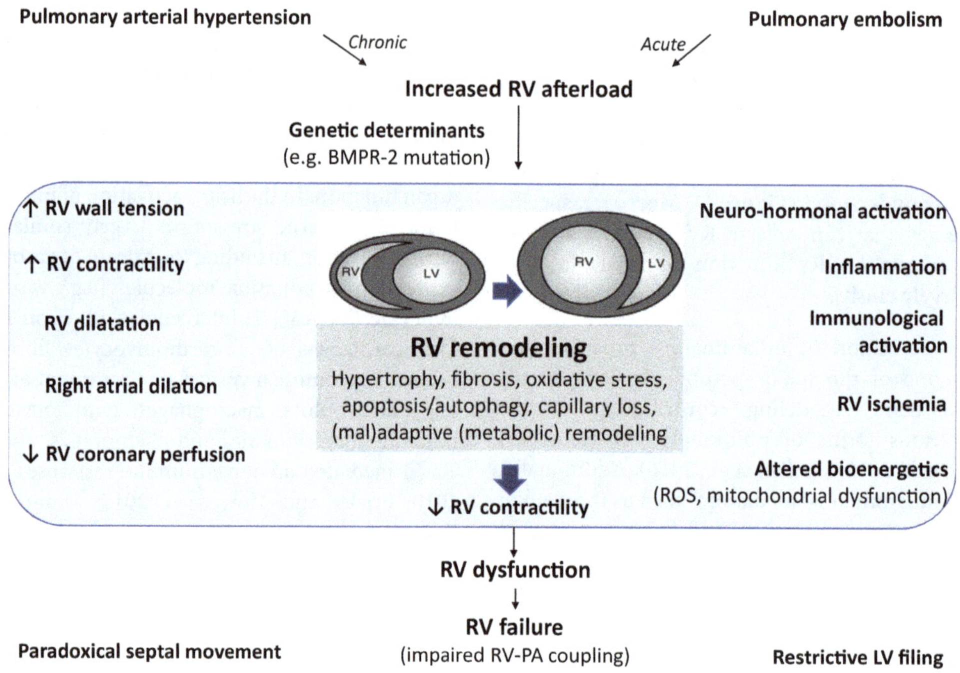

FIGURE 1 | Pathophysiology of right ventricular (RV) failure implicating activation of inflammatory and immune processes. Pulmonary arterial hypertension (as well as acute pulmonary embolism) induces an increased afterload for the RV resulting in RV remodeling. The structural and functional changes during the development of RV failure can be characterized clinically, as summarized on the left hand. RV dysfunction is also probably due the activation of other pathophysiological mechanisms (summarized on the right hand) leading to multiple cellular changes, such as oxidative stress, apoptosis, inflammation, fibrosis, and metabolic remodeling. These factors also contribute to RV dysfunction and subsequent RV failure (characterized by altered coupling between the RV and the pulmonary circulation). The cellular changes are either the result of chronic RV pressure overload or the effect of circulating factors released from the sick lung circulation. RV, right ventricle; BMPR-2, bone morphogenetic protein type 2 receptor; ROS, reactive oxygen species; PA, pulmonary artery; LV, left ventricle.

(Kapadia et al., 1995), cardiac endothelial cells (Liu et al., 2014) and fibroblasts, resident macrophages (Pinto et al., 2016) and infiltrated inflammatory cells, as well as by extra-cardiac tissues (e.g., adipose tissue). In PAH patients, increased levels of circulating pro-inflammatory cytokines (e.g., IL-1β, TNF-α) have been correlated to the severity of the disease (Humbert et al., 1995; Dolenc et al., 2014), which also reinforces the vicious circle between inflammation and RV failure.

IL-1 Signaling Pathway

In persistent RV failure induced by acute pulmonary artery banding, IL-1β was overexpressed in the RV, mainly in the vessels and myocardial infiltrating cells, rather than in cardiac cells themselves (Dewachter et al., 2015). This was associated with decreased expression of IL-33, a cardio-protective cytokine of the IL-1 family, and of ST2, a soluble decoy receptor regulating negatively the IL-1/IL-33 signaling (Dewachter et al., 2015). Overexpression of IL-1α and−1β was also reported in experimental RV failure on chronic systemic-to-pulmonary shunting in pigs (Rondelet et al., 2012), while IL-33 expression did not change (Belhaj et al., 2013). Pro-inflammatory cytokines (such as IL-1β and TNF-α) act as acute-phase mediators after tissue injury. In the heart, they mediate negative inotropic effects and promote myocardial hypertrophy and cell death (Bujak and Frangogiannis, 2009). Mechanistically, IL-1β-induced negative inotropic effects were mediated by inducible nitric oxide (NO)-synthase activation and peroxynitrite production, which can interfere with the excitation-contraction coupling, leading to a rapid and reversible contractile dysfunction (Finkel et al., 1992; Van Tassell et al., 2013). In addition, it was demonstrated that IL-1β (as well as IL-6) were able to reduce the expression of sarco/endoplasmic reticulum calcium (Ca^{2+})-ATPase in cardiomyocytes (Thaik et al., 1995), suggesting abnormalities of Ca^{2+} handling underlying these negative inotropic effects. IL-1β promotes cardiac hypertrophy through insulin-like growth factor-1 release from cardiac fibroblasts, via a paracrine mechanism involving signal transducer and activator of transcription3 (STAT3) activation (Honsho et al., 2009). In cardiomyocytes, IL-1β-induced apoptosis was reported to be mediated by the activation of inducible NO-synthase and the upregulation of Bcl2 homologous antagonist/killer (Bak) and B-cell lymphoma-extra-large (Bcl-XL) (Ing et al., 1999). In addition, IL-1β directly induced cardiomyocyte growth in a NO-independent manner (Thaik et al., 1995). On the other hand, IL-1β also contributed to fibrotic processes, stimulating the release of matrix metalloproteinases in cardiac fibroblasts, through the inhibition of the endoglin signaling and the activation of the bone morphogenetic protein (BMP) pathway (Saxena et al., 2013). IL-1β, has also been shown to impair cardiac energy

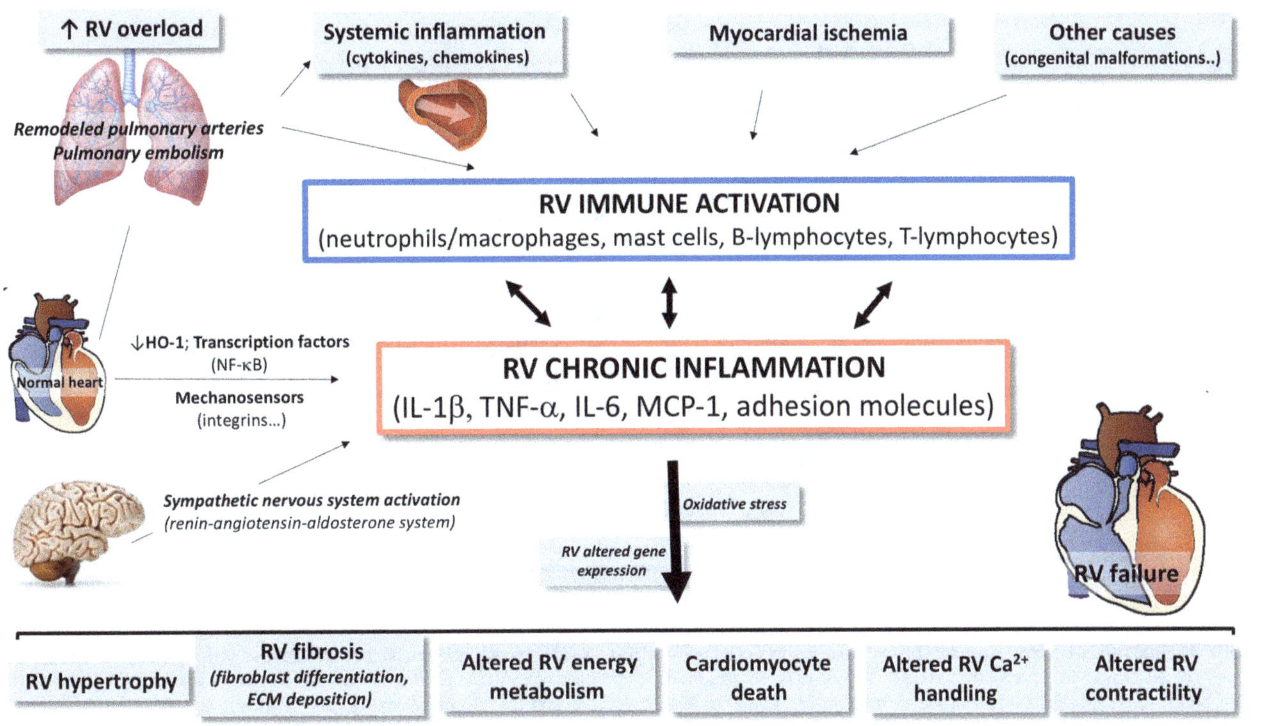

FIGURE 2 | Schematic overview of the contribution of immune and inflammatory mediators and cells in the pathogenesis of right ventricular (RV) dysfunction/failure. In presence of pulmonary arterial hypertension or pulmonary embolism, circulating inflammatory mediators originating from the pulmonary vasculature may trigger or contribute to local activation of inflammatory processes in the RV. Inflammation in the RV is characterized by activation of immune processes, implying expansion and activation of different cell types and by up-regulation of cytokines, chemokines, and cell adhesion molecules contributing to chronic inflammatory status. Through this upregulation of immune and inflammatory processes, mediators contribute to the development of RV failure. RV, right ventricle; HO-1, heme oxygenase-1; NF-κB, nuclear factor kappa B; IL, interleukin; TNF, tumor necrosis factor; MCP, monocyte chemoattractant protein; ECM, extracellular matrix.

metabolism, increasing myocardial oxygen demand adding to the detrimental effects of myocardial contractile performance in a context of oxygen supply limitation (Hofmann et al., 2007). Therefore, upregulation of IL-1β could contribute to the pathogenesis of RV failure by decreasing RV contractility, inducing cardiomyocyte death and altered supply in metabolic energy.

TNF-α Signaling Pathway

RV failure induced by transient pulmonary artery banding was associated with a RV increase in TNF-α expression, whereas circulating serum levels of TNF-α remained undetectable after pulmonary artery banding (Dewachter et al., 2010), suggesting local early expression of this pro-inflammatory cytokine in this experimental model. A local increased expression of TNF-α was also observed in experimental brain death-induced RV dysfunction (Belhaj et al., 2016) and tightly correlated to the prediction to develop RV failure early after heart transplantation (Birks et al., 2000). Expression of TNF-α was increased in the failing RV after 6-month systemic-to-pulmonary shunting in pigs, together with increased circulating serum TNF-α levels (Rondelet et al., 2012). Early activation of inflammatory processes, characterized by an increase in TNF-α and myeloperoxidase expression, was also observed in RV dysfunction in rats developing severe PH induced by monocrotaline injection (Campian et al., 2010). In patients with advanced heart failure, myocardial expression of TNF-α was abundantly increased (Torre-Amione et al., 1996), probably contributing to maladaptive mechanisms implicated in the development of cardiac hypertrophy and dysfunction (Frieler and Mortensen, 2015; Mann, 2015; Prabhu and Frangogiannis, 2016). In these patients, high circulating TNF-α levels were tightly correlated to myocardial fibrosis, inflammation, as well as ventricular dilatation and mortality (Kubota et al., 2000b). This is consistent with experimental data showing that TNF-α contributes to substantial cardiac remodeling. In cardiomyocytes, TNF-α induced the activation of apoptosis (Chandrasekar et al., 2004), through the activation of nuclear factor-κB (NF-κB) signaling (Glezeva and Baugh, 2014). TNF-α induced cardiomyocyte hypertrophy, through mechanisms dependent on the interaction between cell integrin and the extracellular matrix (Yokoyama et al., 1997) and the activation of AKT/NF-κB and JNK pathways (Higuchi et al., 2006). In cardiac fibroblasts, TNF-α induced proliferation and collagen production through the suppression of miR-29 (Venkatachalam et al., 2009). Experimentally, TNF-α has been shown to contribute to systolic and diastolic dysfunction (Kubota et al., 2000a; Dibbs et al., 2003) and increased arrhythmogenesis (Lee et al., 2007). In mice,

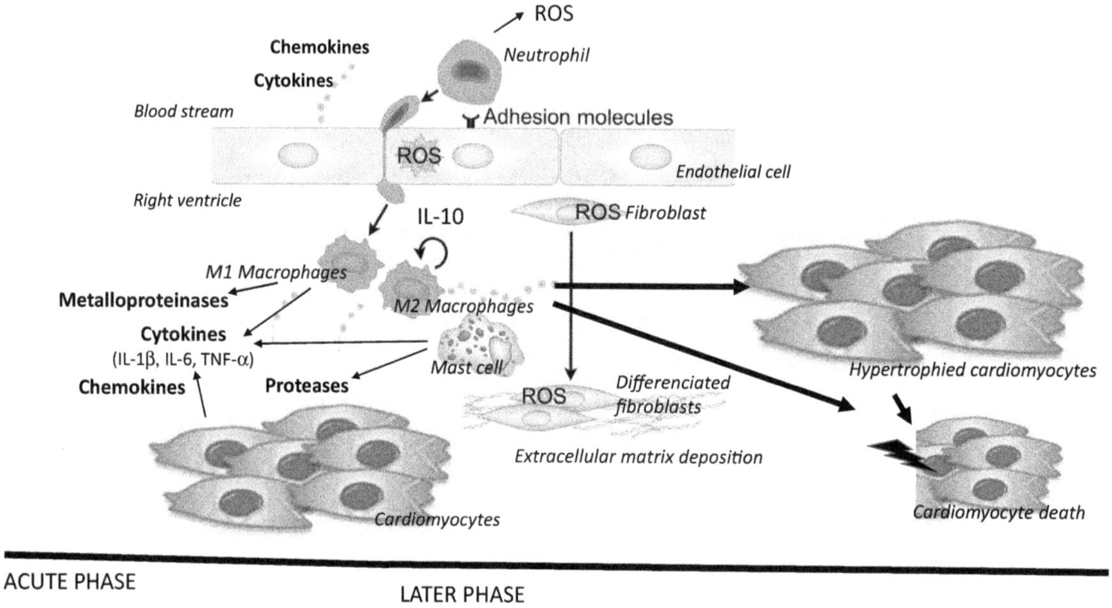

FIGURE 3 | Hypothetical schematic cellular and molecular insights of immune cells and inflammatory mediators on the pathogenesis of right ventricular failure, more precisely on cardiomyocyte hypertrophy and death, as well as on fibrosis. Immune and inflammatory cells are myocardial resident cells or are coming from the blood stream, adhere to endothelial cells and invade the myocardium. Cytokines (e.g., IL-1β, IL-6, and TNF-α), chemokines (e.g., MCP-1), and enzymes (e.g., metalloproteinases and proteases, such as chymase) released by these cells promote cardiomyocyte hypertrophy, fibroblast differentiation/activation, deposition of extracellular matrix and cardiomyocyte apoptosis. Acute-phase inflammatory and immune mediators are represented in red, while late-phase mediators after myocardial injury are represent in blue. ROS, reactive oxygen species; IL, interleukin; TNF, tumor necrosis factor.

cardiomyocyte-specific overexpression of TNF-α induced dilated cardiomyopathy characterized by ventricular hypertrophy and dilatation, myocardial infiltration of inflammatory cells, fibrosis and cardiomyocyte apoptosis, together with reduced ejection fraction (Kubota et al., 1997). In contrast, TNF-α-deficient mice subjected to pressure overload were protected against cardiac hypertrophy, fibrosis and dysfunction (Sun et al., 2007). Interestingly, TNF-α (as well as IL-1β) downregulated the expression of Ca^{2+}-regulating genes, including sarcoplasmic reticulum Ca^{2+} ATPase (Wu et al., 2011) and Ca^{2+}-release channels (Thaik et al., 1995), responsible for direct negative inotropic effects (Yokoyama et al., 1993; Duncan et al., 2007). This shows the contribution of inflammation in Ca^{2+} imbalance and cardiac remodeling, leading to a vicious circle observed in heart failure (Tschöpe and Lam, 2012). Moreover, TNF-α also altered the activity of β-adrenergic receptors, leading to the uncoupling of these receptors from the adenylyl cyclase (Gulick et al., 1989; Chung et al., 1990). In RV failure, TNF-α could, therefore, contribute to altered RV contractility and remodeling, through a Ca^{2+} imbalance responsible for ventriculo-arterial uncoupling. Moreover, it has been suggested that estrogen could alter inflammatory cell-induced synthesis of TNF-α, preventing the induction of cardiac fibroblasts that leads to adverse remodeling of the extracellular matrix (McLarty et al., 2013). This could, at least partly, explain why estrogen contributes to RV function improvement in different experimental models of PH (Frump et al., 2015; Liu et al., 2017).

IL-6 Signaling Pathway

In experimental RV failure, increased expression of IL-6 in the RV was inversely correlated to RV adaptation to increased afterload [assessed by the ratio between the pulmonary arterial elastance (Ea) and the end-systolic elastance (Ees)], while RV expressions of binding- (IL-6R) and signal transducing (gp130)-subunits of the IL-6 receptor remained unchanged (Dewachter et al., 2015). This is well-known that IL-1 and TNF-α are able to induce IL-6 release in different cell types (Zhang et al., 1990), which suggests that IL-6 has direct negative inotropic effects (Yu et al., 2005), but can also potentate these of IL-1 and TNF-α (Maass et al., 2002). Therefore, increased RV expression in IL-6, IL-1β, and TNF-α could contribute to the amplified activation of inflammatory processes in the setting of RV failure. Circulating IL-6 levels were increased in RV failure on acutely increased afterload (Dewachter et al., 2015), which also probably contributes to the perpetuation of the inflammatory state and to the acceleration of the progression of global heart failure (as already described in the setting of LV failure). High circulating levels of CRP and IL-6 were independently associated to increased RV mass and volume (Harhay et al., 2013). High circulating levels of IL-6 have been reported in patients with severe PAH (Humbert et al., 1995), predicting negatively their survival and outcome (Soon et al., 2010). In contrast, RV expression of IL-6 did not change in RV failure induced by 6-month systemic-to-pulmonary shunting in pigs (Rondelet et al., 2012). Therefore, IL-6 could play a role in the transition from acute to chronic inflammation in RV failure. Moreover, IL-6 has also been incriminated in the pathogenesis of cardiac hypertrophy and dysfunction (Frieler and Mortensen, 2015; Mann, 2015; Prabhu and Frangogiannis, 2016), through the activation of the Ca^{2+}/calmodulin-dependent protein kinase II and STAT3 pathways (Kunisada et al., 1996). Experimentally, infusion of IL-6 in rats was able to induce cardiac hypertrophy, inflammation, fibrosis and diastolic dysfunction (Meléndez et al., 2010), whereas IL-6 genetic deletion ameliorated angiotensin II- (Coles et al., 2007; Ma et al., 2012) and norepinephrine-induced cardiac hypertrophy and fibrosis (Meier et al., 2009). Downregulation of IL-6 expression reduced inflammation and reversed altered glucose metabolism induced by high fat diet in mice, through the inhibition of suppressor of cytokine signaling-3 signaling and the upregulation of insulin receptor substrate-1 signaling (Ko et al., 2009). This suggests that chronic inflammation may contribute to cardiac dysfunction through metabolic perturbations that can impair cardiac energetic production in response to metabolic stress. Overexpression of the signal transducer gp130 was shown to be sufficient to induce cardiomyocyte hypertrophy and to mediate IL-6 effects (Ancey et al., 2003), through the activation of STAT3 signaling (Kunisada et al., 1998) and the GRB2-associated-binding protein 1-Src homology 2 domain-containing phosphatase2 interaction (Nakaoka et al., 2003). Therefore, IL-6 could also be implicated in the development of RV remodeling in RV failure, but its precise role should be confirmed for the RV.

IL-10 Signaling Pathway

In RV failure on acutely increased afterload, the pro-inflammatory status (described above) is reinforced by the downregulation of anti-inflammatory cytokine IL-10 (Dewachter et al., 2015), leading to increased pro-inflammatory ratio of IL-6/IL-10 both in the RV and in the serum. Macrophages are the major source of IL-10, a cytokine that mediates its anti-inflammatory effects, through the inhibition of the synthesis of various inflammatory molecules such as interferon-γ, IL-1, IL-6, and TNF-α (Anker and von Haehling, 2004). Therefore, IL-10 is usually called a neutralizer of inflammation and a tissue protective cytokine. However, expression of IL-10 did not change in the failing RV in an experimental model of systemic-to pulmonary shunting in pigs (Rondelet et al., 2012), suggesting a role mainly in the acute phase of inflammation. The role of IL-10 in heart failure is not well established. In experimental myocardial infarction, myocardial IL-10 expression was decreased (Kaur et al., 2006). Circulating IL-10 levels were diminished in patients with heart failure (Stumpf et al., 2003), while it has been reported that elevated levels of IL-10 and TNF-α was associated with an increased risk of mortality (Amir et al., 2010). These data are conflicting. Nevertheless, IL-10 is considered as a cardio-protective cytokine and increased levels of IL-10 in heart failure may be seen as a compensatory mechanism to counter deleterious effects of cytokines, such as TNF-α or IL-6.

MCP-1 (Endothelium-Derived CC Chemokine Ligand 2; CCL-2) Signaling Pathway

Expressions of MCP-1 and its receptor CCR2 were increased in the failing RV in two experimental models of RV failure on acute increase in afterload (Watts et al., 2006; Dewachter et al., 2015). Increased expression of MCP-1 (as well as other chemokines) has been described in the pressure-overloaded RV following pulmonary artery banding and linked to altered expression of small leucine-rich proteoglycans by cardiac cells (e.g., fibroblasts), probably contributing to matrix remodeling (Waehre et al., 1985) and inflammation regulation (Iozzo and Schaefer, 2010; Moreth et al., 2010). Circulating levels of MCP-1 were increased in patients with PAH (Sanchez et al., 2007) and with heart failure (Kohno et al., 2008). However, the precise mechanistic role played by MCP-1 in heart failure remains elusive. We know that chemokines are, at least, able to promote myocardial infiltration and activation of leukocytes in the failing heart. Via its receptor CCR2, MCP-1 induced cardiomyocyte apoptosis, therefore contributing to ventricular dysfunction (Zhou et al., 2006). Interestingly, myocardial expression of MCP-1 increased during the early phases of myocardial infarction (Maekawa et al., 2004; Hayasaki et al., 2006) and inhibition of MCP-1 prevents ventricular remodeling after myocardial infarct (Hayashidani et al., 2003). Moreover, targeted deletion of MCP-1 in mice was shown to improve survival, attenuate LV dilatation and reduce contractile dysfunction after coronary occlusion (Hayashidani et al., 2003). In contrast, myocardial overexpression of MCP-1 was associated with altered contractile function associated with myocardial infiltration of leukocytes, mainly macrophages (Kolattukudy et al., 1998). Moreover, MCP-1 also induced the release of pro-inflammatory cytokines (Wrigley et al., 2011), such as IL-1β and IL-6, participating to a "cytokine cascade" leading to the amplification of inflammatory processes in RV failure.

CELLULAR REGULATORS OF INFLAMMATION

Heme Oxygenase (HO)-1

Expression of HO-1 was decreased in the failing RV following acute (Dewachter et al., 2015) and chronic increase in afterload (Belhaj et al., 2013), with a tight correlation between RV expression of HO-1 and RV-pulmonary artery coupling (assessed by the Ees/Ea ratio) (Belhaj et al., 2013; Dewachter et al., 2015), suggesting a functional role of HO-1 in maintaining RV systolic function. This stress-inducible enzyme plays crucial roles in the control of inflammation and cytoprotective processes (Otterbein et al., 1999). Indeed, HO-1 catalyzes heme degradation into carbon monoxide, biliverdin and iron (Tenhunen et al., 1968). Through the biological activities of its metabolite products, activation of HO-1 contributes to cell defense, through reduced oxidative stress and inhibition of the activation of inflammatory and apoptotic processes. Moreover, carbon monoxide is an effective vasodilator which is also able to inhibit platelet aggregation, reduce leucocyte adhesion, cellular apoptosis, and pro-inflammatory cytokine production. Therefore, a decrease in HO-1 expression may lead to an increase in pro-inflammatory cytokine expression (Constantin et al., 2012) in the failing RV. Moreover, there were inverse relations between HO-1 expression and RV neutrophil and macrophage infiltration, as well as with RV pro-apoptotic

Bax/Bcl-2 ratio (Dewachter et al., 2015), which strongly suggests a potential mechanistic link between downregulated HO-1 expression and inflammation and apoptosis in RV failure. In chronic hypoxia-exposed mice, administration of mesenchymal cells overexpressing HO-1 was associated with reduced RV hypertrophy, limited infarcted zones and decreased RV systolic pressure to normal values (Liang et al., 2011). In contrast, in the same experimental PH model, downregulation of HO-1 was shown to induce severe RV dilatation and dysfunction, together with cardiac inflammation, fibrosis, and apoptosis (Yet et al., 1999). However, expression of HO-1 was respectively increased and decreased in the RV of experimental models of RV pressure overload (Katayose et al., 1993) and RV failure (Bogaard et al., 2009b). This suggests variable HO-1 expression depending on the stress-induced cardiomyocyte damage and the progression of RV failure. In RV failure, we could speculate that downregulated HO-1 expression could impair its physiological implication in the control of inflammation activation in RV failure. However further studies are necessary to confirm that.

NF-κB

In an inflammatory experimental model of PH, cardiac specific inhibition of the major inflammatory transcription factor NF-κB, prevented RV hypertrophy and remodeling, despite the presence of PH, mainly through the restored expression of BMP signaling members, and the reduced inflammatory phenotype (including reduced expression of IL-6 and cell adhesion molecules) (Kumar et al., 2012). Activation of NF-κB signaling also plays regulates cardiomyocyte hypertrophy, promoting cardiomyocyte growth and expression of fetal sarcomeric genes, whereas its inhibition reduces cardiac growth *in vivo* (Kawano et al., 2005; Zelarayan et al., 2009; Liu et al., 2012). Mechanistically, the cross-talk between NF-κB and nuclear factor of activated T-cells (NFAT) seems to be critical to promote cardiomyocyte growth (Liu et al., 2012). In addition, cardiac expression of peroxisome proliferator-activated receptor gamma coactivator-1α, a master regulator of mitochondrial function (Shah et al., 2016), has been shown to be inhibited by chronic inflammatory activation, through a NF-κB-dependent mechanism, suggesting that chronic activation also impairs mitochondrial metabolic regulation. However, the precise role of NF-κB in the progression of RV failure remains unknown. Activation of NF-κB has been associated to the development of heart failure in both humans and experimental models. Myocardial levels of NF-κB were increased in patients with advanced heart failure (Frantz et al., 2003). In contrast, in patients with advanced heart failure with LV assist device, the number of NF-κB immune-positive myocardial cells decreased (Grabellus et al., 2002), suggesting that activation of NF-κB signaling seems to involve a complex cellular response to heart failure.

Cellular Mechanosensing

In heart failure, wall stress increases, exposing cardiac cells to increasing biomechanical strain. Mechanosensitive adhesion proteins, including integrins, and cadherins, transduce these mechanical signals, and can stimulate inflammation (Schroer and Merryman, 2015). It has been described, in stretched cardiomyocytes and in hemodynamic-overloaded myocardium, increased secretion of TNF-α and IL-6, together with increased expression of atrial natriuretic peptide (Yoshida et al., 2014). Upon mechanical stretch, cardiac fibroblasts, rather than cardiomyocytes themselves, can be activated, secreting more chemokines and inflammatory cytokines (such as IL-1β), but also extracellular matrix components (Lindner et al., 2014). This contributes to recruit further monocytes by allowing transendothelial migration into cardiac tissue (Lindner et al., 2014). Mechanical strain induce in macrophages the activation of inflammatory processes, leading to increased expression of TNF-α, IL-6, and metalloproteinases acting on the extracellular matrix (Pugin et al., 1998) and increased expression of scavenger receptors (Sakamoto et al., 2001). Moreover, macrophages submitted to mechanical strain are more prone to entry the cell cycle (Sager et al., 2016), suggesting increased wall tension observed in right heart failure could participate to local macrophage proliferation. Strong similarities suggest that all these phenomena could be of importance in RV failure, but still remain unexplored.

INFLAMMATORY AND IMMUNE CELLS

In heart failure, the inflammatory/immune component includes infiltrated neutrophils/monocytes, macrophages, dendritic cells, and lymphocytes, but also cardiac resident cells such as cardiomyocytes, fibroblasts, and endothelial cells (**Figure 2**). All these cells are responsible for local cardiac expression and release of inflammatory mediators (**Figure 3**).

After injury, circulating immune cells, which come from lymphoid organs (spleen and bone marrow), are directed to sites of injury, adhere (or come close) to endothelial cells, invade the myocardium and release a variety of inflammatory molecules (e.g., cytokines and chemokines), acting locally, and promoting chemotaxis of other inflammatory cells. These released cytokines induce the activation of inflammatory processes, mediating multiple interactions between circulating and cardiac cells (Kim et al., 2014). These complex communications result in cardiac remodeling through matrix deposition (mainly collagen) and remodeling, cardiomyocyte apoptosis and differentiation. In addition, we know that inflammatory cells activate cardiac fibroblasts leading to adverse deposition of extracellular matrix, which contributes to the pathobiology of heart failure.

Innate Immune Cells

Dendritic Cells

Acting as sentinels, immature dendritic cells patrol the blood and peripheral tissue to detect foreign and pathogenic antigens, as well as tissue damage and inflammation. This leads to antigen phagocytosis by dendritic cells, which then expresses the maturation marker CD83 and class I and II major histocompatibility complexes. Mature antigen-presenting dendritic cells migrate to secondary lymphoid tissue, where they present antigens to naïve helper and cytotoxic T-cells and prime them (Banchereau et al., 2000). According to their hematopoietic origin, dendritic cells can be divided into myeloid and plasmacytoid dendritic cells, inducing a Th1 and Th2-biased immune response respectively. Furthermore, specialized cardiac dendritic cells have been found in the human heart (Zhang et al., 1993; Yokoyama et al., 2000), and further characterized as a subtype of dendritic cells expressing human leukocyte antigen-DR (but not S100, CD1a, CD21, CD23, and CD35) (Yokoyama et al., 2000). This different surface marker profile compared to ordinary dendritic cells has led to the hypothesis that dendritic cells could change their phenotype depending on the local environment. In various cardiovascular diseases (as well as in hypoxic conditions), dendritic cells play a central role in mediating immunological effects (Yilmaz et al., 2009; Kretzschmar et al., 2015; Rohm et al., 2016). In end-stage heart failure, elevated numbers of dendritic cells have been identified, with a marked increase in myeloid dendritic cells and a concomitant decrease in plasmacytoid dendritic cells (Athanassopoulos et al., 2004, 2009). This suggests a systemic Th1 polarization in these patients. In contrast, lower circulating myeloid and plasmacytoid dendritic cell counts have been described in decompensated heart failure (Sugi et al., 2011). In idiopathic PAH patients, decreased percentage of monocyte-derived dendritic cells has been observed in the peripheral blood, suggesting a Th1 reaction in these patients (Wang et al., 2009). However, the presence and the potential role of dendritic cells have not been considered yet in RV failure.

Mast Cells

Mast cells are granulocytes that develop in the bone marrow and migrate, with the blood stream, to different tissue, where they differentiate and mature. Upon inflammatory stimuli, cardiac mast cells degranulate, releasing a broad spectrum of mediators, including histamine, leukotrienes, growth factors, vasoactive substances, proteases, and cytokines (i.e., IL-1, TNF-α). The secretion of mast cell content is responsible for local inflammation. During the last decade, the possible role of cardiac mast cells has emerged in the pathogenesis of various cardiovascular diseases (Levick et al., 2011). Indeed, increased number of mast cells has been documented in hypertensive and failing LV (Batlle et al., 2006) and described as playing an important role in LV fibrosis, hypertrophy and failure (Stewart et al., 2003; Levick et al., 2008; Zhang et al., 2011 Therapy with mast cell stabilizer reduced fibrosis and preserved LV wall mass in experimental fulminant myocarditis in rats (Mina et al., 2013). Prolonged pressure overload on the RV induced by pulmonary artery banding was associated with increased mast cell density in the RV (Olivetti et al., 1989 This probably results from proliferation and maturation of resident immature cardiac mast cells (Forman et al., 2006; Li et al., 2012), as well as from recruitment of mast cell progenitors followed by further maturation and differentiation in the RV (Frangogiannis et al., 1998; Ngkelo et al., 2016 Despite the presence of RV hypertrophy, mast cell density was not affected in the RV of 3-month-old rats born at high altitude (Rakusan et al., 1990). Mast cells also contribute to cardiac hypertrophy and fibrosis by synthesizing and secreting pro-hypertrophic and pro-fibrotic cytokines (e.g., TNF-α and IL-6) and growth factors [e.g., transforming growth factor (TGF)-β and basic fibroblast growth factor] (Gordon and Galli, 1990; Gordon et al., 1990; Shiota et al., 2003; Sun et al., 2007; Meléndez et al., 2010). In addition, mast cells can also promote tissue fibrosis, stimulating proliferation, maturation and synthesis of collagen in cardiac fibroblasts (Liao et al., 2010). Upon their degranulation, masts cells release very high levels of proteases (e.g., chymases and tryptases) which can activate the proliferation and the synthesis of matrix protein in fibroblasts (Cairns and Walls, 1997; Akers et al., 2000). Inhibition of these proteases was shown to prevent the development of cardiac fibrosis and improve LV dysfunction in experimental models of LV disease (Matsumoto et al., 2003; Kanemitsu et al., 2006). Therefore, inhibition of mast cell proteases might be an original strategy to manage cardiac function. In the hypertrophied RV induced by pressure overload, the expressions of mast cell proteases (i.e., chymases-2,-4,-5,-6 and exopeptidase CPA3) were upregulated (Luitel et al., 2017). Moreover, a mast cell stabilizing compound was tested in chronic hypoxia exposed rats, showing significant reduced RV hypertrophy and lung mast cell hyperplasia (Kay et al., 1981). This should be further explored in RV failure.

Neutrophils/Monocytes and Macrophages

Upon tissue damage, monocytes massively leave the blood stream to differentiate into macrophages in tissues. There, they patrol to eliminate dead cells or pathogens, using phagocytosis and destroying foreign bodies by enzymatic digestion. Macrophages also reside in many healthy tissues, with a substantial tissue-specific heterogeneity among each macrophage population. In the heart, 6–8% of non-cardiomyocytes are cardiac resident macrophages (Pinto et al., 2016), with a dynamic balance between classically-activated macrophages (M1-like cells) and alternatively-activated macrophages (M2-like cells) depending on the activation stimulus. M1 macrophages are known to display a cytotoxic and pro-inflammatory phenotype characterized by strong pathogen and debris clearance and pro-inflammatory cytokine (i.e., IL-6, TNF-α, IL-1β, IL-12, and IL-23) secretion. In contrast, M2 macrophages suppress immune and inflammatory responses (through the release of anti-inflammatory IL-10 and TGF-β), and participate in tissue remodeling and scar formation (Frantz and Nahrendorf, 2014). Deriving from local cardiac progenitors, M2 macrophages have been shown to be the major steady-state cardiac macrophage population, even if their specific functions remain largely unknown. However, these cells may have typical tissue resident macrophage roles, including guarding against infection/insult, but also probably regulating cardiac metabolism, contraction, extracellular matrix deposition, and survival of cardiomyocytes (Frantz and Nahrendorf, 2014). In experimental models of myocardial infarction (Swirski et al., 2009) and chronic heart failure (Ismahil et al., 2014), activation and migration of monocytes to the heart have been described and tightly linked to the activity of angiotensin II (Leuschner et al., 2010). In the early inflammatory steps after myocardial injury, M1 macrophages are predominantly present, while during the later remodeling phase, M2 macrophages are mostly present.

M1 macrophages probably act to clear debris, dead cardiac cells and neutrophils in order to allow tissue regeneration. This initial phase is followed by a proliferation phase during which M2 macrophages participate to myocardial mechanical stability through the regulation of angiogenesis and myofibroblast activity (Nahrendorf et al., 2007). The presence of sequential biphasic M1/M2 macrophage response seems to be crucial for wound healing and for a stable myocardial scar after cardiac injury (van Amerongen et al., 2007; Frantz et al., 2013). However, overabundant pro-inflammatory macrophages are also harmful. Indeed, massive recruitment of macrophages to the heart in response to cardiac injury has a prominent role in the development of myocardial remodeling, hypertrophy and fibrosis (Zhang et al., 2011; Frieler and Mortensen, 2015; Mann, 2015; Prabhu and Frangogiannis, 2016). During the progression of the pulmonary hypertensive disease, the role, dynamics and composition of M1/M2 macrophage populations in the RV are currently largely undefined. Most data are descriptive and come from *post-mortem* histological analysis of RV obtained after fatal pulmonary thromboembolism. They showed RV inflammatory infiltrate predominantly comprised of macrophages, T cells (Begieneman et al., 2008; Orde et al., 2011), neutrophils and macrophages (Iwadate et al., 2003). In experimental pulmonary embolism in rats, early and acute RV damage was associated with infiltration of mononuclear cells with characteristics of M1 phenotype. In the later phase, RV contractile function was reduced together with RV infiltration of mononuclear cells with M2 phenotype and collagen deposition beginning scar formation. This strongly suggests that neutrophil response corresponds to the early acute phase of inflammatory events, while macrophages are present during the proliferative phase and extracellular matrix deposition, changing from M1 to M2 phenotype (Watts et al., 2008). In an experimental model of persistent RV failure on acute increase in afterload, RV extravascular macrophage number was increased and tightly correlated to the coupling of the RV to the pulmonary circulation (assessed by the Ees/Ea ratio) (Dewachter et al., 2015), suggesting a potential mechanistic link between RV macrophage infiltration and RV dysfunction. Ischemia, which can be present in RV failure, induces the recruitment of macrophages (through MCP-1 release) (Kai et al., 2005). This could, at least partly, explain why RV dysfunction after pulmonary embolism was associated with increased expression of MCP-1 and C-C motif chemokine ligand 3 (CCL3 or MIP-1α), as well as RV infiltration with neutrophil and monocyte/macrophage (Watts et al., 2006). In the hypertrophied RV, increased number of activated macrophages contributes to the release of a variety of pro-inflammatory cytokines (e.g., MCP1 and metalloproteinases), that contribute to the pathogenesis of RV failure. To date, cardiac macrophages have never been therapeutically targeted. Crucial to maintain the steady sate and defending against infection, specific population of macrophages should be targeted to avoid collateral damage. During inflammatory processes, monocyte recruitment, which is tightly regulated by interaction between CCL2 and CCR2, could be reduced using silencing of the chemokine CCR2 with nanoparticles, as already experimentally tested in experimental myocardial infarction (Majmudar et al., 2013). It should be interesting to evaluate this further in RV failure.

Adaptive Immune Cells

B-Lymphocytes

B-lymphocytes are able to differentiate into antibody-producing plasma B-cells, which play crucial roles in cell-mediated immune regulation through antigen presentation, cytokine release, differentiation of T-effector cells, and collaboration with antigen-presenting dendritic cells. In PAH patients, a distinct gene expression profile of their peripheral blood B-lymphocytes has been identified (Ulrich et al., 2008b), suggesting activation of B-cells in these patients. Moreover, antibodies directed against pulmonary endothelial cells and fibroblasts have been found in PAH, suggesting a role of B-cells in the pathogenesis of PAH (Tamby et al., 2005, 2006). However, the role played by these cells in the pathogenesis of RV failure remains unknown.

T-Lymphocytes

T-lymphocytes play a central role in cell-mediated immunity and include different types regarding their activity. T helper cells type 1 (Th1) are mainly pro-inflammatory and induce macrophage activation, while T helper cells type 2 (Th2) are predominantly anti-inflammatory through the release of multiple anti-inflammatory cytokines, such as IL-4,-10,-13. Treg cells control the balance between Th1 and Th2 responses, and are implicated in the control of autoimmunity. Tregs not only control other T-cells but also regulate monocytes, macrophages, dendritic cells, natural killer cells and B-cells. In heart failure, the presence of circulating CD4+ T-cells (expressing inflammatory cytokines) tightly correlates with altered LV function (Satoh et al., 2006; Fukunaga et al., 2007), and probably contributes to the transition from cardiac adaptation to heart failure. B- and T-lymphocyte-deficient mice submitted to chronic pressure overload had preserved systolic function, reduced myocardial fibrosis and macrophage infiltration (Laroumanie et al., 2014). In contrast, increased number of CD4+ T-cells have been reported early after coronary occlusion in mice (Hofmann et al., 2012), probably contributing to wound healing just after ischemic injury. Moreover, CD4+ T-cell deficient mice presented impaired wound healing with extracellular matrix disorganization in the ischemic zone (Hofmann et al., 2012). This strongly suggests protective adaptive immune responses early after myocardial insult, which seem to be detrimental at latter stages. Altered Treg function has been identified in patients with PAH (Tamosiuniene et al., 2011; Huertas et al., 2012) and in patients with PAH associated to HIV, systemic sclerosis, systemic lupus erythematosus, Hashimoto's thyroiditis, Sjögren's syndrome, and the anti-phospholipid syndrome (Speich et al., 1991; Covas et al., 1992; Mandl et al., 2004; Bonelli et al., 2009; Radstake et al., 2009). Moreover, higher numbers of circulating Treg cells have been shown in PAH patients, suggesting altered immune control by CD4+ T-lymphocytes (Ulrich et al., 2008a). However, the proportion of these cells in the hypertrophied/failing RV remains to be investigated in PAH, as well as their role in the pathogenesis of RV failure.

Resident Cardiac Cells

Endothelial Cells

In cardiac endothelial cells, pro-inflammatory cytokines induce the expression of adhesion molecules (Tamaru et al., 1998), promote subsequent endothelial binding of immune cells and platelets (Zakrzewicz et al., 1997) and transendothelial migration (Woodfin et al., 2009). In an experimental model of RV failure induced by transient pulmonary artery banding, RV expression of VCAM-1 increased, while expression of ICAM-1 did not change (Dewachter et al., 2015). This was associated to increased RV expression of cytokines and chemokines, together with RV infiltration of neutrophils and macrophages, indicating an early immune response. RV dysfunction associated to brain death was also associated to increased expression of ICAM-1,-2, and VCAM-1 in the RV (Stoica et al., 2005; Belhaj et al., 2016), suggesting endothelial activation, which persists in the post-operative period, even in the absence of acute rejection. On the other hand, we also know that cytokines induce the apoptosis of cardiac endothelial cells and increase endothelial generation of reactive oxygen species (ROS), which induce the production of plasminogen activator inhibition-1 and of collagen by cardiac endothelial cells (Chandrasekar et al., 2004).

INFLAMMATION AS POTENTIAL THERAPEUTIC TARGET IN RIGHT HEART FAILURE

Even if inflammatory processes are activated in RV failure, the precise role of inflammation is yet to be deciphered in this morbid condition. Indeed, it remains unknown if inflammation in the RV could be a key transition step from RV adaptation to failure or if RV activation of inflammatory processes could be a mere bystander and a normal consequence to the primary processes involved in the pathogenesis of RV failure. In addition, whether a myocardial inflammatory process is exclusively maladaptive or whether it may be protective in allowing the heart to properly respond to metabolic stress remains elusive in RV failure. It was previously demonstrated that after acute myocardial injury, an acute inflammatory phase is important to remove damaged tissue and to induce the repair mechanisms that lead to scar formation (Frieler and Mortensen, 2015; Mann, 2015; Prabhu and Frangogiannis, 2016). Suppression of this acute inflammatory phase was proven to be detrimental and to impair post-infarction remodeling (van Amerongen et al., 2007; Frantz et al., 2013). Therefore, further studies should be focused on elucidating the various phases implicated in the pathogenesis of RV inflammation, and trying to dissect the mediators and cellular components that are important in each of these phases. On the other hand, we also know that clinical trials evaluating specific anti-inflammatory treatment in heart failure, despite a strong pathobiological background also present in this condition, were, so far, quite disappointing (Glezeva and Baugh, 2014; Hartman et al., 2018), which makes one wonder if the appropriate signals are being targeted.

While the activation of inflammatory processes has been obviously identified in RV failure secondary to PH, targeting some of them may prove ineffective or offer an unacceptable risk-to-benefit ratio. For example, while TNF-α appears to be clearly implicated in the pathogenesis of RV failure, as well as of PAH, antagonizing this cytokine was not convincing with mixed pre-clinical results (Henriques-Coelho et al., 2008; Wang et al., 2013) and it is known to predispose patients to severe infectious complications such as tuberculosis. In PAH patients, clinical studies targeting such inflammatory mediator and evaluating the effects on RV function have not yet been performed. Moreover, we know that currently approved drugs used to treat PAH patients, which did not primarily target inflammation, have been shown to present some anti-inflammatory effects in pre-clinical and clinical studies (Stasch et al., 2011; Stitham et al., 2011; Fontoura et al., 2014; Dewachter et al., 2015). However, there is a paucity of data evaluating the effects of these drugs on the RV *per se*. Therefore, this is really difficult to discriminate the potential beneficial RV effects of these drugs vs. those observed in the pulmonary circulation. In an experimental model of acute RV failure on pulmonary embolism, selective anti-inflammatory therapy targeted at neutrophil chemoatractants present beneficial effects on RV function, reducing RV inflammation and damage (Zagorski et al., 2007).

Right heart failure is associated with an increase in sympathetic nervous system tone and an activation of the renin-angiotensin-aldosterone system, both resulting in fluid retention and vascular and myocardial remodeling. In patients with severe PAH, we also know that neuro-humoral activation is associated with a decreased survival (Ciarka et al., 2010; de Man et al., 2013a,b). The activation of the adrenergic nervous system and the regulation of the production of cytokines are tightly linked. Indeed, the activation of β2-receptors reduced TNF-α expression, while its increased anti-inflammatory IL-10 production (Ng and Toews, 2016). Conversely, α1,2- adrenergic stimulation increased expression of TNF-α and reduced in IL-10 (Spengler et al., 1990). We could therefore speculate that blocking the renin-angiotensin system may induce anti- inflammatory effects and may therefore result in reduced structural and functional alterations in the RV.

CONCLUSIONS AND FUTURE PERSPECTIVES

In conclusion, the role of inflammation in the development of RV failure appears to be significant. This is true for both RV failure on acute and chronic increase in afterload. However, more effort is needed to understand the mechanisms promoting this pathologic process and how to modulate it in order to develop new therapeutic interventions aiming at the reduction of RV failure and mortality in PAH patients. Moreover, it seems that inflammation and RV failure are strongly interconnected and mutually reinforce each other. Therefore, the inflammatory processes should be counteracted at early stages to stop the vicious circle existing between inflammation and heart failure. As illustrated in **Figure 1**, it may be that RV failure is not a uniform disease but a clinical syndrome, where different pathways play different important roles. More frequent RV failure in patients with PAH due to chronic inflammatory disorders compared to patients with idiopathic PAH, might be a potential RV affection secondary to systemic inflammation. But if so, the question arises why the LV becomes not altered under these conditions.

Based on the results of experimental and translational studies presented here, we could speculate that a better understanding of the pathogenesis of RV failure will open the door for new therapeutic targets. Probably, different stimuli at various stages in the development of RV failure trigger inflammation, ROS generation, mitochondrial metabolism alteration and induction of cell death. Therefore, it is important to point out key regulators of these signaling pathways. Inflammation and ROS generation may not necessarily be harmful in RV failure, and may even play a protective role depending on the trigger (acute or chronic increase in afterload) and the context. However, uncontrolled or excessive exposure of tissues to intense inflammatory signals may be detrimental. The relevance in the control of inflammation warrants further investigation in RV failure to evaluate if the use of anti-inflammatory therapy to improve RV function might be useful.

AUTHOR CONTRIBUTIONS

All authors listed have made a substantial, direct and intellectual contribution to the work, and approved it for publication.

REFERENCES

Akers, I. A., Parsons, M., Hill, M. R., Hollenberg, M. D., Sanjar, S., Laurent, G. J., et al. (2000). Mast cell tryptase stimulates human lung fibroblast proliferation via protease-activated receptor-2. *Am. J. Physiol. Lung Cell Mol. Physiol.* 278, L193–L201. doi: 10.1152/ajplung.2000.278.1.L193

Amir, O., Rogowski, O., David, M., Lahat, N., Wolff, R., and Lewis, B. S. (2010). Circulating interleukin-10: association with higher mortality in systolic heart failure patients with elevated tumor necrosis factor-alpha. *Isr. Med. Assoc. J.* 12, 158–162.

Ancey, C., Menet, E., Corbi, P., Fredj, S., Garcia, M., Rücker-Martin, C., et al. (2003). Human cardiomyocyte hypertrophy induced *in vitro* by gp130 stimulation. *Cardiovasc. Res.* 59, 78–85. doi: 10.1016/S0008-6363(03)00346-8

Anker, S. D., and von Haehling, S. (2004). Inflammatory mediators in chronic heart failure: an overview. *Heart* 90, 464–470. doi: 10.1136/hrt.2002.007005

Athanassopoulos, P., Balk, A. H., Vaessen, L. M., Caliskan, K., Takkenberg, J. J., Weimar, W., et al. (2009). Blood dendritic cell levels and phenotypic characteristics in relation to etiology of end-stage heart failure: implications for dilated cardiomyopathy. *Int. J. Cardiol.* 131, 246–256. doi: 10.1016/j.ijcard.2007.10.031

Athanassopoulos, P., Vaessen, L. M., Maat, A. P., Balk, A. H., Weimar, W., and Bogers, A. J. (2004). Peripheral blood dendritic cells in human end-stage heart failure and the early post-transplant period: evidence for systemic Th1 immune responses. *Eur. J. Cardiothorac. Surg.* 25, 619–626. doi: 10.1016/j.ejcts.2004.01.032

Banchereau, J., Briere, F., Caux, C., Davoust, J., Lebecque, S., Liu, Y. J., et al. (2000). Immunobiology of dendritic cells. *Annu. Rev. Immunol.* 18, 767–811. doi: 10.1146/annurev.immunol.18.1.767

Batlle, M., Roig, E., Perez-Villa, F., Lario, S., Cejudo-Martin, P., Garcia-Pras, E., et al. (2006). Increased expression of the renin-angiotensin system and mast cell density but not of angiotensin-converting enzyme II in late stages of human heart failure. *J. Heart Lung Transplant.* 25, 1117–1125. doi: 10.1016/j.healun.2006.04.012

Begieneman, M. P., van de Goot, F. R., van der Bilt, I. A., Vonk Noordegraaf, A., Spreeuwenberg, M. D., Paulus, W. J., et al. (2008). Pulmonary embolism causes endomyocarditis in the human heart. *Heart* 94, 450–456. doi: 10.1136/hrt.2007.118638

Belhaj, A., Dewachter, L., Kerbaul, F., Brimioulle, S., Dewachter, C., Naeije, R., et al. (2013). Heme oxygenase-1 and inflammation in experimental right ventricular failure on prolonged overcirculation-induced pulmonary hypertension. *PLoS ONE* 8:e69470. doi: 10.1371/journal.pone.0069470

Belhaj, A., Dewachter, L., Rorive, S., Remmelink, M., Weynand, B., Melot, C., et al. (2016). Roles of inflammation and apoptosis in experimental brain death-induced right ventricular failure. *J. Heart Lung Transplant.* 35, 1505–1518. doi: 10.1016/j.healun.2016.05.014

Birks, E. J., Owen, V. J., Burton, P. B., Bishop, A. E., Banner, N. R., Khaghani, A., et al. (2000). Tumor necrosis factor-alpha is expressed in donor heart and predicts right ventricular failure after human heart transplantation. *Circulation* 102, 326–331. doi: 10.1161/01.CIR.102.3.326

Bogaard, H. J., Abe, K., Vonk Noordegraaf, A., and Voelkel, N. F. (2009a). The right ventricle under pressure: cellular and molecular mechanisms of right-heart failure in pulmonary hypertension. *Chest* 135, 794–804. doi: 10.1378/chest.08-0492

Bogaard, H. J., Natarajan, R., Henderson, S. C., Long, C. S., Kraskauskas, D., Smithson, L., et al. (2009b). Chronic pulmonary artery pressure elevation is insufficient to explain right heart failure. *Circulation* 120, 1951–1960. doi: 10.1161/CIRCULATIONAHA.109.883843

Bonelli, M., Savitskaya, A., Steiner, C. W., Rath, E., Smolen, J. S., and Scheinecker, C. (2009). Phenotypic and functional analysis of CD4+ CD25- Foxp3+ T cells in patients with systemic lupus erythematosus. *J. Immunol.* 182, 1689–1695. doi: 10.4049/jimmunol.182.3.1689

Bujak, M., and Frangogiannis, N. G. (2009). The role of IL-1 in the pathogenesis of heart disease. *Arch. Immunol. Ther. Exp.* 57, 165–176. doi: 10.1007/s00005-009-0024-y

Cairns, J. A., and Walls, A. F. (1997). Mast cell tryptase stimulates the synthesis of type I collagen in human lung fibroblasts. *J. Clin. Invest.* 99, 1313–1321. doi: 10.1172/JCI119290

Campian, M. E., Hardziyenka, M., de Bruin, K., van Eck-Smit, B. L., de Bakker, J. M., Verberne, H. J., et al. (2010). Early inflammatory response during the development of right ventricular heart failure in a rat model. *Eur. J. Heart Fail.* 12, 653–658. doi: 10.1093/eurjhf/hfq066

Chandrasekar, B., Vemula, K., Surabhi, R. M., Li-Weber, M., Owen-Schaub, L. B., Jensen, L. E., et al. (2004). Activation of intrinsic and extrinsic proapoptotic signaling pathways in interleukin-18-mediated human cardiac endothelial cell death. *J. Biol. Chem.* 279, 20221–20233. doi: 10.1074/jbc.M313980200

Chen, G. Y., and Nuñez, G. (2010). Sterile inflammation: sensing and reacting to damage. *Nat. Rev. Immunol.* 10, 826–837. doi: 10.1038/nri2873

Chung, M. K., Gulick, T. S., Rotondo, R. E., Schreiner, G. F., and Lange, L. G. (1990). Mechanism of cytokine inhibition of beta-adrenergic agonist stimulation of cyclic AMP in rat cardiac myocytes. Impairment of signal transduction. *Circ. Res.* 67, 753–763. doi: 10.1161/01.RES.67.3.753

Ciarka, A., Doan, V., Velez-Roa, S., Naeije, R., and van de Borne, P. (2010). Prognostic significance of sympathetic nervous system activation in pulmonary arterial hypertension. *Am. J. Respir. Crit. Care Med.* 181, 1269–1275. doi: 10.1164/rccm.200912-1856OC

Coles, B., Fielding, C. A., Rose-John, S., Scheller, J., Jones, S. A., and O'Donnell, V. B. (2007). Classic interleukin-6 receptor signaling and interleukin-6 trans-signaling differentially control angiotensin II-dependent hypertension, cardiac signal transducer and activator of transcription-3 activation, and vascular hypertrophy *in vivo*. *Am. J. Pathol.* 171, 315–325. doi: 10.2353/ajpath.2007.061078

Condliffe, R., Kiely, D. G., Peacock, A. J., Corris, P. A., Gibbs, J. S., Vrapi, F., et al. (2009). Connective tissue disease-associated pulmonary arterial hypertension in the modern treatment era. *Am. J. Respir. Crit. Care Med.* 179, 151–157. doi: 10.1164/rccm.200806-953OC

Constantin, M., Choi, A. J., Cloonan, S. M., and Ryter, S. W. (2012). Therapeutic potential of heme oxygenase-1/carbon monoxide in lung disease. *Int. J. Hypertens.* 2012:859235. doi: 10.1155/2012/859235

Covas, M. I., Esquerda, A., García-Rico, A., and Mahy, N. (1992). Peripheral blood T-lymphocyte subsets in autoimmune thyroid disease. *J. Investig. Allergol. Clin. Immunol.* 2, 131–135.

de Man, F. S., Handoko, M. L., Guignabert, C., Bogaard, H. J., and Vonk-Noordegraaf, A. (2013b). Neurohormonal axis in patients with pulmonary arterial hypertension: friend or foe? *Am. J. Respir. Crit. Care Med.* 187, 14–19. doi: 10.1164/rccm.201209-1663PP

de Man, F. S., Tu, L., Handoko, M. L., Rain, S., Ruiter, G., François, C., et al. (2013a). Dysregulated renin-angiotensin-aldosterone system contributes to pulmonary arterial hypertension. *Am. J. Respir. Crit. Care Med.* 186, 780–789. doi: 10.1164/rccm.201203-0411OC

Dewachter, C., Belhaj, A., Rondelet, B., Vercruyssen, M., Schraufnagel, D. P., Remmelink, M., et al. (2015). Myocardial inflammation in experimental acute right ventricular failure: effects of prostacyclin therapy. *J. Heart Lung Transplant.* 34, 1334–1345. doi: 10.1016/j.healun.2015.05.004

Dewachter, C., Dewachter, L., Rondelet, B., Fesler, P., Brimioulle, S., Kerbaul, F., et al. (2010). Activation of apoptotic pathways in experimental acute afterload-induced right ventricular failure. *Crit. Care Med.* 38, 1405–1413. doi: 10.1097/CCM.0b013e3181de8bd3

Dibbs, Z. I., Diwan, A., Nemoto, S., DeFreitas, G., Abdellatif, M., Carabello, B. A., et al. (2003). Targeted overexpression of transmembrane tumor necrosis factor provokes a concentric cardiac hypertrophic phenotype. *Circulation* 108, 1002–1008. doi: 10.1161/01.CIR.0000085203.46621.F4

Dolenc, J., Šebeštjen, M., Vrtovec, B., KoŽelj, M., and Haddad, F. (2014). Pulmonary hypertension in patients with advanced heart failure is associated with increased levels of interleukin-6. *Biomarkers* 19, 385–390. doi: 10.3109/1354750X.2014.918654

Duncan, D. J., Hopkins, P. M., and Harrison, S. M. (2007). Negative inotropic effects of tumour necrosis factor-alpha and interleukin-1beta are ameliorated by alfentanil in rat ventricular myocytes. *Br. J. Pharmacol.* 150, 720–726. doi: 10.1038/sj.bjp.0707147

Finkel, M. S., Oddis, C. V., Jacob, T. D., Watkins, S. C., Hattler, B. G., and Simmons, R. L. (1992). Negative inotropic effects of cytokines on the heart mediated by nitric oxide. *Science* 257, 387–389. doi: 10.1126/science.1631560

Fontoura, D., Oliveira-Pinto, J., Tavares-Silva, M., Leite, S., Vasques-Nóvoa, F., Mendes-Ferreira, P., et al. (2014). Myocardial and anti-inflammatory effects of chronic bosentan therapy in monocrotaline-induced pulmonary hypertension. *Rev. Port. Cardiol.* 33, 213–222. doi: 10.1016/j.repc.2013.09.016

Forman, M. F., Brower, G. L., and Janicki, J. S. (2006). Rat cardiac mast cell maturation and differentiation following acute ventricular volume overload. *Inflamm. Res.* 55, 408–415. doi: 10.1007/s00011-006-6016-z

Frangogiannis, N. G. (2014). The inflammatory response in myocardial injury, repair, and remodelling. *Nat. Rev. Cardiol.* 11, 255–265. doi: 10.1038/nrcardio.2014.28

Frangogiannis, N. G., Perrard, J. L., Mendoza, L. H., Burns, A. R., Lindsey, M. L., Ballantyne, C. M., et al. (1998). Stem cell factor induction is associated with mast cell accumulation after canine myocardial ischemia and reperfusion. *Circulation* 98, 687–698. doi: 10.1161/01.CIR.98.7.687

Frantz, S., Fraccarollo, D., Wagner, H., Behr, T. M., Jung, P., Angermann, C. E., et al. (2003). Sustained activation of nuclear factor kappa B and activator protein 1 in chronic heart failure. *Cardiovasc. Res.* 57, 749–756. doi: 10.1016/S0008-6363(02)00723-X

Frantz, S., Hofmann, U., Fraccarollo, D., Schäfer, A., Kranepuhl, S., Hagedorn, I., et al. (2013). Monocytes/macrophages prevent healing defects and left ventricular thrombus formation after myocardial infarction. *FASEB J.* 27, 871–881. doi: 10.1096/fj.12-214049

Frantz, S., and Nahrendorf, M. (2014). Cardiac macrophages and their role in ischaemic heart disease. *Cardiovasc. Res.* 102, 240–248. doi: 10.1093/cvr/cvu025

Friedberg, M. K., and Redington, A. N. (2014). Right versus left ventricular failure: differences, similarities, and interactions. *Circulation* 129, 1033–1044. doi: 10.1161/CIRCULATIONAHA.113.001375

Frieler, R. A., and Mortensen, R. M. (2015). Immune cell and other noncardiomyocyte regulation of cardiac hypertrophy and remodeling. *Circulation* 131, 1019–1030. doi: 10.1161/CIRCULATIONAHA.114.008788

Frump, A. L., Goss, K. N., Vayl, A., Albrecht, M., Fisher, A., Tursunova, R., et al. (2015). Estradiol improves right ventricular function in rats with severe angioproliferative pulmonary hypertension: effects of endogenous and exogenous sex hormones. *Am. J. Physiol. Lung Cell Mol. Physiol.* 308, L873–L890. doi: 10.1152/ajplung.00006.2015

Fukunaga, T., Soejima, H., Irie, A., Sugamura, K., Oe, Y., Tanaka, T., et al. (2007). Expression of interferon-gamma and interleukin-4 production in CD4+ T cells in patients with chronic heart failure. *Heart vessels* 22, 178–183. doi: 10.1007/s00380-006-0955-8

Galiè, N., Palazzini, M., and Manes, A. (2010). Pulmonary arterial hypertension: from the kingdom of the near-dead to multiple clinical trial meta-analyses. *Eur. Heart J.* 31, 2080–2086. doi: 10.1093/eurheartj/ehq152

Glezeva, N., and Baugh, J. A. (2014). Role of inflammation in the pathogenesis of heart failure with preserved ejection fraction and its potential as a therapeutic target. *Heart Fail. Rev.* 19, 681–694. doi: 10.1007/s10741-013-9405-8

Gordon, J. R., Burd, P. R., and Galli, S. J. (1990). Mast cells as a source of multifunctional cytokines. *Immunol. Today* 11, 458–464. doi: 10.1016/0167-5699(90)90176-A

Gordon, J. R., and Galli, S. J. (1990). Mast cells as a source of both preformed and immunologically inducible TNF-alpha/cachectin. *Nature* 346, 274–276. doi: 10.1038/346274a0

Grabellus, F., Levkau, B., Sokoll, A., Welp, H., Schmid, C., Deng, M. C., et al. (2002). Reversible activation of nuclear factor-kappaB in human end-stage heart failure after left ventricular mechanical support. *Cardiovasc. Res.* 53, 124–130. doi: 10.1016/S0008-6363(01)00433-3

Gulick, T., Chung, M. K., Pieper, S. J., Lange, L. G., and Schreiner, G. F. (1989). Interleukin 1 and tumor necrosis factor inhibit cardiac myocyte beta-adrenergic responsiveness. *Proc. Natl. Acad. Sci. U.S.A.* 86, 6753–6757. doi: 10.1073/pnas.86.17.6753

Harhay, M. O., Tracy, R. P., Bagiella, E., Barr, R. G., Pinder, D., Hundley, W. G., et al. (2013). Relationship of CRP, IL-6, and fibrinogen with right ventricular structure and function: the MESA-right ventricle study. *Int. J. Cardiol.* 168, 3818–3824. doi: 10.1016/j.ijcard.2013.06.028

Hartman, M. H. T., Groot, H. E., Leach, I. M., Karper, J. C., and van der Harst, P. (2018). Translational overview of cytokine inhibition in acute myocardial infarction and chronic heart failure. *Trends Cardiovasc. Med.* doi: 10.1016/j.tcm.2018.02.003. [Epub ahead of print].

Hayasaki, T., Kaikita, K., Okuma, T., Yamamoto, E., Kuziel, W. A., Ogawa, H., et al. (2006). CC chemokine receptor-2 deficiency attenuates oxidative stress and infarct size caused by myocardial ischemia-reperfusion in mice. *Circ. J.* 70, 342–351. doi: 10.1253/circj.70.342

Hayashidani, S., Tsutsui, H., Shiomi, T., Ikeuchi, M., Matsusaka, H., Suematsu, N., et al. (2003). Anti-monocyte chemoattractant protein-1 gene therapy attenuates left ventricular remodeling and failure after experimental myocardial infarction. *Circulation* 108, 2134–2140. doi: 10.1161/01.CIR.0000092890.29552.22

Henriques-Coelho, T., Brandão-Nogueira, A., Moreira-Gonçalves, D., Correia-Pinto, J., and Leite-Moreira, A. F. (2008). Effects of TNF-alpha blockade in monocrotaline-induced pulmonary hypertension. *Rev. Port. Cardiol.* 27, 341–348.

Higuchi, Y., Chan, T. O., Brown, M. A., Zhang, J., DeGeorge, B. R. Jr., Funakoshi, H., et al. (2006). Cardioprotection afforded by NF-κB ablation is associated with activation of Akt in mice overexpressing TNF-alpha. *Am. J. Physiol. Heart Circ. Physiol.* 290, H590–H598. doi: 10.1152/ajpheart.00379.2005

Hofmann, U., Beyersdorf, N., Weirather, J., Podolskaya, A., Bauersachs, J., Ertl, G., et al. (2012). Activation of CD4+ T lymphocytes improves wound healing and survival after experimental myocardial infarction in mice. *Circulation* 125, 1652–1663. doi: 10.1161/CIRCULATIONAHA.111.044164

Hofmann, U., Heuer, S., Meder, K., Boehler, J., Lange, V., Quaschning, T., et al. (2007). The proinflammatory cytokines TNF-alpha and IL-1 beta impair economy of contraction in human myocardium. *Cytokine* 39, 157–162. doi: 10.1016/j.cyto.2007.07.185

Honsho, S., Nishikawa, S., Amano, K., Zen, K., Adachi, Y., Kishita, E., et al. (2009). Pressure-mediated hypertrophy and mechanical stretch induces IL-1 release and subsequent IGF-1 generation to maintain compensative hypertrophy by affecting Akt and JNK pathways. *Circ. Res.* 105, 1149–1158. doi: 10.1161/CIRCRESAHA.109.208199

Huertas, A., Tu, L., Gambaryan, N., Girerd, B., Perros, F., Montani, D., et al. (2012). Leptin and regulatory T-lymphocytes in idiopathic pulmonary arterial hypertension. *Eur. Respir. J.* 40, 895–904. doi: 10.1183/09031936.00159911

Humbert, M., Monti, G., Brenot, F., Sitbon, O., Portier, A., Grangeot-Keros, L., et al. (1995). Increased interleukin-1 and interleukin-6 serum concentrations in severe primary pulmonary hypertension. *Am. J. Respir. Crit. Care Med.* 151, 1628–1631. doi: 10.1164/ajrccm.151.5.7735624

Humbert, M., Morrell, N. W., Archer, S. L., Stenmark, K. R., MacLean, M. R., Lang, I. M., et al. (2004). Cellular and molecular pathobiology of pulmonary arterial hypertension. *J. Am. Coll. Cardiol.* 43, 13S–24S. doi: 10.1016/j.jacc.2004.02.029

Ing, D. J., Zang, J., Dzau, V. J., Webster, K. A., and Bishopric, N. H. (1999). Modulation of cytokine-induced cardiac myocyte apoptosis by nitric oxide, Bak, and Bcl-x. *Circ. Res.* 84, 21–33. doi: 10.1161/01.RES.84.1.21

Iozzo, R. V., and Schaefer, L. (2010). Proteoglycans in health and disease: novel regulatory signaling mechanisms evoked by the small leucine-rich proteoglycans. *FEBS J.* 277, 3864–3875. doi: 10.1111/j.1742-4658.2010.07797.x

Ismahil, M. A., Hamid, T., Bansal, S. S., Patel, B., Kingery, J. R., and Prabhu, S. D. (2014). Remodeling of the mononuclear phagocyte network underlies chronic inflammation and disease progression in heart failure: critical importance of the cardiosplenic axis. *Circ. Res.* 114, 266–282.

doi: 10.1161/CIRCRESAHA.113.301720

Iwadate, K., Doi, M., Tanno, K., Katsumura, S., Ito, H., Sato, K., et al. (2003). Right ventricular damage due to pulmonary embolism: examination of the number of infiltrating macrophages. *Forensic Sci. Int.* 134, 147–153. doi: 10.1016/S0379-0738(03)00138-5

Kai, H., Kuwahara, F., Tokuda, K., and Imaizumi, T. (2005). Diastolic dysfunction in hypertensive hearts: roles of perivascular inflammation and reactive myocardial fibrosis. *Hypertens. Res.* 28, 483–490. doi: 10.1291/hypres.28.483

Kanemitsu, H., Takai, S., Tsuneyoshi, H., Nishina, T., Yoshikawa, K., Miyazaki, M., et al. (2006). Chymase inhibition prevents cardiac fibrosis and dysfunction after myocardial infarction in rats. *Hypertens. Res.* 29, 57–64. doi: 10.1291/hypres.29.57

Kapadia, S., Lee, J., Torre-Amione, G., Birdsall, H. H., Ma, T. S., and Mann, D. L. (1995). Tumor necrosis factor-alpha gene and protein expression in adult feline myocardium after endotoxin administration. *J. Clin. Invest.* 96, 1042–1052. doi: 10.1172/JCI118090

Kasper, W., Konstantinides, S., Geibel, A., Tiede, N., Krause, T., and Just, H. (1997). Prognostic significance of right ventricular afterload stress detected by echocardiography in patients with clinically suspected pulmonary embolism *Heart* 77, 346–349. doi: 10.1136/hrt.77.4.346

Katayose, D., Isoyama, S., Fujita, H., and Shibahara, S. (1993). Separate regulation of heme oxygenase and heat shock protein 70 mRNA expression in the rat heart by hemodynamic stress. *Biochem. Biophys. Res. Commun.* 191, 587–594. doi: 10.1006/bbrc.1993.1258

Kaur, K., Sharma, A. K., and Singal, P. K. (2006). Significance of changes in TNF-alpha and IL-10 levels in the progression of heart failure subsequent to myocardial infarction. *Am. J. Physiol. Heart Circ. Physiol.* 291, H106–H113. doi: 10.1152/ajpheart.01327.2005

Kawano, S., Kubota, T., Monden, Y., Kawamura, N., Tsutsui, H., Takeshita, A., et al. (2005). Blockade of NF-κB ameliorates myocardial hypertrophy in response to chronic infusion of angiotensin II. *Cardiovasc. Res.* 67, 689–698. doi: 10.1016/j.cardiores.2005.04.030

Kawut, S. M., Taichman, D. B., Archer-Chicko, C. L., Palevsky, H. I., and Kimmel, S. E. (2003). Hemodynamics and survival in patients with pulmonary arterial hypertension related to systemic sclerosis. *Chest* 123, 344–350. doi: 10.1378/chest.123.2.344

Kay, J. M., Suyama, K. L., and Keane, P. M. (1981). Mast cell stabilizing compound FPL 55618 reduces right ventricular hypertrophy and lung mast cell hyperplasia in chronically hypoxic rats. *Experientia* 37, 75–76. doi: 10.1007/BF01965579

Kim, E. J., Kim, S., Kang, D. O., and Seo, H. S. (2014). Metabolic activity of the spleen and bone marrow in patients with acute myocardial infarction evaluated by 18f-fluorodeoxyglucose positron emission tomograpic imaging. *Circ. Cardiovasc. Imaging* 7, 454–460. doi: 10.1161/CIRCIMAGING.113.001093

Ko, H. J., Zhang, Z., Jung, D. Y., Jun, J. Y., Ma, Z., Jones, K. E., et al. (2009). Nutrient stress activates inflammation and reduces glucose metabolism by suppressing AMP-activated protein kinase in the heart. *Diabetes* 58, 2536–2546. doi: 10.2337/db08-1361

Kohno, T., Anzai, T., Naito, K., Sugano, Y., Maekawa, Y., Takahashi, T., et al. (2008). Angiotensin-receptor blockade reduces border zone myocardial monocyte chemoattractant protein-1 expression and macrophage infiltration in post-infarction ventricular remodeling. *Circ. J.* 72, 1685–1692. doi: 10.1253/circj.CJ-08-0115

Kolattukudy, P. E., Quach, T., Bergese, S., Breckenridge, S., Hensley, J., Altschuld, R., et al. (1998). Myocarditis induced by targeted expression of the MCP-1 gene in murine cardiac muscle. *Am. J. Pathol.* 152, 101–111.

Kreit, J. W. (2004). The impact of right ventricular dysfunction on the prognosis and therapy of normotensive patients with pulmonary embolism. *Chest* 125, 1539–1545. doi: 10.1378/chest.125.4.1539

Kretzschmar, D., Rohm, I., Schäller, S., Betge, S., Pistulli, R., Atiskova, Y., et al. (2015). Decrease in circulating dendritic cell precursors in patients with peripheral artery disease. *Mediators Inflamm.* 2015:450957. doi: 10.1155/2015/450957

Kubota, T., Bounoutas, G. S., Miyagishima, M., Kadokami, T., Sanders, V. J., Bruton, C., et al. (2000a). Soluble tumor necrosis factor receptor abrogates myocardial inflammation but not hypertrophy in cytokine-induced cardiomyopathy. *Circulation* 101, 2518–2525. doi: 10.1161/01.CIR.101.21.2518

Kubota, T., McTiernan, C. F., Frye, C. S., Slawson, S. E., Lemster, B. H., Koretsky, A. P., et al. (1997). Dilated cardiomyopathy in transgenic mice with cardiac-specific overexpression of tumor necrosis factor-alpha. *Circ. Res.* 81, 627–635. doi: 10.1161/01.RES.81.4.627

Kubota, T., Miyagishima, M., Alvarez, R. J., Kormos, R., Rosenblum, W. D., Demetris, A. J., et al. (2000b). Expression of proinflammatory cytokines in the failing human heart: comparison of recent-onset and end-stage congestive heart failure. *J. Heart Lung Transplant.* 19, 819–824. doi: 10.1016/S1053-2498(00)00173-X

Kuhn, K. P., Byrne, D. W., Arbogast, P. G., Doyle, T. P., Loyd, J. E., and Robbins, I. M. (2003). Outcome in 91 consecutive patients with pulmonary arterial hypertension receiving epoprostenol. *Am. J. Respir. Crit. Care Med.* 167, 580–586. doi: 10.1164/rccm.200204-333OC

Kumar, S., Wei, C., Thomas, C. M., Kim, I. K., Seqqat, R., Kumar, R., et al. (2012). Cardiac-specific genetic inhibition of nuclear factor-kappaB prevents right ventricular hypertrophy induced by monocrotaline. *Am. J. Physiol. Heart Circ. Physiol.* 302, H1655–H1666. doi: 10.1152/ajpheart.00756.2011

Kunisada, K., Hirota, H., Fujio, Y., Matsui, H., Tani, Y., Yamauchi-Takihara, K., et al. (1996). Activation of JAK-STAT and MAP kinases by leukemia inhibitory factor through gp130 in cardiac myocytes. *Circulation* 94, 2626–2632. doi: 10.1161/01.CIR.94.10.2626

Kunisada, K., Tone, E., Fujio, Y., Matsui, H., Yamauchi-Takihara, K., and Kishimoto, T. (1998). Activation of gp130 transduces hypertrophic signals via STAT3 in cardiac myocytes. *Circulation* 98, 346–352. doi: 10.1161/01.CIR.98.4.346

Laroumanie, F., Douin-Echinard, V., Pozzo, J., Lairez, O., Tortosa, F., Vinel, C., et al. (2014). CD4+ T cells promote the transition from hypertrophy to heart failure during chronic pressure overload. *Circulation* 129, 2111–2124. doi: 10.1161/CIRCULATIONAHA.113.007101

Lee, S. H., Chen, Y. C., Chen, Y. J., Chang, S. L., Tai, C. T., Wongcharoen, W., et al. (2007). Tumor necrosis factor-alpha alters calcium handling and increases arrhythmogenesis of pulmonary vein cardiomyocytes. *Life Sci.* 80, 1806–1815. doi: 10.1016/j.lfs.2007.02.029

Leuschner, F., Panizzi, P., Chico-Calero, I., Lee, W. W., Ueno, T., Cortez-Retamozo, V., et al. (2010). Angiotensin-converting enzyme inhibition prevents the release of monocytes from their splenic reservoir in mice with myocardial infarction. *Circ. Res.* 107, 1364–1373. doi: 10.1161/CIRCRESAHA.110.227454

Levick, S. P., Gardner, J. D., Holland, M., Hauer-Jensen, M., Janicki, J. S., and Brower, G. L. (2008). Protection from adverse myocardial remodeling secondary to chronic volume overload in mast cell deficient rats. *J. Mol. Cell. Cardiol.* 45, 56–61. doi: 10.1016/j.yjmcc.2008.04.010

Levick, S. P., Meléndez, G. C., Plante, E., McLarty, J. L., Brower, G. L., and Janicki, J. S. (2011). Cardiac mast cells: the centrepiece in adverse myocardial remodelling. *Cardiovasc. Res.* 89, 12–19. doi: 10.1093/cvr/cvq272

Li, J., Lu, H., Plante, E., Meléndez, G. C., Levick, S. P., and Janicki, J. S. (2012). Stem cell factor is responsible for the rapid response in mature mast cell density in the acutely stressed heart. *J. Mol. Cell Cardiol.* 53, 469–474. doi: 10.1016/j.yjmcc.2012.07.011

Liang, O. D., Mitsialis, S. A., Chang, M. S., Vergadi, E., Lee, C., Aslam, M., et al. (2011). Mesenchymal stromal cells expressing heme oxygenase-1 reverse pulmonary hypertension. *Stem Cells* 29, 99–107. doi: 10.1002/stem.548

Liao, C. H., Akazawa, H., Tamagawa, M., Ito, K., Yasuda, N., Kudo, Y., et al. (2010). Cardiac mast cells cause atrial fibrillation through PDGF-A-mediated fibrosis in pressure-overloaded mouse hearts. *J. Clin. Invest.* 120, 242–253. doi: 10.1172/JCI39942

Libby, P. (2007). Inflammatory mechanisms: the molecular basis of inflammation and disease. *Nutr. Rev.* 65, S140–S146. doi: 10.1301/nr.2007.dec.S140-S146

Lindner, D., Zietsch, C., Tank, J., Sossalla, S., Fluschnik, N., Hinrichs, S., et al. (2014). Cardiac fibroblasts support cardiac inflammation in heart failure. *Basic Res. Cardiol.* 109:428. doi: 10.1007/s00395-014-0428-7

Liu, A., Philip, J., Vinnakota, K. C., Van den Bergh, F., Tabima, D. M., Hacker, T., et al. (2017). Estrogen maintains mitochondrial content and function in the right ventricle of rats with pulmonary hypertension. *Physiol. Rep.* 5:e13157. doi: 10.14814/phy2.13157

Liu, Q., Chen, Y., Auger-Messier, M., and Molkentin, J. D. (2012). Interaction between NFkappaB and NFAT coordinates cardiac hypertrophy and pathological remodeling. *Circ. Res.* 110, 1077–1086. doi: 10.1161/CIRCRESAHA.111.260729

Liu, Y., Lian, K., Zhang, L., Wang, R., Yi, F., Gao, C., et al. (2014). TXNIP mediates NLRP3 inflammasome activation in cardiac microvascular endothelial cells as a novel mechanism in myocardial ischemia/reperfusion injury. *Basic Res. Cardiol.* 109:415. doi: 10.1007/s00395-014-0415-z

Luitel, H., Sydykov, A., Schymura, Y., Mamazhakypov, A., Janssen, W., Pradhan, K., et al. (2017). Pressure overload leads to an increased accumulation and activity of mast cells in the right ventricle. *Physiol Rep* 5:e13146. doi: 10.14814/phy2.13146

Ma, F., Li, Y., Jia, L., Han, Y., Cheng, J., Li, H., et al. (2012). Macrophage-stimulated cardiac fibroblast production of IL-6 is essential for TGF beta/Smad activation and cardiac fibrosis induced by angiotensin II. *PLoS ONE* 7:e35144. doi: 10.1371/journal.pone.0035144

Maass, D. L., White, J., and Horton, J. W. (2002). IL-1beta and IL-6 act synergistically with TNF-alpha to alter cardiac contractile function after burn trauma. *Shock* 18, 360–366. doi: 10.1097/00024382-200210000-00012

Maekawa, Y., Anzai, T., Yoshikawa, T., Sugano, Y., Mahara, K., Kohno, T., et al. (2004). Effect of granulocyte-macrophage colony-stimulating factor inducer on left ventricular remodeling after acute myocardial infarction. *J. Am. Coll. Cardiol.* 44, 1510–1520. doi: 10.1016/j.jacc.2004.05.083

Majmudar, M. D., Keliher, E. J., Heidt, T., Leuschner, F., Truelove, J., Sena, B. F., et al. (2013). Monocyte-directed RNAi targeting CCR2 improves infarct healing in atherosclerosis-prone mice. *Circulation* 127, 2038–2046. doi: 10.1161/CIRCULATIONAHA.112.000116

Mandl, T., Bredberg, A., Jacobsson, L. T., Manthorpe, R., and Henriksson, G. (2004). CD4+ T-lymphocytopenia–a frequent finding in anti-SSA antibody seropositive patients with primary Sjogren's syndrome. *J. Rheumatol.* 31, 726–728.

Mann, D. L. (2002). Inflammatory mediators and the failing heart: past, present, and the foreseeable future. *Circ. Res.* 91, 988–998. doi: 10.1161/01.RES.0000043825.01705.1B

Mann, D. L. (2015). Innate immunity and the failing heart: the cytokine hypothesis revisited. *Circ. Res.* 116, 1254–1268. doi: 10.1161/CIRCRESAHA.116.302317

Matsumoto, T., Wada, A., Tsutamoto, T., Ohnishi, M., Isono, T., and Kinoshita, M. (2003). Chymase inhibition prevents cardiac fibrosis and improves diastolic dysfunction in the progression of heart failure. *Circulation* 107, 2555–2558. doi: 10.1161/01.CIR.0000074041.81728.79

McLarty, J. L., Li, J., Levick, S. P., and Janicki, J. S. (2013). Estrogen modulates the influence of cardiac inflammatory cells on function of cardiac fibroblasts. *J. Inflamm. Res.* 6, 99–108. doi: 10.2147/JIR.S48422

Meier, H., Bullinger, J., Marx, G., Deten, A., Horn, L. C., Rassler, B., et al. (2009). Crucial role of interleukin-6 in the development of norepinephrine-induced left ventricular remodeling in mice. *Cell Physiol. Biochem.* 23, 327–334. doi: 10.1159/000218180

Meléndez, G. C., McLarty, J. L., Levick, S. P., Du, Y., Janicki, J. S., and Brower, G. L. (2010). Interleukin 6 mediates myocardial fibrosis, concentric hypertrophy, and diastolic dysfunction in rats. *Hypertension* 56, 225–231. doi: 10.1161/HYPERTENSIONAHA.109.148635

Mina, Y., Rinkevich-Shop, S., Konen, E., Goitein, O., Kushnir, T., Epstein, F. H., et al. (2013). Mast cell inhibition attenuates myocardial damage, adverse remodeling, and dysfunction during fulminant myocarditis in the rat. *J. Cardiovasc. Pharmacol. Ther.* 18, 152–161. doi: 10.1177/1074248412458975

Moreth, K., Brodbeck, R., Babelova, A., Gretz, N., Spieker, T., Zeng-Brouwers, J., et al. (2010). The proteoglycan biglycan regulates expression of the B cell chemoattractant CXCL13 and aggravates murine lupus nephritis. *J. Clin. Invest.* 120, 4251–4272. doi: 10.1172/JCI42213

Naeije, R., Brimioulle, S., and Dewachter, L. (2014). Biomechanics of the right ventricle in health and disease (Grover Conference series). *Pulm. Circ.* 4, 395–406. doi: 10.1086/677354

Nahrendorf, M., Swirski, F. K., Aikawa, E., Stangenberg, L., Wurdinger, T., Figueiredo, J. L., et al. (2007). The healing myocardium sequentially mobilizes two monocyte subsets with divergent and complementary functions. *J. Exp. Med.* 204, 3037–3047. doi: 10.1084/jem.20070885

Nakaoka, Y., Nishida, K., Fujio, Y., Izumi, M., Terai, K., Oshima, Y., et al. (2003). Activation of gp130 transduces hypertrophic signal through interaction of scaffolding/docking protein Gab1 with tyrosine phosphatase SHP2 in cardiomyocytes. *Circ. Res.* 93, 221–229. doi: 10.1161/01.RES.0000085562.48906.4A

Ng, T. M., and Toews, M. L. (2016). Impaired norepinephrine regulation of monocyte inflammatory cytokine balance in heart failure. *World J. Cardiol.* 8, 584–589. doi: 10.4330/wjc.v8.i10.584

Ngkelo, A., Richart, A., Kirk, J. A., Bonnin, P., Vilar, J., Lemitre, M., et al. (2016). Mast cells regulate myofilament calcium sensitization and heart function after myocardial infarction. *J. Exp. Med.* 213, 1353–1374. doi: 10.1084/jem.20160081

Olivetti, G., Lagrasta, C., Ricci, R., Sonnenblick, E. H., Capasso, J. M., and Anversa, P. (1989). Long-term pressure-induced cardiac hypertrophy: capillary and mast cell proliferation. *Am. J. Physiol.* 257, H1766–H1772. doi: 10.1152/ajpheart.1989.257.6.H1766

Orde, M. M., Puranik, R., Morrow, P. L., and Duflou, J. (2011). Myocardial pathology in pulmonary thromboembolism. *Heart* 97, 1695–1699. doi: 10.1136/hrt.2011.226209

Otterbein, L. E., Kolls, J. K., Mantell, L. L., Cook, J. L., Alam, J., and Choi, A. M. (1999). Exogenous administration of heme oxygenase-1 by gene transfer provides protection against hyperoxia-induced lung injury. *J. Clin. Invest.* 103, 1047–1054. doi: 10.1172/JCI5342

Overbeek, M. J., Lankhaar, J. W., Westerhof, N., Voskuyl, A. E., Boonstra, A., Bronzwaer, J. G., et al. (2008). Right ventricular contractility in systemic sclerosis-associated and idiopathic pulmonary arterial hypertension. *Eur. Respir. J.* 31, 1160–1166. doi: 10.1183/09031936.00135407

Overbeek, M. J., Mouchaers, K. T., Niessen, H. M., Hadi, A. M., Kupreishvili, K., Boonstra, A., et al. (2010). Characteristics of interstitial fibrosis and inflammatory cell infiltration in right ventricles of systemic sclerosis-associated pulmonary arterial hypertension. *Int. J. Rheumatol.* 2010:604615. doi: 10.1155/2010/604615

Pinto, A. R., Ilinykh, A., Ivey, M. J., Kuwabara, J. T., D'Antoni, M. L., Debuque, R., et al. (2016). Revisiting cardiac cellular composition. *Circ. Res.* 118, 400–409. doi: 10.1161/CIRCRESAHA.115.307778

Prabhu, S. D., and Frangogiannis, N. G. (2016). The Biological basis for cardiac repair after myocardial infarction: from inflammation to fibrosis. *Circ. Res.* 119, 91–112. doi: 10.1161/CIRCRESAHA.116.303577

Pugin, J., Dunn, I., Jolliet, P., Tassaux, D., Magnenat, J. L., Nicod, L. P., et al. (1998). Activation of human macrophages by mechanical ventilation *in vitro*. *Am. J. Physiol.* 275, L1040–L1050. doi: 10.1152/ajplung.1998.275.6.L1040

Rabinovitch, M. (2012). Molecular pathogenesis of pulmonary arterial hypertension. *J. Clin. Invest.* 122, 4306–4313. doi: 10.1172/JCI60658

Radstake, T. R., van Bon, L., Broen, J., Wenink, M., Santegoets, K., Deng, Y., et al. (2009). Increased frequency and compromised function of T regulatory cells in systemic sclerosis (SSc) is related to a diminished CD69 and TGFbeta expression. *PLoS ONE* 4:e5981. doi: 10.1371/journal.pone.0005981

Rakusan, K., Sarkar, K., Turek, Z., and Wicker, P. (1990). Mast cells in the rat heart during normal growth and in cardiac hypertrophy. *Circ. Res.* 66, 511–516. doi: 10.1161/01.RES.66.2.511

Ribeiro, A., Lindmarker, P., Juhlin-Dannfelt, A., Johnsson, H., and Jorfeldt, L. (1997). Echocardiography Doppler in pulmonary embolism: right ventricular dysfunction as a predictor of mortality rate. *Am. Heart J.* 134, 479–487. doi: 10.1016/S0002-8703(97)70085-1

Rohm, I., Aderhold, N., Ratka, J., Goebel, B., Franz, M., Pistulli, R., et al. (2016). Hypobaric hypoxia in 3000 m altitude leads to a significant decrease in circulating plasmacytoid dendritic cells in humans. *Clin. Hemorheol. Microcirc.* 63, 257–265. doi: 10.3233/CH-152035

Rondelet, B., Dewachter, C., Kerbaul, F., Kang, X., Fesler, P., Brimioulle, S., et al. (2012). Prolonged overcirculation-induced pulmonary arterial hypertension as a cause of right ventricular failure. *Eur. Heart J.* 33, 1017–1026. doi: 10.1093/eurheartj/ehr111

Sager, H. B., Hulsmans, M., Lavine, K. J., Moreira, M. B., Heidt, T., Courties, G., et al. (2016). Proliferation and recruitment contribute to myocardial macrophage expansion in chronic heart failure. *Circ. Res.* 119, 853–864. doi: 10.1161/CIRCRESAHA.116.309001

Sakamoto, H., Aikawa, M., Hill, C. C., Weiss, D., Taylor, W. R., Libby, P., et al. (2001). Biomechanical strain induces class a scavenger receptor expression in human monocyte/macrophages and THP-1 cells: a potential mechanism of increased atherosclerosis in hypertension. *Circulation* 104, 109–114. doi: 10.1161/hc2701.091070

Sanchez, O., Marcos, E., Perros, F., Fadel, E., Tu, L., Humbert, M., et al. (2007). Role of endothelium-derived CC chemokine ligand 2 in idiopathic pulmonary arterial hypertension. *Am. J. Respir. Crit. Care Med.* 176, 1041–1047. doi: 10.1164/rccm.200610-1559OC

Satoh, S., Oyama, J., Suematsu, N., Kadokami, T., Shimoyama, N., Okutsu, M., et al. (2006). Increased productivity of tumor necrosis factor-alpha in helper T cells in patients with systolic heart failure. *Int. J. Cardiol.* 111, 405–412. doi: 10.1016/j.ijcard.2005.08.021

Saxena, A., Chen, W., Su, Y., Rai, V., Uche, O. U., Li, N., et al. (2013). IL-1 induces proinflammatory leukocyte infiltration and regulates fibroblast phenotype in the infarcted myocardium. *J. Immunol.* 191, 4838–4848. doi: 10.4049/jimmunol.1300725

Schoepf, U. J., Kucher, N., Kipfmueller, F., Quiroz, R., Costello, P., and Goldhaber, S. Z. (2004). Right ventricular enlargement on chest computed tomography: a predictor of early death in acute pulmonary embolism. *Circulation* 110, 3276–3280. doi: 10.1161/01.CIR.0000147612.59751.4C

Schroer, A. K., and Merryman, W. D. (2015). Mechanobiology of myofibroblast adhesion in fibrotic cardiac disease. *J. Cell Sci.* 128, 1865–1875. doi: 10.1242/jcs.162891

Seta, Y., Shan, K., Bozkurt, B., Oral, H., and Mann, D. L. (1996). Basic mechanisms in heart failure: the cytokine hypothesis. *J. Card. Fail.* 2, 243–249. doi: 10.1016/S1071-9164(96)80047-9

Shah, T., Joshi, K., Mishra, S., Otiv, S., and Kumbar, V. (2016). Molecular and cellular effects of vitamin B12 forms on human trophoblast cells in presence of excessive folate. *Biomed. Pharmacother.* 84, 526–534. doi: 10.1016/j.biopha.2016.09.071

Shimano, M., Ouchi, N., and Walsh, K. (2012). Cardiokines: recent progress in elucidating the cardiac secretome. *Circulation* 126, e327–e332. doi: 10.1161/CIRCULATIONAHA.112.150656

Shiota, N., Rysä, J., Kovanen, P. T., Ruskoaho, H., Kokkonen, J. O., and Lindstedt, K. A. (2003). A role for cardiac mast cells in the pathogenesis of hypertensive heart disease. *J. Hypertens.* 21, 1935–1944. doi: 10.1097/00004872-200310000-00022

Soon, E., Holmes, A. M., Treacy, C. M., Doughty, N. J., Southgate, L., Machado, R. D., et al. (2010). Elevated levels of inflammatory cytokines predict survival in idiopathic and familial pulmonary arterial hypertension. *Circulation* 122, 920–927. doi: 10.1161/CIRCULATIONAHA.109.933762

Speich, R., Jenni, R., Opravil, M., Pfab, M., and Russi, E. W. (1991). Primary pulmonary hypertension in HIV infection. *Chest* 100, 1268–1271. doi: 10.1378/chest.100.5.1268

Spengler, R. N., Allen, R. M., Remick, D. G., Strieter, R. M., and Kunkel, S. L. (1990). Stimulation of alpha-adrenergic receptor augments the production of macrophage-derived tumor necrosis factor. *J. Immunol.* 145, 1430–1434.

Stasch, J. P., Pacher, P., and Evgenov, O. V. (2011). Soluble guanylate cyclase as an emerging therapeutic target in cardiopulmonary disease. *Circulation* 123, 2263–2273. doi: 10.1161/CIRCULATIONAHA.110.981738

Stewart, J. A. Jr., Wei, C. C., Brower, G. L., Rynders, P. E., Hankes, G. H., Dillon, A. R., et al. (2003). Cardiac mast cell- and chymase-mediated matrix metalloproteinase activity and left ventricular remodeling in mitral regurgitation in the dog. *J. Mol. Cell Cardiol.* 35, 311–319. doi: 10.1016/S0022-2828(03)00013-0

Stitham, J., Midgett, C., Martin, K. A., and Hwa, J. (2011). Prostacyclin: an inflammatory paradox. *Front. Pharmacol.* 2:24. doi: 10.3389/fphar.2011.00024

Stoica, S. C., Atkinson, C., Satchithananda, D. K., Charman, S., Goddard, M., Redington, A. N., et al. (2005). Endothelial activation in the transplanted human heart from organ retrieval to 3 months after transplantation: an observational study. *J. Heart Lung Transplant.* 24, 593–601. doi: 10.1016/j.healun.2004.01.021

Stumpf, C., Lehner, C., Yilmaz, A., Daniel, W. G., and Garlichs, C. D. (2003). Decrease of serum levels of the anti-inflammatory cytokine interleukin-10 in patients with advanced chronic heart failure. *Clin. Sci.* 105, 45–50. doi: 10.1042/CS20020359

Sugi, Y., Yasukawa, H., Kai, H., Fukui, D., Futamata, N., Mawatari, K., et al. (2011). Reduction and activation of circulating dendritic cells in patients with decompensated heart failure. *Int. J. Cardiol.* 147, 258–264. doi: 10.1016/j.ijcard.2009.09.524

Sun, M., Chen, M., Dawood, F., Zurawska, U., Li, J. Y., Parker, T., et al. (2007). Tumor necrosis factor-alpha mediates cardiac remodeling and ventricular dysfunction after pressure overload state. *Circulation* 115, 1398–1407. doi: 10.1161/CIRCULATIONAHA.106.643585

Swirski, F. K., Nahrendorf, M., Etzrodt, M., Wildgruber, M., Cortez-Retamozo, V., Panizzi, P., et al. (2009). Identification of splenic reservoir monocytes and their deployment to inflammatory sites. *Science* 325, 612–616. doi: 10.1126/science.1175202

Tamaru, M., Tomura, K., Sakamoto, S., Tezuka, K., Tamatani, T., and Narumi, S. (1998). Interleukin-1beta induces tissue- and cell type-specific expression of adhesion molecules *in vivo*. *Arterioscler. Thromb. Vasc. Biol.* 18, 1292–1303. doi: 10.1161/01.ATV.18.8.1292

Tamby, M. C., Chanseaud, Y., Humbert, M., Fermanian, J., Guilpain, P., Garcia-de-la-Peña-Lefebvre, P., et al. (2005). Anti-endothelial cell antibodies in idiopathic and systemic sclerosis associated pulmonary arterial hypertension. *Thorax* 60, 765–772. doi: 10.1136/thx.2004.029082

Tamby, M. C., Humbert, M., Guilpain, P., Servettaz, A., Dupin, N., Christner, J. J., et al. (2006). Antibodies to fibroblasts in idiopathic and scleroderma-associated pulmonary hypertension. *Eur. Respir. J.* 28, 799–807. doi: 10.1183/09031936.06.00152705

Tamosiuniene, R., Tian, W., Dhillon, G., Wang, L., Sung, Y. K., Gera, L., et al. (2011). Regulatory T cells limit vascular endothelial injury and prevent pulmonary hypertension. *Circ. Res.* 109, 867–879. doi: 10.1161/CIRCRESAHA.110.236927

Tenhunen, R., Marver, H. S., and Schmid, R. (1968). The enzymatic conversion of heme to bilirubin by microsomal heme oxygenase. *Proc. Natl. Acad. Sci U.S.A.* 61, 748–755. doi: 10.1073/pnas.61.2.748

Thaik, C. M., Calderone, A., Takahashi, N., and Colucci, W. S. (1995). Interleukin-1 beta modulates the growth and phenotype of neonatal rat cardiac myocytes. *J. Clin. Invest.* 96, 1093–1099. doi: 10.1172/JCI118095

Torre-Amione, G., Kapadia, S., Lee, J., Durand, J. B., Bies, R. D., Young, J. B., et al. (1996). Tumor necrosis factor-alpha and tumor necrosis factor receptors in the failing human heart. *Circulation* 93, 704–711. doi: 10.1161/01.CIR.93.4.704

Tschöpe, C., and Lam, C. S. (2012). Diastolic heart failure: what we still don't know. Looking for new concepts, diagnostic approaches, and the role of comorbidities. *Herz* 37, 875–879. doi: 10.1007/s00059-012-3719-5

Ulrich, S., Nicolls, M. R., Taraseviciene, L., Speich, R., and Voelkel, N. (2008a). Increased regulatory and decreased CD8+ cytotoxic T cells in the blood of patients with idiopathic pulmonary arterial hypertension. *Respir. Int. Rev. Thorac Dis.* 75, 272–280. doi: 10.1159/000111548

Ulrich, S., Taraseviciene-Stewart, L., Huber, L. C., Speich, R., and Voelkel, N. (2008b). Peripheral blood B lymphocytes derived from patients with idiopathic pulmonary arterial hypertension express a different RNA pattern compared with healthy controls: a cross sectional study. *Respir. Res.* 9:20. doi: 10.1186/1465-9921-9-20

van Amerongen, M. J., Harmsen, M. C., van Rooijen, N., Petersen, A. H., and van Luyn, M. J. (2007). Macrophage depletion impairs wound healing and increases left ventricular remodeling after myocardial injury in mice. *Am. J. Pathol.* 170, 818–829. doi: 10.2353/ajpath.2007.060547

Van Linthout, S., Miteva, K., and Tschöpe, C. (2014). Crosstalk between fibroblasts and inflammatory cells. *Cardiovasc. Res.* 102, 258–269. doi: 10.1093/cvr/cvu062

Van Tassell, B. W., Seropian, I. M., Toldo, S., Mezzaroma, E., and Abbate, A. (2013). Interleukin-1beta induces a reversible cardiomyopathy in the mouse. *Inflamm. Res.* 62, 637–640. doi: 10.1007/s00011-013-0625-0

Venkatachalam, K., Venkatesan, B., Valente, A. J., Melby, P. C., Nandish, S., Reusch, J. E., et al. (2009). WISP1, a pro-mitogenic, pro-survival factor, mediates tumor necrosis factor-alpha (TNF-alpha)-stimulated cardiac fibroblast proliferation but inhibits TNF-alpha-induced cardiomyocyte death. *J. Biol. Chem.* 284, 14414–14427. doi: 10.1074/jbc.M809757200

Voelkel, N. F., Tamosiuniene, R., and Nicolls, M. R. (2016). Challenges and opportunities in treating inflammation associated with pulmonary hypertension. *Exp. Rev. Cardiovasc. Ther.* 14, 939–951. doi: 10.1080/14779072.2016.1180976

Vonk Noordegraaf, A., Westerhof, B. E., and Westerhof, N. (2017). The relationship between the right ventricle and its load in pulmonary hypertension. *J. Am. Coll. Cardiol.* 69, 236–243. doi: 10.1016/j.jacc.2016.10.047

Vonk-Noordegraaf, A., Haddad, F., Chin, K. M., Forfia, P. R., Kawut, S. M., Lumens, J., et al. (2013). Right heart adaptation to pulmonary arterial hypertension: physiology and pathobiology. *J. Am. Coll. Cardiol.* 62, D22–D33. doi: 10.1016/j.jacc.2013.10.027

Waehre, A., Vistnes, M., Sjaastad, I., Nygård, S., Husberg, C., Lunde, I. G., et al. (1985). Chemokines regulate small leucine-rich proteoglycans in the extracellular matrix of the pressure-overloaded right ventricle. *J. Appl. Physiol.* 112, 1372–1382. doi: 10.1152/japplphysiol.01350.2011

Wang, Q., Zuo, X. R., Wang, Y. Y., Xie, W. P., Wang, H., and Zhang, M. (2013). Monocrotaline-induced pulmonary arterial hypertension is attenuated by TNF-alpha antagonists via the suppression of TNF-alpha expression and NF-κB pathway in rats. *Vasc. Pharmacol.* 58, 71–77. doi: 10.1016/j.vph.2012.07.006

Wang, W., Yan, H., Zhu, W., Cui, Y., Chen, J., Wang, X., et al. (2009). Impairment of monocyte-derived dendritic cells in idiopathic pulmonary arterial hypertension. *J. Clin. Immunol.* 29, 705–713. doi: 10.1007/s10875-009-9322-8

Watts, J. A., Gellar, M. A., Obraztsova, M., Kline, J. A., and Zagorski, J. (2008). Role of inflammation in right ventricular damage and repair following experimental pulmonary embolism in rats. *Int. J. Exp. Pathol.* 89, 389–399. doi: 10.1111/j.1365-2613.2008.00610.x

Watts, J. A., Zagorski, J., Gellar, M. A., Stevinson, B. G., and Kline, J. A. (2006). Cardiac inflammation contributes to right ventricular dysfunction following experimental pulmonary embolism in rats. *J. Mol. Cell Cardiol.* 41, 296–307. doi: 10.1016/j.yjmcc.2006.05.011

Woodfin, A., Voisin, M. B., Imhof, B. A., Dejana, E., Engelhardt, B., and Nourshargh, S. (2009). Endothelial cell activation leads to neutrophil transmigration as supported by the sequential roles of ICAM-2, JAM-A, and PECAM-1. *Blood* 113, 6246–6257. doi: 10.1182/blood-2008-11-188375

Wrigley, B. J., Lip, G. Y., and Shantsila, E. (2011). The role of monocytes and inflammation in the pathophysiology of heart failure. *Eur. J. Heart Fail.* 13, 1161–1171. doi: 10.1093/eurjhf/hfr122

Wu, C. K., Lee, J. K., Chiang, F. T., Yang, C. H., Huang, S. W., Hwang, J. J., et al. (2011). Plasma levels of tumor necrosis factor-alpha and interleukin-6 are associated with diastolic heart failure through downregulation of sarcoplasmic reticulum Ca2+ ATPase. *Crit. Care Med.* 39, 984–992. doi: 10.1097/CCM.0b013e31820a91b9

Yet, S. F., Perrella, M. A., Layne, M. D., Hsieh, C. M., Maemura, K., Kobzik, L., et al. (1999). Hypoxia induces severe right ventricular dilatation and infarction in heme oxygenase-1 null mice. *J. Clin. Invest.* 103, R23–R29. doi: 10.1172/JCI6163

Yilmaz, A., Fuchs, T., Dietel, B., Altendorf, R., Cicha, I., Stumpf, C., et al. (2009). Transient decrease in circulating dendritic cell precursors after acute stroke: potential recruitment into the brain. *Clin. Sci.* 118, 147–157. doi: 10.1042/CS20090154

Yokoyama, H., Kuwao, S., Kohno, K., Suzuki, K., Kameya, T., and Izumi, T. (2000). Cardiac dendritic cells and acute myocarditis in the human heart. *Jpn. Circ. J.* 64, 57–64. doi: 10.1253/jcj.64.57

Yokoyama, T., Nakano, M., Bednarczyk, J. L., McIntyre, B. W., Entman, M., and Mann, D. L. (1997). Tumor necrosis factor-alpha provokes a hypertrophic growth response in adult cardiac myocytes. *Circulation* 95, 1247–1252. doi: 10.1161/01.CIR.95.5.1247

Yokoyama, T., Vaca, L., Rossen, R. D., Durante, W., Hazarika, P., and Mann, D. L. (1993). Cellular basis for the negative inotropic effects of tumor necrosis factor-alpha in the adult mammalian heart. *J. Clin. Invest.* 92, 2303–2312. doi: 10.1172/JCI116834

Yoshida, T., Friehs, I., Mummidi, S., del Nido, P. J., Addulnour-Nakhoul, S., Delafontaine, P., et al. (2014). Pressure overload induces IL-18 and IL-18R expression, but markedly suppresses IL-18BP expression in a rabbit model. IL-18 potentiates TNF-alpha-induced cardiomyocyte death. *J. Mol. Cell Cardiol.* 75, 141–151. doi: 10.1016/j.yjmcc.2014.07.007

Yu, X. W., Liu, M. Y., Kennedy, R. H., and Liu, S. J. (2005). Both cGMP and peroxynitrite mediate chronic interleukin-6-induced negative inotropy in adult rat ventricular myocytes. *J. Physiol.* 566, 341–353. doi: 10.1113/jphysiol.2005.087478

Zagorski, J., Gellar, M. A., Obraztsova, M., Kline, J. A., and Watts, J. A. (2007). Inhibition of CINC-1 decreases right ventricular damage caused by experimental pulmonary embolism in rats. *J. Immunol.* 179, 7820–7826. doi: 10.4049/jimmunol.179.11.7820

Zakrzewicz, A., Grafe, M., Terbeek, D., Bongrazio, M., Auch-Schwelk, W., Walzog, B., et al. (1997). L-selectin-dependent leukocyte adhesion to microvascular but not to macrovascular endothelial cells of the human coronary system. *Blood* 89, 3228–3235.

Zelarayan, L., Renger, A., Noack, C., Zafiriou, M. P., Gehrke, C., van der Nagel, R., et al. (2009). NF-κB activation is required for adaptive cardiac hypertrophy. *Cardiovasc. Res.* 84, 416–424. doi: 10.1093/cvr/cvp237

Zhang, J., Yu, Z. X., Fujita, S., Yamaguchi, M. L., and Ferrans, V. J. (1993). Interstitial dendritic cells of the rat heart. Quantitative and ultrastructural changes in experimental myocardial infarction. *Circulation* 87, 909–920. doi: 10.1161/01.CIR.87.3.909

Zhang, W., Chancey, A. L., Tzeng, H. P., Zhou, Z., Lavine, K. J., Gao, F., et al. (2011). The development of myocardial fibrosis in transgenic mice with targeted overexpression of tumor necrosis factor requires mast cell-fibroblast interactions. *Circulation* 124, 2106–2116. doi: 10.1161/CIRCULATIONAHA.111.052399

Zhang, Y. H., Lin, J. X., and Vilcek, J. (1990). Interleukin-6 induction by tumor necrosis factor and interleukin-1 in human fibroblasts involves activation of a nuclear factor binding to a kappa B-like sequence. *Mol. Cell Biol.* 10, 3818–3823. doi: 10.1128/MCB.10.7.3818

Zhou, L., Azfer, A., Niu, J., Graham, S., Choudhury, M., Adamski, F. M., et al. (2006). Monocyte chemoattractant protein-1 induces a novel transcription factor that causes cardiac myocyte apoptosis and ventricular dysfunction. *Circ. Res.* 98, 1177–1185. doi: 10.1161/01.RES.0000220106.64661.71

Permissions

All chapters in this book were first published Frontiers; hereby published with permission under the Creative Commons Attribution License or equivalent. Every chapter published in this book has been scrutinized by our experts. Their significance has been extensively debated. The topics covered herein carry significant findings which will fuel the growth of the discipline. They may even be implemented as practical applications or may be referred to as a beginning point for another development.

The contributors of this book come from diverse backgrounds, making this book a truly international effort. This book will bring forth new frontiers with its revolutionizing research information and detailed analysis of the nascent developments around the world.

We would like to thank all the contributing authors for lending their expertise to make the book truly unique. They have played a crucial role in the development of this book. Without their invaluable contributions this book wouldn't have been possible. They have made vital efforts to compile up to date information on the varied aspects of this subject to make this book a valuable addition to the collection of many professionals and students.

This book was conceptualized with the vision of imparting up-to-date information and advanced data in this field. To ensure the same, a matchless editorial board was set up. Every individual on the board went through rigorous rounds of assessment to prove their worth. After which they invested a large part of their time researching and compiling the most relevant data for our readers.

The editorial board has been involved in producing this book since its inception. They have spent rigorous hours researching and exploring the diverse topics which have resulted in the successful publishing of this book. They have passed on their knowledge of decades through this book. To expedite this challenging task, the publisher supported the team at every step. A small team of assistant editors was also appointed to further simplify the editing procedure and attain best results for the readers.

Apart from the editorial board, the designing team has also invested a significant amount of their time in understanding the subject and creating the most relevant covers. They scrutinized every image to scout for the most suitable representation of the subject and create an appropriate cover for the book.

The publishing team has been an ardent support to the editorial, designing and production team. Their endless efforts to recruit the best for this project, has resulted in the accomplishment of this book. They are a veteran in the field of academics and their pool of knowledge is as vast as their experience in printing. Their expertise and guidance has proved useful at every step. Their uncompromising quality standards have made this book an exceptional effort. Their encouragement from time to time has been an inspiration for everyone.

The publisher and the editorial board hope that this book will prove to be a valuable piece of knowledge for researchers, students, practitioners and scholars across the globe.

List of Contributors

Kelsey Horton, Diana Martinez and Michael J. Katovich
Department of Pharmacodynamics, University of Florida, Gainesville, FL, United States

Anandharajan Rathinasabapathy
Department of Pharmacodynamics, University of Florida, Gainesville, FL, United States
Allergy, Pulmonary and Critical Care Medicine, Vanderbilt University Medical Center, Nashville, TN, United States

Santhi Gladson and James West
Allergy, Pulmonary and Critical Care Medicine, Vanderbilt University Medical Center, Nashville, TN, United States

Alana Horowitz
Department of Pharmacodynamics, University of Florida, Gainesville, FL, United States
Anatomy, University of California at San Francisco, San Francisco, CA, United States

Mohan K. Raizada and Colin Sumners
Department of Physiology and Functional Genomics, University of Florida, Gainesville, FL, United States

Ashok Kumar
Department of Physiology and Functional Genomics, University of Florida, Gainesville, FL, United States
Cardiopulmonary Vascular Biology Lab, Providence VA Medical Center, Brown University, Providence, RI, United States

Thomas Unger
Cardiovascular Research Institute Maastricht School for Cardiovascular Diseases, Maastricht University, Maastricht, Netherlands

Gaurav Bedse
Psychiatry and Behavioral Sciences, Vanderbilt University Medical Center, Nashville, TN, United States

Ulrike M. Steckelings
Department of Cardiovascular and Renal Research, Institute for Molecular Medicine, University of Southern Denmark, Odense, Denmark

Vinayak Shenoy
Department of Pharmacodynamics, University of Florida, Gainesville, FL, United States
Department of Pharmaceutical and Biomedical Sciences, California Health Sciences University, Clovis, CA, United States

Catherine G. Billings, Robert Lewis, Iain J. Armstrong, Judith A. Hurdman, Ian A. Smith, Matthew Austin, Charlie A. Elliot, Athanasios Charalampopoulos and Robin Condliffe
Sheffield Pulmonary Vascular Disease Unit, Sheffield Teaching Hospitals NHS Foundation Trust, Royal Hallamshire Hospital, Sheffield, United Kingdom
Sheffield Pulmonary Vascular Disease Unit, Royal Hallamshire Hospital, Sheffield Teaching Hospitals NHS Foundation Trust, Sheffield, United Kingdom

Ian Sabroe, Allan Lawrie and A. A. Roger Thompson
Department of Infection, Immunity and Cardiovascular Disease, University of Sheffield, Medical School, Sheffield, United Kingdom

David G. Kiely
Sheffield Pulmonary Vascular Disease Unit, Sheffield Teaching Hospitals NHS Foundation Trust, Royal Hallamshire Hospital, Sheffield, United Kingdom
Department of Infection, Immunity and Cardiovascular Disease, University of Sheffield, Medical School, Sheffield, United Kingdom
Insigneo Institute for in Silico Medicine, University of Sheffield, Sheffield, United Kingdom

Nedim Durmus
Department of Environmental Medicine and Division of Pulmonary Medicine, Department of Medicine, New York University School of Medicine, New York, United States

Gabriele Grunig
Department of Environmental Medicine and Division of Pulmonary Medicine, Department of Medicine, New York University School of Medicine, New York, United States
Mirna Analytics LLC, New York, United States

Serhiy Pylawka
Mirna Analytics LLC, New York, United States

Christina A. Eichstaedt, Jeremias Verweyen and Ekkehard Grünig
Thoraxklinik, Heidelberg University Hospital, Heidelberg, Germany

Stephanie Saxer and Silvia Ulrich
Clinic for Pulmonology, University Hospital Zürich, Zurich, Switzerland

Greta Krafsur and Kurt Stenmark
Department of Medicine, University of Colorado, Aurora, CO, United States

Adam T. Braithwaite, Helen M. Marriott and Allan Lawrie
Infection, Immunity and Cardiovascular Disease, University of Sheffield, Medical School, Sheffield, United Kingdom

Latha Ramakrishnan, Sofia L. Pedersen, Quezia K. Toe, Gregory J. Quinlan and Stephen J. Wort
Cardiorespiratory Interface - Vascular Biology, The National Heart and Lung Institute, Faculty of Medicine, Imperial College London, London, United Kingdom

Matthew Chin, Christopher Johns, Benjamin J. Currie, Nicholas Weatherley and Jim M. Wild
Department of Infection, Immunity and Cardiovascular Disease, University of Sheffield, Royal Hallamshire Hospital, Sheffield, United Kingdom

Catherine Hill, Smitha Rajaram and Stephen Bianchi
Sheffield Teaching Hospitals NHS Foundation Trust, Sheffield, United Kingdom

Andrew J. Swift
Department of Infection, Immunity and Cardiovascular Disease, University of Sheffield, Royal Hallamshire Hospital, Sheffield, United Kingdom
Institute for in silico Medicine, Sheffield, United Kingdom

Suhong Wu
Department of Nanomedicine, Houston Methodist Research Institute, Houston, TX, United States

Victor Segura-Ibarra and Jose A. Moran-Guerrero
Department of Nanomedicine, Houston Methodist Research Institute, Houston, TX, United States
Escuela de Ingeniería y Ciencias, Tecnológico de Monterrey, Monterrey, Mexico

Nida Hassan
Department of Nanomedicine, Houston Methodist Research Institute, Houston, TX, United States
McGovern Medical School, The University of Texas Health Science Center at Houston, Houston, TX, United States

Mauro Ferrari
Department of Nanomedicine, Houston Methodist Research Institute, Houston, TX, United States
Department of Medicine, Weill Cornell Medicine, New York, United States

Elvin Blanco
Department of Nanomedicine, Houston Methodist Research Institute, Houston, TX, United States
Department of Cardiology, Houston Methodist DeBakey Heart and Vascular Center, Houston Methodist Hospital, Houston, TX, United States

Ashrith Guha
Department of Cardiology, Houston Methodist DeBakey Heart and Vascular Center, Houston Methodist Hospital, Houston, TX, United States
Houston Methodist J.C. Walter Jr. Transplant Center, Houston Methodist Hospital, Houston, TX, United States

Harry Karmouty-Quintana
Department of Biochemistry and Molecular Biology, McGovern Medical School, The University of Texas Health Science Center at Houston, Houston, TX, United States

Jason M. Young
Edinburgh Medical School, University of Edinburgh, Edinburgh, United Kingdom
Apex (Altitude Physiology Expeditions), Edinburgh, United Kingdom

David R. Williams
Apex (Altitude Physiology Expeditions), Edinburgh, United Kingdom

A. A. Roger Thompson
Apex (Altitude Physiology Expeditions), Edinburgh, United Kingdom
Department of Infection, Immunity and Cardiovascular Disease, University of Sheffield, Sheffield, United Kingdom

Junmei Zhou
Department of Pediatrics, University of Florida, Gainesville, FL, United States

Yuanquing Lu, Marda Jorgensen and Andrew J. Bryant
Division of Pulmonary, Critical Care, and Sleep Medicine, Department of Medicine, College of Medicine, University of Florida, Gainesville, FL, United States

Kenneth E. Lipson
FibroGen, Inc., San Francisco, CA, United States

Edward W. Scott
Department of Molecular Genetics and Microbiology, University of Florida, Gainesville, FL, United States

Anna R. Hemnes
Division of Allergy, Pulmonary and Critical Care Medicine, Vanderbilt University Medical Center, Nashville, TN, United States

Lian Tian, Francois Potus, Danchen Wu, Asish Dasgupta, Kuang-Hueih Chen, Jeffrey Mewburn, Patricia Lima and Stephen L. Archer
Department of Medicine, Queen's University, Kingston, ON, Canada

Athanasios Charalampopoulos
Sheffield Pulmonary Vascular Disease Unit, Royal Hallamshire Hospital, Sheffield Teaching Hospitals NHS Foundation Trust, Sheffield, United Kingdom

Jennifer T. Middleton and Alexander Rothman
Sheffield Pulmonary Vascular Disease Unit, Royal Hallamshire Hospital, Sheffield Teaching Hospitals NHS Foundation Trust, Sheffield, United Kingdom
Department of Infection, Immunity and Cardiovascular Disease, Medical School, University of Sheffield, Sheffield, United Kingdom
Department of Cardiology, Northern General Hospital, Sheffield Teaching Hospitals NHS Foundation Trust, Sheffield, United Kingdom

Robert Lewis
Sheffield Pulmonary Vascular Disease Unit, Royal Hallamshire Hospital, Sheffield Teaching Hospitals NHS Foundation Trust, Sheffield, United Kingdom
Department of Infection, Immunity and Cardiovascular Disease, Medical School, University of Sheffield, Sheffield, United Kingdom

Angshuman Maulik
Department of Infection, Immunity and Cardiovascular Disease, Medical School, University of Sheffield, Sheffield, United Kingdom
Department of Cardiology, Northern General Hospital, Sheffield Teaching Hospitals NHS Foundation Trust, Sheffield, United Kingdom

Andreas Kyriacou
Department of Cardiology, Northern General Hospital, Sheffield Teaching Hospitals NHS Foundation Trust, Sheffield, United Kingdom

Mark Toshner
Department of Medicine, Addenbrooke's Hospital, University of Cambridge, Cambridge, United Kingdom
Royal Papworth Hospital NHS Foundation Trust, Cambridgeshire, United Kingdom

Tinne C. J. Mertens, Ankit Hanmandlu, Scott D. Collum, Ning-Yuan Chen, Tingting Weng Chen Liu Yang Xia, Michael R. Blackburn and Harry Karmouty-Quintana
Department of Biochemistry and Molecular Biology, McGovern Medical School, The University of Texas Health Science Center at Houston, Houston, TX, United States

Ly Tu Carole Phan and Christophe Guignabert
Institut National de la Santé et de la Recherche Médicale UMR_S 999, Le Plessis-Robinson, France
Université Paris-Sud and Université Paris-Saclay, Le Kremlin-Bicêtre, France

Jonathan Davies
Department of Pediatrics, Baylor College of Medicine, Houston, TX, United States

Holger K. Eltzschig
Department of Anesthesiology, McGovern Medical School, The University of Texas Health Science Center at Houston, Houston, TX, United States

Soma S. K. Jyothula and Keshava Rajagopal
Department of Internal Medicine, McGovern Medical School, The University of Texas Health Science Center at Houston, Houston, TX, United States

Ashrith Guha and Brian A. Bruckner
Methodist Debakey Heart and Vascular Center, Houston Methodist Hospital, Houston, TX, United States

Athanasios Charalampopoulos, Peter Hickey, Charlotte Durrington, Charlie Elliot and Ian Sabroe
Sheffield Pulmonary Vascular Disease Unit, Royal Hallamshire Hospital, Sheffield Teaching Hospitals NHS Foundation Trust, Sheffield, United Kingdom

Argen Mamazhakypov, Aleksandar Petrovic, Djuro Kosanovic, Norbert Weissmann, Hossein A. Ghofrani and Ralph T. Schermuly
Excellence Cluster Cardio-Pulmonary System, Universities of Giessen and Marburg Lung Center, German Center for Lung Research, Justus Liebig University of Giessen, Giessen, Germany

Akylbek Sydykov
Excellence Cluster Cardio-Pulmonary System, Universities of Giessen and Marburg Lung Center, German Center for Lung Research, Justus Liebig University of Giessen, Giessen, Germany
Department of Mountain and Sleep Medicine and Pulmonary Hypertension, National Center of Cardiology and Internal Medicine, Bishkek, Kyrgyzstan

Akpay S. Sarybaev
Department of Mountain and Sleep Medicine and Pulmonary Hypertension, National Center of Cardiology and Internal Medicine, Bishkek, Kyrgyzstan

Wei Sun and Stephen Y. Chan
Division of Cardiology, Department of Medicine, Center for Pulmonary Vascular Biology and Medicine, Pittsburgh Heart, Lung, Blood, and Vascular Medicine Institute, University of Pittsburgh School of Medicine and University of Pittsburgh Medical Center, Pittsburgh, PA, United States

Balazs Odler Vasile Foris and Horst Olschewski
Ludwig Boltzmann Institute for Lung Vascular Research, Graz, Austria
Division of Pulmonology, Department of Internal Medicine, Medical University of Graz, Graz, Austria

Anna Gungl and Grazyna Kwapiszewska
Ludwig Boltzmann Institute for Lung Vascular Research, Graz, Austria
Physiology, Otto Loewi Research Center, Medical University of Graz, Graz, Austria

Veronika Müller
Department of Pulmonology, Semmelweis University, Budapest, Hungary

Paul M. Hassoun
Division of Pulmonary & Critical Care Medicine, Johns Hopkins University, Baltimore, MD, United States

Allan Lawrie
Department of Infection, Immunity and Cardiovascular Disease, University of Sheffield, Sheffield, United Kingdom

Robin Condliffe
Pulmonary Vascular Diseases Unit, Royal Hallamshire Hospital, Sheffield, United Kingdom

Peter M. Hickey
Department of Infection, Immunity and Cardiovascular Disease, University of Sheffield, Sheffield, United Kingdom
Pulmonary Vascular Diseases Unit, Royal Hallamshire Hospital, Sheffield, United Kingdom

Anandharajan Rathinasabapathy, Toshio Suzuki, Christy Moore, Sheila Shay, Santhi Gladson, James D. West and Erica J. Carrier
Allergy, Pulmonary and Critical Care Medicine, Vanderbilt University Medical Center, Nashville, TN, United States

Andrew J. Bryant
Pulmonary, Critical Care, and Sleep Medicine, College of Medicine, University of Florida, Gainesville, FL, United States

Shalina Taylor and Marlene Rabinovitch
Department of Pediatrics, Stanford University School of Medicine, Stanford, CA, United States
Vera Moulton Wall Center for Pulmonary Vascular Disease, Stanford University, Stanford, CA, United States

Omar Dirir and A. A. Roger Thompson
Infection, Immunity, and Cardiovascular Disease, University of Sheffield, Sheffield, United Kingdom

Roham T. Zamanian
Vera Moulton Wall Center for Pulmonary Vascular Disease, Stanford University, Stanford, CA, United States
Division of Pulmonary and Critical Care Medicine, Stanford University School of Medicine, Stanford, CA, United States

Laurence Dewachter
Laboratory of Physiology and Pharmacology, Faculty of Medicine, Université Libre de Bruxelles, Brussels, Belgium

Céline Dewachter
Laboratory of Physiology and Pharmacology, Faculty of Medicine, Université Libre de Bruxelles, Brussels, Belgium
Department of Cardiology, Erasmus Academic Hospital, Brussels, Belgium

Index

www.ingramcontent.com/pod-product-compliance
Lightning Source LLC
LaVergne TN
LVHW060514210926
848485LV00005B/1080
* 9 7 8 1 6 3 9 2 7 8 4 0 4 *